Advanced Classification Techniques for Healthcare Analysis

Chinmay Chakraborty
Birla Institute of Technology Mesra, India

A volume in the Advances in Medical Technologies and Clinical Practice (AMTCP) Book Series

IGI Global
DISSEMINATOR OF KNOWLEDGE

Published in the United States of America by
IGI Global
Medical Information Science Reference (an imprint of IGI Global)
701 E. Chocolate Avenue
Hershey PA, USA 17033
Tel: 717-533-8845
Fax: 717-533-8661
E-mail: cust@igi-global.com
Web site: http://www.igi-global.com

Library of Congress Cataloging-in-Publication Data

Names: Chakraborty, Chinmay, 1984- editor.
Title: Advanced classification techniques for healthcare analysis / Chinmay Chakraborty, editor.
Description: Hershey, PA : Medical Information Science Reference, [2019] | Includes bibliographical references.
Identifiers: LCCN 2018036802| ISBN 9781522577966 (hardcover) | ISBN 9781522577973 (ebook)
Subjects: | MESH: Image Interpretation, Computer-Assisted | Classification--methods | Image Processing, Computer-Assisted
Classification: LCC RC78.7.D53 | NLM WN 182 | DDC 616.07/54--dc23 LC record available at https://lccn.loc.gov/2018036802

This book is published in the IGI Global book series Advances in Medical Technologies and Clinical Practice (AMTCP) (ISSN: 2327-9354; eISSN: 2327-9370)

British Cataloguing in Publication Data
A Cataloguing in Publication record for this book is available from the British Library.

All work contributed to this book is new, previously-unpublished material. The views expressed in this book are those of the authors, but not necessarily of the publisher.

For electronic access to this publication, please contact: eresources@igi-global.com.

Advances in Medical Technologies and Clinical Practice (AMTCP) Book Series

Srikanta Patnaik
SOA University, India
Priti Das
S.C.B. Medical College, India

ISSN:2327-9354
EISSN:2327-9370

Mission

Medical technological innovation continues to provide avenues of research for faster and safer diagnosis and treatments for patients. Practitioners must stay up to date with these latest advancements to provide the best care for nursing and clinical practices.

The **Advances in Medical Technologies and Clinical Practice (AMTCP) Book Series** brings together the most recent research on the latest technology used in areas of nursing informatics, clinical technology, biomedicine, diagnostic technologies, and more. Researchers, students, and practitioners in this field will benefit from this fundamental coverage on the use of technology in clinical practices.

Coverage

- Medical Imaging
- E-Health
- Neural Engineering
- Clinical Studies
- Clinical High-Performance Computing
- Medical Informatics
- Clinical Data Mining
- Clinical Nutrition
- Biomedical Applications
- Biomechanics

IGI Global is currently accepting manuscripts for publication within this series. To submit a proposal for a volume in this series, please contact our Acquisition Editors at Acquisitions@igi-global.com or visit: http://www.igi-global.com/publish/.

The Advances in Medical Technologies and Clinical Practice (AMTCP) Book Series (ISSN 2327-9354) is published by IGI Global, 701 E. Chocolate Avenue, Hershey, PA 17033-1240, USA, www.igi-global.com. This series is composed of titles available for purchase individually; each title is edited to be contextually exclusive from any other title within the series. For pricing and ordering information please visit http://www.igi-global.com/book-series/advances-medical-technologies-clinical-practice/73682. Postmaster: Send all address changes to above address.

Titles in this Series

For a list of additional titles in this series, please visit: www.igi-global.com/book-series

Computational Techniques for Dental Image Analysis
K. Kamalanand (Anna University, India) B. Thayumanavan (Sathyabama University Dental College and Hospital, India) and P. Mannar Jawahar (Anna University, India)
Medical Information Science Reference • copyright 2019 • 334pp • H/C (ISBN: 9781522562436) • US $225.00 (our price)

Emerging Trends in the Diagnosis and Intervention of Neurodevelopmental Disorders
Sanjeev Kumar Gupta (All India Institute of Speech and Hearing, India) Srinivasan Venkatesan (All India Institute of Speech and Hearing, India) S.P. Goswami (All India Institute of Speech and Hearing, India) and Rajeev Kumar (Indian Institute of Technology Kharagpur, India)
Medical Information Science Reference • copyright 2019 • 394pp • H/C (ISBN: 9781522570042) • US $265.00 (our price)

Histopathological Image Analysis in Medical Decision Making
Nilanjan Dey (Techno India College of Technology, India) Amira S. Ashour (Tanta University, Egypt) Harihar Kalia (Seemantha Engineering College, India) R.T. Goswami (Techno India College of Technology, India) and Himansu Das (KIIT University, India)
Medical Information Science Reference • copyright 2019 • 340pp • H/C (ISBN: 9781522563167) • US $265.00 (our price)

Healing Through the Arts for Non-Clinical Practitioners
Jenny Bopp (Westtown School, USA) Amy M. Grebe (Zinnia Consulting and Design, USA) and Joanna Hope Denny (Pellisippi State Community College, USA)
Medical Information Science Reference • copyright 2019 • 309pp • H/C (ISBN: 9781522559818) • US $255.00 (our price)

Medical Image Processing for Improved Clinical Diagnosis
A. Swarnambiga (Indian Institute of Technology Madras, India)
Medical Information Science Reference • copyright 2019 • 313pp • H/C (ISBN: 9781522558767) • US $245.00 (our price)

Clinical Costing Techniques and Analysis in Modern Healthcare Systems
Ronald Ma (Austin Health, Australia)
Medical Information Science Reference • copyright 2019 • 265pp • H/C (ISBN: 9781522550822) • US $235.00 (our price)

IGI Global
DISSEMINATOR OF KNOWLEDGE

701 East Chocolate Avenue, Hershey, PA 17033, USA
Tel: 717-533-8845 x100 • Fax: 717-533-8661
E-Mail: cust@igi-global.com • www.igi-global.com

Editorial Advisory Board

List of Reviewers

Table of Contents

Section 2
Analysis of Healthcare

Section 3
Others

Detailed Table of Contents

and heuristic methods, and explains them with example dataset. It also compares these models and their efficiencies with model evaluation techniques and briefs some blended classification models. The goal of this chapter is to provide a comprehensive review of different classification techniques and give a quick refresher on classification models in big data analytics. The comparison of various classification models helps the readers to quickly decide which classification model to choose for the given business scenario.

In recent years, a vast research is concentrated towards the development of electroencephalography (EEG)-based human-computer interface in order to enhance the quality of life for medical as well as nonmedical applications. The EEG is an important measurement of brain activity and has great potential in helping in the diagnosis and treatment of mental and brain neuro-degenerative diseases and abnormalities. In this chapter, the authors discuss the classification of EEG signals as a key issue in biomedical research for identification and evaluation of the brain activity. Identification of various types of EEG signals is a complicated problem, requiring the analysis of large sets of EEG data. Representative features from a large dataset play an important role in classifying EEG signals in the field of biomedical signal processing. So, to reduce the above problem, this research uses three methods to classify through feature extraction and classification schemes.

Abnormal behavior of heart muscles generates irregular heartbeats which are collectively known as arrhythmia. Classification of arrhythmia beats plays a prominent role in electrocardiogram (ECG) analysis. It is widely used in online and long-term patient monitoring systems. This chapter reports a classification technique to recognize normal (N) and five arrhythmia beats (i.e., left bundle branch block [LBBB], right bundle branch block [RBBB], premature ventricular contraction [V], paced [P], and atrial premature contraction [A]). The technique utilizes features of heartbeats extracted by the wavelet multi-resolution analysis. The feature vectors are used to train and test the classifier based on the support vector machine which has been emerged as a benchmark in machine learning classifier. It accomplishes the beat classification very efficiently. ECG records of the MIT-BIH arrhythmia database are utilized to acquire the different types of heartbeats. Performance of the proposed classifier outperforms the contemporary arrhythmia beats classification techniques.

An improved energy-based technique with a Lattice Boltzmann method organizes with the neighborhood and global energy terms, local term propels to pull the frame and constrain it to protest limit, decides noteworthy points of interest not confined to, snappy planning, automation, invariance of exact medical image segmentation, and analysis. Consequently, the worldwide vitality fitting term drives the advancement of the frame at a division of the question limit. The worldwide vitality term relies upon the worldwide division computation, which can better catch drive information of pictures than mixture area-based dynamic shape technique. Both neighborhood and worldwide terms are ordinarily acclimatized to construct a level set strategy to divide pictures with exactness. The level set technique with Boltzmann system uses neighborhood mean, a quality which engages it as far as possible. The proposed chapter gathers gainful purposes of intrigue not stuck just using expedient process, computerization, and right helpful picture partitions.

In the modern era of information technology, machine learning algorithms are used in different domains for boosting the quality of decision making. The correct decision making about the disease diagnosis is one of the applications where these approaches are applied successfully for assisting the doctors. Correct and timely diagnosis of disease is the primary requirement of effective treatment. Today, one of the most leading causes of death is heart disease. This chapter deals with the application of different machine learning algorithms for effective heart disease diagnosis. Diagnosis through the machine learning algorithms involves the three major steps, data preprocessing, feature selection, and classification. The chapter covers the experimental study of performance of SVM, ANN, logistic regression, random forest, KNN, AdaBoost, Naive Bayes, decision tree, SGD, CN2 rule inducer approaches.

This chapter provides significant theoretical and systematic frameworks and the latest empirical research towards the development of an automated cardiovascular disorder diagnostic system with the classifier. This research proposes an accurate non-invasive model of the cardiovascular diseases diagnostic system. This model of diagnostic system support superior mobility with continuous real-time monitoring facility. This monitoring system will uncover a new dimension towards cardiovascular research. A physician will able to monitor several heart patients remotely with this device. Also, they can prescribe proper medicine remotely to the patient in an emergency. The system also has a provision to alert the patient by predicting the specific type of cardiovascular disorder accurately. An automated cardiovascular disorder diagnostic system development focuses towards the prime objective. Another objective is the adoption of modern classification technique for detecting cardiovascular disorders with high accuracy.

In this chapter, different types of image fusion techniques have been studied and evaluated in the medical applications. The ultimate goal of this proposed method is to obtain the fused image without any loss of similar information and preserve all special features present in the input medical images. This method is used to improve the fused image quality for better diagnosis of critical disease analysis. The fused hybrid multimodal medical image should convey better visual description than the individual input images. This chapter proposes the method for multimodal medical image fusion using the hybrid fusion algorithm. The computed tomography, magnetic resonance imaging, positron emission tomography, and single photon emission computed tomography are the input images used for this experimental work. In this chapter, experimental results discovered that the proposed techniques provide better visualization of fused image and gives the superior results compared to various existing traditional algorithms.

An early diagnosis of insomnia can prevent further medical aids such as anger issues, heart diseases, anxiety, depression, and hypertension. Fifteen machine learning algorithms have been applied and 14 leading factors have been taken into consideration for predicting insomnia. Seven performance parameters (accuracy, kappa, the true positive rate, false positive rate, precision, f-measure, and AUC) are used and for implementation. The authors have used python language. The support vector machine is giving higher performance out of all algorithms giving accuracy 91.6%, f-measure is 92.13, and kappa is 0.83. Further, SVM is applied on another dataset of 100 patients and giving accuracy 92%. In addition, an analysis of the variable importance of CART, C5.0, decision tree, random forest, adaptive boost, and XG boost is calculated. The analysis shows that insomnia primarily depends on the factors, which are the vision problem, mobility problem, and sleep disorder. This chapter mainly finds the usages and effectiveness of machine learning algorithms in Insomnia diseases prediction.

Section 3
Others

Foreword

I am delighted to write the foreword for this edited book on *Advanced Classification Techniques for Healthcare Analysis*. This book briefly describes the new engineering tool applied for different diseases diagnosis which can help the health practitioner/doctors to some extent in their diagnosed decision.

Healthcare is the maintenance or improvement of health via the prevention, diagnosis, and treatment of disease, illness, injury, and other physical and mental impairments in human beings. To accomplish this task many data are gathered about a patient. These data are either generated manually by regular and repeated observation or may be by digital means by using various machines. These data are of various type and format. Some are image based; some are text, some are sound, some are electrical signals, etc. To extract the information about a patient from such heterogeneous data is a huge and complicated task and requires many tools and techniques.

To diagnosis a patient can be viewed as a classification problem where based on the available data a person is classified in a disease class. And for such classification the proper extraction of information and proper drawing of inference is very crucial. These classification problems, the way it is handled may turn into a life and death problem. So the accuracy of the inference is of utmost important.

But accuracy cannot be achieved by using a single instance. Knowledge is a learning procedure from previous experiences. There may also be comparison between similar phenomena to find unique quality that isolates them from each other.

Keeping these scenarios in mind this book has been posed. This book handles different form of data for analysis such as image, EEG signals, Ultrasound, manual observations etc. This is one of the unique features of this book which makes it stand apart.

The book describes and explains various classification techniques over various medical data types. It also focuses on the different statistical, evolutionary and hybrid techniques for the decision-making process.

This book provides a window to the field of analysis of medical and healthcare data analysis in a comprehensive way and enumerates the evolutions of such tools and techniques.

In this new age of global interconnectivity and interdependence, it is necessary to provide practitioners, both professionals and students, with state-of-the art knowledge on the frontiers in information processing in the field of healthcare. This book is a good step in that direction.

It is my hope and expectation that this book will provide an effective learning experience and referenced resource for all health professionals.

Bharat Gupta
National Institute of Technology Patna, India

Preface

Advancement in technologies will help in taking a fast decision in diagnosis the medical condition of the patient. Currently, various medical and Information Communication Technology is working on the development of robust classification techniques especially in healthcare data/image analysis. Furtherance in Information and Communication Technology provides improved and eases in the life of patients in term of healthcare at any place, any time. In today's world, a vast amount of medical information is collected and stored in the database daily. There is an important need to analyze this medical data automatically rather than manually because it is a tedious and complex process. The classifier tool is used to analyzing large healthcare data from a different perspective and it helps us to extract and sum up useful information. Here different classification techniques are applied to the specific dataset using different learning tools. It is essential to develop a model which helps to extract useful information and provide decision-making for the diagnosis. Early diagnosis of diseases is a significant requirement in healthcare. The supervised and un-supervised classifiers, machine learning and deep learning techniques play an important role in analyzing medical data. This book will help researchers to get efficient results after knowing the best classifiers for this particular dataset. In this book, an analysis of various classification techniques is done which are used for analyzing medical data. The classification accuracy for the specific disease is mainly focused on this work.

OBJECTIVE

This book aims to focus an insight into classification techniques which broadly deals in delivery of quality, accurate and affordable healthcare. This book focuses to publish the original research outcomes towards medical healthcare using advanced classification techniques. The book will additionally investigate the potential for making faster advances in many scientific disciplines and improving the profitability and success of different enterprises.

BOOK ORGANISATION

The book content is organized as follow:

The book is structured into three main sections: (1) Classification of Health Data, (2) Analysis of Healthcare, and (3) Others. The summary of the chapters is presented here briefly. This book consists of 15 excellent chapters in the field of healthcare technology.

Section 1: Classification of Health Data

Section 1 of this book compromises five chapters that highlight the classifier's performance in various diseases.

Developing an Effective Classification Model for Medical Data Analysis

This chapter constructs the effective classification model for medical data analysis. In particular, nine classification models namely Naïve Bayes, Decision Tree (i.e., J48 and Random Forest), Multilayer Perceptron, Radial Bias Function, K-Nearest Neighbors, Single Conjunctive Rule Learner, Support Vector Machine and Simple logistics have been applied for developing an effective model. Besides, classification models have also been used in conjunction with ensemble learning methods, since ensemble methods significantly increase the predictive outcomes of the classification models. The evaluation of classification models has been measured using accuracy, f-measure, precision and recall metrics. The empirical results revealed that the combination of ensemble learning methods with classification models produces better predictions in comparison with the sole classification model for the medical data.

Synthesis of Classification Models and Review in the Field of Machine Learning

This chapter describes various classification models by its learning mechanism and categorized them into different statistical, probabilistic and heuristic methods and explained them with an example dataset. Compared these model and their efficiencies with model evaluation techniques. Further briefed some blended classification models. The goal of this article is to provide a comprehensive review of different classification techniques and enables the reader to give a quick refresh on classification models in big data analytics and the comparison of various classification models help the reader of this article to quickly decide on what classification model to choose for the given business scenario.

Classification Algorithms for EEG-Based Brain-Computer Interface: A Review

This chapter used to classify EEG signals is a key issue in biomedical research for the identification and evaluation of brain activity. Identification of various types of EEG signals is a complicated problem, requiring the analysis of large sets of EEG data. Representative features from a large dataset play an important role in classifying of EEG signals in the field of biomedical signal processing. So, to reduce the above problem, this research has been three types of methods are focused to classify through using feature extraction and classification schemes.

Arrhythmia ECG Beats Classification Using Wavelet-Based Features and Support Vector Machine Classifier

This chapter reports a classification technique to recognize normal (N) and five arrhythmia beats i.e., left bundle branch block (LBBB), right bundle branch block (RBBB), premature ventricular contraction (V), paced (P), and atrial premature contraction (A). The technique utilizes features of heartbeats extracted by the wavelet multi-resolution analysis. The feature vectors are used to train and test the classifier based on the support vector machine which has been emerged as a benchmark in machine learning classifier. It accomplishes the beat classification very efficiently. ECG records of the MIT-BIH arrhythmia database are utilized to acquire the different types of heartbeats. Performance of the proposed classifier outperforms the contemporary arrhythmia beats classification techniques.

Melanoma Image Classification Based on Multivariate Parametric Statistical Tests of Hypothesis

This chapter proposes a novel method, based on the multivariate parametric statistical tests of hypotheses, which classifies the normal skin lesion images and the various stages of the melanoma images. The melanoma images are categorized into two classes, such as initial stage and advanced stage, based on the degree of aggressiveness of cancer. The region of interest is identified and segmented from the input skin melanoma image. The features, such as HSV color, shape, and texture, are extracted from the region of interest. The features are treated as a feature space, which is assumed to be a multivariate normal random field. The proposed statistical tests are employed to identify and classify the melanoma images. The proposed method yields an average correct classification up to 91.55% for the normal skin lesion versus the initial and the advanced stages of the melanoma images; up to 91.39% for initial stage melanoma versus the normal skin lesion and the advanced stages melanoma; and up to 92.27% for the advanced stage melanoma versus the normal skin lesion and the initial stage melanoma.

Section 2: Analysis of Healthcare

Section 2 of this book compromises six chapters that focus on analyzing the healthcare data over various diseases.

Improvement of Variant Adaptable LSTM Trained With Metaheuristic Algorithms for Healthcare Analysis

In this chapter, adaptable LSTM trained with two optimizing algorithms instead of the backpropagation learning algorithm. The optimization algorithms are Biogeography Based Optimization (BBO) and Genetic Algorithm (GA). Data sets collected locally and another benchmark dataset used as well. Finally, the datasets fed into adaptable LSTM- BBO and LSTM-GA models for classification purposes. The experimental and testing results compared and they are promising. This system helps physicians and doctors to provide proper health treatment for patients with diabetes mellitus.

Medical Image Segmentation and Analysis

The chapter gathers gainful purposes of intrigue not stuck just using expedient process, computerization, and right helpful picture partitions. The worldwide vitality term relies upon the worldwide division computation, which can better catch drive information of pictures than a mixture area based dynamic shape technique. Both neighborhood and worldwide terms are ordinarily acclimatized to construct a level set strategy to divide pictures with exactness. the level set technique with Boltzmann system which uses neighborhood mean a quality which engages it as far as possible.

Heart Disease Diagnosis: A Machine Learning Approach

This chapter deals with the application of different machine learning algorithms for effective heart disease diagnosis. Diagnosis through machine learning algorithms involve the three major steps, data preprocessing, feature selection and classification. The chapter covers the experimental study of the performance of SVM, ANN, Logistic regression, Random Forest, KNN, AdaBoost, Naive Bayes, Decision Tree, SGD, CN2 rule inducer approaches.

Real-Time Cardio Monitoring and Characterization of Diseases Introducing Statistical and Spectrogram Analysis

This chapter intends to provide significant theoretical and systematic frameworks and the latest empirical research on the development of an automated cardiovascular disorder diagnostic system with the classifier. This chapter proposes an accurate non-invasive model of the cardiovascular diseases diagnostic system. This model of diagnostic system support superior mobility with continues real-time monitoring facility. This real-time continues monitoring the heart diseases monitoring system will uncover a new dimension towards cardiovascular research. A physician will able to monitor several heart patients remotely with this device. Also, they can prescribe proper medicine remotely to the patient in the emergency time. The system also has a provision to alert the patient by predicting the specific type of cardiovascular disorder accurately. An automated cardiovascular disorder diagnostic system development focuses on the prime objective. Another objective is the adoption of a modern classification technique for detecting cardiovascular disorder with the high accuracy.

Hybrid Multimodality Medical Image Fusion Using Various Fusion Techniques With Quantitative and Qualitative Analysis

This chapter proposes the multimodal medical image fusion method using the hybrid fusion algorithm. The computed tomography, magnetic resonance imaging, positron emission tomography and single photon emission computed tomography are the input images used for this experimental work. In this chapter, experimental results discovered that the proposed techniques provide better visualization of the fused image and give the superior results compared to various existing traditional algorithms. This method is used to improve the fused image quality for better diagnosis of critical disease analysis. The fused hybrid multimodal medical image should convey a better visual description than the individual input images.

Comparative Study of Various Machine Learning Algorithms for Prediction of Insomnia

This Chapter mainly finds the usages and effectiveness of machine learning algorithms in Insomnia diseases prediction. Fifteen machine learning algorithms have been applied and fourteen leading factors have been taken into consideration for predicting Insomnia. Seven performance parameters (Accuracy, Kappa, the True positive rate, false positive rate, Precision, F-measure, and AUC) are used and for implementation, the authors have used python language. The Support vector machine is giving higher performance out of all algorithms giving accuracy 91.6%, F-measure is 92.13, and Kappa is 0.83. Further, SVM is applied on another dataset of 100 patients and giving accuracy 92%. In addition, an analysis of the variable importance of CART, C5.0, Decision Tree, Random Forest, Adaptive boost and XG Boost is calculated.

Section 3: Others

Section 3 of this book compromises four chapters that introducing different innovative practices for the delivery of healthcare.

Smart Technologies to Build Healthcare Models for Vision Impairment

This chapter highlights the recent and smartly configured technologies for building models and related applications, which could be useful for managing health problems in case of visually challenged ones. Several intelligent systems are analyzed and highlighted that can be utilized for providing sub-optimal cure to the concerned patients who mostly confront problems in the plight of accessing relevant information, thereby receiving severely limited healthcare facilities. This chapter is used to address smart technologies for creating healthcare model for blind patients. One can create and use smart healthcare models for no vision patients. The main idea is to connect them with their smartphones with voice assistant for navigating into the system. Development of smart health apps would help in smoothing the way for a healthy lifestyle for visually impaired patients and assist them in case of severe health issues or emergency.

Despeckling Algorithms for Optical Coherence Tomography Images: A Review

This chapter discusses the Optical Coherence Tomography (OCT) non-invasive imaging technique that is widely used in ophthalmology. The presence of speckle affects the quality of OCT images. Despeckling is necessary to improve its visual quality, and it is an integral part of software packages used for the computerized analysis of OCT. Even though a few methods for despeckling OCT are available in the literature, a cross-comparison of their performance is not known to be available. Here, the techniques available in the literature for despeckling the OCT images have been identified. The results of the despeckling algorithms are compared both qualitatively and quantitatively by concerning the noise suppression capability and feature preservation. Among the available techniques, Iterative Adaptive Unbiased (IAUB) filter is found to be superior as far as its performance regarding despeckling on retinal OCT images.

Advances in Ultrasound Despeckling: An Overview

This chapter is intended to encapsulate various techniques for reducing speckle in medical ultrasound images and improving the image quality for visual inspection and/or computer-assisted diagnosis of ultrasound images. In addition, the chapter surveys the papers published between 2015 and 2018 to highlight the latest trends in the despeckling of ultrasound images. The chapter also presents the performance comparison of a few popular algorithms to despeckle medical ultrasound images.

Prevalence of Musculoskeletal Disorders of Odisha Farmers in Selected Agricultural Tasks: A Critical Analysis During Seeding, Fertilizing, and Weeding of Crops

This chapter presents the extensive review of the literature on the application of Cuckoo search (CS) methodology, its application for the optimization of agricultural pesticide sprayers for maximum efficiency was suggested. In the second phase of study, 75 farmers of Odisha in India were considered to assess their musculoskeletal disorders (MSDs) during seeding, fertilizing and weeding of crops using a standardized Nordic questionnaire with a five-point rating scale i.e. (1 = Very less, 2 =Less, 3 = Nil, 4 = Strong, 5 = Very Strong). Factor analysis was performed for "seeding, fertilizing and weeding characteristics", "economical characteristics", and "tools & equipment characteristics of farmers". Then Pearson correlation coefficient matrix was generated for the seeding, fertilizing and weeding characteristics of farmers, followed by regression analysis for the economic characteristics of farmers.

TARGET AUDIENCE

The target audience is constituted by students of Engineering and allied branches; Engineers, Research Scientists, Academicians, technology developers will benefit from reading this book. This book will be a collective resource with comprehensive knowledge in the field of medical imaging and healthcare technology. Contributions to this publication will be made by innovation and technology management practitioners and academics throughout the world.

Acknowledgment

I would like to acknowledge the help of all the people involved in this project and, more specifically, to the authors and reviewers that took part in the review process. Without their support, this book would not have become a reality.

First, the editors would like to thank each one of the authors for their contributions. Our sincere gratitude goes to the chapter's authors who contributed their time and expertise to this book.

Second, the editor wishes to acknowledge the valuable contributions of the reviewers regarding the improvement of quality, coherence, and content presentation of chapters.

I would like to express my gratitude to the global manager team of IGI global for their suggestions and helps in order to make this work much less painful than it could be.

Thank you finally to the authors who will recognize themselves here, for their participation so precious and especially for their availability which allowed me to realize in good conditions this project.

Chinmay Chakraborty
Birla Institute of Technology Mesra, India
September 2018

Section 1
Classification of Health Data

Chapter 1
Developing an Effective Classification Model for Medical Data Analysis

Naeem Ahmed Mahoto
Mehran University of Engineering and Technology, Pakistan

Abdul Hafeez Babar
Mehran University of Engineering and Technology, Pakistan

ABSTRACT

The sparse nature of medical data makes knowledge discovery and prediction a complex task for analysis. Machine learning algorithms have produced promising results for diversified data. This chapter constructs the effective classification model for medical data analysis. In particular, nine classification models, namely Naïve Bayes, decision tree (i.e., J48 and Random Forest), multilayer perceptron, radial bias function, k-nearest neighbors, single conjunctive rule learner, support vector machine, and simple logistics have been applied for developing an effective model. Besides, classification models have also been used in conjunction with ensemble learning methods, since ensemble methods significantly increase the predictive outcomes of the classification models. The evaluation of classification models has been measured using accuracy, f-measure, precision, and recall metrics. The empirical results revealed that the combination of ensemble learning methods with classification models produces better predictions in comparison with sole classification model for the medical data.

INTRODUCTION

Health is the key element of human life. Healthcare industry is one of the largest and fastest growing industries and is the backbone of our society (Lakshmi, Haritha & Srkit, 2016). The healthcare agencies, equipped with modern technological healthcare services, store information regarding health-related issues (Shah, Meghji & Mahoto, 2018; Mahoto, Shaikh & Ansari, 2014). Thus, everyday massive amount of data is being stored. This data is a great source for finding knowledge discoveries in order to determine disease trends, risk factors, and prediction of severe cases, medical pathways and general health inter-

DOI: 10.4018/978-1-5225-7796-6.ch001

ventions (Mahoto, Shaikh & Chowdhry, 2015; Mahoto, Shaikh & Khuhawar, 2014). Data mining allows discovery of hidden patterns from collected database (Banu & Gomathy, 2014). A main challenge, being faced by healthcare facilities, is delivery service with quality (Palaniappan & Awang, 2008). The quality service provides better and correct treatments to patients and helps in effective recovery processes. Poor diagnostic and treatment decisions may lead to disastrous and thus, are rarely distracted. Data mining techniques have been largely applied in healthcare for several purposes in the existing scientific literature. For instance, medical pathways have been extracted in Antonelli et al. (2012A) and Antonelli et al. (2012B), clustering in Antonelli et al. (2013), classification in (Babar & Mahoto, 2018; Shaikh et al., 2015) and association rule analysis has been carried out in Antonelli et al. (2015).

The World Health Organization (WHO) estimation inspired this study to be carried out, since WHO estimated, till 2030, almost 23.6 million individuals will expire due to severe complications of heart related issues (W.H.O., 2018). The possible reasons behind such a large number may be because people are overloaded with work burden in numerous developing countries. Eventually, many people suffer from mental stress and several other health complications. Therefore, it is an important task to diagnose the health related issues proactively, accurately and efficiently (Jarad, Katkar, Shaikh, & Salve, 2015). Generally, diagnosis is carried out based on medical expert's experience and knowledge. However, discovering the heart related problems based on merely symptoms, physical examination and signs of patient body is the difficult assignment in medical domain. This, being a multifaceted problem, may lead towards wrong hypothesis and unforeseeable effects (Turabieh, 2016). Nowadays, healthcare facilities have provided numerous amounts of medical data about patients, their diseases, diagnosis, and hospital resources, & many other important attributes. The advancement of machine learning field has opened ways for handling such a massive and high-dimensional data.

The classification of medical data helps in predicting and getting insight information of treatment procedures as well as historical outcomes. Several attempts have been made for the development of classification models to address the predictive outcomes of the medical data. However, medical data is inherently complex due to its sparse nature. This leads towards open challenge of predicting medical data. The machine learning algorithms have dealt with medical data and also ensemble-learning methods have been reported in the existing literature. Unfortunately, due to diversified nature of medical data, each algorithm behaves differently with different dataset. Therefore, it would be very likely that an algorithm that outperforms at certain medical data; it may not produce promising results for the other medical dataset. However, the investigation of several classification models for a certain medical data may provide broader picture of each considered classification model, which has been taken into consideration in this chapter.

This chapter aims at developing an efficient classification model, which may help in medical data analysis. Particularly, machine-learning algorithms such as Naïve Bayes (NB), Radial Bias Function (RBF), Decision Tree (DT), Random Forest (RF), Single Conjunctive Rule Learner (SCRL), K-Nearest Neighbor (KNN) and Support Vector Machine (SVM) would be considered for experimental activities. The performance of considered classification algorithms has been measured by exploiting well-established matrices: accuracy, precision, Recall and F-measure.

The rest of this chapter is organized as follows: Section 2 briefly presents related work done in the area of machine learning techniques applied for medical data; Section 3 describes classification models being applied in this chapter. The performance measures being used for evaluation of classification models are reported in section 4. The experimental results and conclusion are described in section 5 and Section 6 respectively.

BACKGROUND

In the last few years, numerous amount of research works has been done for diagnosing medical data (Soni, Ansari, Sharma & Soni, 2011). In this context, several data mining techniques, including association analysis, clustering and classification, have been exploited for extracting potentially interesting information. The comparison of classification algorithms, namely, support vector machine, multilayer perceptron and neural network has been used in (Naraei, Abhari, & Sadeghian, 2016) for coronary disease dataset. The results showed support vector machine performed better than the other classifiers. The two data mining toolkits, namely, WEKA and Rapid Miner have been used to predict the effective accuracies of several classifiers in (Shrivas, 2017); SVM outperformed in comparison with other classifiers.

The study in Dhanasekar and Mala (2016) has built a model for heart disease prediction system by means of stream associative classification and rule mined with decision trees. Another study (Shaikh, Mahoto, Khuhawar, & Memon, 2015) focused on three popular data mining classification algorithms: K-NN, Naïve Bayes and decision tree; it compared the predictive accuracy of highly dispersed cleveland heart disease database, which has been divided into three different scenarios. The K-NN outperformed Naïve Bayes and decision tree classification models (Shaikh et al., 2015). Three classification algorithms: CART, ID3 and Decision Table have been exploited in Chaurasia (2017) using 10-fold cross validation for medical data. The results showed that CART exceeds ID3 and Decision Table methods (Chaurasia, 2017). Likewise, the study in (Lakshmi et al., 2016) considered 10 classification algorithms - Random Forest, Rule Induction, CHAID, Neural Network, K-NN, Decision Stump, Decision Tree, Naïve Bayes and SVM; it discovered that Naïve Bayes and SVM performed better for prediction and detection of heart disease (Lakshmi et al., 2016). Another similar study compared performance of Naïve Bayes, K-NN and Decision List; Naïve Bayes produced better outcomes (Jarad, Katkar, Shaikh, & Salve, 2015).

This chapter considers higher number of classification models, which cover larger domain of supervised learning approaches. The considered classification models are Decision Tree (DT), Naïve Bayes (NB), Random Forest (RF), Radial Bias function (RBF), K-Nearest Neighbors (KNN), Single Conjunctive Rule Learner (SCRL), Support Vector Machine (SVM), and Multilayer Perceptron (MLP), which have been applied over medical data. The aim of the study is developing an effective classification model; therefore, ensemble-learning methods have also been exploited in aggregation to classification models. Subsequently, the experimental results describe the broader spectrum of a supervised learning algorithm for high-dimensional data (i.e. medical data) analysis.

CLASSIFICATION MODEL FOR MEDICAL DATA ANALYSIS

This section describes medical dataset, classification models and ensemble methods used in this study. The details are reported in the following.

Dataset

The medical data, specially, cleveland heart disease dataset has been obtained from the online repository (UCI Machine Learning Repository, 2018). The dataset contains 76 attributes, which possess numeric and nominal value. The preprocessing phase significantly reduced the number of attributes and 14 related attributes have been used for this study. The considered attributes are reported in Table 1.

Table 1. The Cleveland disease dataset - attributes

Serial#	Attributes	Description (unit)	Type	Values
1	Age	Patient's age (years)	Numeric	Integer values
2	Sex	Sex of patient	Nominal	1=Male or 0=Female
3	Cp	Chest Pain Type	Nominal	1=typical type, 2=typical type angina, 3=non-angina pain, 4=asymptomatic
4	Trestbps	Resting Blood Pressure (mm Hg)	Numeric	Integer values
5	Chol	Serum Cholesterol (mg/dl)	Numeric	Integer values
6	Fbs	Fasting Blood Sugar	Nominal	1=FBS>120 mg/dl and 0=FBS<120 mg/dl
7	Restecg	Resting electrocardiographic results	Nominal	0=normal, 1=having ST-T wave abnormality 2=showing definite left ventricular hypertrophy
8	Thalach	Maximum heart rate of patient	Numeric	Integer values
9	Exang	Exercise induced angina	Nominal	1=yes and 0=no
10	Oldpeak	The ST depression induced	Numeric	Integer values
11	Slope	The slope of the peak exercise ST segment	Nominal	
12	Ca	Number of major vessels (0-3) colored by fluoroscopy	Numeric	Integer values
13	Thal	Defect Type	Nominal	3=normal, 6=fixed defect 7=reversible defect
14	Num (predicted Value)	Diagnosis of heart disease (angiographic disease status)	Nominal	0=has no heart disease and 1=has heart disease

Classification Models

The classification is considered one of the challenging tasks in the emerging data science activities. In recent years, a number of impressive studies have reported use of classification algorithms for several application domains. Furthermore, analysis of classification methods, their performance evaluation, their comparison with other different classification algorithms in solving complex and real-world problems have remained as focused area in medicine, engineering, and business domains. Classification is a classical machine learning that falls into supervised learning category. It is a model discovering a process that is used for dividing the data into several classes corresponding to some constraints (Akinola & Oyabugbe, 2015). Machine learning algorithms have been successfully employed in prediction of health-related disease (Shaikh et al., 2015). Machine learning algorithms namely, Rule-based method (e.g., Single Conjunctive Rule Learner), Decision Tree (e.g., C4.5), perceptron-based (e.g., Multilayer Perceptron), instance-based (e.g., K-Nearest Neighbors algorithm), statistical learning method (e.g., Naïve Bayes classifier), and support vector machine are widely employed in heart disease prediction system. The considered classification models are described in the following.

Decision Tree: J48

J48, a simple C4.5 decision tree classification algorithm, is mostly used for classification problems. The algorithm constructs a tree to devise classification process. After the construction of tree, it is applied to each ordered set of data and produces classification outcomes for such set of ordered data (Dunham, 2006; Salzberg, 1994). The working mechanism of Decision Tree based classification algorithms is simple; it applies divide and conquer strategy. The tree comprises of decision nodes and leafs, where nodes represent the attributes of the given dataset and leaf represents the class label that is assigned by the classification model (Sahu & Mahtre, 2015; J. Ross, 1993).

Naïve Bayes

NB, a statistical learning algorithm, relies on Bayes' Theorem. This algorithm possesses semantics for representation probabilistic knowledge, and learning probabilities knowledge (Han, Pei, & Kamber, 2011). NB focuses on class conditional autonomy inference that helps to remove the required complexities of computational rate. Therefore, it can rate well and can clearly make use of a numerous number of the domain, inclusive of disease prediction. The algorithm produces great accuracy and speediness on large-scale datasets. The Naïve Bayes is considered as one of the efficient classification algorithm. The basic idea of computing probabilities are given in the *Equation 1* below (Shatovskaya et al., 2006):

$$P\left(\frac{C_i}{X}\right) = \frac{P\left(\frac{X}{C_i}\right)P\left(C_i\right)}{P\left(X\right)} \tag{1}$$

where $\boldsymbol{P(X)}$ represents probability occurrences of instance $\boldsymbol{X}$, $\boldsymbol{P(C_i)}$ shows the probability occurrences of class $\boldsymbol{C_i}$, and $\boldsymbol{P(X/C_i)}$ presents probability generating instance $\boldsymbol{X}$ given $\boldsymbol{C_i}$. This algorithm also furnishes the corresponding results to another classification algorithm including decision trees and neural networks (John & Langley, 1995).

K-Nearest Neighbor

K-NN algorithm is a simple classification method. This algorithm keeps storage of all the possible cases/facts and assigns labels/classes to unknown cases/facts based on resemblances/distance functions. The similarity/distance functions, which are amongst popular ones, are given in the following Equations 2-4:

$$\text{Euclidean}_{\mathrm{E}(x,y)} = \sqrt{\sum_{i=1}^{m}\left(x_i - y_i\right)^2} \tag{2}$$

$$\text{Manhatton}_{\mathrm{M}(x,y)} = \sqrt{\sum_{i=1}^{m}\left|x_i - y_i\right|} \tag{3}$$

$$\text{Chebyshev}_{\mathrm{Ch}(x,y)} = \max_{i=1}\left|x_i - y_i\right| \tag{4}$$

The x_i and y_i in the Equations (2-4) represent the coordinate positions of the data points (i.e., cases/facts). Those cases (i.e., data points), which are close to others based on similarity computed using distance measurements, are called a "neighbors". K-NN detects out a new case or unidentified data points by means of previously identified data points (also referred to as nearest neighbors), and assigns the class label to data points (Han et al., 2011; Tomar & Agarwal, 2013). Multiple nearest neighbors play a role in the classification of data points. The learning of K-NN has been observed as slow (it is also known as Lazy Learner) (Han et al., 2011).

MultiLayer Perceptron

MLP algorithm (Chitra & Seenivasagam, 2013) is feed-forward ANN (artificial neural network), which applies backpropagation to classify instances for supervised learning problems. The MLP algorithm comprises multiple layers of simple, two-state and neurons, which intermingle using weighted networks (i.e., connections). In between input and output layer, there can be any number of hidden layers in the MLP. The weights of the neurons are the computations (i.e., measurements) of degree of correlations among the neurons being connected. This method is good in predicting disease but it also consumes more time in determining the input features for constructing network (Chitra & Seenivasagam, 2013).

Radial Bias Function

RBF is a machine learning classification algorithm. The architecture of Radial Bias Function (Moody & Darken, 1989) offers a simple as well as powerful distance learning system that has been broadly utilized and has produced numerous success for numerical data (Alexandridis, Chondrodima, & Sarimveis, 2013). The Radial Bias Function is an interpolation technique in a given multi-dimensional space. The certain improvements in the interpolation technique lead towards neural models based on radial bias functions, which are also known as radial basis networks. The goal of RBF is to determine an interpolation function that replies on certain number of representatives acquired from data quantification instead of dataset size. Unfortunately, RBF is inadequate to deal with categorical data.

Single Conjunctive Rule Learner

SCRL, also known as inductive learning, is well-established machine learning algorithm. The aim of rule induction is basically to influence a set of rules from data that apprehend all induce knowledge enclosed by that data (Cohen, 1995). Rule-induction classifiers are ordinarily formed of the assigning of a rule on a testing sample, set off by matching attribute values at the left-hand side of the rule (Langley & Sage, 1994). Numerous normal forms of rule can be ordinarily ordered. The first rule, that fires with ordered rules, governed the classification outputs and stops the classification process.

Random Forest

RF classification model is one of the algorithms that could be used for both classification as well as regression tasks. RF is builds a 'forest' by constructing several decision trees at training time, and by producing the class by a vote of an individual tree of the forest. It works same as Decision Tree, but this algorithm builds a forest of decision trees with the location of attributes chosen as random. This algorithm produces accurate and stable prediction due to its nature of merging decision tress. It has also advantages of computing efficiency, increasing the predictive accuracy without significant increase of computational cost. This algorithm can also predict higher dimensional variables (Li, Wu, & Ye, 2015).

Support Vector Machine

SVM algorithm classifies both linear as well as non-linear data (Vapnik, 2013). SVM also can be used for classification as well as regression predictions. SVM is based on concepts of decision planes (also called hyperplanes), which define decision boundaries. A hyerplane detaches boundaries of objects belonging to different other class labels (Joachims, 1998). The working mechanism of SVM plots each item of the given dataset as a point in the n-dimensional space (n is the number of attributes/features of data point). The value of each data item is considered as the value of coordinate system. The SVM performs classification in order to find hyperplane of the n-dimensional space data points. The SVM is determined to the discovery of optimal decision boundary (i.e., hyperplane) that effectively separates several class labels.

Simple Logistics

SL is the classification method that is applied for constructing a linear logistic regression model. SL is considered as special case of linear regression, where outcome variable is categorical. SL predicts the probability of occurrences of a certain event. This prediction is formulated by fitting data to a logistic function. It computes the probability of outcomes of dependent variables (Freitas & Lavington, 1997).

Ensemble Learning Methods

Ensemble-learning method is an inspired research path of machine learning (Onan, 2016; Ranawana & Palade, 2006). The central concept behind ensemble methods is merging decisions from a set of a weak learning algorithm (base learners) for acquiring better accuracy and robustness of classification models. Ensemble method in conjunction with classification model produces better in comparison with a single base-line learner. There are significant statistical, adaptive and representational grounds that emphasize building manifold classification systems (Rokach, 2010). Ensemble-learning methods can be openly attributed to two groups, based on utilized formation in constructing of ensembles, dependent and independent methods (Kuncheva, 2004). The base-line learner's outcomes are employed to accumulate the next classification model in independent method. Thus, the result achieved in the earlier iterations can be assigned in acquiring knowledge of later iterations. Furthermore, the base-line learner's independent methods are built impartially and the outcomes of such learning algorithm are merged through a grouping approach such as meta-learning or mainstream voting schemes (Breiman, 1996). The dependent methods, as name suggests, rely on the outcomes of the base learner. This study has adopted five ensemble methods for building effective classification model. These ensemble methods are AdaBoost, Bagging, Dagging, RandomSubSpace and Voting algorithms. The details of these methods are discussed as under.

AdaBoost

Boosting algorithm, widely used ensemble learning method, increases anticipated performance of weak classification models. It combines several imprecise classification rules into a single and highly accurate rule. The main concept of boosting is to expand the predictive performance of a classification model by compounding several training samples. Applying such boosting algorithm results in a better accuracy rate of a classification model.

Bagging

Bagging (BootStrap aggregating), another ensemble method, focuses on constructing a robust compound classification model with a greater predictive outcomes by merging the trained classification models on several training sets (Breiman, 1996). The training examples for each classifier are chosen by sampling with the replacement and are referred to as bootstrap samples. This approach has been repeatedly shown to offer high-level results in patent scenarios. This approach is not effective for decreasing the bias but can decrease the variance due to specific random aspects of the training data.

Dagging

Dagging method practices disjoint data points, unlike Bagging which uses bootstrapping (Ting & Witten, 1997). The algorithm is efficient when independent classification models have inadequate time complexity. Dagging method strengthens weak classification models by merging, usually, by voting schemes.

RandomSubSpace

The RandomSubSpace combines numerous classification models that are trained using arbitrarily selected features (Ho, 1998). This method focuses on avoiding overfitting, at the same time improving the predictive performance. A robust classification model is built by bagging method to combine the weak learners, which have been trained on several samples of the training set. This is merely binding for the RandomSubSpace method. Besides, several samples are needed for feature selection.

Voting

Voting can be termed as the easiest way of combining several base-line classification models. The combination of weak learners' outcomes can be carried out in numerous ways. The voting, weighted voting, Naïve Bayes and combination of other several classification models comes within the popular ways of combination approach (Kuncheva, 2004).

EVALUATION INDEXING AND VALIDATION

Evaluation Indexing

To evaluate the performance of considered classification models and ensemble methods, the well-established evaluation indexing (i.e., metrics/measures) have been applied, namely, accuracy, precision, recall and F-measure.

Accuracy is widely employed metric for evaluating performance of classification models. It is the ratio of true positive and true negative over the total number of data points in a given dataset as defined in Equation 5.

$$Accuracy = \left(\frac{TN + TP}{TP + FP + FN + TN}\right) * 100 \tag{5}$$

where true negative is represented as TN, true positive as TP, false positive as FP, and false negative is termed as FN.

Precision is the ratio of TP over total sum of TP and FP as defined in Equation 6.

$$Precision = \left(\frac{TP}{TP + FP}\right) \tag{6}$$

Recall is the ratio of TP over summation of TP and FN as defined in Equation 7.

$$Recall = \frac{TP}{TP + FN} \tag{7}$$

F-measure **is** another evaluation metrics that aggregates precision and recall values into a single value (Sannino & De Pietro, 2011) as defined in Equation 8.

$$F - measure = 2 * \frac{precision * recall}{precision + recall} \tag{8}$$

Validation

The classification is a supervised learning method. The classification models are trained using training dataset, and as a result these learned classification models predict testing dataset. This chapter has applied two well-known validation techniques (i.e., cross-validation and split percentage) for segmenting given dataset into training as well as testing portions. The details of these techniques are reported in the following.

- **Cross-Validation:** Cross-validation technique is used for partitioning the original dataset into a training set to train classification model and rest of data is exploited to test the developed model. Cross-validation technique splits the given training data into different disjoint parts with equal size. All parts are chosen as the testing data at their turns, while the other remaining portion of data is applied as training data. The classification model, constructed using training data, is employed in predicting suitable class labels for testing data. The whole process is iterated; the process stops when all parts are covered once. Finally, prediction accuracies over all the blinded tests are merged to obtain an inclusive performance estimation (Zengyou, 2015). K-fold cross-validation method runs iterations for K times, and the first K-1 times are used for training; and final fold is for testing. Finally, average value of model against each of the fold is finalized.

- **Split Percentage:** Split Percentage is a technique used to split the sample data into training (Split percentage) set to construct classification model and rest of percentage data is used to test the developed model. This technique is beneficial, when learning algorithm is slow. Dataset can be split into several samples percentage training and testing such as 20-80%, 30-70%, 40-60%, 50-50%, 60-40%, 70-30%, 80-20%. For example, 20-80% shows that 20% of the given dataset has been used as training dataset, whilst 80% remaining dataset has been used for testing the classification model.

EXPERIMENTAL RESULTS

To analyze medical data, several experiments has been carried out using considered classification models as well as combination of classification models and ensemble-learning methods. The experiments have been performed using popular data mining tool – Waikato Environment for Knowledge Analysis (WEKA) version 3.8 (I. H. Witten, 2016) on a PC having 2.5GHz Intel processor, 8 GB RAM (Random Access Memory). The default parameters of each considered classification model are assigned in WEKA to obtain predictive outcomes, since default parameters have performed well (Amancio et al., 2014).

The performance of each considered classification model with and without ensemble learning methods has been measured using both validation techniques: 1) K-fold cross-validation and 2) split percentage. In k-fold cross-validation, the original considered dataset is randomly divided into 10 and 20 mutually exclusive folds. Training and testing process is repeatedly applied 10 and 20 times respectively and each part is tested and trained ten and twenty times. The average results for 10-fold and 20-fold are reported respectively in Table 2. In split percentage technique, the original dataset is divided into different percentage training and testing value such as 20-80%, 30-70%, 40-60%, 50-50%, 60-40%, 70-30% and 80-20%. The average results for split percentage are also reported in Table 2.

Table 2. Performance of several classification models

Classification Model Name	Cross-Validation		Split Percentage (Training% - Testing%)						
	10-Fold	20-Fold	20-80	30-70	40-60	50-50	60-40	70-30	80-20
J48	77.77	80.19	73.14	80.66	77.47	70.19	73.55	76.92	**85.24**
Naïve Bayes	83.49	82.83	81.40	83.01	86.26	83.44	85.12	85.71	**86.88**
K-NN	83.16	82.50	81.81	83.01	85.16	**85.43**	85.12	84.61	85.24
MLP	80.85	82.50	77.66	83.49	78.57	84.10	80.99	**85.71**	85.24
RBF	83.82	83.16	80.57	83.96	84.06	85.43	**85.95**	84.61	83.60
RF	83.16	81.84	80.99	84.90	81.31	79.47	82.64	84.61	**88.52**
SCRL	69.96	71.28	73.55	71.22	69.78	73.50	75.20	**79.12**	78.68
SVM	84.15	83.82	83.05	84.43	84.06	81.45	84.29	**85.71**	81.96
Simple Logistics	83.16	83.49	83.47	81.60	83.51	83.44	82.64	**86.81**	83.60

The first part of this study inspects the effectiveness of base classification model (i.e., in the absence of ensemble learning method) using 10-fold, 20-fold and several split percentage portions. The higher classification prediction outcomes have been observed with split percentage technique with values: 70% training and 30% testing (70-30%) for several models as reported in Table 2. Though, some of the models have outperformed using 80-20%, for instance, J48 (85.24% accuracy) and NB (86.88% accuracy). Thus, it has been concluded in the experimental results that split percentage technique produces better predictive outcomes for the considered base classification models.

Another analysis has been carried out in the experimental results for the considered classification models, when these are applied in presence of ensemble-learning methods. The split percentage technique since produced better outcomes using 70-30% ratio. Therefore, 70-30% has been applied in presence of each considered ensemble method. The performance of each classification model in combination of ensemble method is reported in Table 3. It has been observed that presence of ensemble methods significantly increased the performance of classification models. For instance, J48 as base learning model produced 76.92% with 70-30% split percentage technique. The presence of ensemble methods has improved its performance upto 84.61% using dagging ensemble method. Though, the same ensemble method has also decreased performance of other model such as NB (from 85.71% as base-line to 83.51% with dagging method). Generally, the presence of ensemble methods has increased performance of the models.

The experimental results in Table 3 reports that Decorate ensemble-learning method has effectively enhanced performance of higher number of classification models. The highest accuracy rate of 89.11% has been observed for MLP in presence of Decorate ensemble method. RBF being second having 89.01% and SVM with 86.81% accuracy rate as third.

The other evaluation metrics such as precision, recall and f-measures are reported in Table 4. The time to build the classification model has also been reported in Table 4 for each model. The Decorate ensemble method significantly improved performance of several classification models; therefore, the precision, recall, f-measure and timing have been computed to compare the outcomes with and without decorate ensemble method. Table 4 shows that presence of ensemble method also increases the time for construction classification model. The models such as J48, NB, K-NN and SCRL took less than a second in building model. However, MLP consumed 1.13 seconds as a base-line classification model

Table 3. Performance of classification models with split percentage 70-30% (i.e., 70% training- 30% testing)

Classification Model Name	Base-line Accuracy	Bagging	Boosting	Decorate	Voting	RandomSubSpace	Dagging
J48	76.92	80.21	83.51	81.31	76.92	83.51	**84.61**
Naïve Bayes	85.71	85.71	**86.81**	84.61	85.71	84.61	83.51
K-NN	84.61	84.61	84.61	**86.81**	84.61	81.31	84.61
MLP	85.71	84.61	85.71	**89.11**	85.71	82.41	86.81
RBF	84.61	86.81	84.61	**89.01**	84.61	82.41	83.51
RF	**84.61**	**84.61**	82.41	**84.61**	**84.61**	78.02	**84.61**
SCRL	79.12	80.21	**85.71**	75.82	79.12	79.12	76.92
SVM	85.71	85.71	83.51	**86.81**	85.71	83.51	85.71
Simple Logistics	86.81	86.81	86.81	86.81	86.81	**87.91**	86.81

Table 4. Comparison of base-line classification model and presence of ensemble method (decorate) with split percentage (70% training - 30% testing)

Classification Model	Base-line Classification Models					Combination of Ensemble Method (Decorate)				
	Precision	Recall	F-measure	Accuracy (%)	Time (sec)	Precision	Recall	F-measure	Accuracy (%)	Time (sec)
J48	0.74	0.822	0.779	76.92	-	0.804	0.822	0.813	81.31	0.68
NB	**0.833**	0.889	0.86	85.71	-	0.83	0.867	0.848	84.61	1.53
K-NN	**0.833**	0.867	0.848	84.61	-	0.837	0.911	0.872	86.81	6.74
MLP	**0.833**	0.889	0.86	85.71	1.13	**0.872**	0.911	0.891	**89.11**	120.07
RBF	0.83	0.867	0.848	84.61	0.05	0.857	**0.933**	**0.894**	89.01	20.16
RF	0.816	0.889	0.851	84.61	0.05	0.816	0.889	0.851	84.61	8.98
SCRL	0.76	0.844	0.8	79.12	-	0.695	0.911	0.788	75.82	0.48
SVM	0.808	**0.933**	0.866	85.71	0.01	0.824	**0.933**	0.875	86.81	3.47
SL	0.824	**0.933**	**0.875**	**86.81**	0.13	0.824	**0.933**	0.875	86.81	3.61

and almost 120% times, MLP consumed time in presence of decorate ensemble method. Besides, MLP also outperformed all other considered models with 89.11% accuracy rate. This is a trade-off; presence of ensemble methods increases the performance of classification models as well as time to construct the model.

The experimental results can be summarized as split percentage technique performs better for the medical data being used for prediction. Besides, base-line classification models perform effectively in presence of ensemble learning methods with the cost of more time required for developing classification model. Among the considered classification models, as a base-line model Decision Tree based algorithms (i.e., J48 and RF) outperformed in comparison with other models. However, MLP performed quite better in presence of ensemble methods, in particular, with Decorate method. MLP has also taken more time in constructing the model. The possible reason behind such behavior can be the foundation of MLP, which relies on hidden layers for developing the classification model.

CONCLUSION AND FUTURE RESEARCH DIRECTIONS

The chapter investigated nine classification algorithms, namely - Naïve Bayes, Decision Tree (J48 and Random Forest), Multilayer Perceptron, K-Nearest Neighbor, Radial Bias Function, Single Conjunctive Rule Learner, Support Vector Machine, and Simple logistics, when applied over high dimensional dataset (i.e., medical data). Furthermore, cross-validation and split percentage techniques have been employed in the analysis in two case scenarios: 1) Base-line classification model and 2) Base-line classification model in conjunction with ensemble method.

The experimental results revealed that split percentage is better choice for the considered dataset and classification models. In case scenario one, Decision Tree algorithms and Naïve Bayes outperformed the other considered models with split percentage technique (i.e., 70% training -30% testing) having 85.24% and 86.88% accuracy rates respectively.

The combination of ensemble methods significantly enhanced accuracy rates of several classification models including MLP, RBF, SVM, DT and NB. Besides, presence of ensemble methods also took more time in constructing classification model. The presence of Decorate ensemble method effectively increased accuracy rates of classification models. MLP produced the highest accuracy rate of 89.11% using split percentage technique (70% Training – 30% Testing), RBF as second with 89.01% accuracy, and both K-NN and SVM being the third with accuracy rate of 86.81%.

The investigation of how attribute values of considered dataset impact towards performance of classification model would be considered as future directions. For instance, if an attribute has only 2 to 3 possible values and some other attributes may have from 10 to 100 different values; in presence of these varying values of dataset, how does classification model predict. Furthermore, the analysis of each classification model with and without ensemble learning methods for several different medical datasets is also considered as future directions.

REFERENCES

Akinola, S. O., & Oyabugbe, O. J. (2015). Accuracies and training times of data mining classification algorithms: An empirical comparative study. *Journal of Software Engineering and Applications*, *8*(09), 470–477. doi:10.4236/jsea.2015.89045

Alexandridis, A., Chondrodima, E., & Sarimveis, H. (2013). Radial basis function network training using a nonsymmetric partition of the input space and particle swarm optimization. *IEEE Transactions on Neural Networks and Learning Systems*, *24*(2), 219–230. doi:10.1109/TNNLS.2012.2227794 PMID:24808277

Amancio, D. R., Comin, C. H., Casanova, D., Travieso, G., Bruno, O. M., Rodrigues, F. A., & da Fontoura Costa, L. (2014). A systematic comparison of supervised classifiers. *PLoS One*, *9*(4), e94137. doi:10.1371/journal.pone.0094137 PMID:24763312

Antonelli, D., Baralis, E., Bruno, G., Cerquitelli, T., Chiusano, S., & Mahoto, N. A. (2013). Analysis of diabetic patients through their examination history. *Expert Systems with Applications*, *40*(11), 4672–4678. doi:10.1016/j.eswa.2013.02.006

Antonelli, D., Baralis, E., Bruno, G., Chiusano, S., Mahoto, N. A., & Petrigni, C. (2012A). Extraction of medical pathways from electronic patient records. In *Medical Applications of Intelligent Data Analysis: Research Advancements* (pp. 273–289). IGI Global. doi:10.4018/978-1-4666-1803-9.ch018

Antonelli, D., Baralis, E., Bruno, G., Chiusano, S., Mahoto, N. A., & Petrigni, C. (2012B). Analysis of diagnostic pathways for colon cancer. *Flexible Services and Manufacturing Journal*, *24*(4), 379-399.

Antonelli, D., Baralis, E. M., Bruno, G., Cagliero, L., Cerquitelli, T., Chiusano, S. A., . . . Mahoto, N. A. (2015). MeTA: Characterization of medical treatments at different abstraction levels. *ACM Transactions on Intelligent Systems and Technology*, *6*(4), 1-25.

Babar, A. H., Mahoto, N. A. (2018). Comparative Analysis of Classification Models for Healthcare Data Analysis. *International Journal of Computer and Information Technology,* *7*(4), 170-175.

Banu, M. N., & Gomathy, B. (2014). Disease forecasting system using data mining methods. *International Conference on Intelligent Computing Applications (ICICA).* 10.1109/ICICA.2014.36

Breiman, L. (1996). Bagging predictors. *Machine Learning, 24*(2), 123–140. doi:10.1007/BF00058655

Chaurasia, V. (2017). *Early prediction of heart diseases using data mining techniques*. Academic Press.

Chitra, R., & Seenivasagam, V. (2013). Review of heart disease prediction system using data mining and hybrid intelligent techniques. *ICTACT Journal on Soft Computing, 3*(4), 605-609.

Cohen, W. W. (1995). *Fast effective rule induction. In Machine Learning Proceedings 1995* (pp. 115–123). Elsevier. doi:10.1016/B978-1-55860-377-6.50023-2

Dhanasekar, A., & Mala, R. (2016). Analysis of Association Rule for Heart Disease Prediction from Large Datasets. *International Journal of Innovative Research in Science, Engineering and Technology, 5*(10), 18059-18063.

Dunham, M. H. (2006). *Data mining: Introductory and advanced topics*. Pearson Education India.

Freitas, A. A., & Lavington, S. H. (1997). *Mining very large databases with parallel processing* (Vol. 9). Springer Science & Business Media.

Han, J., Pei, J., & Kamber, M. (2011). *Data mining: concepts and techniques*. Elsevier.

Ho, T. K. (1998). The random subspace method for constructing decision forests. *IEEE Transactions on Pattern Analysis and Machine Intelligence, 20*(8), 832–844. doi:10.1109/34.709601

J. Ross Quinlan. (1993). *C4.5: Programs for Machine Learning*. San Francisco, CA: Morgan Kaufmann Publishers Inc.

Jarad, A., Katkar, R., Shaikh, A. R., & Salve, A. (2015). Intelligent Heart Disease Prediction System With MongoDB. *Future, 13*, 14.

Joachims, T. (1998). *Text categorization with support vector machines: Learning with many relevant features*. Paper presented at the European conference on machine learning. 10.1007/BFb0026683

John, G. H., & Langley, P. (1995). Estimating continuous distributions in Bayesian classifiers. *Proceedings of the Eleventh conference on Uncertainty in artificial intelligence*.

Kuncheva, L. I. (2004). *Combining pattern classifiers: methods and algorithms*. John Wiley & Sons. doi:10.1002/0471660264

Lakshmi, M. S., Haritha, D., & Srkit, V. (2016). Heart disease diagnosis using predictive data mining. *International Journal of Computer Science and Information Security*.

Langley, P., & Sage, S. (1994). *Induction of selective Bayesian classifiers. In Uncertainty Proceedings 1994* (pp. 399–406). Elsevier. doi:10.1016/B978-1-55860-332-5.50055-9

Li, L., Wu, Y., & Ye, M. (2015). Experimental comparisons of multi-class classifiers. *Informatica, 39*(1).

Mahoto, N. A., Shaikh, A., & Khuhawar, F. (2014). CliTA: Discovering Knowledge from Clinical Data. *Sindh University Research Journal, 46*(4), 539-546.

Mahoto, N. A., Shaikh, F. K., & Ansari, A. Q. (2014). Exploitation of Clustering Techniques in Transactional Healthcare Data. *Mehran University Research Journal of Engineering & Technology, 33*(1), 77-92.

Mahoto, N. A., Shaikh, F. K., & Chowdhry, B. S. (2015). Innovative Architecture to Enhance Quality of Service for Laboratory Management Information System. In *Laboratory Management Information Systems: Current Requirements and Future* (pp. 242–256). IGI Global. doi:10.4018/978-1-4666-6320-6.ch012

Moody, J., & Darken, C. J. (1989). Fast learning in networks of locally-tuned processing units. *Neural Computation*, *1*(2), 281–294. doi:10.1162/neco.1989.1.2.281

Naraei, P., Abhari, A., & Sadeghian, A. (2016). *Application of multilayer perceptron neural networks and support vector machines in classification of healthcare data.* Paper presented at the Future Technologies Conference (FTC). 10.1109/FTC.2016.7821702

Onan, A. (2016). Classifier and feature set ensembles for web page classification. *Journal of Information Science*, *42*(2), 150–165. doi:10.1177/0165551515591724

Palaniappan, S., & Awang, R. (2008). Intelligent heart disease prediction system using data mining techniques. *IEEE/ACS International Conference on Computer Systems and Applications, AICCSA 2008.* 10.1109/AICCSA.2008.4493524

Ranawana, R., & Palade, V. (2006). Multi-classifier systems: Review and a roadmap for developers. *International Journal of Hybrid Intelligent Systems*, *3*(1), 35–61. doi:10.3233/HIS-2006-3104

Rokach, L. (2010). Ensemble-based classifiers. *Artificial Intelligence Review*, *33*(1-2), 1–39. doi:10.100710462-009-9124-7

Sahu, S., & Mehtre, B. M. (2015). Network intrusion detection system using J48 Decision Tree. *International Conference on Advances in Computing Communication Information*, *2015*, 2023–2026. doi:10.1109/icacci.2015.7275914

Salzberg, S. L. (1994). C4. 5: Programs for machine learning by j. ross quinlan. *Machine Learning*, *16*(3), 235–240. doi:10.1007/BF00993309

Sannino, G., & De Pietro, G. (2011). A smart context-aware mobile monitoring system for heart patients. *IEEE International Conference on Bioinformatics and Biomedicine Workshops (BIBMW).* 10.1109/BIBMW.2011.6112448

Shah, H., Meghji, A. F., & Mahoto, N. A. (2018). Healthcare Services in Developing Countries of the South Asian Region: Present and Future Perspectives. In Design and Development of Affordable Healthcare Technologies. IGI Global. Doi:10.4018/978-1-5225-4969-7.ch001

Shaikh, A., Mahoto, N., Khuhawar, F., & Memon, M. (2015). Performance evaluation of classification methods for heart disease dataset. *Sindh University Research Journal-SURJ (Science Series)*, *47*(3).

Shatovskaya, T., Repka, V., & Good, A. (2006). Application of the Bayesian Networks in the informational modeling. *International conference: Modern problems of radio engineering, telecommunications, and computer science* (p. 108). Lviv-Slavsko, Ukraine: Academic Press.

Shrivas, A. K. & R. K. Y. (2017). An Effective Prediction Factors for Coronary Heart Disease using Data Mining based Classification Technique. *International Journal on Recent and Innovation Trends in Computing and Communication*, *5*(5).

Soni, J., Ansari, U., Sharma, D., & Soni, S. (2011). Predictive data mining for medical diagnosis: An overview of heart disease prediction. *International Journal of Computers and Applications*, *17*(8), 43–48. doi:10.5120/2237-2860

Ting, K. M., & Witten, I. H. (1997). *Stacking bagged and dagged models*. Academic Press.

Tomar, D., & Agarwal, S. (2013). A survey on Data Mining approaches for Healthcare. *International Journal of Bio-Science and Bio-Technology*, *5*(5), 241–266. doi:10.14257/ijbsbt.2013.5.5.25

Turabieh, H. (2016). A Hybrid ANN-GWO Algorithm for Prediction of Heart Disease. *American Journal of Operations Research*, *6*(02), 136–146. doi:10.4236/ajor.2016.62016

UCI Machine Learning Repository. (2018). *Cleveland Heart Disease Dataset*. Retrieved from https://archive.ics.uci.edu/ml/datasets/Heart+Disease

Vapnik, V. (2013). *The nature of statistical learning theory*. Springer science & business media.

W.H.O. (2018). Retrieved from http://www.who.int/mediacentre/factsheets/fs310.pdf

Witten, Hall, & Pal. (2016). *Data Mining: Practical machine learning tools and techniques*. Academic Press.

Zengyou, H. (2015). *Data mining for bioinformatics applications*. Woodhead Publishing.

ADDITIONAL READING

Delen, D., Fuller, C., McCann, C., & Ray, D. (2009). Analysis of healthcare coverage: A data mining approach. *Expert Systems with Applications*, *36*(2), 995–1003. doi:10.1016/j.eswa.2007.10.041

Gosain, A., & Kumar, A. (2009). *Analysis of health care data using different data mining techniques*. Paper presented at the Intelligent Agent & Multi-Agent Systems, 2009. IAMA 2009. International Conference on.

Kaur, H., & Wasan, S. K. (2006). Empirical study on applications of data mining techniques in healthcare. *Journal of Computational Science*, *2*(2), 194–200. doi:10.3844/jcssp.2006.194.200

Kurgan, L. A., Cios, K. J., Tadeusiewicz, R., Ogiela, M., & Goodenday, L. S. (2001). Knowledge discovery approach to automated cardiac SPECT diagnosis. *Artificial Intelligence in Medicine*, *23*(2), 149–169. doi:10.1016/S0933-3657(01)00082-3 PMID:11583923

Lin, F., Chou, S., Pan, S., & Chen, Y. (2001). Mining time dependency patterns in clinical pathways. *International Journal of Medical Informatics*, *62*(1), 11–25. doi:10.1016/S1386-5056(01)00126-5 PMID:11340003

Prather, J. C., Lobach, D. F., Goodwin, L. K., Hales, J. W., Hage, M. L., & Hammond, W. E. (1997). *Medical data mining: knowledge discovery in a clinical data warehouse*. Paper presented at the Proceedings of the AMIA annual fall symposium.

KEY TERMS AND DEFINITIONS

Classification: The process of assigning class label to unknown data points based on learned facts.

Ensemble Learning Method: It is a machine learning technique that allows combination of several base-learning models to produce optimal predictive model.

Knowledge Discovery: The process of extracting useful information from large set of data using sophisticated algorithms/methods.

Machine Learning: It is sub-field of artificial intelligence that often uses statistical techniques to make computers capable enough to "learn" with data.

Supervised Learning: It is a type of machine learning algorithm that uses a known dataset (called the training dataset) to construct a learned model, which makes predictions for unknown datasets (called the testing datasets).

Chapter 2
Synthesis of Classification Models and Review in the Field of Machine Learning

Venkatram Kari
VIT University, India

Geetha Mary Amalanathan
VIT University, India

ABSTRACT

Classification method is an important technique used in machine learning for predictive analytics. Classification enables business to predict future trends and behaviors of an enterprise with the help of their past data. Classification is a supervised learning model, which is built in twostep process, first building the classification model and second predicting the outcome for unknown data. This chapter describes various classification models by learning mechanisms and categorizes them into different statistical, probabilistic, and heuristic methods, and explains them with example dataset. It also compares these models and their efficiencies with model evaluation techniques and briefs some blended classification models. The goal of this chapter is to provide a comprehensive review of different classification techniques and give a quick refresher on classification models in big data analytics. The comparison of various classification models helps the readers to quickly decide which classification model to choose for the given business scenario.

INTRODUCTION

The easy way to understand the data is to distribute the data into different classes on the basis of their data attribute and characteristics. This process of organizing the data is known as classification. It is very difficult to interpret the data which is unorganized, such data can neither be easily compared nor interpreted.

Machine learning models are primarily built in collaboration of two important techniques - Supervised learning (classification & regression), unsupervised learning (clustering). A target function (f) is

DOI: 10.4018/978-1-5225-7796-6.ch002

estimated by classification model which maps input variables (A) to an output variable (B) i.e., B=f(A). Target function f(A) is built from labeled training data and will predict the outcome of unknown data into a categorical value called target class (Jothi, Rashid, & Husain, 2015). Classification is a twostep process (Wahbeh, Al-Radaideh, Al-Kabi, & Al-Shawakfa, 2011), 1) Model construction 2) Predicting the unknown data. Prediction is performed after rigorous testing for acceptance.

Classification objectives - simple to understand, easy to compare and intuitive to interpret by enabling data to represent in brief and simple way. It will summarize the large data into condensed form which is easy to understand. For instance 250 patients' in a hospital classified them on medical problems, status into 100, 70, 50, 30 as self-care, minimum-care, intermediate-care, ICU patients. Now it easy to interpret and compare data. This is motivation for classification & interpret the similarities and dissimilarities among the data visualize and goal to build a function to make distinction data into classes.

At times some important features will be missing in data, eg., patient data without age or tests etc. which are critical for predicting treatment. When attribute values are missing, there are several actions mentioned in the literature. These are 1) Discard the missing value's instances. 2) Acquire missing values 3) Imputation.

LITERATURE REVIEW

Researchers and health care industry practitioners are widely using machine learning and classification models for building decision support system. Tarik A and all has used Artificial Neural Network to classify of diabetic patients to predict the rate of fasting blood sugar and diabetes mellitus and figure out the relations between the FBS and symptoms with prediction rate and identify the impact and symptoms of the patient's health(Tarik A. Rashid, Abdullah, & Abdullah, 2016). Artificial bee colony ABC and genetic algorithm (GA), and back propagation neural network (BPNN) for better prediction of diagnosing diabetes mellitus (DM) (Tarik A Rashid & Abdullah, 2018). It enables decision support system and help physicians to provide patients good health treatments and recommendations for further medication(Tarik A. Rashid, 2016).

Premature Ventricular Contraction Detection on ECG Trace is predicted with classification by Manuel M. Casas and All. Bayesian classification algorithms trained from the patient ECG traces and concluded PVC complexes with 95% accurately. This automated mechanisms enable for the detection of PVC complexes(Casas, Avitia, Gonzalez-Navarro, Cardenas-Haro, & Reyna, 2018). This is a very good achievement to predict the PVC detection based on ECG trace.

Abraham Yosipof & All, in their recent paper build ensemble model -AL Boost for the visualization and identifying of interesting trends, which opens up new opportunities for designing new drugs(Yosipof, Guedes, & García-Sosa, 2018).

Singh and all tried to diagnose the disease by analyzing with pattern matching and neural networks (Singh, Prasad, Das, Poddar, & Choudhury, 2018).

BACKGROUND

A typical classification model is shown in the following diagram Figure 1, with two processes 1) Model construction for known dataset with predefined class labels. Build the model with a training dataset. Validating the model on the validation dataset. 2) Classify the unknown data.

Generalizing the model is an important consideration, it is important because data collected in just a sample and incomplete/ noisy. Goal of the model is to generalize from the training data, so that make accurate predictions for unseen data. Model's performance impacted by overfitting and under fitting, overfitting refers to a model, which get very well trained for known data including noisy data and negatively performance on new data, under fitting model can neither fit to training data nor generalize.

Feature selection is an important process of classification and it is used to identify only the subset of all the features in dataset used for predicting which are important. The purpose this process to simplify the model and perform well as it takes shorter time to train and predict and avoid the curse of dimensionality & reduce the overfitting. Deep (End2End) learning technique learn its tasks and features from data. Artificial Neural networks, convolutional neural networks trains the model by with DNNs, it leads to overfitting and computation time increases in deep learning.

There are numerous applications harness classification models for prediction, typical examples are: credit/ loan approvals – predict the risk based on attributes to approve or deny. A tumor classified as cancerous or benign in Medical diagnosis. Credit card transactions – It is fraudulent or genuine. Web page categorization – Predict it is arts, games, entertainment etc. Machine learning algorithms have been successfully generating very high accuracy and have drawn great significance to use them in healthcare recently. For instance cancer survival groups, intensive care, hospital inpatient, emergency ward admissions etc., (Harper, 2005) are few examples of classification models used in healthcare applications

Classification models categorized based on their learning ability. As depicted in the Figure 2, it can be divided two categories - eager learners and lazy learners.

Lazy learners are exampled based learns, it stores training data with no or little processing and waits for testing. It takes less learning time and long prediction time. It uses many local linear functions effectively and implicitly to form approximations for finding the prediction. It will have multiple hypotheses. KNN classification model, case-based classification models are examples for lazy learners.

Figure 1.

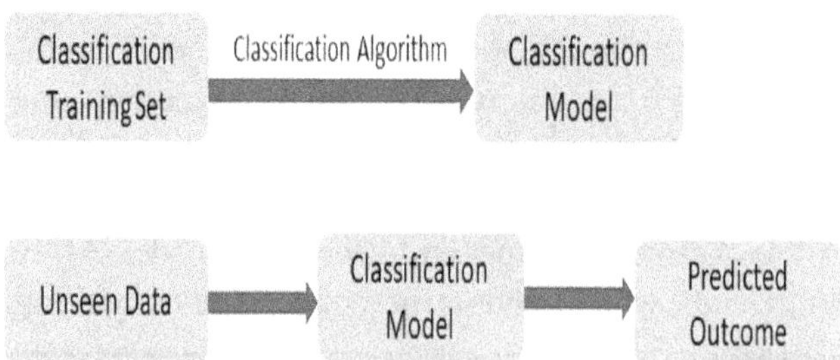

Figure 2.

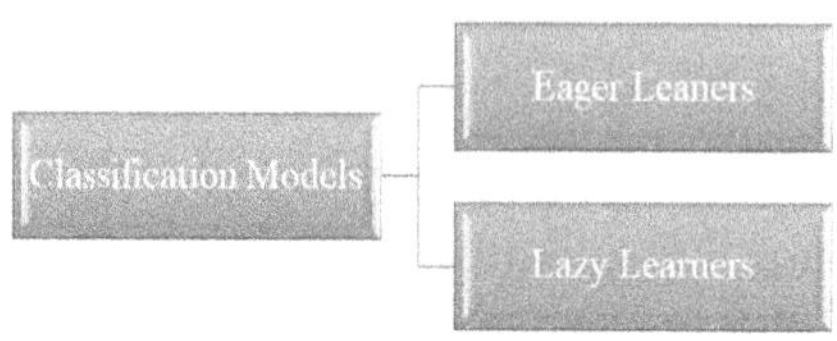

Figure 3.

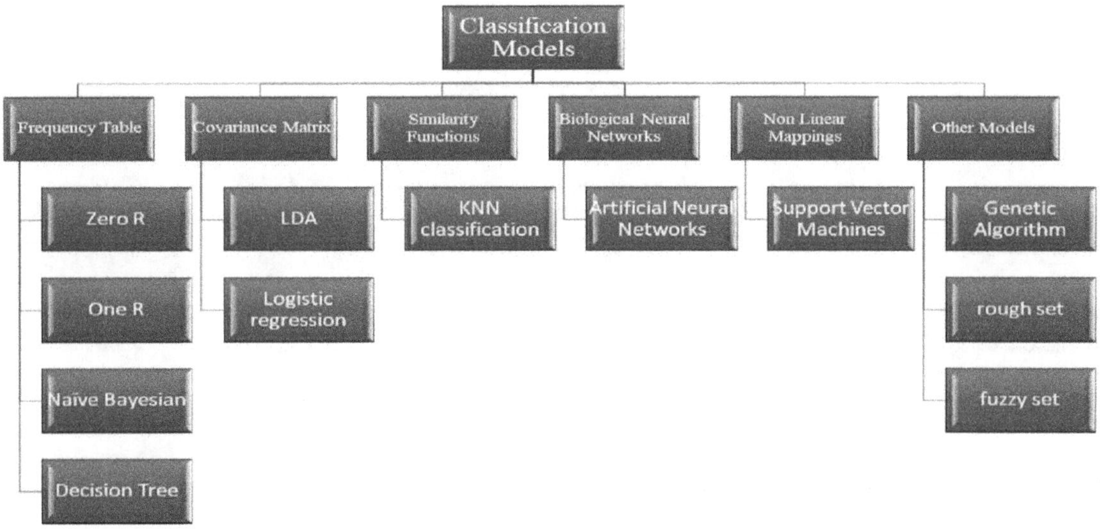

Eager leaners build a target function with general, autonomous and input-independent learning mode during the training. It builds learning model during the training and eager to classify any previously unseen data. It will have single hypothesis which covers total instance of input space. Bayesian, Decision tree induction -rule-based classification, SVM, ANN and association rule-based classification etc are eager learners

Categorizing classification models based on interesting facts are discussed in Figure 3.

As mentioned in the Figure 3, classification models are categorized based on the interesting facts: Classification based on the 1) frequency table – Zero R, One R, Naïve Bayesian, Decision Tree. 2) Covariance matrix – Linear Discriminative Analysis and Logistic regression. 3) Similarity functions – KNN classification. 4) Biological neural networking system –Artificial Neural networks. 5) Nonlinear mappings - support vectors. 6) Other techniques such as genetic algorithm, rough set and fuzzy set.

VARIOUS CLASSIFICATION MODELS AND EVALUATION

Discussed data collection and pre-processing of the data and further discussed various classification algorithms mentioned in Figure 3.

DATA COLLECTION AND PREPROCESSING

There are 43400 patients data (42453 patients without stroke and 947 patients with stroke) collected with 10 attributes collected from the kaggle data source. 17724 male patients, 25665 female patients and 11 others. Age ranging from 3 - 80+ years. All attributes of dataset and their description are shown in Figure 4. Data pre-processing and cleansing is important issue while working on classification models. Missing data replaced by mean of the attributes, some normalized & attributes are converted to categorical.

Figure 4.

#	Predictor	Type of Parameter	Description
1	gender	Categorical	Patient gender – 0,1,2 or Male, Female, Others
2	age	Categorical/ Numerical	Patient age - <=18, 18-60,>60. – 0, 1, 2
3	hypertension	Categorical	Patient is known hypertension or not – 0,1 – No, Yes
4	heart_disease	Categorical	Patient having heart disease – 0, 1 – No, Yes
5	ever_married	Categorical	Patient is Married or not – 0, 1 – No, Yes
6	work type	Categorical	Patient working status – 0, 1, 2, 3 -Child, Never worked or self-employed, Private, Govt employee
7	residence_type	Categorical	Patient residential status – 0, 1 -Rural, Urban
8	avg_glucose_level	Categorical / Numerical	Glucose Levels of the patient - <120, 121-200, >200 – 0, 1, 2
9	bmi	Categorical / Numerical	Patient BMI - <24, >24 – 0, 1
10	smoking_status	Categorical	Patient smoking behavior – 0, 1, 2 - Never, Formerly, Smoker
11	heart_stroke	Categorical	Target Class – 0, 1 – No, Yes

Figure 5.

gender	age	hypertension	heart disease	married	work type	residence type	glucose level	bmi	smoking status	heart stroke
Female	21	No	No	No	Private	Rural	89.44	21.9	smokes	No
Female	61	Yes	No	Yes	Self-employed	Rural	202.21	28.61	never smoked	Yes
Female	18	No	No	No	Private	Rural	111.38	38.4	smokes	No
Female	78	No	No	Yes	Private	Urban	243.5	26.1	never smoked	No
Female	78	Yes	No	Yes	Private	Urban	182.2	30.5	formerly smoked	No
Male	33	No	No	Yes	Self-employed	Urban	229.92	25.9	smokes	No
Female	52	No	No	Yes	Private	Urban	82.24	54.7	formerly smoked	No
Female	51	No	No	Yes	Self-employed	Rural	89.84	29.9	smokes	No
Male	11	No	No	No	children	Rural	90.69	18.6	never smoked	No
Female	48	No	No	Yes	Private	Urban	84.38	27.1	smokes	No

As depicted sample dataset in Figure 5, 10 predictors and a target class label, this is used in this chapter for classification

CLASSIFICATION BASED ON FREQUENCY TABLE

These models - Zero R, One R, Naïve Bayesian, Decision Tree (ID3, ID 4.5) are built based on the frequency table.

Frequency Table is a statistical model to depict how often each attribute value in a set of data occurs. This technique can be used to summarize categorical, nominal, and ordinal data. The frequency of a particular data value occurrences are in the given dataset (Manikandan, 2011).

Table 1. Frequency table to get a patient heart stroke

Patient Get Heart Stroke	
Female	21
Female	61

ZERO R CLASSIFIER

ZeroR or Zero Rule model (Sierra, Lazkano, Irigoien, Jauregi, & Mendialdua, 2011), predicts outcome with no predictor, and it is the simplest classification model. It relies solely on the target and ignores all predictors (Kachroo, Melek, & Kurian, 2013). It predicts the outcome of majority category (Wahbeh, Al-Radaideh, Al-Kabi, & Al-Shawakfa, 2011). It is ideally considered to benchmark for other classification.

There are two target classes No Stroke (0) and Yes Stroke (1). As shown in the Table 1, frequency table for the stroke dataset, No Stroke (0) is more frequent value. Hence it is always predicts class No stroke (0).

Now predict the outcome for the following unseen data: gender: Male (0), Age =80, hypertension=0, heart disease =1, married = yes (0), Work type: Not working (1), residence type: Rural (0), average glucose: 105.92, BMI=32.5, smoking: 0

The model always predict that that patient no risk.

ONE R CLASSIFIER

One R is a classification technique with one primary predictor. This is simple but often yields better results compared to ZeroR (Kachroo et al., 2013). It generates a rule for each predictor and select the best rule which has smallest error (Nevill-Manning, Holmes, & Witten, 1995) . The rule with lowest error rate is the rule used for prediction.

As shown in Figure 6 for each attribute value and its corresponding frequencies are given. Decision is made based on the accuracy.

Confusion matrix gives four measurements - True Positives –TP, True Negatives – TN, False Positives – FP and False Negative (FN) (Patro & Patra, 2015). The accuracy of the model is calculated as shown in the Equation 1:

$$\frac{True\ Positives + True\ Negatives}{\#total\ events} \quad (1)$$

Since all the attributes predicts No (0) and highest accurate predictor is also predict No(0). Outcome for the data: gender: Male (0), Age =80, hypertension=0, heart disease =1, married = yes (0), Work type: Not working (1), residence type: Rural (0), average glucose: 105.92, BMI=32.5, smoking: 0 hypertension =0 accuracy is having highest among all other attribute values so the prediction is no risk(0).

Figure 6.

Predictor	Attribute Value	Frequency Table		Accuracy
		Stroke		
		No Stroke (0)	Stroke (1)	
gender	Male (0)	17276	448	0.9747235
	Female (1)	25166	499	0.9805572
	Other (2)	11	0	1
age	<18	8039	0	1
	18-60	24107	127	0.9947594
	>60	10307	820	0.9263054
hypertension	No (0)	38784	555	0.9858919
	Yes(1)	3669	392	0.9034721
heart disease	No (0)	40767	571	0.986187
	Yes (1)	1686	376	0.8176528
married	No (0)	15512	194	0.987648
	Yes (1)	26941	753	0.97281

Predictor	Attribute Value	Frequency Table		Accuracy
		Stroke		
		No Stroke (0)	Stroke (1)	
work Type	Children (0)	8039	0	1
	Not working (1)	22734	436	0.9811826
	Private (2)	5203	113	0.9787434
	Govt (3)	6477	398	0.9421091
residence type	Rural (0)	21199	445	0.97944
	Urban (1)	21254	502	0.9769259
glucose level	<120	34393	409	0.9882478
	121-200	5264	166	0.9694291
	>200	2796	372	0.8825758
bmi	<24	30593	839	0.9733075
	>24	11860	108	0.9909759
smoking status	Never (0)	22358	340	0.9850207
	Formerly (1)	13151	273	0.9796633
	Smoker(2)	6944	334	0.9541083

NAÏVE BAYESIAN CLASSIFIER

The Naive Bayesian (Bayesian) are statistical classifiers built on Bayes theorem (Qin, Xia, Prabhakar, & Tu, 2009) and it is a powerful probabilistic representation of predictors. It builds model with independence assumptions among predictors, hence reduces computational cost. It is linear, easy and simple and efficient model (Raschka, 2014), hence it is widely used as it yields better prediction over other methods(Domingos & Pazzani, 1997).

Bayes theorem calculates posterior probability, mentioned Equation 2.

$$\left(\frac{\text{conditional probability} - \text{prior probability}}{\text{evidence}}\right) \tag{2}$$

The model predicts the class (c) given the predictor (x) called $P\left(\frac{c}{X}\right)$ this is derived from P(c), P(X), and $P\left(\frac{X}{c}\right)$ where P(c) is prior probability of the class c, $P\left(\frac{X}{c}\right)$ is likelihood. Probability of predictor given the class and P(x) prior probability of predictor(Wang, Garrity, Tiedje, & Cole, 2007). Since there is no effect to probability of predictor x on given class(class conditional independence), helps in simplifying the model as depicted in the Equation 3.

$$P\left(\frac{c}{X}\right) = \frac{P\left(\frac{X}{c}\right) * P\left(c\right)}{P\left(X\right)} \tag{3}$$

Predictor of the given class c is independent of each other attribute hence it is simplified as shown in Equation 4.

$$P\left(\frac{c}{X}\right) = P\left(\frac{x1}{c}\right) * P\left(\frac{x2}{c}\right) * P\left(\frac{x3}{c}\right) * \ldots * P\left(\frac{xn}{c}\right) * P\left(c\right) \tag{4}$$

Now posterior probability $P\left(\frac{c}{X}\right)$ is calculated from frequency table, then transform it into likely hood table with the formula $p\left(\frac{x}{c}\right)$. Calculate posterior probability for all the target classes and given class using Naïve Bayesian algorithm. The class gets highest posterior probability will be the predicted outcome.

Likely hood table for all attributes in the dataset is given in the Figure 7. For each predictor values in the dataset frequency table is created for target classes. Accuracy of the outcome for each attribute and likelihood values for each of the attribute are described in the table. Calculate the posterior probability of any unseen data using the Naïve Bayesian algorithm.

Predict the outcome class for the following unseen test data:

Gender: Male (0), Age =80, hypertension=0, heart disease =1, married = yes (0), Work type: Not working (1), residence type: Rural (0), Average glucose: 105.92, BMI=32.5, Smoking: 0

Finding the posterior probability for the data set is given as below Equation 5:

P (gender=male) * P(age =80) * P(hypertension=no) * P(heart disease = yes) * P(married=yes) * P (Work type = not working) * P(residence type = rural) * P (average glucose = 105.92) * P(BMI=32.5) * P (smoking=no) --- (5)

Figure 7.

Predictor	Attribute Value	Frequency table(stroke)		Accuracy	Likelihood	
		No (0)	Yes (1)		No (0)	Yes (1)
gender	Male (0)	17276	448	0.974723539	0.406944	0.473073
	Female (1)	25166	499	0.980557179	0.592797	0.526927
	Other (2)	11	0	1	0.000259	0
age	<18	8039	0	1	0.189362	0
	18-60	24107	127	0.994759429	0.567852	0.134108
	>60	10307	820	0.926305383	0.242786	0.865892
hypertension	No (0)	38784	555	0.985891863	0.913575	0.586061
	Yes(1)	3669	392	0.903472051	0.086425	0.413939
heart disease	No (0)	40767	571	0.986187043	0.960285	0.602957
	Yes (1)	1686	376	0.817652764	0.039715	0.397043
married	No (0)	15512	194	0.987648033	0.365392	0.204857
	Yes (1)	26941	753	0.972809995	0.634608	0.795143

Predictor	Attribute Value	Frequency table(stroke)		Accuracy	Likelihood	
		No (0)	Yes (1)		No (0)	Yes (1)
work type	Children (0)	8039	0	1	0.189362	0
	Not working (1)	22734	436	0.981182564	0.53551	0.460401
	Private (2)	5203	113	0.978743416	0.122559	0.119324
	Govt (3)	6477	398	0.942109091	0.152569	0.420275
residence type	Rural (0)	21199	445	0.97944003	0.499352	0.469905
	Urban (1)	21254	502	0.976925905	0.500648	0.530095
glucose level	<120	34393	409	0.988247802	0.810143	0.43189
	121-200	5264	166	0.969429098	0.123996	0.17529
	>200	2796	372	0.882575758	0.065861	0.392819
bmi	<24	30593	839	0.973307457	0.720632	0.885956
	>24	11860	108	0.990975936	0.279368	0.114044
smoking status	Never (0)	22358	340	0.985020707	0.526653	0.359029
	Formerly (1)	13151	273	0.97966329	0.309778	0.288279
	Smoker(2)	6944	334	0.954108272	0.163569	0.352693

Transform the numerical data into categorical data for the attributes which are not in categorical form. In this case need to transform age, average glucose and BMI into categorical as shown in the likelihood and frequency tables. So the posterior probability calculation is changed as below Equation 6

P(Gender=0) * P(age>60) * P(Hypertension=0) * P(Heart disease =1) * P(married=1)

* P(Work type=1) * P(Residence Type=0) * P(average glucose <120) * P(bmi>24)

* P(smoking=0) --- (6)

Calculations for posterior probability for output class – Stroke Yes (1) calculated as per the Equation 7

$$P\left(gender > \frac{0}{yes}\right) * P\left(age = \frac{>18}{Yes}\right) * P\left(Hypertension < \frac{0}{yes}\right) * P\left(Heart\,disease = \frac{1}{Yes}\right) * \\ P(married > \frac{0}{yes}) * P(work\,type = \left(\frac{1}{yes}\right) * P\left(residence = \frac{1}{yes}\right) * P(average\,glucose > \frac{80}{yes}) * \\ P(bmi = (> \frac{24}{yes}) * P\left(smoking = \frac{0}{yes}\right) \tag{7}$$

⇨ 0.473073 * 0.865892 * 0.586061 * 0.397043 * 0.795143 * 0.460401 * 0.469905 * 0.43189018 * 0.359029

⇨ 0.002542533

Calculations for posterior probability for output class – No Stroke (0) as per Equation 8

$$P\left(gender > \frac{0}{No}\right) * P\left(age = \frac{>18}{No}\right) * P\left(Hypertension < \frac{0}{No}\right) * P\left(Heart\,disease = \frac{1}{No}\right) * \\ P(married > \frac{0}{No}) * P(work\,type = \left(\frac{1}{No}\right) * P\left(residence = \frac{1}{No}\right) * P(average\,glucose > \frac{80}{No}) * \\ P(bmi = (> \frac{24}{No}) * P\left(smoking = \frac{0}{No}\right) \tag{8}$$

⇨ 0.406944 * 0.242786 *0.913575 * 0.039715 * 0.634608 * 0.53551 * 0.499352 * 0.810143 * 0.526653

⇨ 0.000259551

Now normalize the result for both target classes Yes and No scenarios

P(yes)=0. 002542533/(0. 002542533+0. 000259551)

⇨ 0.907372156

P(No)=0. 000259551/(0. 002542533+0. 000259551)

⇨ 0.092627844

P(No)< P(Yes), Hence as per the model, the patient has a risk of stroke. The outcome is Stroke -Yes. Hence the model predicts that there is a risk of heart stroke to the patient.

DECISION TREE INDUCTION

CART – classification and regression trees are widely used models in the Healthcare industry. Decision tree induction is the learning model of a decision tree from class-labeled training tuples (Qin et al., 2009). Decision tree builds classification models in the form of a tree like structures. It breaks down the dataset into smaller datasets and a decision tree is developed incrementally while it break down the data. Finally it looks like a tree with some decision nodes and some leaf nodes. A decision node is a node having two or more branches, which are essentially options to that node at that point in time. Leaf node is a node, which represents a class label (decision). Root Node is the topmost decision node in the tree (Pradhan, Taneja, Dixit, & Suhag, 2017). Decision trees can handle both categorical and numerical data. The Decision Tree - DT design in the literature was based on the algorithm Classification And Regression Trees – CART. In this algorithm the training process dataset is divided in the recursive manner to the split the data into subsets with an optimal split point achieved.

Several of decision tree model available in the modern literature, however all these models are evolved from ID3 based algorithm. In this chapter discussed two important models such as 1) ID3 and 2) C4.5. ID3, C4.5 generates classifiers expressed as decision trees, however these will construct classifiers in more comprehensible ruleset forms (Wu et al., 2008). The core of decision tree is based an algorithm called ID3 algorithm which was invented by J R Quinlan, it is a top down greedy approach to construct the decision tree with no backtracking model. ID3 algorithm uses Entropy and Information Gain, where entropy is homogeneity of the data and Information gain is the gain of choosing the predictor to construct the decision trees.

Attribute selection for ID3 algorithm uses Information gain. Information gain (Fan et al., 2011) calculation is mentioned below. There are two types of entropies, Entropy for a target E(T) class is calculated as below Equation 9. Entropy for attribute E(T,X) for a given class is calculated as below Equation 10. From these two information gain or loss is calculated.

$$Entropy\ is\ calculated\ as: E\left(T\right) = \sum_{i=1}^{n} - P_i log_2 P_i \tag{9}$$

$$E\left(T,X\right)=\sum_{c\varepsilon X}P\left(c\right)*E\left(c\right) \tag{10}$$

Information gain is calculated with the Equation 11:

Gain (T, X) = E(T) – E(T,X) --- (11).

This enables decrease in the entropy after data set is split on the given attribute. Highest information gain (Chen, Han, & Yu, 1996) is most homogeneous, so most homogeneous predictor is picked and continue until entire tree covering all the samples.

As discussed above first calculate entropy for target classes. Entropy – Stroke E(T) = E(stroke)

$$=> E\left(42453,947\right)=-\frac{42453}{43400}log\frac{42453}{43400}-\frac{947}{43400}log\frac{947}{43400}$$

= 0.978179724 * -0.031134028- 0.021820276 * -0.120408362

= 0.15154239

Calculate the entropy for each attribute in the dataset. This can be achieved by sum of entropy for the split of the attribute is by adding entropy of each value proportionally. Entropy for all the attributes calculated and shown in Figure 8.

Calculate information gain from the entropies calculated for target class label and all attributes.

Figure 8.

Probability and Entropy		Frequency Table (Stroke)			Probability		Entropy
Predictor	Attribute value	No (0)	Yes (1)	Total	No(0)	Yes(1)	
Gender	Male (0)	17276	448	17724	0.974723539	0.025276461	0.069475
	Female (1)	25166	499	25665	0.980557179	0.019442821	0.081785
	Other (2)	11	0	11	1	0	0
			Entropy of Gender				0.15126
Age	<18	8039	0	8039	1	0	0
	18-60	24107	127	24234	0.994759429	0.005240571	0.02638
	>60	10307	820	11127	0.926305383	0.073694617	0.097313
							0.123693
Hyper Tension	No (0)	38784	555	39339	0.985891863	0.014108137	0.096931
	Yes(1)	3669	392	4061	0.903472051	0.096527949	0.042846
							0.139776
Heart Disease	No (0)	40767	571	41338	0.986187043	0.013812957	0.100129
	Yes (1)	1686	376	2062	0.817652764	0.182347236	0.032554
							0.132683
Married	No (0)	15512	194	15706	0.987648033	0.012351967	0.034745
	Yes (1)	26941	753	27694	0.972809995	0.027190005	0.114922
							0.149667

Probability and Entropy		Frequency Table (Stroke)			Probability		Entropy
Predictor	Attribute value	No (0)	Yes (1)	Total	No(0)	Yes(1)	
Work Type	Children (0)	8039	0	8039	1	0	0
	Not working (1)	22734	436	23170	0.981182564	0.018817436	0.085479
	Private (2)	5203	113	5316	0.978743416	0.021256584	0.021604
	Govt (3)	6477	398	6875	0.942109091	0.057890909	0.060047
							0.167131
Residence Type	Rural (0)	21199	445	21644	0.97944003	0.02055997	0.0721
	Urgan (1)	21254	502	21756	0.976925905	0.023074095	0.079389
							0.151489
Glucose Level	<120	34393	409	34802	0.988247802	0.011752198	0.073932
	121-200	5264	166	5430	0.969429098	0.030570902	0.024679
	>200	2796	372	3168	0.882575758	0.117424242	0.038097
							0.136708
BMI	<24	30593	839	31432	0.973307457	0.026692543	0.12857
	>24	11860	108	11968	0.990975936	0.009024064	0.020476
							0.149045
Smoking	Never (0)	22358	340	22698	0.985020707	0.014979293	0.058699
	Formerly (1)	13151	273	13424	0.97966329	0.02033671	0.044332
	Smoker(2)	6944	334	7278	0.954108272	0.045891728	0.045057
							0.148088

Calculation of Information gain for Gender

Entropy for attribute gender:

$$= P(Male) * E(17276, 448) + P(Female) * E(25166, 499) + P(\text{Others}) * \text{E}(11, 0)$$

=0.408387097 * 0.051211189 + 0.591359447 * 1.008361286 + 0.000253456 * 0

= 0.617217961

$$Information\ gain : G(T, X) = E(T) - E(T, X) \tag{12}$$

Here information gain for Gender = 0.15154239-0.151260141 = 0.151260141

Similarly information gain for all the attributes are calculated and shown in the following Table 2

Finally after calculating the information gain the decision tree is created and the largest information gain is achieved is the decision node selected. Then divide the dataset by its branches, further do repeat the same process on every branch until it reaches the decision tree.

The decision tree for the stroke data set is depicted in the following Figure 9. It is a very easy for any person to read and understand the decision trees and infer the outcomes based on the decision tree.

Predict the outcome class for the following unseen test data using decision tree model shown in the Equation 13:

P(gender=male) * P(age =80) * P(hypertension=no) * P(heart disease = yes) * P(married=yes)

* P (Work type = not working) * P(residence type = rural) * P (average glucose = 105.92)

* P(BMI=32.5) * P (smoking=no) (13)

Table 2. Information gain for each attribute in stroke dataset

Attribute	Information Gain
Gender	0.0002822
Age	0.0278490
Hypertension	0.0117662
Heart disease	0.0188590
Married	0.0018749
Work Type	-0.0155883
Residence Type	0.0000534
Glucose Levels	0.0148347
BMI	0.0024970
Smoking	0.0034545

Figure 9.

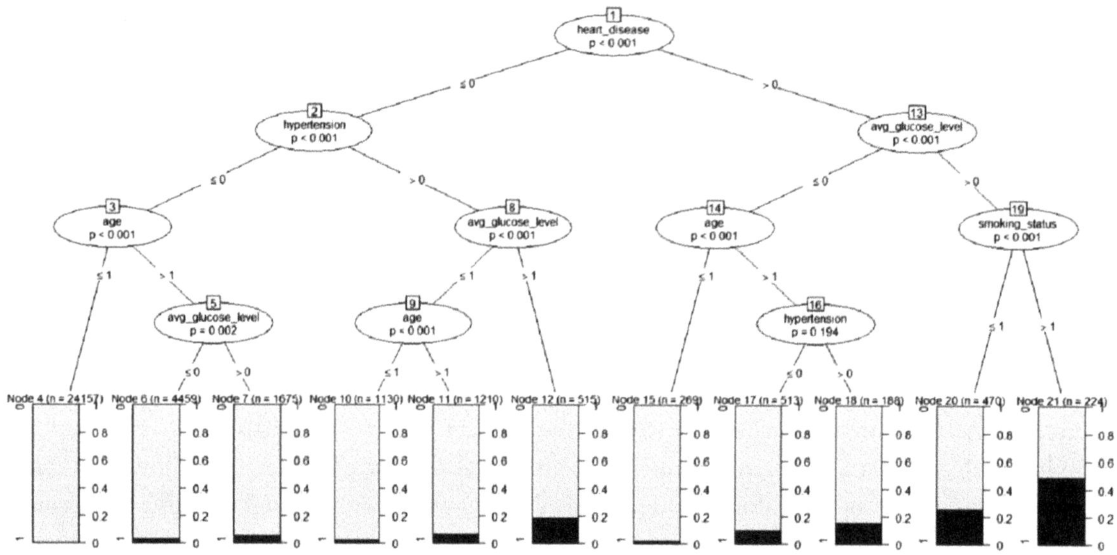

With decision tree the outcome for the above unseen data is that patient has risk to get stroke.

C4.5 is an algorithm used to produce a decision tree which is an expansion of prior ID3 calculation. As per the studies, C 4.5 has good combination of speed with low error rate (Dobre, Abdi, Bar-Ness, & Su, 2007). Construct decision trees based on ID3 or C4.5 methods for attribute selection. However we have few more methods Gini Index, CART, MDL etc.

The split optimization criterion used in this Decision Tree (DT) model is the Gini Index or Gini's Diversity Index (GDI), which is a measure of node impurity. DT can be used for classification and regression problems, however finding an optimal binary split for a continuous predictor is far less computationally intensive than for a categorical predictor with multiple levels (Shaikhina et al., 2017).

When decision tree constructed, the tree may over fit to the training data, it may have too many branches as it is considering the anomalies due to noise or outlier while constructing the model. Decision tree is fits its model very specific to the training data and can't predict accurately for unseen data. This can be addressed by using a method call tree pruning. Pruning is a Machine Learning (ML) technique is to reduce the size of a DT and prevents over fitting problem. Pruning is achieved by means of removing some of the nodes that have least impact on the overall classification performance. So it is essential to apply pruning to achieve the quality of the prediction model and significant performance improvements (Shaikhina et al., 2017). Decision trees are instable due to data volatility.

Decision trees are more popular as it has the inherent features like faster learning speed, convert the decision tree to decision rules and human understandable formats, easy to compare and SQL queries to access databases. Rainforest is one decision tree algorithm built to improve the scalability aspect with the help of AVC – Attribute, Value and Class Label (Gehrke, Ramakrishnan, & Ganti, 1998). Other models are Random forests – RF, which are also called as Bagged Decision Trees which are involved in construction of multiple DTs via bootstrap aggregation or bagging. Random Forest addresses the volatility issues or not being notoriously instable for changes in the training data set and improves the robustness of predictions (Shaikhina et al., 2017).

CLASSIFICATION BASED ON COVARINACE MATRIX

There are two famous classification methods built based on covariance matrix. 1) Linear discriminant analysis and 2) Logistic regression

Linear Discriminant Analysis: LDA Classifier

Linear Discriminant Analysis - LDA is the most popular discriminant analysis method, which is usually applied for pattern recognition and dimensionality reduction. This method discriminant analysis seeks to statistically distinguish between two or more target classes and this technique uses least squares methods to separate data into two or more groups (Harper, 2005). In this method a discriminant vector by maximizing the ratio of the between-class scatter measure to the within-class scatter measure (Shao & Sang, 2017). This method is built based on the covariance matrix. Data is shown in the Table 2 will be used to train and predict the classifier.

There are two important matrices used (1. Deviation matrix (a), 2. Covariance matrix (€)) in building the LDA

Generating the deviation matrix (a): a= A-Average matrix or mean matrix of A

$$a = A - \left[I\right] A \left(\frac{1}{\# Rows}\right) \tag{14}$$

$$\text{Covariance matrix } € = a\,\mathrm{T} * \, a \text{---} \tag{15}$$

Covariance matrix is a matrix with diagonal elements represents variance of the attributes and off diagonal elements are covariance against to other attributes

Mean / average vectors for the target classes for No and Yes for each attribute in stroke dataset has depicted in the following Table 3.

Covariance matrix is calculated from the above mean vector and presented below Figure 10. It is a square matrix of 10X10 as there are 10 predictors in the stroke database.

Linear discrimination coefficients calculated as shown below:

LDA is based upon the concept of searching for a linear combination of predictors, which best separates two target classes. Fisher defined something called a scoring function to capture the notion of reparability. He defined the scoring Equation 16

Table 3. Mean vector for target class labels

	Gender	Age	Hyper tension	Heart Disease	Married	Work Type	Residence Type	Glucose Levels	BMI	Smoking Status
Mean for No	1.5955	1.0526	0.0865	0.0392	0.6339	1.2345	0.4986	0.2529	0.2805	0.6386
Mean for Yes	1.5148	1.8609	0.4261	0.4157	0.7896	1.9583	0.5252	0.9617	0.1183	0.9930

$$Z = \beta_1 x_1 + \beta_2 x_2 + \ldots + \beta_2 x_2 \tag{16}$$

$$Scoring\ function\ defined\ as\ S\left(\beta\right) = \frac{\beta^T \mu_1 - \beta^T \mu_2}{\beta^T C \beta} \tag{17}$$

$$S\left(\beta\right) = \frac{Z_1 - Z_2}{varianc\ of\ Z\ in\ group} \tag{18}$$

Now as per the scoring function defined above, need to identify the linear coefficients to maximize the score. So for making the maximizing the score, define a Equation 19

$$\beta = C^{-1}\left(\mu_1 - \mu_2\right) \tag{19}$$

This model coefficients are built based on C, $\mu_{1,}\mu_2$

Where β – Linear model coefficients, $\mu_{1,}\mu_2$ - mean vectors, C is pooled covariance matrix

Effectiveness of LDA is calculated Mahalanobis distance between the two groups, the distance can be inferred as if distance is greater than 3 - the two group are at least 3 standard deviations apart. So the overlap between two groups are quite small as it is over 3 and the misclassification is quite less and we can consider the LDA model is efficient.

Figure 10.

	gender	age	hypertension	heart disease	married	work type	residence type	glucose levels	bmi	smoking status
Gender		0.04	-0.02	-0.08	0.03	0.04	0	-0.04	0.05	0.04
Age	0.04		0.24	0.23	0.61	0.6	0	0.21	-0.42	0.38
Hyper tension	-0.02	0.24		0.12	0.17	0.16	0	0.15	-0.14	0.08
Heart disease	-0.08	0.23	0.12		0.12	0.13	0	0.14	-0.08	0.11
Married	0.03	0.61	0.17	0.12		0.46	0	0.13	-0.38	0.3
Work Type	0.04	0.6	0.16	0.13	0.46		-0.01	0.13	-0.34	0.29
Residence Type	0	0	0	0	0	-0.01		0	0	0
Glucose Levels	-0.04	0.21	0.15	0.14	0.13	0.13	0		-0.13	0.09
BMI	0.05	-0.42	-0.14	-0.08	-0.38	-0.34	0	-0.13		
Smoking	0.04	0.38	0.08	0.11	0.3	0.29	0	0.09	-0.23	

Table 4. Coefficients of linear discriminants

Attribute	LDA Coefficient
Gender	-0.02859502
Age	0.62665072
Hyper tension	1.1350743
Heart disease	3.06904603
Married	-0.61437085
Work Type	0.09421032
Residence Type	0.06141875
Glucose Levels	0.62937792
BMI	0.18560868
Smoking	0.01847326

Mahalanobis distance (△) calculated as follows Equation 20.

$$\sqrt{\beta^T\left(\mu_1 - \mu_2\right)} \tag{20}$$

Now we can predict the new or unknown data set with the following Equation 21.

$$\beta^T(x - \frac{(\mu_2 + \mu_2)}{2}) \text{ ---} \tag{21}$$

$$if\ \beta^T(x - \frac{(\mu_2 + \mu_2)}{2}) > log\left(\frac{p\left(c1\right)}{p\left(c2\right)}\right) \text{ then it belongs to class C1 otherwise it belongs class C2}$$

Using the above equation LDA Coefficients can be calculated. Table 4, shows LDA coefficients for all the attributes – gender, age, hypertension, marital status, work type, residence type, average glucose levels, BMI, smoking status in the stroke database.

Hence with this LDA coefficients mentioned above, the algorithm can predict the outcome using linear discriminant Equation 22.

$$\beta^T(x - \frac{(\mu_2 + \mu_2)}{2}) \text{ ---} \tag{22}$$

P (gender=male) * P(age =80) * P(hypertension=no) * P(heart disease = yes) * P(married=yes) * P (Work type = not working) * P(residence type = rural) * P (average glucose = 105.92) * P(BMI=32.5) * P (smoking=no).

$$\beta^T(x - \frac{(\mu_2 + \mu_2)}{2}) =>$$

β^T = [-0.02859502, 0.62665072, 1.1350743, 3.06904603, -0.61437085, 0.09421032, 0.06141875, 0.62937792, 0.18560868, 0.01847326]

$x - \frac{(\mu_2 + \mu_2)}{2} =$ [0.01429751,-0.31332536,-0.56753715,-1.534523015, 0.307185425,-0.04710516, -0.030709375 , -0.31468896, -0.09280434, -0.00923663]

$$\beta^T(x - \frac{(\mu_2 + \mu_2)}{2}) = 5.210947318$$

$$log\left(\frac{p(c1)}{p(c2)}\right) = \log (0.978179723502304 / 0.0218202764976959) = 5.48636$$

$if\ \beta^T(x - \frac{(\mu_2 + \mu_2)}{2}) < log\left(\frac{p(c1)}{p(c2)}\right)$ hence the outcome is No.

Hence the model predicts that there is no risk of heart stroke to the patient.

Logistic Regression: LR Classifier

Logistic regression is a statistical method, which models a binary classifiers (Algamal, Lee, Al-Fakih, & Aziz, 2017), it predicts the probability of an outcome that can only have two values (i.e. a dichotomy). The regression function has a nonlinear relationship with the linear combination of the descriptors. Logistic regression is a model built based on the covariance matrix. This model work with both categorical and numerical predictors. Logistic regression is extended further in case the predicted outcome is having more than two categories. If categories are nominal we can use multi nominal logistic regression, or if they are ordinal in nature we can use ordered logistic regression models.

Logistic regression gives a curve called logistic curve which will have boundaries 0 and 1. It is similar to linear regression where linear regression predicts the real numbers whereas logistic regression predicts one class out of two classes such as Yes or No. In logistic regression logistic curve is constructed with natural algorithms of odds of the target variable.

Logistic regression model is given as below Equation 23

$$log\left(\frac{p}{1-p}\right) = a + bX \text{ (in case of one independent variable) ----} \quad (23)$$

$$=> \frac{p}{1-p} = e^{a+bX}$$

$$=> p = \frac{1}{1+e^{-(a+bX)}}$$

In case of multiple variables the statement would be something the below Equation 24

$$log\left(\frac{p}{1-p}\right) = a + b_1x_1 + b_2x_2 + \ldots + b_nx_n \tag{24}$$

$$=> p = \frac{1}{1+e^{-(a+b_1x_1+b_2x_2+\ldots+b_nx_n)}}$$

In the above equation variable 'a' is one can move the logistic curve left to right and variables ' $b_1, b_2, \ldots, b_n$ ' used to change the slope of the logistic curve.

There are lots of similarities between linear regression and logistic regression. In case of linear regression, least square regression used to estimate coefficients for the best fit of a line. In logistic regression, it uses maximum likelihood estimation (MLE) to obtain the model coefficients. After this initial function is estimated, the process will be repeated until Look Likelihood -LL substantially does not change.

Here we are going to optimize the likelihood of the training data with respect to the parameters β. where β is vector of coefficients of the curve, i.e., $b_1, b_2, \ldots, b_n$.

Likelihood is the probability of training data for given the set of parameters. In other words it is a function of parameter given as below Equation 25.

$$\beta_1 = \beta_0 + [X^TWX]X^T(y-\mu) \text{---} \tag{25}$$

Where β_1 is later vector of logistic regression coefficients
Where β_0 is prior vector of logistic regression coefficients
Where X is vector of predictors or attributes
Where W is a square matrix of order n (# attributes) with elements $n_i\Pi_i(1-\Pi_i)$

μ is a vector of length n, with elements $\mu_i = n_i\Pi_i$

Some important terms in this model evaluation are 'Pseudo R – Squared', 'model chi-square' these two defined as: Pseudo R – Squared is a value used to indicate the acceptability of the regression model and model chi-square is a value which is the difference between likelihood ratio of baseline and likelihood ratio of reduced model.

Table 5. Deviance residuals

Min	IQ	Median	3Q	Max
-1.0889	-0.1791	-0.0841	-0.0806	3.3855

Look likelihood Ratio test provides a way to compare the likelihood of the data with another data, usually these data is compared between full data vs intercept data i.e., restricted data as shown in the Equation 26.

$$LL = \sum_{i=1}^{n} y_i \ln(\mathrm{p}_i) + (1 - y_i) \ln\left(1 - p_i\right) \tag{26}$$

where p is the logistic model predicted probability and y is the predicted value

$$L\left(\beta_0, \beta_1\right) = \sum_{i=1}^{n} p\left(x_i\right)^{y_i} p\left(1 - x_i\right)^{(1-y_i)} \tag{27}$$

Identify statistically significant attributes and use only those attributes for performing this logistic regression model. Those attributes having low confidence levels will not make any sense to add them in the model hence attributes are ignored while modeling the logistic regression. Deviance residual is useful for determining how the individual points are not well fit by the model. The models deviance residuals are shown in Table 5. So this model mean of deviance residual is -0.0841 and Min, Inter Quartile, 3rd Quartile and Max given.

The main interest of logistic regression is often prediction. Coefficients mentioned in Table 6 are derived from the above function using R program is depicted in the following table – Table 5 and Table 6

(Dispersion parameter for binomial family taken to be 1)

Null deviance : 7392.3 on 34811 degrees of freedom
Residual deviance : 5317.4 on 34807 degrees of freedom
AIC : 5327.4

Table 6. Coefficients

	Estimate	Std. Error	z Value	Pr(>lzl)
Intercept	-7.85507	0.19632	-40.012	< 2e-16 ***
Age	2.1911	0.1067	20.535	< 2e-16 ***
Heart disease	1.72159	0.08432	20.418	< 2e-16 ***
Glucose Levels -1	0.6424	0.10702	6.003	1.94e-09 ***
Glucose Levels -2	1.51869	0.0897	16.931	< 2e-16 ***

Number of Fisher Scoring iterations: 25

$$y = e^{(a+b_1x_1+b_2x_2+b_3x_3)}$$

where a, b_1, b_2 *and* b_3 are -7.85507, 2.1911, 1.72159, 0.6424/ 1.51869

Now with this coefficients, it is possible to predict the outcomes using the above function by plugging in these values.

P(gender=male) * P(age =80) * P(hypertension=no) * P(heart disease = yes) * P(married=yes) * P (Work type = not working) * P(residence type = rural) * P (average glucose = 105.92) * P(BMI=32.5) * P (smoking=no).

$$y = e^{(-7.85507+2.1911*2+1.72159*1+0*0)} = 0.173551655$$

$$substitute\ the\ y\ value\ here\ldots p = \frac{1}{1+y}$$

$$p = \frac{1}{1+0.173551655} = 0.852114175$$

Hence this model predicts that the patient has risk for heart stroke

CLASSIFICATION BASED ON SIMILARITY MEASURES

Similarity-based classifiers estimate the class label of a test dataset based on the similarities between the validation dataset and a set of labeled training data. It is majorly used in the field of computer vision, bioinformatics, information retrieval, natural language processing, and other fields. Similarity functions may be asymmetric and fail to satisfy the other mathematical properties required for metrics or inner products KNN classifier is one of the important classifiers built based on similarity functions.

K Nearest Neighbourhood: KNN Classifier

K nearest neighborhood algorithm is a simple and straight forward instance based algorithm(Kachroo et al., 2013). It is based on the similarities of the predictors (Cover & Hart, 1967) based on some distance function. (Derrac, Chiclana, García, & Herrera, 2016). It uses an algorithm called "Closest Point Search"(AL-Nabi & Ahmed, 2013) and it is widely used technique in statistical estimations and pattern recognitions(Pradhan et al., 2017). It is as a non-parametric technique (Li, Liu, & Li, 2017; Maillo, Ramírez, Triguero, & Herrera, 2017) lazy learning and intuitive model, which can be used for both classification and regression problems.

A simple implementation of KNN regression is to calculate the average of the numerical target of the K nearest neighbors. Another approach uses an inverse distance weighted average of the K nearest neighbors. KNN regression uses the same distance functions as KNN classification.

Distance measure functions: Identify distance between two variables, continuous variable can be measured Euclidean (Phyu, 2009), Manhattan (Phyu, 2009), Minkowski (Phyu, 2009). Generally Euclidean distance is most common one used and are depicted in Equations 28, 29 & 30.

Distance functions used in KNN for identifying distance between two vectors for numerical continuous variables:

$$\text{Manhattan}: \sum_{i=1}^{k} \left| x_i - y_i \right| \tag{29}$$

$$\text{Minkowski}: \left(\sum_{i=1}^{k} \left(\left| x_i - y_i \right| \right)^q \right)^{1/q} \tag{30}$$

Categorical variables distance measured using Hamming distance, it checks if both variables are similar or not. It returns zero if same else one.

Hamming distance function is shown in the following Equations 31:

$$D_H = \sum_{i=1}^{k} \left| x_i - y_i \right| \tag{31}$$

$$x = y \Rightarrow D = 0$$

$$x \neq y \Rightarrow D = 1$$

Table 7, shows distance between two attribute values.

In the KNN algorithm, K is an arbitrary number, an optimal for the given dataset and calculate the distance of K nearby data points. Large K value is yields precise predictions and reduces noise. The optimal K for most datasets is square root of the no of observations in the data set.

Table 7. distance function using Hamming distance function

Attribute Value 1	Attribute Value 2	Distance
Male	Male	0
Male	Female	1

There is a serious issues in measuring distances, if we have data of mixture of continuous and categorical variables or variables have different measures. The issue is drawback of calculating the distance measures directly from the training data. For an instance two independent variables salary and age, Salary will have higher influence as the salary is a big number compared to age. To solve the issue need to standardize the values salary and age. Equation 32 shown below used for standardization.

$$\text{Standardized value of } x = \frac{x - min}{max - min} \quad (32)$$

pred <- knn(training,testing, training$stroke, k=255)

k-NN algorithm with k=255, the algorithm predicted No stroke, as there are having majority of neighbor records are classified as No stroke in the training set. So the model will predict the outcome as No Stroke.

There are few more distance functions can be used in KNN.

Locally weighted regression: Calculate the distance based on Constructs local approximation.

Case-based reasoning: Symbolic representations and knowledge-based inference. In this similarities are not based on the distance, however it is derived based on a symbolic descriptions.

CLASSIFICATION BASED ON BIOLOGICAL NEURAL NETWORKS: ARTIFICIAL NEURAL NETWORKS: ANN CLASSIFIER

Artificial neural network is a classification technique which has been built based on the biological networks (Qin et al., 2009) used in our brain nerves system. It seems, if the sum of these signals received from each other neurons crosses certain threshold, then only a response will be sent back. This response will be sent through something called axon. With this analogy artificial neural networks are built in the computer-based analytics. Artificial neural network is a set of connected input/output units where each connection has a weight associated with it. ANN is composed of nodes (artificial neurons), all the nodes connected each other. If the value of the connection is high then the strength of the connection is strong. For each node there will be a function built to which takes some inputs and gives an output. There are

Figure 11.

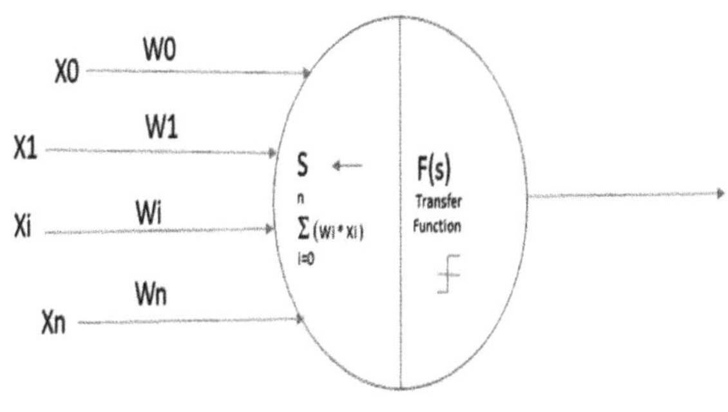

three types of neurons in the field of Artificial Neural networks 1) Input Node 2) Hidden Node and 3) Output Node. Input nodes are the nodes which will take input from the predicted attributes with an associated transform function and produces a result. A perceptron is an artificial neuron, which received several inputs. It sums those inputs and check the results and further produce the output. It is used for classification of any linearly separable data classes. It is often used for binary classification.

As mentioned in the Figure 11, a perceptron can take n weighted inputs and sum all the inputs with its weights Ex. $S = bias + W_1X_1 + W_2X_2 .... + +W_nX_n$. If the sum is crossing some threshold it will transform the inputs into output by its transformation function (Prasad, Belwin Edward, & Ravi).

As we shown above Figure 5, a perceptron has n weighted inputs and summation process to calculate the sum of inputs and activation function - transfer function based on the sum of waited inputs are greater than some adjustable threshold value.

For instance if $bias + W_1X_1 + W_2X_2 .... + +W_nX_n > T$ then class 1

Else then class 0

Transfer/activate function translates the input signals to output signals. Typically four types of the transfer functions are used, 1) threshold, 2) sigmoid, 3) piecewise linear and 4) The Gaussian.

- **Threshold/Unit Step:** The output is set to one class based sum of the inputs and threshold.
- **Sigmoid:** Is of two types 1) logistic and 2) tangential. Logistic function range from 0 to 1, Tangential function ranging from -1 to +1.
- **Piecewise Linear:** The output is proportional to the total weighted output. It ranges from 0 to 1.
- **Gaussian Function:** Bell-shaped curves used for continuous variable.
- **Linear:** Linear function to output based on the weighted sum inputs of the neuron.

As depicted in Figure 12, ANN has types of nodes - Input, Output and Hidden nodes. Input nodes takes the numerically expressed data. It passes through the activation function and presented to hidden nodes. Hidden nodes are intermediate nodes which also have activation functions, it will present the output to the output node. The output nodes then reflect the input in a meaningful way to the outside world.

As depicted in the Figure 13, for each training tuple, the weights are modified to minimize the mean squared error between the network's prediction and the actual target value. Modifications are made in

Figure 12.

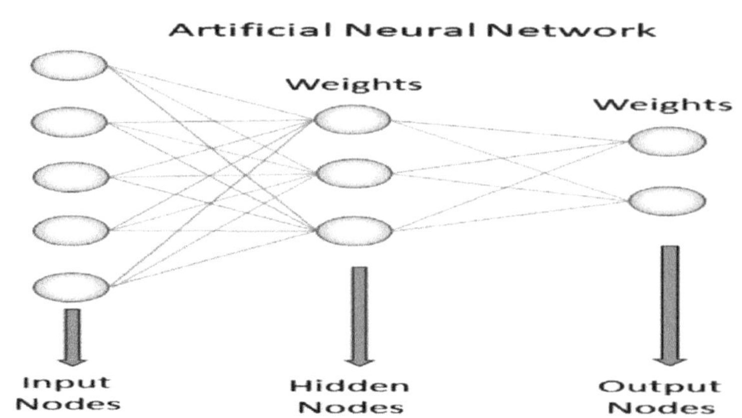

Figure 13.

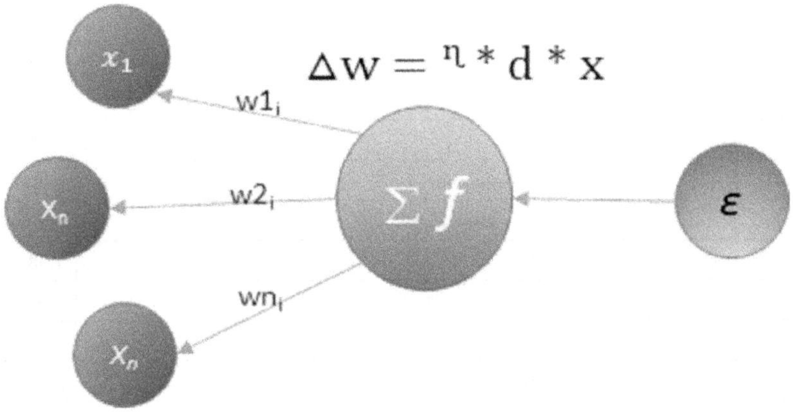

the "backwards" direction: from the output layer, through each hidden layer down to the first hidden layer. This is called backpropagation.

As shown in Figure 14, 8 input nodes, one hidden node and output node are present in ANN. Output from all the 8 inputs are calculated. Input is calculated as: Bias value + sum of all the attribute value and its coefficient mentioned in the below figure. Then calculate the output using sigmoid function $\frac{1}{1+Exp^{-input}}$. Same is given to next hidden node (Node 9). At hidden node weighted sum of the input is calculated and output is generated as sigmoid function and the same is given to output node (Node 10), similarly output values are calculated as mentioned above.

Figure 14.

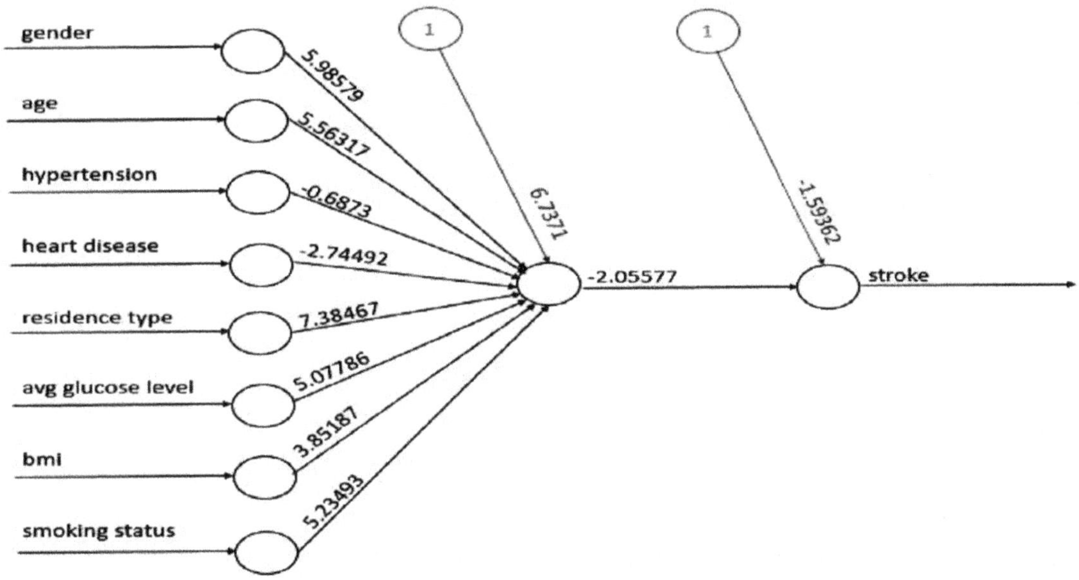

Table 8. Distance function using Hamming distance function

Node # (Type)	Attribute	Coefficient
	Bias	6.7373
Node 1 (Input)	gender	5.98579
Node 2 (Input)	age	5.56317
Node 3 (Input)	hypertension	-0.6873
Node 4 (Input)	heart disease	2.74492
Node 5 (Input)	Residence type	7.38467
Node 6 (Input)	avg glucose level	5.07786
Node 7 (Input)	bmi	3.85187
Node 8 (Input)	smoking status	5.23493
Node 9 (Hidden)	Hidden	-2.05577
	Bias	-1.59362
Node 10 (Output)	Output	

All the node details and attribute name and coefficients as per the above ANN diagram is mentioned in the Table 8. With the help of the below table any outcome for given unseen data can be easily calculated.

P(gender=male) * P(age =80) * P(hypertension=no) * P(heart disease = yes) * P(married=yes) * P (Work type = not working) * P(residence type = rural) * P (average glucose = 105.92) * P(BMI=32.5) * P (smoking=no).

Input from Node 1 to 8 + Bias = 6.7373 + 0 * 5.98579 + 0.78 * 5.56317 + 0 * -0.6873 + 1 * -2.74492 + 0 * 7.38467 + 0.15496717 * 5.07786 + 0.2571429 * 3.85187 + 0 * 5.23493 =10.10903522

$$Exp^{\left(-input1-8\right)+Bias} = Exp^{\left(-10.10903522\right)} = 4.07101E - 05$$

$$\frac{1}{1+Exp^{-input}} = 0.999959292$$

Hidden Node input: 0.999959292 *-2.05577 =-2.055686313

$$Exp^{\left(-hidden\ node\right)+Bias} = Exp^{\left(--2.055686313\right)} = 7.812197645$$

$$\frac{1}{1+Exp^{-hidden\ node}} = 0.113479071$$

This is the output, since the output 0.113479071 <0.5 it is classified as no Stroke to the patient.

As per the above diagram and ANN prediction, model predicted outcome is patient is not having risk of getting heart stroke.

CLASSIFICATION BASED ON NON LINEAR MAPPINGS: SUPPORT VECTOR MACHINES: SVM CLASSIFIER

SVM built based on statistical learning and gives promising empirical results in many practical applications starting from handwritten digit recognition to text categorization(Qin et al., 2009). SVM used in classification (Archana & Elangovan, 2014) and regression problems. As illustrated in Figure 15, SVM can identify a hyperplane to split the optimal hyperplane as wide as possible to have a max distance between observation and hyperplane (Pradhan et al., 2017) between two datasets. The vectors defined on the hyperplane are called support vectors. SVM efficiently separates both linearly & non linearly separable observations by means of kernel functions (Prakash, Chakravarthy, & Kaveri, 2015).

Linear SVM is defined as: xi. xj

Non-linear SVM is defined with a function: $\varnothing\left(x_i\right).\varnothing(x_j)$

Figure 15.

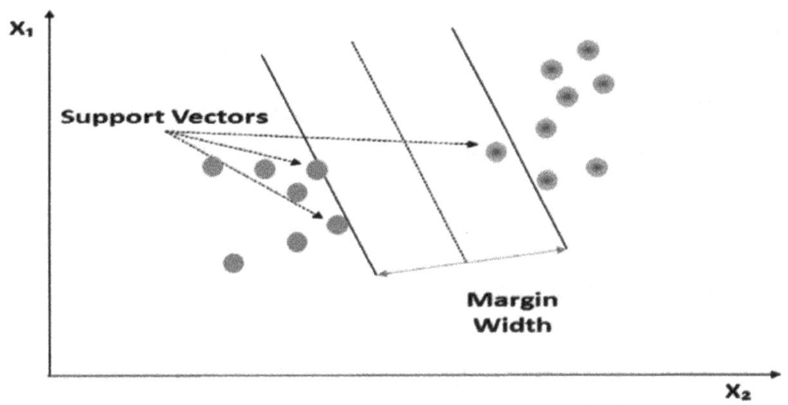

Figure 16.

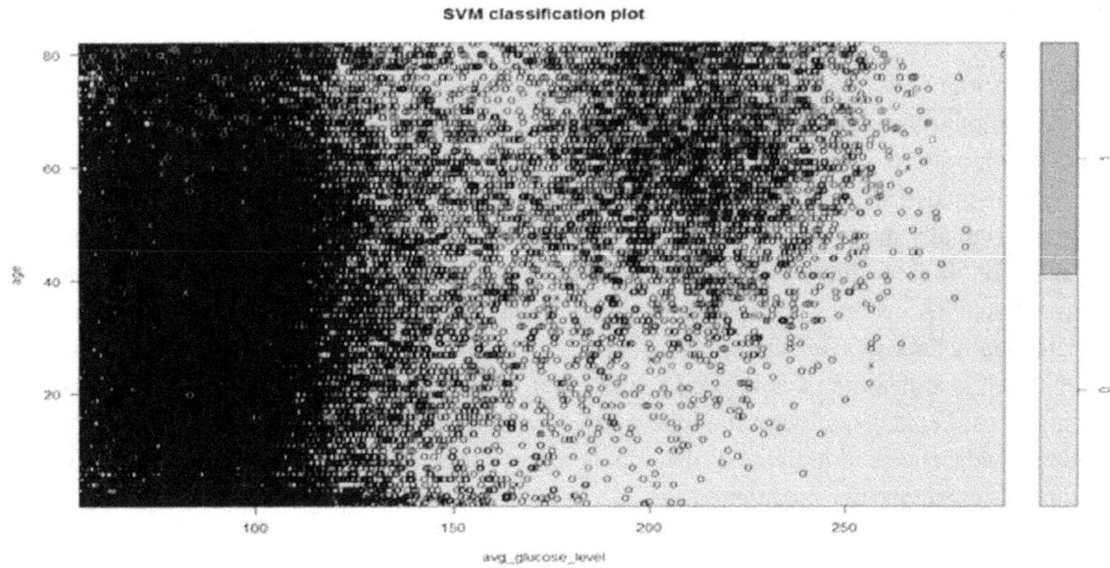

Kernel function: k(x_i . x_j)

As depicted in Figure 16, 4443 'x' symbols are support vectors, in this 3343 belongs to Class 0 and 1091 belongs to class 1.

From this we can observed that the model is built with Radial Kernel function, with SVM type as classification model with two different classes No and Yes. It has total 13 support vectors 4 of them belongs No class and 9 of them belongs to Yes class.

We can tune the model with different combinations of epsilon and cost parameters.

Example: - tmodel <- tune(svm, tab~.,data=tabdata,
ranges = list(epsilon = seq(0,1,0.1), cost = 2^(1:7)))

In the above we have given epsilon value starting from 0 to 1 with an increment of 0.1 and cost up to 128. So there will be 1408 validations to be done to tune the model.

The model can be tuned with the above mentioned variables and bring in the best model to generate support vector machines. The best model can be achieved with the different epsilon values and cost functions.

With this model, the above we can predict any unknown samples. When tried to predict the outcome for this sample: P(gender=male) * P(age =80) * P(hypertension=no) * P(heart disease = yes) * P(married=yes) * P (Work type = not working) * P(residence type = rural) * P (average glucose = 105.92) * P(BMI=32.5) * P (smoking=no) using support vector machine, it predicted Yes. Which means the patient have chances to get stroke.

CLASSIFICATION BASED ON OTHER FEATURES

Classification models developed based on different other features such as biological evolution, rough set theory, fuzzy sets etc., are discussed below

Genetic Algorithm

Genetic Algorithm is developed based on an analogy to biological evolution. It is often applied in search and optimization techniques. It built using evolutionary computing based on the analogy survival of the fittest. This algorithm is robust because it eliminates expensive redesigning. Also it is capable of self-repairing, self-guided and can reproduce as in genetics. It is a heuristic solution-search or optimization technique, originally motivated by the Darwinian principle (McCall, 2005) of evolution through (genetic) selection. It uses a highly abstract version of evolutionary processes to evolve solutions to given problems. Each GA operates on a population of artificial chromosomes. These are strings in a finite alphabet (usually binary). Each chromosome represents a solution to a problem and has a fitness, a real number which is a measure of how good a solution it is to the particular problem. Usually, it has the following steps: 1) Computation of the fitness value for the current population 2) the choice of the best individuals 3) the choice of individuals that will compose the new population and 4) the use of selected individuals to create the new population

Rough Sets

Rough set method is another classification technique in data mining. A suite of methodologies that is useful for characterization of data that is not accurate has been provided by rough set theory. One of the main aspects in rough set methods is providing a formal framework for automated transformation of data into knowledge for changing the modules. Rough set theory (RST) was introduced by Pawlak in 1982 (Riza et al., 2014) as a methodology for data analysis based on the approximation of concepts in information systems. Rough sets are used to approximately or "roughly" define equivalent classes. Rough Set theory (RST), which is a mathematical approach for addressing vagueness and uncertainty (Liu et al., 2017). A rough set for a given class C is approximated by two sets: a lower approximation (certain to be in C) and an upper approximation (cannot be described as not belonging to C).

Fuzzy Sets

Fuzzy classification is derived by the process of grouping the elements with help of fuzzy sets. Fuzzy sets are the sets whose membership functions defined by fuzzy logic. Fuzzy logic is an approach of computing based on degree of truth rather binary such as 0 or 1 / true or false etc. It works on the approximation rather based on actual count. In most of the real life scenarios it is required to approximate, so fuzzy logic is used. It is built with membership function and member ship values (degree of truth) which ranges between 0.0 and 1.0 to represent the degree of membership. Fuzzy concepts can be characterized in terms of fuzzy predicates (properties) which are combined by means of generalized logical connectives (Hüllermeier, 2011). In fact, one should recognize that gradualism is not only advantageous for expressing the concept itself, but also for modelling the qualifying properties.

HYBRID CLASSIFIERS

This section focuses on the blended classification models or combining classifiers. There is no thumb rule to suggest a best classifier for problem at hand. This leads the researchers to think of ensemble the classification models to yield better results. For instance, Random Forest can use for features selection and model can built using ANN or SVM.

Combination of some classifiers to give a collective prediction. Use of multiple classification models to predict for the same dataset and prediction is decided by majority of the predictions. So the class maximum votes will be winning class and will the outcome. It can be fine-tuned by weighted predictions are combined to predict the result using this blended classification model.

Another technique of blended classification can be used is hybrid classification models. For instance, a hybrid classifier combines Bayesian Network algorithm uses KNN distance based algorithm. Lazkano and Sierra proposed network structure obtained from the data set using Nearest Neighborhood is used in combination of Bayesian Network (Sierra et al., 2011).

Blended algorithms are present in recent versions of machine learning tools such as weka (Hall et al., 2009) like Bayesian logistic regression (BLR) method widely used in text categorization, which is a combination of Bayesian and logistic models. Similarly, Naïve Bayes classification and Decision tree can be blended.

Table 9. Validation framework: Representation of Confusion matrix

		Predicted	
		Class 0	**Class 1**
Actual	**Class 0**	*a*	*b*
		True Negatives	*False Positive*
		Rejections are correct	*False Alarm*
	Class 1	*c*	*d*
		False Negative	*True Positive*
		Over look	*Positive correct*

Xiao Liu and all proposed a Hybrid Classification System Based for heart disease diagnosis with ensemble classification method of C4.5 and Naïve Bayes and Bayesian Neural Networks (BNN) methods. It seems ensemble classification method gave better performance than the individual C4.5 classifier and the other two classifiers (Liu et al., 2017).

Cagatay CATAL and Mehmet NANGIR in their recent paper "A Sentiment Classification Model Based On Multiple Classifiers" built a hybrid classifier with Naive Bayes, SVM, and Bagging for sentiment classification. As per the results, multiple classifiers and meta classifier (Bagging algorithm) improved the performance of a component of the model (Catal & Nangir, 2017).

The hybrid algorithms consistently produce a lower average error than the base algorithms it combines, but at a higher computational cost. It has to be wisely decided based on this tradeoff.

RESLUTS AND RECOMMENDATIONS

This section details about how to assess classification performance. The performance of the model is usually calculated using accuracy and error rate. Accuracy is the percent of correct classifications in the validation dataset. Error rate is the percent of the inaccurate classifications in the validation set. Performance measures calculated from the confusion matrix/ contingency table.

The confusion matrix depicted in Table 9, talks about the TN-true negatives – 'a' – which represents the records rejections correctly by model, FP - false positives – 'b'– wrongly alarmed by the classification model, FN -false negatives – 'c'- overlooked by the classification model and true positives correctly classified as positive. Model is evaluated based on below measures.

$$\text{Accuracy} = (a + d)/(a + b + c + d) = (TN + TP)/\text{total} \text{ ----} \quad (32)$$

$$\text{True positive rate (Sensitivity)} = d/(c + d) = TP/\text{actual positive} \text{ ----} \quad (33)$$

$$\text{True negative rate (Specificity)} = a/(a + b) = TN/\text{actual negative} \text{ ----} \quad (34)$$

Table 10. Model performance metrics

	Accuracy	Sensitivity	Specificity
Zero R	0.978624174	#DIV/0!	0.978624174
One R	0.978624174	#DIV/0!	0.978624174
Naive Bayesian	0.962145356	0.044198895	0.975244402
Decision Tree	0.978701904	0.515151515	0.979894015
Random Forest	0.978235523	0.469879518	0.981536536
LDA	0.950097163	0.174067496	0.985612096
LR	0.978546444	0.482758621	0.979666563
KNN	0.974547941	1	0.974544073
ANN	0.974970851	#DIV/0!	0.974970851
SVM	0.979479207	0.72	0.979984424

Predicted positive value (Precision) = d/(b + d) = TP/predicted positive ---- (35)

False positive rate (False alarm) = b/(a + b) = FP/actual negative = 1 – specificity ---- (36)

False negative rate = c/(c + d) = FN/actual positive ---- (37)

Above mentioned classification model performance metrics for the given data set has been evaluate and shown in the below table: Table 10 for reference. Accuracy of the model, sensitivity and specificity of the model is calculated as per the above mentioned equations.

Stroke data is not a balanced, as dataset has 97.8% of the data No stroke (0) and only 2.2% data stroke (1). Hence prediction would be biased hence most of the models did not perform well. This can be addressed by over sampling - adding 97% additional samples of class 1 by duplicating the same data multiple times. Otherwise can also do under sampling. This is roughly opposite to the over sampling technique to addressed biased dataset.

Figure 17 depicts the pros and cons of classification models discussed in this chapter and various comparisons.

FUTURE WORK

The advantages of AI have been extensively discussed in the field of healthcare industry. Sophisticated classification algorithms with help of AI on large volume of healthcare data - tests, X-Rays, CT scans etc., and can obtain foresights from them, assist doctors in decision making. Cardiologists and radiologists in the future should only look at the most complicated cases where human supervision is needed. Genetics and genomics look for mutations and links to disease from the information in DNA. With the help of AI, body scans can spot cancer and vascular diseases early and predict the health issues people might face

Figure 17.

Method	Advantage	Limitation	Accuracy	Train/Test	Remarks
Zero R	Very Simple Support discrete, continuous	No predictors contribution, No predictive power.	Low	Fast/Fast	No predictors Contribution
One R	Simple to build Support discrete, continuous	Predict with one predictor	Moderately Low	Fast/Fast	Predict based on the best rule with smallest error
Novie Bayesian	Easy to build No complicated iterative parameter estimation Support large data sets & Better performance	Zero frequency problem Numerical variables to be transformed as categorical	Moderate	Fast/Fast	Better predictor contribution Independence assumption among predictors
DT (ID3 & C 4.5)	Top down approach Easy to interpret & implement Support discrete, continuous	Over fitting Missing values	Moderate	Fast/Fast	Unstable tend to over fit Greedy approach with no back track
LDA	Mathematically robust Better accuracy	Old algorithm	Moderately High	Fast/Fast	Correlation varies from -1 to 1, 1 & -1 are highest contributions in either directions and 0 being no contribution
Logistic Regression	Easy to compute Can handle non-linear attributes	Stability requires much more data	Moderately High	Fast/Fast	Logistic regression predicts based on logistic curve – constructed with natural algorithm of odds of target variable
KNN	Classes need not to be linearly separable Zero learning process cost Robust against noisy data Multi model class	Expensive on large datasets Performance depends on # of dimensions Locality sensitive	Moderate	Fast/Depends on N	Based on similarity measure Accuracy depends on value of N, Better results for higher N
ANN	Easy to implement Wide range of problems can be solved	High processing time Slow learning	High	Slow/Fast	Non linear model Based on biological neural networks Can't interpret the relationship between input & output
SVM	High accuracy Works well with non linearly separable data	High complex and expensive model	Very High	Slow/Slow	Kernel function SVM gain flexibility, Kernel with non linear transformation requires no assumptions. Lack of transparency due to non parametric technique
Generic Algorithm	Easy to implement Low memory requirement	Randomized Can get stuck on local maxima	High	Fast/Fast	Randomized heuristic technique

based on their genetics. AI/ ML models can learn from the healthcare data of a country and highlight mistakes in treatments, workflow inefficiencies and helps area healthcare systems avoid unnecessary patient hospitalizations. Achieving above is not simple and straightforward with existing classification algorithms and need to build more sophisticated hybrid, ensemble and deep learning classification models.

CONCLUSION

This chapter highlights various classification techniques, methods used in the machine learning. Classification is to describe the important data classes from the dataset. This review describes various statistical, probabilistic & heuristic methods based on frequency table, covariance matrix, similarity functions and others features. Comparison of various methods with advantages, limitations along with efficiency are discussed. Naïve Bayesian algorithm is simple and no complicated iterative parameter model but outperforms compared to other. Decision tree models are based on J. R. Quinlan's ID3 algorithm and can easily interpretable. Random Forest is the multitude of decision trees model, which can give accurate results. LDA and Logistic regression are mathematically robust and yield moderately accurate results. KNN algorithm can be able to classify even nonlinear data, can give accurate prediction when use high K values. ANN is based on biological neural networks and it is a back-tracking propagation to improve the accuracy of the model. SVM classifies by identifying the hyperplane that maximizes margin among the classes. Other models like genetic algorithm, fuzzy sets and rough sets etc along with hybrid and ensemble models. Ensemble models gives a better accuracy and discussed different ways to synthesize them to get a better result. The conclusion of this chapter is there are quite a many classification algorithms existing based on size of data and problem statement one has to take a wise decision to select the classification models and ensemble them to gain better accuracy.

REFERENCES

AL-Nabi, D. A., & Ahmed, S. S. (2013). Survey on classification algorithms for data mining: Comparison and evaluation. *International Journal of Computer Engineering and Intelligent Systems*, *4*(8), 18–27.

Algamal, Z. Y., Lee, M. H., Al-Fakih, A. M., & Aziz, M. (2017). High-dimensional QSAR classification model for anti-hepatitis C virus activity of thiourea derivatives based on the sparse logistic regression model with a bridge penalty. *Journal of Chemometrics*, *31*(6), e2889. doi:10.1002/cem.2889

Archana, S., & Elangovan, K. (2014). Survey of classification techniques in data mining. *International Journal of Computer Science and Mobile Applications*, *2*(2), 65–71.

Casas, M. M., Avitia, R. L., Gonzalez-Navarro, F. F., Cardenas-Haro, J. A., & Reyna, M. A. (2018). Bayesian Classification Models for Premature Ventricular Contraction Detection on ECG Traces. *Journal of Healthcare Engineering*, *7*. doi:10.1155/2018/2694768 PMID:29861881

Chen, M.-S., Han, J., & Yu, P. S. (1996). Data mining: An overview from a database perspective. *IEEE Transactions on Knowledge and Data Engineering*, *8*(6), 866–883. doi:10.1109/69.553155

Cover, T., & Hart, P. (1967). Nearest neighbor pattern classification. *IEEE Transactions on Information Theory*, *13*(1), 21–27. doi:10.1109/TIT.1967.1053964

Derrac, J., Chiclana, F., García, S., & Herrera, F. (2016). Evolutionary fuzzy k-nearest neighbors algorithm using interval-valued fuzzy sets. *Information Sciences*, *329*, 144–163. doi:10.1016/j.ins.2015.09.007

Dobre, O. A., Abdi, A., Bar-Ness, Y., & Su, W. (2007). Survey of automatic modulation classification techniques: Classical approaches and new trends. *IET Communications*, *1*(2), 137–156. doi:10.1049/iet-com:20050176

Domingos, P., & Pazzani, M. (1997). On the optimality of the simple Bayesian classifier under zero-one loss. *Machine Learning*, *29*(2), 103–130. doi:10.1023/A:1007413511361

Fan, R., Zhong, M., Wang, S., Zhang, Y., Andrew, A., Karagas, M., ... Moore, J. (2011). Entropy-based information gain approaches to detect and to characterize gene-gene and gene-environment interactions/correlations of complex diseases. *Genetic Epidemiology*, *35*(7), 706–721. doi:10.1002/gepi.20621 PMID:22009792

Gehrke, J., Ramakrishnan, R., & Ganti, V. (1998). *RainForest-A framework for fast decision tree construction of large datasets*. Paper presented at the VLDB.

Hall, M., Frank, E., Holmes, G., Pfahringer, B., Reutemann, P., & Witten, I. H. (2009). The WEKA data mining software: an update. *ACM SIGKDD Explorations Newsletter, 11*(1), 10-18.

Harper, P. R. (2005). A review and comparison of classification algorithms for medical decision making. *Health Policy (Amsterdam)*, *71*(3), 315–331. doi:10.1016/j.healthpol.2004.05.002 PMID:15694499

Hüllermeier, E. (2011). Fuzzy sets in machine learning and data mining. *Applied Soft Computing*, *11*(2), 1493–1505. doi:10.1016/j.asoc.2008.01.004

Kachroo, S., Melek, W. W., & Kurian, C. (2013). *Evaluation of predictive learners for cancer incidence and mortality*. Paper presented at the E-Health and Bioengineering Conference (EHB). 10.1109/EHB.2013.6707388

Li, Z., Liu, G., & Li, Q. (2017). Nonparametric Knn estimation with monotone constraints. *Econometric Reviews*, 1–19. doi:10.1080/07474938.2017.1310080

Liu, X., Wang, X., Su, Q., Zhang, M., Zhu, Y., Wang, Q., & Wang, Q. (2017). A Hybrid Classification System for Heart Disease Diagnosis Based on the RFRS Method. *Computational and Mathematical Methods in Medicine*. PMID:28127385

Maillo, J., Ramírez, S., Triguero, I., & Herrera, F. (2017). kNN-IS: An Iterative Spark-based design of the k-Nearest Neighbors classifier for big data. *Knowledge-Based Systems*, *117*, 3–15. doi:10.1016/j.knosys.2016.06.012

McCall, J. (2005). Genetic algorithms for modelling and optimisation. *Journal of Computational and Applied Mathematics*, *184*(1), 205–222. doi:10.1016/j.cam.2004.07.034

Nevill-Manning, C. G., Holmes, G., & Witten, I. H. (1995). The development of Holte's 1R classifier. *Proceedings of the Second New Zealand International Two-Stream Conference.*

Patro, V. M., & Patra, M. R. (2015). *A Novel Approach to Compute Confusion Matrix for Classification of n-Class Attributes with Feature Selection*. doi:10.14738/tmlai.32.1108

Phyu, T. N. (2009). Survey of classification techniques in data mining. *Proceedings of the International MultiConference of Engineers and Computer Scientists.*

Pradhan, L., Taneja, N. A., Dixit, C., & Suhag, M. (2017). *Comparison of Text Classifiers on News Articles*. Academic Press.

Prakash, S., Chakravarthy, T., & Kaveri, E. (2015). Statistically weighted reviews to enhance sentiment classification. *Karbala International Journal of Modern Science*, *1*(1), 26–31. doi:10.1016/j.kijoms.2015.07.001

Prasad, A., Belwin Edward, J., & Ravi, K. (n.d.). A review on fault classification methodologies in power transmission systems: Part—I. *Journal of Electrical Systems and Information Technology*. doi:10.1016/j.jesit.2017.01.004

Qin, B., Xia, Y., Prabhakar, S., & Tu, Y. (2009). *A rule-based classification algorithm for uncertain data*. Paper presented at the Data Engineering, 2009. ICDE'09. IEEE 25th International Conference on.

Raschka, S. (2014). *Naive bayes and text classification i-introduction and theory*. arXiv preprint arXiv:1410.5329

Rashid, T. A., & Abdullah, S. M. (2018). A Hybrid of Artificial Bee Colony, Genetic Algorithm, and Neural Network for Diabetic Mellitus Diagnosing. *ARO-The Scientific Journal of Koya University*, *6*(1), 55–64. doi:10.14500/aro.10368

Rashid, T. A., Abdullah, S. M., & Abdullah, R. M. (2016). *An Intelligent Approach for Diabetes Classification*. Cham: Prediction and Description.

Riza, L. S., Janusz, A., Bergmeir, C., Cornelis, C., Herrera, F., Śle¸zak, D., & Benítez, J. M. (2014). Implementing algorithms of rough set theory and fuzzy rough set theory in the R package "RoughSets". *Information Sciences*, *287*, 68–89. doi:10.1016/j.ins.2014.07.029

Shaikhina, T., Lowe, D., Daga, S., Briggs, D., Higgins, R., & Khovanova, N. (2017). Decision tree and random forest models for outcome prediction in antibody incompatible kidney transplantation. *Biomedical Signal Processing and Control*. doi:10.1016/j.bspc.2017.01.012

Shao, G., & Sang, N. (2017). Regularized max-min linear discriminant analysis. *Pattern Recognition*, *66*, 353–363. doi:10.1016/j.patcog.2016.12.030

Sierra, B., Lazkano, E., Irigoien, I., Jauregi, E., & Mendialdua, I. (2011). K Nearest Neighbor Equality: Giving equal chance to all existing classes. *Information Sciences*, *181*(23), 5158–5168. doi:10.1016/j.ins.2011.07.024

Singh, P. P., Prasad, S., Das, B., Poddar, U., & Choudhury, D. R. (2018). Classification of Diabetic Patient Data Using Machine Learning Techniques. Singapore: Academic Press. doi:10.1007/978-981-10-7386-1_37

Tarikm, A. R. (2016). Decision Support System for Diabetes Mellitus through Machine Learning Techniques. *International Journal of Advanced Computer Science and Applications*, *7*(7). doi:10.14569/IJACSA.2016.070724

Wahbeh, A. H., Al-Radaideh, Q. A., Al-Kabi, M. N., & Al-Shawakfa, E. M. (2011). A comparison study between data mining tools over some classification methods. *International Journal of Advanced Computer Science and Applications*, *8*(2), 18–26.

Wang, Q., Garrity, G. M., Tiedje, J. M., & Cole, J. R. (2007). Naive Bayesian classifier for rapid assignment of rRNA sequences into the new bacterial taxonomy. *Applied and Environmental Microbiology*, *73*(16), 5261–5267. doi:10.1128/AEM.00062-07 PMID:17586664

Wu, X., Kumar, V., Ross Quinlan, J., Ghosh, J., Yang, Q., Motoda, H., ... Steinberg, D. (2008). Top 10 algorithms in data mining. *Knowledge and Information Systems*, *14*(1), 1–37. doi:10.100710115-007-0114-2

Yosipof, A., Guedes, R. C., & García-Sosa, A. T. (2018). Data Mining and Machine Learning Models for Predicting Drug Likeness and Their Disease or Organ Category. *Frontiers in Chemistry*, *6*, 162. doi:10.3389/fchem.2018.00162 PMID:29868564

Chapter 3 Classification Algorithms for EEG-Based Brain-Computer Interface: A Review

Sravanth Kumar Ramakuri
VNR Vignana Jyothi Institute of Engineering and Technology, India

Chinmay Chakraboirty
Birla Institute of Technology Mesra, India

Anudeep Peddi
VNR Vignana Jyothi Institute of Engineering and Technology, India

Bharat Gupta
National Institute of Technology Patna, India

ABSTRACT

In recent years, a vast research is concentrated towards the development of electroencephalography (EEG)-based human-computer interface in order to enhance the quality of life for medical as well as nonmedical applications. The EEG is an important measurement of brain activity and has great potential in helping in the diagnosis and treatment of mental and brain neuro-degenerative diseases and abnormalities. In this chapter, the authors discuss the classification of EEG signals as a key issue in biomedical research for identification and evaluation of the brain activity. Identification of various types of EEG signals is a complicated problem, requiring the analysis of large sets of EEG data. Representative features from a large dataset play an important role in classifying EEG signals in the field of biomedical signal processing. So, to reduce the above problem, this research uses three methods to classify through feature extraction and classification schemes.

DOI: 10.4018/978-1-5225-7796-6.ch003

INTRODUCTION

EEG signal illustrates the electrical movement of the brain. They are exceptionally arbitrary in nature and might include valuable data about the brain state. EEG signals are profoundly non-Gaussian, non-stationary and have a non-linear nature. Electroencephalography is a non-invasive procedure utilized to analyze brain associated diseases and side effects. It assists in diagnosing numerous neurological sicknesses, for example, epilepsy, tumor, cerebrovascular sores, depression and issues related with shock. EEG traces are distinctive for various brain actions. The brain action of an anomalous individual can undoubtedly be recognized from an ordinary individual utilizing signal preparing strategies.

EEG signals are exceptionally client-specific, and in that capacity, most existing BCI frameworks are aligned particularly for every client. This training informationset ought to have EEG signals registered while the client played out each psychological undertaking of interest quite a lot of times, as indicated by given commands. The registered EEG signals will be applied as mental state cases with a specific end goal to locate the best adjustment parameters for this client. EEG is the most well-known technique for recording brain signals in people since it is protected, inexpensive, simple to utilize, and for the reason that it has a elevated temporal resolution (of the order of milliseconds) portrayed by Yoshida et al. (2015). EEG electrodes, put on the scalp, are capable of either "passive" or "active". Metallic passive electrodes are associated with an amplifier by a wire. Active electrodes contain an inherent preamplifier to construct them less responsive to ecological noise and cable actions. The two kinds of electrodes require gel or saline fluid to work, keeping in mind the end goal to lessen the skin-electrode contact resistance. This keeps their utilization for extended periods, for example, an entire day, for the reason that the gel dries with time, making the resistances toincrease and the signals to debase. Consequently, dry electrodes are as of now being created and tried for BCI. Notwithstanding a low spatial resolution, (at best the inter-distance connectingelectrodes is 1-2 cm) and a shortsignal-to-noise proportion, this arrangement gives numerous favourable circumstances for extensive use.

There are modern medical devices for imaging techniques used for human being they are Electrocardiography (ECG) utilized in support of heart, Electromyography (EMG) utilized in support of muscular contractions, Electroencephalography (EEG) utilized in support of brain activity, Magneto encephalography (MEG) also used for brain activity, Magnetic Resonance Imaging (MRI) and many more such devices are used for various diagnosis of human described by Joseph and Bronzino (2000). The EEG machine is used on the scalp of the brain to diagnose various activities in different lobes of the human brain.

Murugappan et al. (2007) composed a competent attainment protocol for obtaining the EEG signals under audio-visual initiation condition. The EEG data has been gathered from 6 strong subjects with inside an age set of 21-27 utilizing 63 biosensors. From the subjective investigation on every emotion, three emotions have been related to higher understanding. Subsequent to preprocessing the signals, distinct wavelet change is utilized to remove the EEG parameters. The feature vectors got from the above feature extraction technique on 63 biosensors create an information network for emotion classification. Here, we have utilized Fuzzy C-Means (FCM) and Fuzzy k-Means (FKM) grouping strategies for ordering the emotions. We have additionally examined the execution of FCM and FKM on decreased number of 24 biosensors revealed in Figure 1. At long last, it looked at the execution of clustering the distinct emotions utilizing FCM and FKM on both 64 biosensors and 24 biosensors. Results affirm the likelihood of utilizing wavelet change based feature extraction for evaluating the human emotions from EEG signal, and of choosing an insignificant number of channels for emotion acknowledgment test.

Figure 1. 24 Channel electrode placements for EEG recording

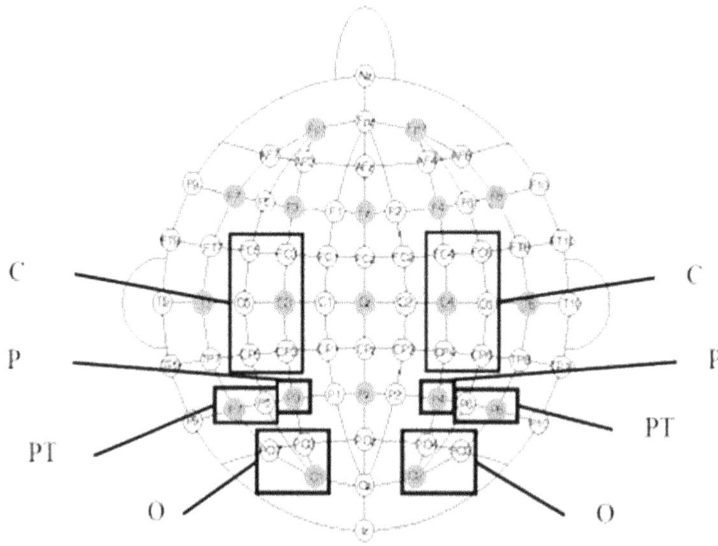

Suleiman et al (2007) proposed feature extraction techniques for EEG signal for BCI applications. BCI is composed utilizing electroencephalogram (EEG) signals where the subjects need to consider just a solitary mental assignment. EEG signals are recorded from 16 channels and concentrated amid a few mental and motor errands. Features are extricated from those signals utilizing a few techniques: Time Analysis, Frequency Analysis, Time Frequency Analysis and Time-Frequency-Space Analysis. Separated EEG features are characterized utilizing a mock neural network prepared with the back engendering algorithm. Classification rates that achieve 99% between two errands and 96% between three errands utilizing Space-Time-Frequency-Analysis and Time Frequency-Analysis are acquired.

Alharbi et al (2016) presented a solitary preliminary classification for the Electroencephalography (EEG) signals evoked by RGB colors. It explores distinctive feature extraction strategies to discover the best technique which can be utilized with hues dataset. These strategies are: Event-Related Spectral Perturbations (ERSP), Target mean, Auto Regressive and EMD residual. It utilized another feature choice algorithm, which centers on choosing the best features by examining the conduct of EEG parts that show up due to the presented shading. It presented a correlation between the classification consequences of utilizing all separated features, the results of utilizing the chosen features by the proposed algorithm and the consequences of utilizing the chosen features by recursive feature elimination algorithm, which is utilized by comparative investigation. The algorithm is demonstrated with all the explored feature extraction strategies as the classification certainties are expanded. Support Vector Machine (SVM) is utilized as a part of the classification procedure. The best feature extraction strategy that gives the most noteworthy classification exactness and can be utilized with continuous BCI frameworks are target mean and EMD residual, as their efficiency is high and the calculation time is low.

Robinson et al (2016) plans to conquer the protection issues emerging from the exchange of unprocessed EEG data by anchoring the unprocessed EEG data through encryption and by giving just the significant features related to a specific application, when asked. Feature is a particular trademark estimation of a pattern segment. EEG signal processing relates essentially to feature extraction. Consequently the business locales the genuine however regularly disregarded issue of security which rises in connection with the use of brain rushes of a man.

Braack et al (2013) executed in feature extraction of EEG signal is Principal Component Analysis (PCA). It is a basic, nonparametric method in removing data from befuddles data and communicates it in their shared trait and contrasts. PCA will change the data by pivot, where it will discover the route in the data with most deviation. The first axis comparing to the primary segment is turned to the course where the difference of the data is the most. At that point, the following segment will be opposite to the main segment with the most fluctuation and so on.

Zhang et al (2017) demonstrates a model-based Field Programmable Gates Array (FPGA) outline for real-time feature removal of Electroencephalogram (EEG) signals, which can be utilized for brainwaves bands classification to record and distinguish mental status in Brain Computer Interface (BCI) applications and awareness contemplates. A model-based outline approach is utilized to execute Short-time Fourier Transform (STFT) and concentrate 20 frequency feature elements for classification. These 20 features are isolated into 5 bunches relating to 5 distinct brainwaves bands. Each feature is characterized as the normal power range of various contiguous frequency components. A hardware model is composed utilizing Xilinx System Generator and actualized on FPGA. Fixed-point is utilized as opposed to floating-point to increment working velocity for meeting timing necessity of the ongoing framework. The outline is executed on a Xilinx Zedboard at 50MHz clock rate, and can be utilized for up to 128-channel EEG signals feature extraction at 250 Hz sample rate.

Pattnaik et al (2016) concentrated on the removal of features of EEG motor exercises utilizing Discrete Wavelet Transform (DWT) and ordered the signal for utilizing Artificial Neural Network (ANN) for separating left and right hand symbolism development and the stream of this work was appeared in Figure 2. Two arrangements of feature vectors are taken from beta rhythm as contribution to the Feed-forward neural network classifier. We watched that three information feature vectors like mean, standard deviation and peak power accomplished better classification execution effect of 80.71% contrasted with two input feature vector which is of 78.57%.

Mangalagowri et al (2016) are examined the EEG signals and feature extraction is finished by utilizing "db4" wavelet with multilevel decay. 10 genuine human subjects genuine EEG tests are gathered utilizing standard International 10-20 Electrode placement framework which is set over a whole scalp of human subject and it is disintegrated into 5 distinctive EEG bands utilizing Discrete wavelet Transform

Figure 2. Flow diagram of DWT with ANN scheme

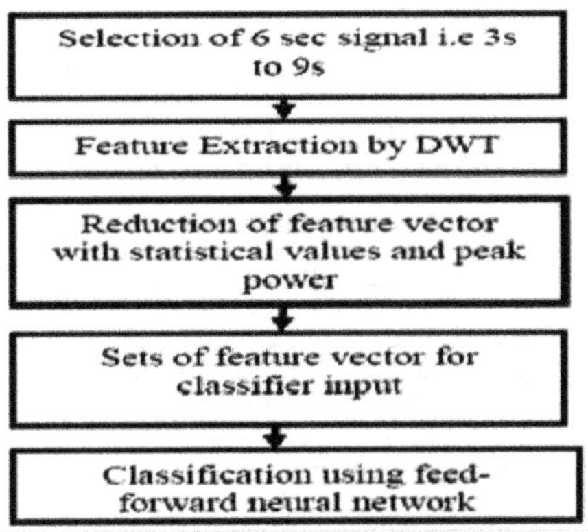

(DWT).Emotion detection is the assignment of emotional state like perceiving a man's joy, fear, outrage, perplexity or duplicity crosswise over both voice and non voice channels. Emotion detection depends on an arrangement of customary features which are extricated like energy, power spectral density, from the EEG signals for grouping emotions and to recognize the force level of various bands of EEG signal. Feature extraction comes about are acquired by utilizing "Bior 5.5" and "db4" wavelet for signal decay and to acquire the exact frequency bands and feature Classification is carried out by getting an exactness of 75% for ordinary patient and 65% for irregular patient.

Aris et al (2016) decide the quantity of EEG practices existed amid eyes shut. The EEG signals when before and after stretch test were chosen and processed into the EEG features known as asymmetry index (AsI). Keeping in mind the end goal to decide the number EEG practices, the cluster focuses of the EEG features are tried utilizing subtractive clustering (SC) and the general procedure of this plan was revealed in Figure 3. The most extreme number of three clusters focuses was distinguished and Fuzzy C-Means (FCM) was utilized to isolate the data features into comparative gathering. With a specific end goal to test which clusters number gives most elevated classification, the FCM was executed independently for three clusters and two clusters. In this manner, the k-Nearest Neighbor (k-NN) was utilized to order the three clusters and two clusters and the classification rates are distinguished. The classification results demonstrated that the quantity of two clusters provide elevated classification rate which was 100%.

Cososchi et al (2006) presents an approach that utilizes self-sorting out fuzzy neural network based time series prediction that executes EEG feature extraction in the time domain only. EEG is registered from two electrodes put on the scalp over the motor cortex. EEG signals coming from every electrode are anticipated by a solitary fuzzy neural network. Features got from the mean squared error of the forecasts and from the mean squared of the anticipated signals are separated from EEG data using a sliding window. The design of the two auto arranging fuzzy neural networks is a network with multi sources of info and single output.

Pang et al (2016) utilized the t-CWT strategy which depended on the continuous wavelet transform (CWT) and Student's t-test for extricating ERN features. In the analysis, EEG was registered from 5 electrode destinations (Fz, FC1, Cz, FCz and FC2) amid a maintained consideration explore in 10 subjects. We utilized a support vector machine for classification. Additionally, the algorithm gives completely

Figure 3. Flow Chart of the FCM with KNN process

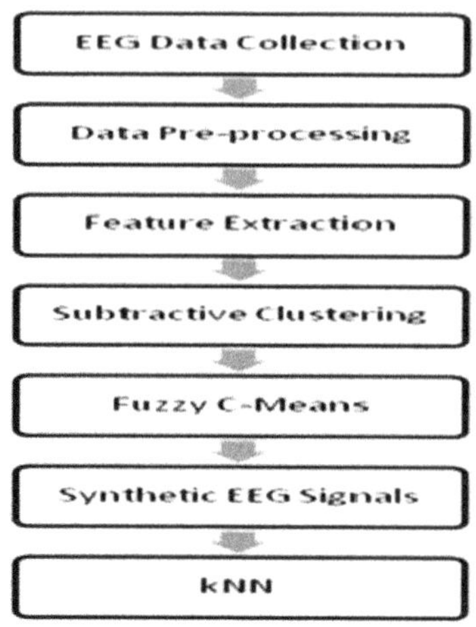

Figure 4. Main components of the EEG monitoring model

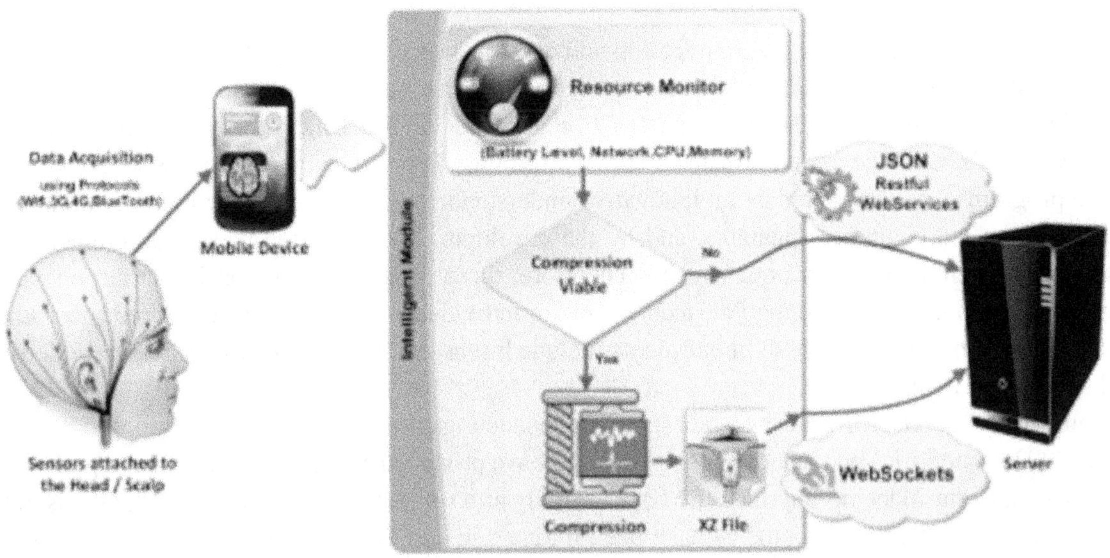

automated detection and evaluation strategies for extricating the most discriminative. ERP elements are between two intellectual states and are specific reasonable for arranging single-preliminary ERPs. The features removed by the algorithm can be translated as far as signal attributes that are adding to the effectiveness of classification, providing another technique for brain movement examination.

Sakai et al (2013) displayed the KNMF algorithm, which receives a powerful requirement to arrange motor symbolism EEG data. The requirement is set to enhance the disfavor between two classes amid motor symbolism assignments, which can augment the energy distinction between the source networks, disintegrated from the input spectral EEG signal, of the target and non-target classes. Classification was carried out utilizing the LD technique. To survey the proposed strategy, the IDIAP database was utilized. After deteriorations from the input information network were accomplished utilizing the proposed strategy, the energy contrast between source frameworks of the target and non-target classes was really enlarged. Accordingly, the classification precision of the proposed technique was roughly 4% higher than that of KNMF without a requirement, which infers the adequacy of applying imperative in expanding the discriminability among two classes. As far as circumstance mindfulness, this shows KNMF_ID can be utilized to recognize shrouded brain states.

Salazar-Varas et al (2015) utilized a feature removal technique for multiclass EEG signals in view of their pairwise intelligibilities. The consistency gives a feeling of the brain's connectivity, and it is significant as various locales of the brain must impart between each other for the mix of tactile data and the model was exposed in Figure 4. For our situation, the procedure of feature determination is advanced in the logic that only those measurably huge and possibly discriminative intelligibilities at a particular frequency are utilized, which brings about a feature vector of decreased measurement. Subsequently, those features are grouped through Mahalanobis distance classifier and the performance is assessed by the kappa coefficient. The EEG coherence determination and classification technique can give great productivity rates, and with the upside of choosing an optimal blend of features without the need of earlier learning about the psychological undertaking. It shows the applicability of the technique through numerical illustrations utilizing genuine EEG data from psychological assignments.

REVIEW ON EEG SIGNAL GENERATION

"Brain computer interfaces for communication and control" was proposed by Wolpaw et al. (2002). For several years, people have wondered that electrophysiological measures or other electroencephalographic activities might give an innovative non-muscular channel for transferring commands and messages to the outside BCI. Over the period of past 15 years, prolific BCIs investigation programs have increased. These programs are encouraged by an innovative understanding of brain roles, by the initiation of potential low-priced computer apparatus, and by the developing identification of the requirements and potentials of individuals with impairments. Therefore, these programs focus on initiating innovative enhancive communication and regulate technology for individuals who suffer from rigorous neuromuscular impairments. Some of these impairments include brainstem stroke, amyotrophic lateral sclerosis, and spinal cord damage.

Current advancement in brain interfaces, such as connecting cortex to machinery is proposed by Donoghue (2002). Scientific and technological progresses have produced extensive interest in the probability of making a Brain-Machine Interface (BMI), especially as a support to the paralyzed individuals in the communication sector. Developments have been initiated in identifying neural signals and converting them into control signals which can regulate devices. Moreover, he also projected systems that make use of outside derived neural signals as a command device, and increase the potentials of more supple systems which directly utilize intra cortical recording are analyzed.

Schwartz et al. (2004) projected "Control Neural prosthetics". Cortical signals that depend on three aspects are used in this control of prostheses. The three aspects include: arrays of chronic microelectrode, mining algorithms, and prosthetic effectors. Chronic arrays of microelectrodes are enduringly fixed in the cerebral cortex. These chronic arrays should record groups of single and multi-unit activities for a long duration. Data comprising velocity and position correlates of live movement requirements are to be mined constantly in actual time from the recorded activities.

"BCI technology: a review of the first international meeting" is designed by Wolpaw et al. (2000). This writing provides a summary of the initial worldwide meeting dedicated to BCI research and advancement. Recent BCIs utilize EEG (Electroencephalographic) activity that is recorded at the scalp or single segment activity that is recorded from inside cortex to regulate the cursor motion, or manage a neuron prosthesis.

Dornhege et al. (2007) developed a concept of 'Toward BCI'. The main objective of Wadsworth centre BCI program is to build up Electroencephalographic BCI systems that could supply rigorously impaired people with a substitute means of control and/or communication. It is displayed that individuals with or without motor impairments can study to regulate sensory motor paces that are recorded from the scalp. This regulation is performed to move the cursor in single or multi-dimensions, and moreover, P300 event associated potential is utilised to regulate signal to create discrete preferences. In general, the current research specifies that there are various approaches that may supply substitutes for people with rigorous motor impairments. Presently, we are assessing the effectiveness and practicality of BCI communication system for a routine purpose by such people in their houses.

Carey (2002) projected a system in which he explained the functioning of the brain. Picard and Klein (2002), in this work, explained the following aspects. The EEG linear characteristics in the clinical treatments are proved to be efficient, the nonlinear approaches such as entropy, and these brain facts are well-recognized in brain signal processing with nonlinear signals. The segmental dimension is a theory nonlinear approach that uses brain conditions such as concentration levels, pain levels etc. for quantification. Two well-recognized approaches known as box counting are used to recognize concentration degrees with neuron criticism of patients and it has superior efficiency.

Serhani et al (2015) utilized a novel way joining both EEG pressure and portable asset accessibility assessment to lift and spare energy for longer observing episode. The principle center of our approach lies in creating and executing an algorithm, which assesses on the fly the pressure cost and accessible assets on the cell phone to choose whether to completely/incompletely pack the input EEG data or not. We tentatively assessed and tried the adequacy of our method utilizing both offline and online data registered by the Emotiv EEG device. The acquired results demonstrate that approach fundamentally spares versatile battery and handling power to adapt to significant health circumstances.

Zabidi et al (2012) portrays the STFT examination of EEG signals acquired amid composing and envisioned writing. The EEG signal is sifted utilizing a band pass channel with a frequency scope of 8-30 Hz before the STFT was processed. The width of the Hamming window utilized as a part of the STFT calculation was shifted to get the ideal width. The consequences of the STFT analysis demonstrated that the frequency components of the EEG signals acquired from composing are the same as that got amid envisioned writing.

Cuesta–Frau et al (2017) evaluates the performance of first generation entropy metrics, featured by the well known and widely used Approximate Entropy (ApEn) and Sample Entropy (SampEn) metrics, and what can be considered an evolution from these, Fuzzy Entropy (FuzzyEn), in the Electroencephalogram (EEG) signal classification context. The study uses the commonest artifacts found in real EEGs, such as white noise, and muscular, cardiac, and ocular artifacts and the example of artifacts are showed in Figure 5. Using two different sets of publicly available EEG records, and a realistic range of amplitudes for interfering artifacts, this work optimizes and assesses the robustness of these metrics against artifacts in

Figure 5. Example of EOG, EMG, and spike artifacts. All the signals were amplitude-normalized for visualization purposes

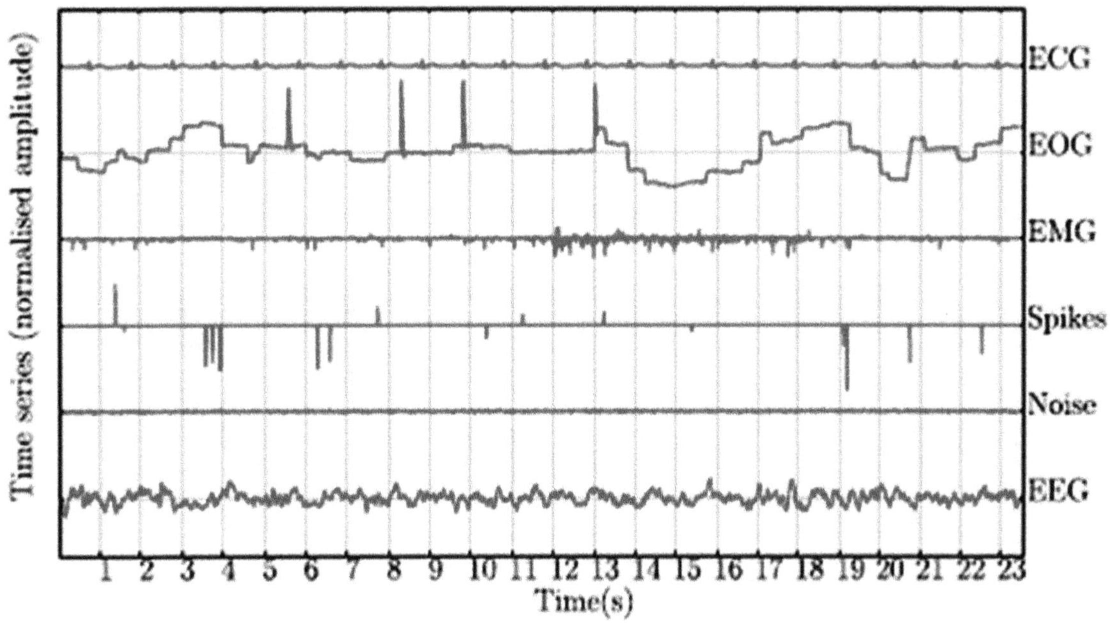

class segmentation terms probability. The results show that the qualitative behaviour of the two datasets is similar, with SampEn and FuzzyEn performing the best, and the noise and muscular artifacts are the most confounding factors. On the contrary, there is a wide variability as regards initialization parameters. The poor performance achieved by ApEn suggests that this metric should not be used in these contexts.

Nguyen et al (2017) explores the effect of epilepsy on EEG-based cryptographic key generation frameworks. Epilepsy is one of the brain issues that includes in the EEG signal and subsequently it might have affect on the framework. On the other hand, this issue has not been explored. To take care of this issue, it utilized a framework for cryptographic key generation from EEG signals was demonstrated in Figure 6, and analyzes it with the Australian EEG dataset. It utilized parametric range appraise system for feature exaction, and arranged a mistake rectification quantization procedure that is helpful for a noisy data, for example, EEG. It accomplishedexperiments on two groupsof subjects, epileptic and non-epileptic to explore the effect of epilepsy on the achievement rate of the framework. Exploratory outcomes demonstrate that epilepsy really affects the performance of the framework.

Liu et al (2017) quantified the complexity features of EEG signals simulated by single neural mass model based on the modified permutation-entropy algorithm. The statistical analysis results prove that there are huge contrasts between the unpredictability features of ordinary EEG signals and epileptiform spikes signals, and demonstrate that the signals can be recognized under various lengths of time series, embedding dimensions and delay times. Along these lines, we reason that the changed stage entropy is a successful multifaceted nature measure to evaluate the EEG signals. In the meantime, it demonstrates that the changed permutation-entropy is more compelling to recognize the EEG signals with various rhythm contrasted with the permutation-entropy and Rényi permutation-entropy.

Dolezal et al (2006) focussed on the classification of right index finger development course using the movement-related EEG signal. The EEG database we utilized was initially registered for a physiological study. This examination depicts technique and procedure of non-development related (resting) EEG signal generation alongside the achieved new classification outcomes including the false caution rate. Artificial EEG signal was created by AR modelling. The AR model parameters were evaluated from short sections (3 sec) of inactive EEG already available in the database utilizing the autocorrelation strategy.

Figure 6. EEG-based cryptographic key generation system

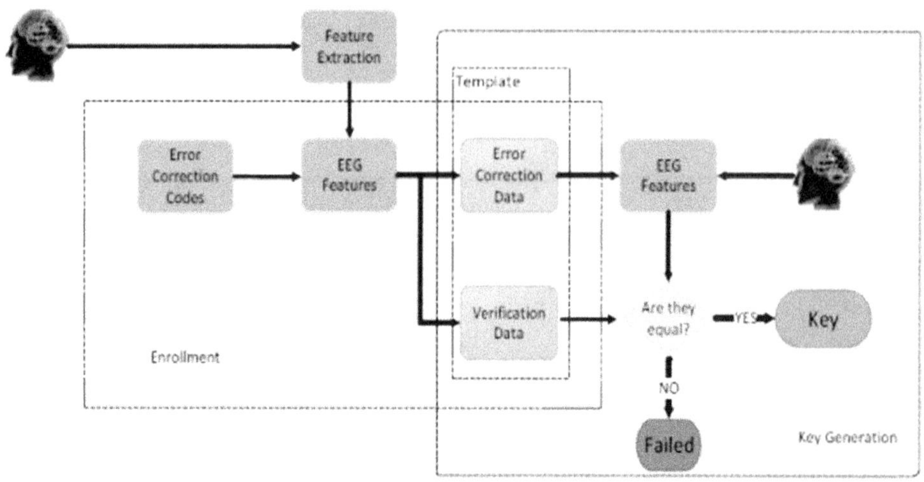

The outcomes demonstrated the framework ought to have the capacity to recognize movement-related and inactive EEG without noteworthy issues.

Koya et al (2015) utilized EEG electrodes which offer new open doors in the advancement of new bio restorative gadgets to create discourse signals for speaking debilitated people. The outline and miniaturized scale manufactured fractal electrodes are exceptionally helpful in getting brain data dependably which is only an effective Brain computer interface which does not require any solid action. A fractal measurement EEG gadget might be utilized to frame an array of EEG signal factors which might be mapped to the speech signals created by a healthy subject. The mapping and connection between the brain signals with the speech created might be firmly correlated with adequate algorithms. These relations will give essential understanding of brain signal to speech connection. A model is utilized to create speech signals from the EEG signals. A wavelet bundles based algorithm is proposed to discover the examples in EEG signals which are mapping with the speech words. The model is extremely valuable for speaking debilitated people specifically and additionally helpful for different applications.

Bawane et al (2014) represents a novel strategy utilizing Self Organizing Feature Map (SOFM) to group left-hand movement imagination, right-hand movement imagination, and word creation from EEG. Welch's periodogram, a power spectrum density (PSD) evaluation which is powerful preprocessing strategy fit for handling both the noisy and non-stationary natures of EEG signals is utilized for feature removal. Additionally, it characterizes the PSD feature utilizing SOFM. SOFM is orchestrated purposely in a particular fashion and prepared with variable learning rate to group different mental assignments under discussion. A classification precision acquired utilizing SOFM is contrasted and other existing procedures.

Almonacid et al (2016) presents the impact of the electing procedure to improve the classification rates in motor symbolism of brain– computer interface (BCI) frameworks. The motor symbolism is the three-class issue of left-hand movement imagination, right-hand movement imagination, and word generation. An algorithm in view of neural networks and fuzzy theory (S-dFasArt) is utilized to characterize unconstrained mental behaviours from electroencephalogram signals, so as to work a non-invasive BCI. This algorithm permits acquiring a few expectation models. The voting among these forecast outcomes enhances the achievement rates of the classifier technique. The quantity of models and the measure of the data set have been examined acquiring some proposal rules for professionals and a change of over 12% can be normal.

Atkinson et al (2016) presented an EEG feature-based emotion acknowledgment strategy. Distinct to other methodologies, the methodology utilizes the mRMR feature choice technique as a signal preprocessing move in order to enhance the perceptive precision of a SVM emotion classifier in light of two-dimension emotions model (i.e., Valence and Arousal).Also, contrasted with state-of-the-art emotion recognition techniques, our technique manages a higher number of emotion classes (i.e., 8) on a standard DEAP dataset, which creates the issue further sensible however in the meantime, the training job turns out to be all the more demanding. Well ordered procedure of this plan was depicted in Figure 7. Moreover, the request which joins feature determination and kernel classifiers utilizes multi-label classifiers to concurrently perceive a more extensive arrangement of emotion classes in view of a dimensional emotion display.

Siuly et al (2012) applied a hybrid algorithm to enhance the classification achievement rate of MI-based electroencephalogram (EEG) signals in BCIs and it was demonstrated in Figure 8. This plan builds up a novel cross-relationship based feature extractor, which is helped with a least square support vector machine (LS-SVM) for two-class MI signals acknowledgment. To confirm the adequacy of the proposed

Figure 7. Step by step process of SVM scheme

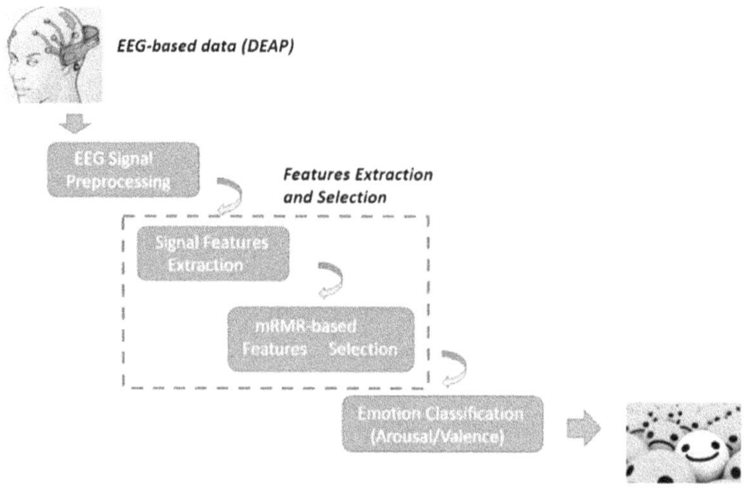

classifier, it substitutes the LS-SVM classifier by a logistic regression classifier and a kernellogisticregression classifier, independently, with similar features extricated from the cross-relationship method for the classification. The proposed suggestion is tried on datasets, IVa and IVb of BCI Competition III. The performances of those techniques are assessed with classification precision through a 10-fold cross-validation system. It additionally evaluates the performance of the proposed strategy by contrasting it with eight newly revealed algorithms. Investigational outcomes on the two datasets demonstrate that the proposed LS-SVM classifier gives a change contrasted with the logistic regression and kernel logistic regression classifiers. The outcomes additionally demonstrate that the proposed suggestion beats the most as of late announced eight techniques and accomplishes a 7.40% change over the best outcomes of the other eight examinations.

Orhan et al (2011) presented a multilayer perceptron neural network (MLPNN) based classification mock-up as a diagnostic choice support component in the epilepsy treatment. EEG signals were decayed into frequency sub-bands utilizing discrete wavelet transform (DWT). The wavelet coefficients were clustered utilizing the K-means algorithm for every frequency sub-band. The likelihood conveyances were processed by dissemination of wavelet coefficients to the clusters, and then utilized as inputs to the MLPNN form. It directed five distinct examinations to assess the performance of the projected form in the

Figure 8. MI-based electroencephalogram (EEG) signals in BCIs

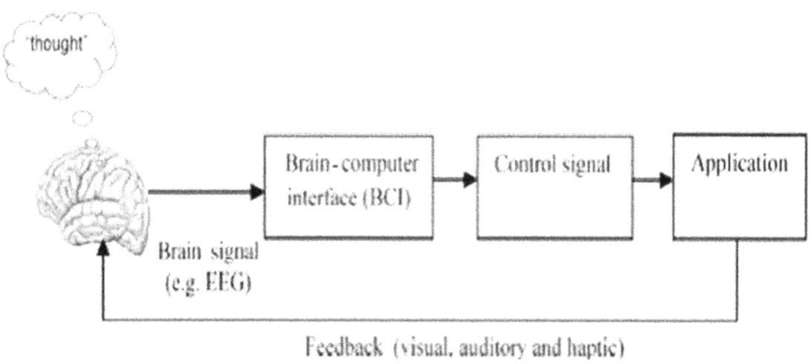

classifications of various blends of solid sections, epileptic seizure free fragments and epileptic seizure portions. It demonstrated that the projected form brought about attractive classification exactness rates.

Müller et al (2004) talked about variable selection techniques and their application to EEG data. These methods are a striking element of the BBCI online input framework. Note that in spite of the fact that machine learning algorithms were at first constantly tried offline, it is the dominance of picking the 'right' unpredictability for a learning issue that influences the subsequent classifiers to sum up and in this manner renders them helpful in genuine BCI criticism tests. Specifically, the change in perspective far from subject training to individualization and adjustment ('let the machines that learn') of the signal handling and classification algorithm to the particular brain 'under examination' holds the way to the achievement of the BBCI. Having the capacity to utilize (B) BCI for untrained subjects significantly upgrades and widens the range of handy applications in human-computer interfacing.

Rejer et al (2017) presents the results of the experiment that was performed in order to test our strategy for applying ICA for a 4-channel EEG data recorded for motor imagery brain computer interface. Five subjects, untrained in motor imagery paradigm took part in the experiment. According to our results the mean classification accuracy increased after applying ICA from 67% to 76% (for 10-second time window) and from 66% to 77% (for reduced 7-second time window).

Valeriani et al (2017) demonstrates a hybrid collaborative Brain Computer Interface (cBCI) to enhance group-based acknowledgment of target faces in swarmed scenes recorded from observation cameras. The cBCI utilizes a mix of neural features extricated from EEG and reaction times to gauge the choice certainty of the clients. Group opinions are then acquired by measuring singular reactions as per these certainty gauges. Results acquired with 10 members show that the proposed cBCI enhances choice blunders by up to 7% over customary cooperative choices in light of dominant part. Also, the certainty gauges acquired by the cBCI are more precise and vigorous than the certainty detailed by the members after every choice. These outcomes demonstrate that cBCIs can be a powerful means of human growth in practical situations.

Almonacid et al (2016) demonstrates the impact of the electing methodology to upgrade the classification rates in motor symbolism of brain– computer interface (BCI) frameworks. The motor symbolism is the three-class issue of left-hand movement imagination, right-hand movement imagination, and word generation. An algorithm in view of neural networks and fuzzy theory (S-dFasArt) is utilized to categorize unconstrained mental behaviours from electroencephalogram signals, with the aim of to handle a noninvasive BCI. This algorithm permits getting a few forecast models. The voting among these forecast outcomes enhances the achievement rates of the classifier strategy. The quantity of models and the span of the data set have been examined acquiring some suggestion rules for specialists and a change of over 12% can be normal.

Li et al (2017) utilized just a single intracranial electrode to execute an online BCI for quick typing. At the point when the subject went to the virtual button containing visual movement boosts, conspicuous reactions were inspired at the stereo-EEG (SEEG) electrodes inside the fMRI characterized middle temporal (MT) location, which were made out of motion-onset visual evoked potential (mVEP) around 200 ms post-stimulus and a power increment at the high gamma (70-100 Hz) frequency level. In the online BCI research by means of surgical epilepsy patients, by joining mVEP and high gamma characteristics together and utilizing smart stopping methodology, single SEEG electrode supported a speed of BCI composing up to 14 characters for every moment. The discoveries show the practicality of executing an insignificantly intrusive intracranial BCI with just a single electrode for quick typing.

Alam et al (2017) demonstrates primary outcomes of preparing real EEG signals utilizing Empirical Mode Decomposition (EMD) for potential applications in Motor Imagery based Brain-Computer Interface (MI-BCI) frameworks. The EEG signals, generally described as boisterous, nonlinear and non-stationary, can process the non-stationary, can be treated utilizing EMD to get signal components (natural mode capacities IMFs) in the physiologically significant frequency areas for MI-BCI applications. The disintegrated signal components, IMFs, can be additionally prepared to remove pertinent features for classification and invigoration of MI exercises for translating to actionable signals for remote activity of gadgets.

Naraballobh et al (2015) concentrated on watched and examined the EEG-based signal and connected the statistic way to deal with the noteworthy distinction of every specific brainwave frequency band while giving the two diverse acoustic stimuli. The two stimuli are binaural beat and instrumental unwinding music which initiated the psychological state similarly. In addition, this examination is relied upon to support the pattern of the consequence of EEG from another exploration. The feeling of anxiety estimated by DASS survey is an essential factor for state of subjects before the trial and is influenced to the results of acoustic stimulus. Connect the EEG meaning with the investigational outcomes, the subjects with ordinary feeling of anxiety are disadvantage the nonexistent and concentrated unwinding for both tuning in to the binaural beat and unwinding music.

EEG SIGNAL CLASSIFICATION METHODS

Emotion is an important issue between human to human communications. In our daily life, emotions play an important role for interacting people. The famous philosopher Aristotle stated that emotions are great feeling and powerful aspect in human to human communication which is based on powerful potential on gain and pleasure (Picard & Klein, 2002; Chew, 2009). Human-computer systems, the information received by human from system is through skin, eyes, ears, and nose etc. and this message is transferred in brain system. This information entered into the computer is through cameras, tracking systems based sensors, and biofeedback sensors. Then based on algorithms, the information system applications are processed.

These emotions are decided to the human behavior status. Emotions are creating that person/subject feelings to the outside world and also its link up to the brain controlled the different types of processed work. Emotions are described that in different methods, these basic emotions are characterized by different colors relates eight basic, emotions to evolutionary valuable properties, and based thereupon he claims these to be the basic emotions. The user's inner feelings are revealed using EEG emotional recognitions and used in treatment or user emotion-enabled or used for applications in real time. The algorithm of emotion recognition consists of two parts: feature classification and extraction. For rcal-time application, the faster algorithms need to be developed for recognizing more emotions with few electrodes.

Murugappan et al. (2007) using 64 biosensors and 24 biosensors of offline data and extract the band spectra features than classify using FCM, FKM with accuracy level 73% with positive/negative emotions, In 2013, his research divide emotions in happy, surprise, neutral, disgust and classify using K-nearest neighbour at accuracy level observed in 91%.

Kemp et al. (2002) extract the features using Fast Fourier Transform using band spectra and resulting emotions classify using neural network and classify emotions in valance (positive/negative) accuracy will be 68.5%, next these emotions states are developed (Zhang et al., 2009) they extract the features using

PCA and separated these emotions by dividing into subclasses negative and positive states classifying through kernel support vector machine (SVM) and improved accuracy level 73%,

The biggest risk in the classification of MI EEG signals emerges because of the way that the brain signals that are recorded are little in amplitude. In this way, events, for example, eye blink, eye movement, muscular movements, teeth crushing and heart rhythm interfere with the EEG signal bringing about a signal having low Signal to Noise Ratio (SNR). This prevents the decoding framework to effectively decode the user feelings. Classifiers, for example, Support Vector Machine (SVM), K-Nearest Neighbors (KNN), Random Forest (RF), and so on...have been investigated for classification of EEG signals.

Support vector machines (SVMs) classification strategy is based on improvements in computational learning hypothesis. On account of their exactness and capacity to manage with a huge amount of predictors, they have more consideration in biomedical applications. Most of the past classifiers isolate classes utilizing hyperplanes that divide the classes, utilizing a level plane, inside the indicator space. SVMs widen the idea of hyperplane division to data that can't be isolated directly, by mapping the indicators onto another, higher-dimensional space in which they can be isolated straightly.

A few researchers have also focused on employing deep learning for EEG signal classification. A deep belief network (DBN) is employed for classification of emotions utilizing EEG signals. Differential entropy characteristics are extricated from multichannel EEG signals and utilized for preparing the deep belief network. A hidden markov model (HMM) is additionally incorporated to the yield of the DBN with the intention to catch a solid emotional stage exchanging with higher exactness. The DBN technique performed better in correlation with the best in class strategies. A deep learning technique for classification of EEG data in view of motor symbolism has been exhibited in Tomasevic et.al (2012). The authors utilized the strategy for EEG based left and right hand motor symbolism undertakings. They initially trained a weak classifier by DBN using certain single channel data and then combined the trained weak classifiers using the AdaBoost algorithm.

Classification of EEG signal for human computer interaction using neural network trained with back propagation algorithm described by Das et.al (2016). Initially, the EEG de-noising has been done using time-domain regression method and AR model was used for feature extraction. They also used probabilistic neural network for classification.

EEG signals classification as focal and non-focal had been additionally done in light of various techniques for epileptogenic focus identification portrayed by Sharma et.al (2014).The statistically optimal void filters are utilized as a building obstruct for the detection of comparative seizures, while crafted by in view of evaluating the sharpness of the waveform. It removes the vital characteristics of the EEG signals. Second, pick and fabricate a suitable classifier to categorize the signals. Caffe structure with three distinct models (LeNet, AlexNet, and GoogLeNet) is utilized as a part of the proposed DNN to categorize focal and non-focal EEG signals. Feature extraction stage is actualized utilizing convolution and pooling layers, while the classification procedure is performed utilizing completely associated and delicate max classifiers.

The marginalized discrete wavelet transform (mDWT) portrayals can uncover characteristics related to the transient character of the EEG signals, the mDWT coefficients have been regularly applied as a part of EEG signal classification depicted in Ma et.al (2016). In EEG signal classification, the SVM-based classifier has been exhibited as an effective device. However, SVM-based techniques do not abuse the non negativity and the sum-to-one nature of the mDWT coefficients portrayed by ma et.al (2012). So as to catch such properties, we connected the Dirichlet appropriation to demonstrate the mDWT coefficients' basic circulation. For the mDWT coefficients from commonly free channels, it is normal to apply the alleged super-Dirichlet circulation. Super-Dirichlet conveyance based classifier to categorize the EEG signals with mDWT portrayal. The performance of the classifier is better than the SVM-based classifier.

A novel EEG signal classification technique is anticipated, which depends on DWT, the measurement lessening (based on ICA, PCA and LDA) and SVM classification. The method of the framework can be outlined as follows. The features figured with measurable features parameter from time–frequency domain utilizing DWT. The framework removes the features applying ICA, PCA and LDA algorithm to diminish the dimensionality. This progression is executed to expel the insignificant features which are repetitive and even debase the performance of the classifier. The classification procedure for epileptic seizure detection is completed utilizing SVM-based classification.

The high classification exactness of the SVM classifier provides bits of knowledge into the features utilized for characterizing the EEG signals. The conclusion drawn in the applications showed that the DWT coefficients are the characteristics, which will correspond to the EEG signals, and by the utilization of these features a decent refinement between classes can be acquired.

`SVM is applied for classification, which creates the classification of huge high-dimensional spare data set in superb classification speed and impact, Experimental outcomes demonstrate that the planned technique can incredibly lessen dimensionality in the feature space and accomplishes better classification precision, which contrasted with the viability of the ordinary algorithm. In addition, the classification is quicker than some normal techniques, for example, KNN and BP.

Gao et al (2012) utilized Harmony Search (HS)-based BP neural networks for the classification of the epileptic electroencephalogram (EEG) signals. It is familiar that the angle descent-based learning technique can bring about local optima in the preparation of BP neural networks, which may altogether influence their estimation performances. Two HS technique is connected at this point to improve the weights in the BP neural networks for the classification of the epileptic EEG signals. Imitations have shown that the classification exactness of the BP neural networks can be amazingly enhanced by the HS technique based preparing.

Figure 9. EEG based on sparse auto-encoder and SVM process

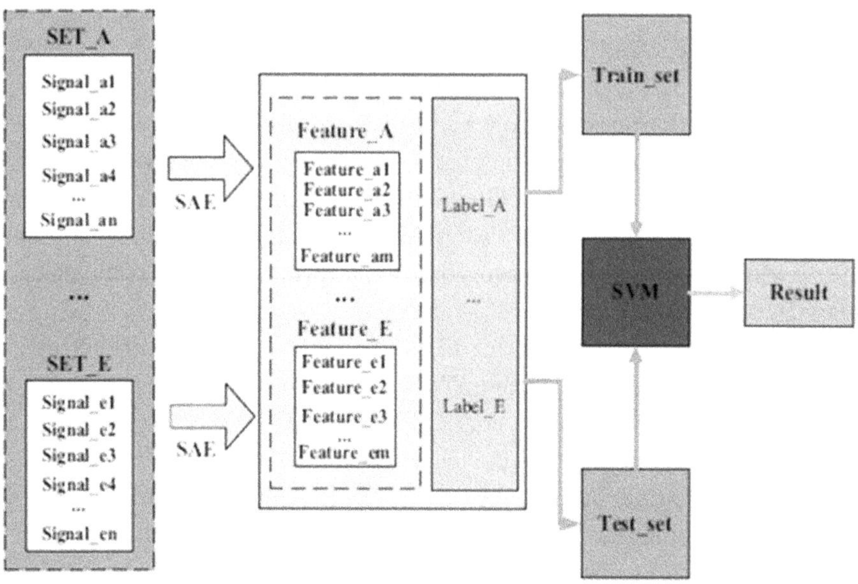

Figure 10. the overall process of ICA with SVM

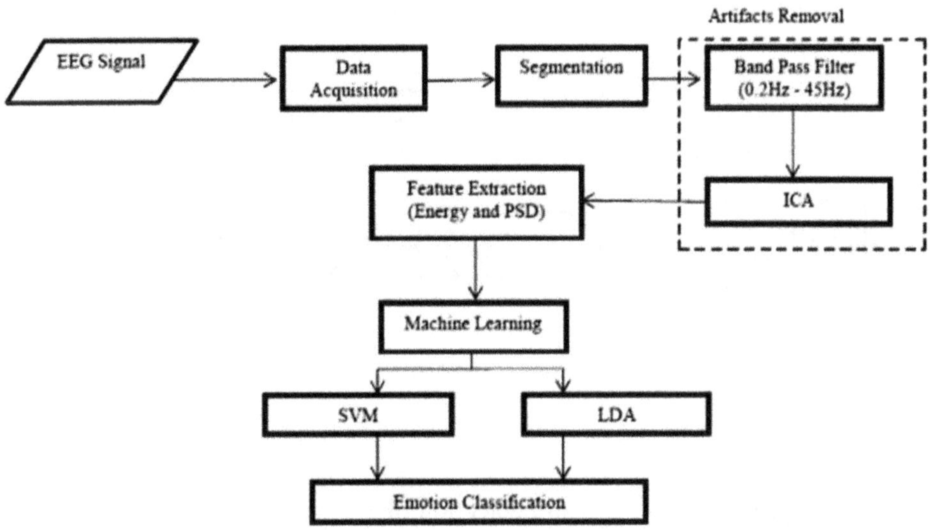

Wang et al (2012) utilized the Adaptive Neuro-Fuzzy Inference System (ANFIS) for the classification of the epileptic electroencephalogram (EEG) signals. The ANFIS joins the adjustment ability of the neural networks and the fuzzy logic-based subjective approach together. A given input/output data set is sent to develop a fuzzy derivation framework, whose enrolment work parameters are prepared utilizing a back engendering algorithm in blend with a minimum squares technique. In any case, the preparation strategy sometimes may prompt nearby optima. It utilized new technique of hybrid training algorithm in view of the combination of the ANFIS and Harmony Search (HS), HS-ANFIS, which is embraced to tune every one of the parameters of the ANFIS.

Bhardwaj et al (2015) utilized a model derived from an Independent Component Analysis (ICA), Support Vector Machine (SVM) and linear discriminant analysis is complete and the entire procedure of this plan was shown in Figure 10. The general pattern which is seen from the test outcomes is that the precision increments with increase in number of preparing tests. From the class-wise precision analysis, it is watched that the Happy and pitiful emotions are perceived with best exactness. SVM can perceive upbeat and miserable emotions with a precision of 87.5% and 92.5% separately while the exactness tumbled to 82.5% and 87.5% individually on account of LDA. Likewise the SVM model is better when contrasted with LDA as a classifier.

Guo et al (2017) proposes a new suggestion with a joined classifier to perceive human emotion states derived from electroencephalogram (EEG) signal. The goal is to accomplish high precision utilizing the consolidated classifier formed, which arranges the extricated features computed from time domain features and Discrete Wavelet Transform (DWT). Two imaginative outlines are engaged with this task: a new variable is set up as another feature and a consolidated SVM and HMM classifier is produced. The outcome demonstrates that the combined features raise the precision by 5% on valence axis and 1.5% on arousal axis. The joined classifier can enhance the precision by 3% contrasting and SVM classifier. One of the imperative applications for high precision emotion classification framework is putting forth a powerful apparatus for clinicians to analyze emotion related mental diseases and the framework created to fill such need.

Figure 11. Principle diagram of GA-SVM

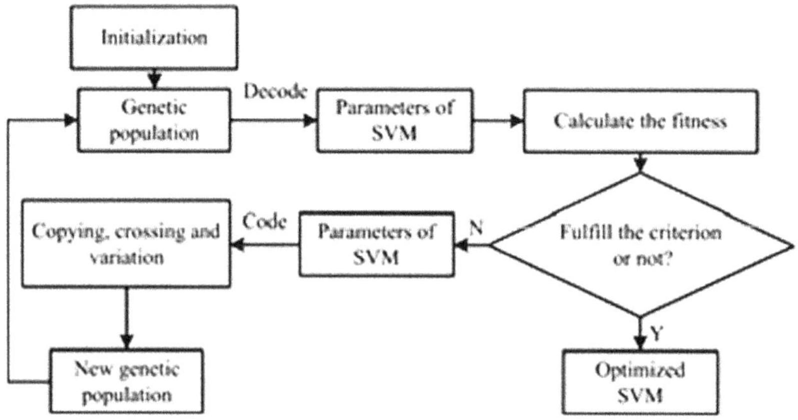

Zhang et al (2017) presents a new seizure detection plot in view of LMD. In view of the fact that EEGs are non-linear and non-stationary signals, LMD, a data-dependent strategy, is connected to disintegrate the crude EEG into a progression of PFs. Nine parameters are removed from the initial five PFs and five classifiers are utilized for five classification goals, separately. Investigational results demonstrate that the deteriorated PFs are of extraordinary significance in segregating distinctive kind of EEG records, and GA-SVM beats the other four classifiers and the rule of this plan was illustrated in Figure 11. Moreover, important features are chosen from the blended features of the initial five PFs and crude EEG, they are then sustained into the GA-SVM for additional classification. The profoundly stable classification comes about show the viability of the proposed strategy, and the proposed technique can deal with all basic clinical cases.

Martín et al (2017) utilized a supervised filter process for developmental multi-target feature choice for classification issues in high-dimensional feature space, which is assessed by examination with wrapper approaches for a similar application. The filter process in view of an arrangement of label-aided utility capacities is contrasted and wrapper approaches utilizing the precision and speculation properties in the successful looking of the most satisfactory subset of features through a transformative multi-objective optimization plan. The target application relates to a brain-computer interface (BCI) classification undertaking derived from linear discriminant analysis (LDA) classifiers, where the properties of multi-resolution analysis (MRA) for signal analysis in temporal and spectral domains have been utilized to remove features from electroencephalogram (EEG) signals.

Ubeda et al (2013) portrays a novel technique for classification for a Brain–Computer Interface (BCI) in light of a standardized cross-connection of EEG maps which stand for the psychological action of the brain and the classification procedure was demonstrated in Figure 12. An improvement protocol has been intended to pick the principle parameters of the classifier with a specific end goal to expand the exactness on the classification. This protocol has been tried with the registers given by IDIAP Research Institute to BCI Competition 2003.Three distinctive mental assignments in light of motor imagery are executed in these sessions. The information have been prepared and tried with the classifier to acquire the optimal achievement rate and dependability. Keeping that in mind, the improvement protocol has been connected to choose the appropriate parameters for the classification. The outcomes are exceptionally acceptable and demonstrate that this sort of classification can be effectively presented in an ongoing BCI.

Figure 12. Classification algorithm. FR: optimal frequency. TI: time interval

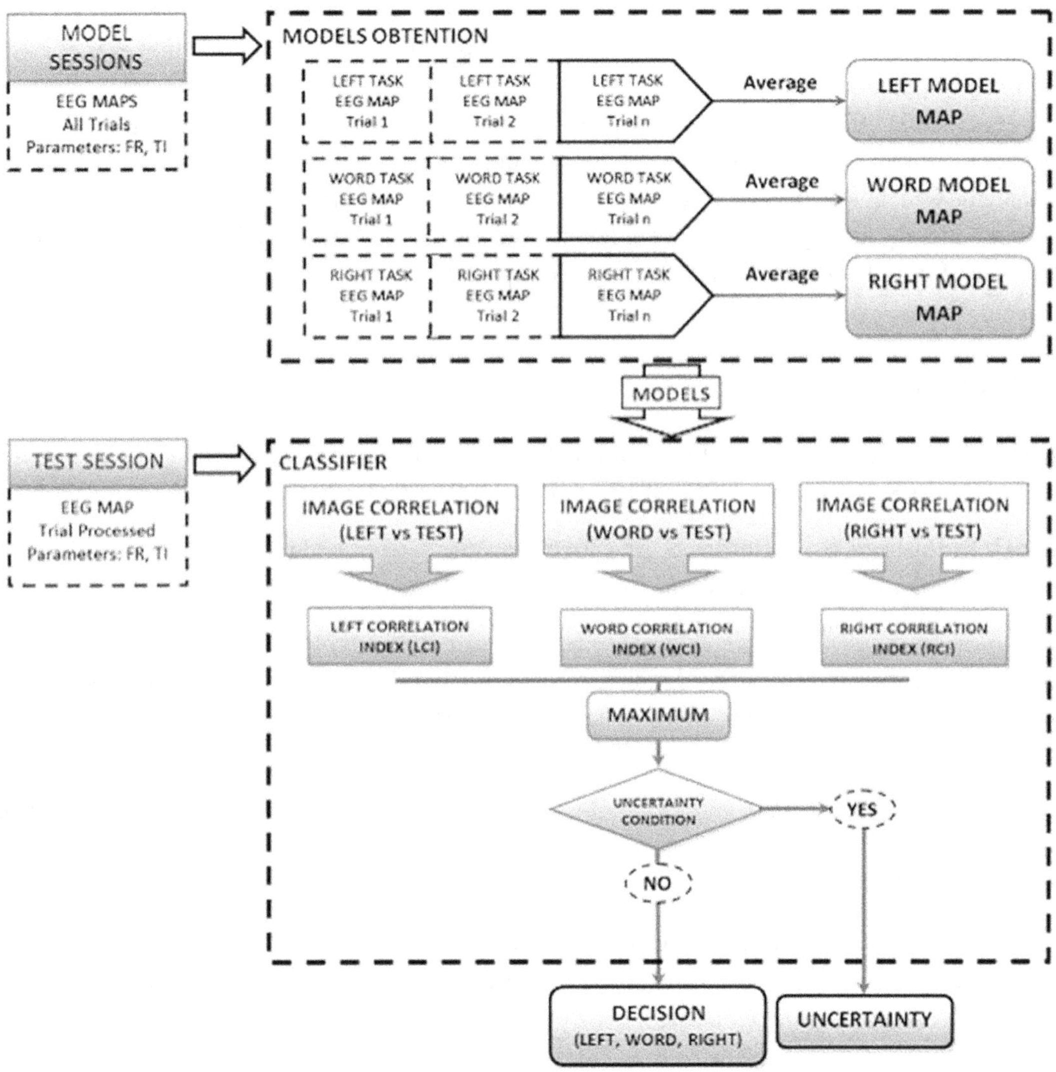

Baig et al (2017) give a complete investigation of the importance of developmental algorithm in choosing the best features for EEG signals. The BCI rivalry III, dataset IVa has been utilized to assess the technique. Exploratory outcomes exhibit that the projected strategy executes well with Support Vector Machine (SVM) classifier, with a normal classification exactness of over 95% with at least 10 features. We likewise introduce a correlation of Differential Evolution (DE) with other developmental algorithms, and the outcomes demonstrate the prevalence of DE which suggests that, with the choice of good seeking algorithm.

Shukla et al (2015) tended to the issue of detecting and transmitting EEG signals over wireless body area network (WBAN). Compressed sensing (CS) methods are utilized abundantly to this last part. In any case, every single earlier method focus on piecemeal recreation of EEG signals from singular channels. From nowhere, we demonstrate how inter-channel relationship can be misused to accomplish better remaking. It used to show the multi-channel signal troupe as (1) a low-rank grid, (2) a row-sparse matrix (in transform domain) and (3) a blend of the two. Enhanced signal reproduction is not the main objective of this work; our approach can likewise lessen the aggregate energy necessity of the EEG sensor hubs by a noteworthy quantity. Earlier procedures could just lessen transmission energy; however our strategy can diminish acquisition energy and wipe out the handling energy required for pressure.

Park et al (2017) offers a novel feature extraction strategy called symmetrical feature was projected. The normal outcomes demonstrated that the new feature compose has bring down performance as far as power than the CSP however has a vigorous characteristic for invariant EEG data contrasted and the past CSP power band. By joining the CSP power feature and the novel symmetrical feature, the classification performance of a BCI framework can be altogether upgraded.

REFERENCES

Alam, M. D. E., & Samanta, B. (2017). Empirical mode decomposition of EEG signals for brain computer interface. In SoutheastCon, 2017. IEEE. doi:10.1109/SECON.2017.7925341

Alharbi, E. T., Rasheed, S., & Buhari, S. M. (2016). Feature selection algorithm for evoked EEG signal due to RGB colors. In *Image and Signal Processing, BioMedical Engineering and Informatics (CISP-BMEI), International Congress on*. IEEE.

Almonacid, M., Ibarrola, J., & Cano-Izquierdo, J.-M. (2016). Voting strategy to enhance multimodel EEG-based classifier systems for motor imagery BCI. *IEEE Systems Journal*, *10*(3), 1082–1088. doi:10.1109/JSYST.2014.2360433

Almonacid, M., Ibarrola, J., & Cano-Izquierdo, J.-M. (2016). Voting strategy to enhance multimodel EEG-based classifier systems for motor imagery BCI. *IEEE Systems Journal*, *10*(3), 1082–1088. doi:10.1109/JSYST.2014.2360433

Aris, S. A. M., Jalil, S. Z. A., Bani, N. A., Kaidi, H. M., & Muhtazaruddin, M. N. (2016). EEG features extraction and k-NN classification during eyes closed. In *Biomedical Engineering and Sciences (IECBES), 2016 IEEE EMBS Conference on*. IEEE.

Atkinson, J., & Campos, D. (2016). Improving BCI-based emotion recognition by combining EEG feature selection and kernel classifiers. *Expert Systems with Applications*, *47*, 35–41. doi:10.1016/j.eswa.2015.10.049

Bawane, M. N., & Bhurchandi, K. M. (2014). Classification of Mental Task Based on EEG Processing Using Self Organising Feature Map. In *Intelligent Human-Machine Systems and Cybernetics (IHMSC), 2014 Sixth International Conference on* (Vol. 2). IEEE.

Bhardwaj, A., Gupta, A., Jain, P., Rani, A., & Yadav, J. (2015). Classification of human emotions from EEG signals using SVM and LDA Classifiers. In *Signal Processing and Integrated Networks (SPIN), 2015 2nd International Conference on*. IEEE.

Cososchi, S., Stungaru, R., Ungureanu, A., & Ugunureanu, M. (2006). EEG features extraction for motor imagery. In *Engineering in Medicine and Biology Society, 2006. EMBS'06. 28th Annual International Conference of the IEEE*. IEEE. 10.1109/IEMBS.2006.260004

Cuesta–Frau, D., Miro-Martinez, P., Nunez, J. J., Oltra-Crespo, S., & Molina Pico, A. (2017). Noisy EEG signals classification based on entropy metrics. Performance assessment using first- and second-generation statistics. *Computers in Biology and Medicine, 87*, 141–151. doi:10.1016/j.compbiomed.2017.05.028 PMID:28595129

Dolezal, J., Stastny, J., & Sovka, P. (2006). Modelling and recognition of movement related EEG signal. In *Applied Electronics, 2006. AE 2006. International Conference on*. IEEE.

Gao, X. Z., Wang, J., Tanskanen, J. M. A., Bie, R., & Guo, P. (2012). BP neural networks with harmony search method-based training for epileptic EEG signal classification. In *Computational Intelligence and Security (CIS), 2012 Eighth International Conference on*. IEEE.

Guo, K., Candra, H., Yu, H., Li, H., Hung, T., & Su, S. W. (2017). EEG-based emotion classification using innovative features and combined SVM and HMM classifier. In *Engineering in Medicine and Biology Society (EMBC), 2017 39th Annual International Conference of the IEEE*. IEEE.

Koya, J. R., & Rao, S. P. V. M. (2015). Nano-fractal Electrodes Use in Electroencephalography (EEG) Array Generation to Map with Speech Signals. *Procedia Materials Science, 10*, 693–698. doi:10.1016/j.mspro.2015.06.072

Li, D., Han, H., Xu, X., Ling, Z., & Hong, B. (2017). Minimally invasive brain computer interface for fast typing. In *Neural Engineering (NER), 2017 8th International IEEE/EMBS Conference on*. IEEE.

Liu, X., Wang, G., Gao, J., & Gao, Q. (2017). A Quantitative Analysis for EEG Signals Based on Modified Permutation-Entropy. *IRBM, 38*(2), 71–77. doi:10.1016/j.irbm.2017.02.001

Mangalagowri, S. G., & Prasanna Raj, P. C. (2016). EEG feature extraction and classification using feed forward backpropogation algorithm for emotion detection. In *Electrical, Electronics, Communication, Computer and Optimization Techniques (ICEECCOT), 2016 International Conference on*. IEEE.

Martín-Smith, P., Ortega, J., Ascenio-Cubero, J., Gan, J. Q., & Ortiz, A. (2017). A supervised filter method for multi-objective feature selection in EEG classification based on multi-resolution analysis for BCI. *Neurocomputing, 250*, 45–56. doi:10.1016/j.neucom.2016.09.123

Müller, K.-R., Krauledat, M., Dornhege, G., Curio, G., & Blankertz, B. (2004). *Machine learning techniques for brain-computer interfaces*. Retrieved from: http://doc.ml.tu-berlin.de/bbci/publications/MueKraDorCurBla04.pdf

Murugappan, M., Rizon, M., Nagarajan, R. & Yaacob, S. (2007). EEG feature extraction for classifying emotions using FCM and FKM. *International Journal of Computers and Communications, 1*(2), 21-25.

Naraballobh, J., Thanapatay, D., Chinrungrueng, J., & Nishihara, A. (2015). Effect of auditory stimulus in EEG signal using a Brain-Computer Interface. In *Electrical Engineering/Electronics, Computer, Telecommunications and Information Technology (ECTI-CON), 2015 12th International Conference on*. IEEE.

Nguyen, D., Tran, D., Sharma, D., & Ma, W. (2017). Investigating the Impact of Epilepsy on EEG-Based Cryptographic Key Generation Systems. *Procedia Computer Science, 112*, 177–185. doi:10.1016/j.procs.2017.08.015

Orhan, U., Hekim, M., & Ozer, M. (2011). EEG signals classification using the K-means clustering and a multilayer perceptron neural network model. *Expert Systems with Applications*, *38*(10), 13475–13481. doi:10.1016/j.eswa.2011.04.149

Pang, Z., Li, J., Ji, H., & Li, M. (2016). A new approach for EEG feature extraction for detecting error-related potentials. In *Progress in Electromagnetic Research Symposium (PIERS)*. IEEE.

Pattnaik, S., Dash, M., & Sabut, S. K. (2016). DWT-based feature extraction and classification for motor imaginary EEG signals. In *Systems in Medicine and Biology (ICSMB), 2016 International Conference on*. IEEE.

Rejer, I., & Górski, P. (2017). Independent component analysis in a motor imagery brain computer interface. In *Smart Technologies, IEEE EUROCON 2017-17th International Conference on*. IEEE.

Robinson, V., & Varghese, E. B. (2016). A novel approach for ensuring the privacy of EEG signals using application-specific feature extraction and AES algorithm. In *Inventive Computation Technologies (ICICT), International Conference on* (Vol. 2). IEEE.

Sakai, M. (2013). Kernel Nonnegative Matrix Factorization with Constraint Increasing the Discriminability of Two Classes for the EEG Feature Extraction. In *Signal-Image Technology & Internet-Based Systems (SITIS), 2013 International Conference on*. IEEE.

Salazar-Varas, R., & Gutiérrez, D. (2015). Feature extraction for multi-class BCI using EEG coherence. In *Neural Engineering (NER), 2015 7th International IEEE/EMBS Conference on*. IEEE.

Serhani, M. A., El Menshawy, M., Benharref, A., & Navaz, A. N. (2015). Real time EEG compression for energy-aware continous mobile monitoring. In *Microelectronics (ICM), 2015 27th International Conference on*. IEEE.

Siuly, S., & Li, Y. (2012). Improving the separability of motor imagery EEG signals using a cross correlation-based least square support vector machine for brain–computer interface. *IEEE Transactions on Neural Systems and Rehabilitation Engineering*, *20*(4), 526–538. doi:10.1109/TNSRE.2012.2184838 PMID:22287252

Suleiman, A.-B. R., & Fatehi, T. A.-H. (2007). Features extraction techniqes of EEG signal for BCI applications. Faculty of Computer and Information Engineering Department College of Electronics Engineering, University of Mosul.

terBraack, E. M., de Jonge, B., & van Putten, M. J. A. M. (2013). Reduction of TMS induced artifacts in EEG using principal component analysis. *IEEE Transactions on Neural Systems and Rehabilitation Engineering*, *21*(3), 376–382. doi:10.1109/TNSRE.2012.2228674 PMID:23359012

Ubeda, A., Ianez, E., Azor'in, J. M., Sabater-Navarro, J. M., & Fernandez, E. (2013). Classification method for BCIs based on the correlation of EEG maps. *Neurocomputing*, *114*, 98–106. doi:10.1016/j.neucom.2012.08.040

Valeriani, D., Cinel, C., & Poli, R. (2017). Augmenting Group Performance in Target-Face Recognition via Collaborative Brain-Computer Interfaces for Surveillance Applications. 2017 *8th International IEEE/EMBS Conference on Neural Engineering (NER)*.

Wang, J., Gao, X. Z., Tanskanen, J. M. A., & Guo, P. (2012). Epileptic EEG Signal Classification with ANFIS based on Harmony Search Method. In *Computational Intelligence and Security (CIS), 2012 Eighth International Conference on*. IEEE.

Yan, B., Wang, Y., Li, Y., Gong, Y., Guan, L., & Yu, S. (2016). An EEG signal classification method based on sparse auto-encoders and support vector machine. In *Communications in China (ICCC), 2016 IEEE/CIC International Conference on*. IEEE.

Zabidi, A., Mansor, W., Lee, Y. K., & Che Wan Fadzal, C. W. N. F. (2012). Short-time Fourier Transform analysis of EEG signal generated during imagined writing. In *System Engineering and Technology (ICSET), 2012 International Conference on*. IEEE.

Zhang, L. (2017). Real-time feature extraction for multi-channel EEG signals time-frequency analysis. In *Neural Engineering (NER), 2017 8th International IEEE/EMBS Conference on*. IEEE.

Zhang, T., & Chen, W. (2017). LMD based features for the automatic seizure detection of EEG signals using SVM. *IEEE Transactions on Neural Systems and Rehabilitation Engineering*, *25*(8), 1100–1108. doi:10.1109/TNSRE.2016.2611601 PMID:27662677

Chapter 4
Arrhythmia ECG Beats Classification Using Wavelet-Based Features and Support Vector Machine Classifier

Chandan Kumar Jha
Indian Institute of Technology Patna, India

Maheshkumar H. Kolekar
Indian Institute of Technology Patna, India

ABSTRACT

Abnormal behavior of heart muscles generates irregular heartbeats which are collectively known as arrhythmia. Classification of arrhythmia beats plays a prominent role in electrocardiogram (ECG) analysis. It is widely used in online and long-term patient monitoring systems. This chapter reports a classification technique to recognize normal (N) and five arrhythmia beats (i.e., left bundle branch block [LBBB], right bundle branch block [RBBB], premature ventricular contraction [V], paced [P], and atrial premature contraction [A]). The technique utilizes features of heartbeats extracted by the wavelet multi-resolution analysis. The feature vectors are used to train and test the classifier based on the support vector machine which has been emerged as a benchmark in machine learning classifier. It accomplishes the beat classification very efficiently. ECG records of the MIT-BIH arrhythmia database are utilized to acquire the different types of heartbeats. Performance of the proposed classifier outperforms the contemporary arrhythmia beats classification techniques.

INTRODUCTION

In recent years, the incidence and prevalence of cardiovascular diseases (CVD) have gained an expanding growth. As per the recent report of WHO, the overall death rates due to CVD have decreased but the burden of heart diseases still remains at peak (Martis *et al.*, 2013). Among many complications of CVD, atrial and ventricular arrhythmias are one of them which occur due to the abnormal electrical activity

DOI: 10.4018/978-1-5225-7796-6.ch004

of heart muscles. Abnormal behavior of heart muscles generates different abnormal cardiac rhythms which are collectively known as arrhythmia. Ventricular fibrillation and flutter are some arrhythmia types which are life-threatening. It results in medical emergencies lead to cardiac arrest, hemodynamic collapse and sudden cardiac death (Huikuri *et al.*, 2001).

The electrical activity of heart muscles could be monitored non-invasively using Electrocardiogram (ECG). Due to the small amplitude and duration, it is difficult to interpret the concealed information present in the ECG data. Therefore, a computer-assisted diagnostic tool could help the physicians in their practice and interpretation. The computer-assisted diagnosis tools can play a major role in the cardiovascular disease management (Hadhoud *et al.,* 2006). These tools are based on many classifiers such neural network (Gutiérrez-Gnecchi *et al.*, 2017), support vector machine (Übeyli, *et al.*, 2007; Kolekar *et al.*, 2015), deterministic learning (Dong *et al.*, 2017), hidden Markov model (Liang *et al.*, 2014; Dash *et al.*, 2017), Bayesian network (de Oliveira *et al.* 2011; Kolekar *et al.*, 2015; Kolekar *et al.*, 2011), linear discriminant analysis (Yeh *et al.*, 2009) etc. These classifiers are widely used for arrhythmia beat classification. A classifier based on the generalized linear model and the auto-regressive model was developed in (Ge *et al.,* 2002) which claims 93.2% classification accuracy for six types of arrhythmia beats. A neuro-fuzzy technique with Hermite coefficients was used in (Linh *et al.,* 2003) to classify ECG beats with 96% accuracy. In (Martis *et. al*, 2009), a Gaussian mixture model-based classification scheme was proposed for normal and abnormal ECG with 94% accuracy. An automated screening tool based on support vector machine classifier was proposed in (Martis *et al., 2012)* to distinguish normal and abnormal ECG beats with 95.6% accuracy.

In Table 1, different arrhythmia beats classifiers and features they used are shown. Generally, classifiers used in computer-assisted diagnosis tools use temporal, morphological, statistical and spectral features (Mar *et al.*, 2011, de Chazal *et al.,* 2006) of ECG beats for proper classification. First, a minicomputer system (Fancott *et. al*, 1980) was developed in 1980 for 24 h monitoring of heart patients. This system utilized the temporal features of ECG to classify three types of beats. The morphological and RR-interval based features of ECG were used in (Melgani *et al.*, 2008) to distinguish normal and five arrhythmia beats using particle swarm optimization. A higher order spectral features based classification scheme for

Table 1. Different arrhythmia beats classifier and features

Literature	Classifier	Features	Classes
Acir *et. al.*, 2005	Least-square SVM	Temporal + spectral	6
Melgani *et al.*, 2008	SVM	Temporal + morphological	6
Chua *et. al.*, 2009	SVM	Higher order spectral	5
Kutlu *et. al.*, 2012	Neural network	Higher order statistics	5
Martis *et. al.*, 2013	SVM	Spectral+PCA	5
Martis *et. al.*, 2013	Least-square SVM	Spectral+PCA	5
Mert *et. al*, 2014	Decision tree	Temporal	6
Khalaf *et. al.*, 2015	SVM	Spectral correlation	5
Thomas *et. al.*, 2015	Artificial neural network	DWT + morphological	5
Shadmand *et. al.*, 2016	Optimized block based neural network	Hermite coefficients + temporal	5
Li *et. al.*, 2017	Regression neural network	Morphological	5

five types of ECG beats was presented in (Martis *et al.*, 2013) using least-square support vector machine classifier. In this technique, PCA was used for dimensionality reduction of bi-spectrum features. In (Raj *et al.*, 2018), an arrhythmia beats classification method was proposed based on DCT based discrete orthogonal Stockwell transform (Jha *et al.*, 2018) based features. In this method, the dimension of the features was reduced using PCA. Classification methods based on temporal and morphological features cannot decipher subtle changes and hidden complexities of the ECG signal. Hence, multi-resolution wavelet transform based features are utilized in the classification scheme presented in this chapter. Utilizing these features, the multi-class support vector machine classifier efficiently distinguishes normal and five types of arrhythmia ECG beats.

MULTI-RESOLUTION WAVELET TRANSFORM

In the field of biomedical signal processing, many potential transforms such as Hilbert transform, Walsh transform, short-time Fourier transform, and wavelet transform are used. Since multi-resolution wavelet transform localizes the signal in time-frequency space properly (Pal *et al.*, 2010). Hence it is widely used in bio-medical signal denoising, classification and compression (Jha *et al.*, 2015; Motinath *et al.*, 2016; Jha *et al.*, 2016; Jha *et al.*, 2017). Discrete wavelet transform (DWT) is implemented using low-pass and high-pass filter banks. The low-pass and high-pass filters of DWT are obtained using a weighted sum of the dilated and shifted version of scaling function. As mentioned in (Sahoo *et al.*, 2017), the wavelet function of the wavelet transform is defined as:

$$\phi(t) = \frac{1}{\sqrt{a}}\phi\left(\frac{t-b}{a}\right) \tag{1}$$

where a, and b are dilation and translation parameters respectively. For DWT, discrete values of a and b are chosen as $a = 2^{-m}$ and $b = n.2^{-m}$, where m and n are integer values. Wavelet function for DWT is obtained by putting discrete values of a and b in Equation (1).

$$\phi_{m,n}(t) = 2^{-\frac{m}{2}}\phi(2^{-m}t - n) \tag{2}$$

Using $\phi_{m,n}(t)$, DWT of a discrete-time signal $x(t)$ can be expressed as:

$$X_{DWT} = \int_{-\infty}^{+\infty} x(t)\phi_{m,n}(t)dt \tag{3}$$

The obtained X_{DWT} values are known as DWT coefficients. For simplicity, DWT is implemented using high pass and low pass filter banks. The impulse response of high pass filter g and low pass filter h are related by:

$$g(L-n-1)=(-1)^{n}h(n) \tag{4}$$

where L denotes the length of the filter. Filtering and sub-sampling operation of DWT is expressed by:

$$y_{high}(k)=\sum_{n} x(n)g(-n+2k) \tag{5}$$

$$y_{low}(k)=\sum_{n} x(n)h(-n+2k) \tag{6}$$

Coefficients obtained by $y_{high}(k)$ and $y_{low}(k)$ are known as detail and approximate coefficients respectively. These coefficients are used for time-frequency representation of the discrete signal $x(n)$.

MULTICLASS SUPPORT VECTOR MACHINE

Multiclass support vector machine (MSVM) is used to solve *k*-class pattern recognition problems. In MSVM, a decision function is constructed by considering all classes at once. In binary classification using support vector machine, a hyperplane is constructed to separate the two classes labeled as $y \in \{-1,+1\}$. The distance between the hyperplane and the nearest point is chosen such that it is maximal. This generates the following optimization problem (Weston *et al.*, 1998): minimize

$$\phi(\omega,\xi)=\frac{1}{2}((\omega.x_{i})+b)\geq 1-\xi_{i},\ i=1,\ldots,1 \tag{7}$$

$$\xi_{i}\geq 0,\ \text{i=1,...,l}$$

There is a dual solution to this problem: quadratic form (8) should be maximizing under constraints (9) and (10).

$$W(\alpha)=\sum_{i=1}^{l}\alpha_{i}-\frac{1}{2}\sum_{i,j=1}^{l}y_{i}y_{j}\alpha_{i}\alpha_{j}K(x_{i},x_{j}) \tag{8}$$

with constraints,

$$0\leq\alpha_{i}\leq C,\ \text{i=1,2,...,l} \tag{9}$$

$$\sum_{i=1}^{l} \alpha_i y_i = 0 \tag{10}$$

It gives the decision function,

$$f(x) = sign\left[(\sum_{i=1}^{l} \alpha_i y_i K(x, x_i) + b \right] \tag{11}$$

where $K(x, x_i)$ is known as the kernel function. In MSVM, optimization problem (7) is generalized as:
minimize

$$\phi(\omega, \xi) = \frac{1}{2} \sum_{i=1}^{m} \left(\omega_m . \omega_m \right) + C \sum_{i=1}^{l} \sum_{m \neq y_i} \xi_i^m \tag{12}$$

with constraints,

$$(\omega_{y_i} . x_i) + \mathrm{b}_{y_i} \geq (\omega_m . x_i) + b_m + 2 - \xi_i^m$$

$$\xi_i^m \geq 0, \ \mathrm{i=1,2,..,l} \quad \mathrm{m} \in \left\{ 1, 2, \ldots, k \right\} \setminus y_i$$

It gives the decision function:

$$f(x) = \arg \ \max_k \left[(\omega_i . x) + b_i \right], \ i = 1, 2, \ldots, k \tag{13}$$

This decision function is further optimized. In MSVM, different Kernel functions such as linear, sigmoid, Gaussian radial basis function (RBF) are utilized. In this chapter, RBF is utilized in the kernel of MSVM to classify different arrhythmia ECG beats. The Gaussian RBF is expressed as (Franc *et al.*, 2002)

$$k(x, x_i) = e^{-\frac{\left\| (x - x_i) \right\|^2}{2\sigma}} \tag{14}$$

where, x and x_i are feature vectors and σ is the variance.

METHODOLOGY

The methodology of the proposed arrhythmia ECG beats classification scheme is shown in Figure 1 using block diagram. The proposed scheme involves the following steps: pre-processing, R-peak detection, beat segmentation, wavelet multi-resolution analysis (WMRA) based features extraction, and classification

Figure 1. Block diagram of the proposed classification scheme

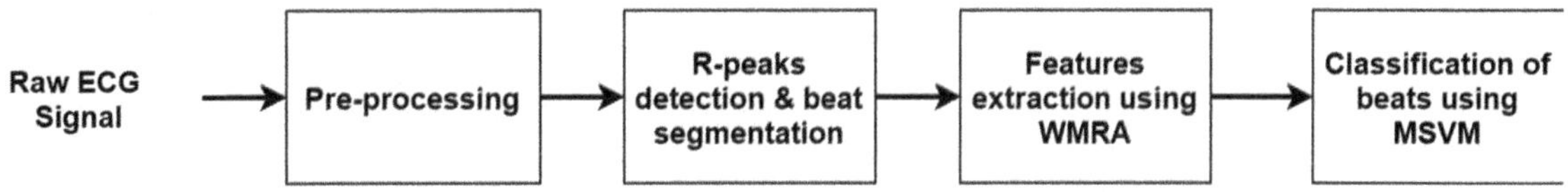

using MSVM. First, the raw ECG signals are acquired from the MIT-BIH arrhythmia database (Moody *et al.*, 2001). These signals consist many ECG beats including normal (N) and different arrhythmia such as left bundle branch block (LBBB), right bundle branch block (RBBB), atrial premature contraction (A), premature ventricular contraction (V) and paced (P).

Pre-Processing

The raw ECG signal obtained from the MIT-BIH arrhythmia database is pre-processed using different filtering techniques to remove high-frequency noises such as muscle noise, electrode movement, and power line interference. Savitzky-Golay filtering of polynomial order 5 and window length 21 is used for high-frequency noise removal. A third-order high-pass Butterworth filter is used to eliminate baseline noise. Waveforms of ECG signals during pre-processing of record no. 108 and 118 of the MIT–BIH arrhythmia database are shown in Figure 2 and Figure 3.

R-Peaks Detection and Beat Segmentation

For segmentation of beats, detection of R-peaks is necessary. A standard Pan –Tompkins algorithm (Pan *et al.*, 1985) is utilized to detect R-peaks. Steps of the Pan-Tomkins algorithm used for R-peaks detection

Figure 2. Pre-processing of ECG record no. 108 of the MIT-BIH arrhythmia database

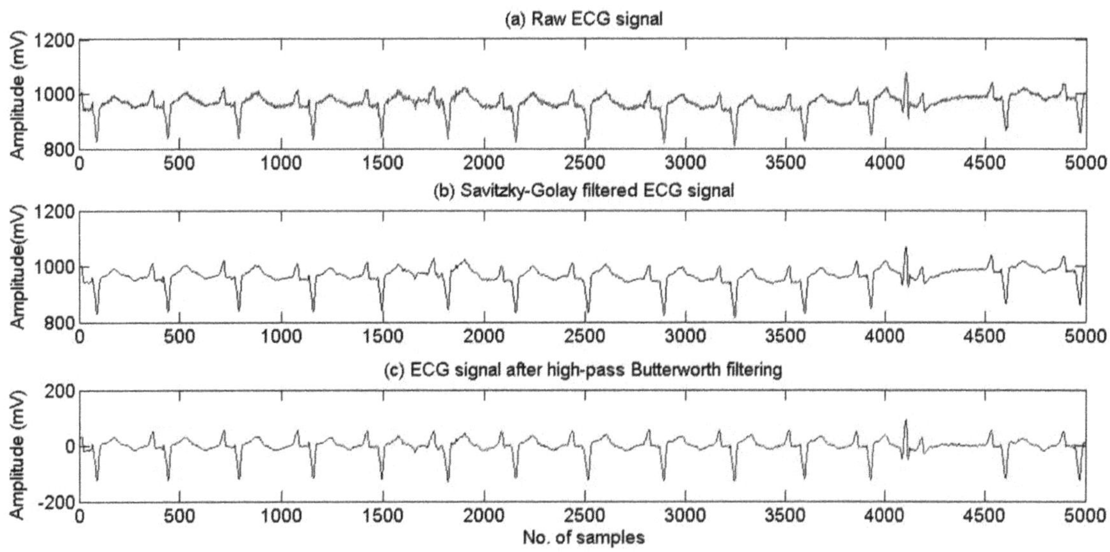

Figure 3. Pre-processing of ECG record no. 118 of the MIT-BIH arrhythmia database

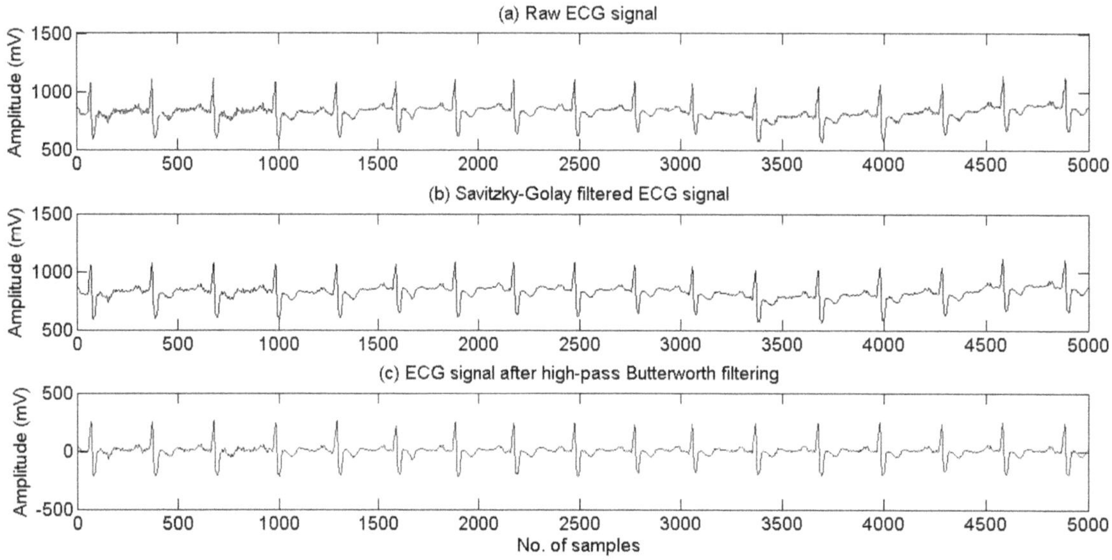

Figure 4. R-peaks detection in ECG signal

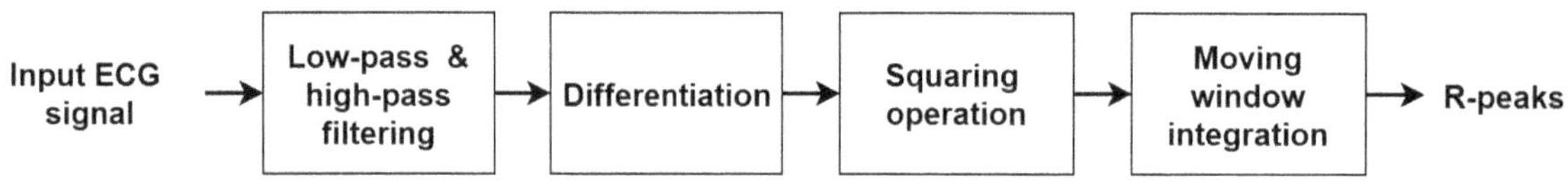

are summarized in Figure 4 using block diagram. First, second-order low-pass filtering is performed on the input ECG signal. The transfer function of the filter is:

$$H(z) = \frac{(1 - z^{-6})^2}{(1 - z^{-1})^2} \tag{15}$$

The low-pass filtered ECG signal is passed through a high-pass filter with transfer function:

$$H(z) = \frac{(-1 + 32z^{-16} + z^{-32})}{(1 + z^{-1})} \tag{16}$$

After filtering, the QRS-complex slope information is achieved using derivative operation. For this, the signal is differentiated using five-point derivative with the transfer function:

$$H(z) = \frac{(-z^{-2} + -2z^{-1} + 2z + z^2)}{8T} \tag{17}$$

where, the sampling period of the signal is T. After differentiation, point by point squaring operation of the signal is carried out. This operation is represented by the equation:

$$y(nT) = [x(nT)]^2 \tag{18}$$

where the input ECG signal is $x(nT)$. The slope of the R-wave with the information of waveform feature is obtained by moving window integration. It is calculated by:

$$y(nT) = \frac{\left[x(nT-(N-1)T) + x(nT-(N-2)T) + \ldots + x(nT)\right]}{N} \tag{19}$$

where, N is the number of samples in the integration window. After moving-window integration, a threshold operation is applied which provides information of R-peaks in the signal. After R-peaks detection, segmentation of ECG beats is performed by selection of 103 samples before the R-peak and 153 samples after the R-peak. Figure 5 depicts the R-peak detection and beat-segmentation of ECG record no. 121 of the MIT-BIH arrhythmia database.

Features Extraction Using WMRA

After beat segmentation, features of each ECG beat are extracted using WMRA. Feature extraction and selection process are elaborated in Figure 6. In WMRA, each ECG beat is decomposed up to 4th level using "bior6.8" mother wavelet. In Figure 6, approximate coefficients are shown by A_1, A_2, A_3, and A_4

Figure 5. R-peaks detection and beat segmentation in the record no. 121 of the MIT-BIH arrhythmia database

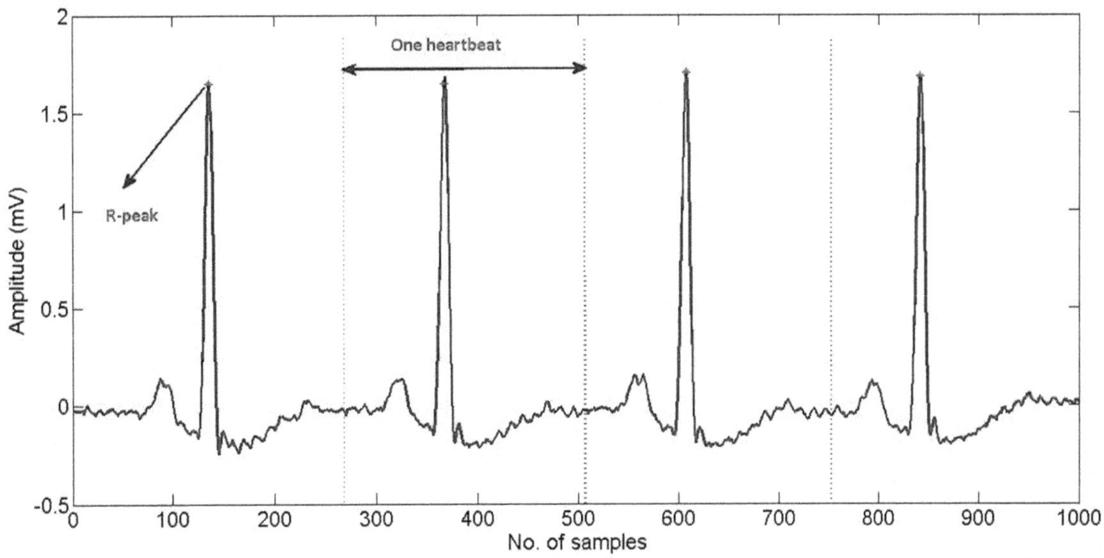

Figure 6. Features extraction and selection process

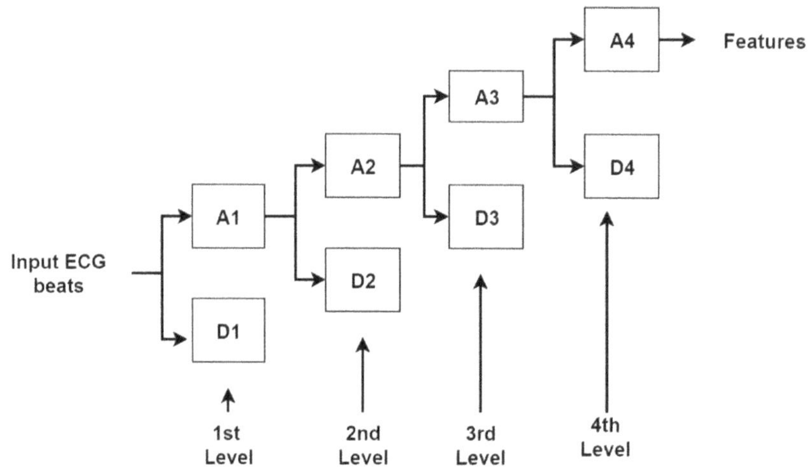

while detail coefficients are shown by D_1, D_2, D_3, and D_4. At each decomposition level, the approximate and detail coefficients are decimated by 2. Approximate coefficients A_4 obtained at the 4th level of decomposition are selected as features for classification of each ECG beat.

Classification Using MSVM

Features of ECG beats are further utilized for classification. Total 5320 beats are obtained from different ECG records of the MIT-BIH arrhythmia database. These records are: 100, 101, 103, 105, 107, 108, 111, 112, 113, 114, 115, 117, 118, 121, 122, 123, 124, 202, 205, 207, 210,219, 230 and 231. The selected beats are of six different types: normal (N), left bundle branch block (LBBB), right bundle branch block (RBBB), atrial premature contraction (A), premature ventricular contraction (V) and paced (P). Number of these beats are 3210, 730, 100, 210, 380 and 380 respectively. Number of training and testing beats used for proposed classification technique is detailed in Table 2. WMRA features of 2660 beats are utilized to train the MSVM classifier. The classifier is tested with features of 2660 beats. In MSVM classifier, "one against all" is used for testing of each class of beats.

Table 2. Distribution of different types of training and testing beats

Types	Number of training beats	Number of testing beats
Normal	1605	1605
Left bundled block	365	365
Right bundled block	345	345
Premature ventricular contraction	90	90
Paced	105	105
Atrial premature contraction	50	50
Total	2660	2660

Performance of the MSVM classifier is evaluated using the following performance metrics (Jha, *et al., 2018):* accuracy, sensitivity, and specificity.

Accuracy is defined as the total number of true events detected by the classifier.

$$Accuracy = \frac{TP + TN}{P + N} \times 100\% \tag{20}$$

Sensitivity is also called the true positive rate. It is defined as the ability of the classifier to detect the true positive events.

$$Sensitivity = \frac{TP}{TP + FN} \times 100\% \tag{21}$$

Specificity is also called the true negative rate. It is defined as the ability of the classifier to detect the true negative events.

$$Specificity = \frac{TN}{TN + FP} \times 100\% \tag{22}$$

where, P, N, TP, TN, FP and FN indicates total positive, total negative, true positive, true negative, false positive and false negative events respectively.

RESULTS AND DISCUSSION

After classification, the performance of the classifier for each class is determined. Table 1 depicts the performance in terms of accuracy, sensitivity, and specificity. Overall accuracy, sensitivity, and specificity of six types of beats are 99.42%, 94.63%, and 99.85% respectively. Table 4 shows the comparison of the performance of the proposed classification scheme with the existing arrhythmia beats classifiers published recently. Classifiers used for comparison are based on deterministic learning, regression neu-

Table 3. Performance of the MSVM classifier

Beat Types	Accuracy (%)	Sensitivity (%)	Specificity (%)
Normal	99.06	98.94	99.24
Left bundled block	99.17	94.52	99.91
Right bundled block	99.02	92.75	99.96
Atrial premature contraction	99.85	92.00	100.0
Premature ventricular contraction	99.66	95.26	100.0
Paced	99.74	94.29	99.96
Overall	99.42	94.63	99.85

Table 4. Performance of the proposed classifier

Literature	Classifier	Features	Classes	Accuracy (%)
Dong *et al.*, 2017	Deterministic learning	Temporal	5	97.78
Li *et. al.*, 2017	Regression neural network	Morphological	5	99.40
Lin *et. al.*, 2014	Linear discriminant analysis	Morphological	6	94.03
Zhu *et. al.*, 2014	SVM, Neural network	Morphological	3	92.85
Zadeh *et. al.*, 2012	SVM, Neural network	Morphological	3	97.14
Acir *et. al.*, 2005	SVM	Temporal and spectral	6	95.20
Proposed	SVM	WMRA	6	99.42

ral network, linear discriminant analysis, SVM, and neural network. All these classifiers use temporal, morphological and/ or spectral features. After the performance comparison of the proposed classifier, it is found that the proposed classifier offers better accuracy than others.

CONCLUSION

This chapter presents arrhythmia beats classification technique to distinguish normal (N) beats and five different arrhythmia beats: left bundle branch block (LBBB), right bundle branch block (RBBB), atrial premature contraction (A), premature ventricular contraction (V), and paced (P). The classification technique utilizes WMRA based features of ECG beats and MSVM classifier. Features of 2660 ECG beats are used to train the classifier while for testing features of 2660 beats are utilized. Average accuracy, sensitivity, and specificity offered by the proposed classifier are 99.42%, 94.63%, and 99.85% respectively. The proposed classification technique outperforms many recently published arrhythmia beats classifier. Performance of The presented classification scheme can be used in computer-aided diagnostic tools for the assistance of cardiologists.

ACKNOWLEDGMENT

This publication was an outcome of the R&D work undertaken a project under the Visvesvaraya Ph.D. Scheme of Ministry of Electronics & Information Technology, Government of India, being implemented by Digital India Corporation.

REFERENCES

Acır, N. (2005). Classification of ECG beats by using a fast least square support vector machines with a dynamic programming feature selection algorithm. *Neural Computing & Applications*, *14*(4), 299–309. doi:10.100700521-005-0466-z

Chua, C. K., Chandran, V., Acharya, R. U., & Min, L. C. (2009). Cardiac health diagnosis using higher order spectra and support vector machine. *The Open Medical Informatics Journal*, *3*(1), 1–8. doi:10.2174/1874431100903010001 PMID:19603098

Coast, D. A., Stern, R. M., Cano, G. G., & Briller, S. A. (1990). An approach to cardiac arrhythmia analysis using hidden Markov models. *IEEE Transactions on Biomedical Engineering*, *37*(9), 826–836. doi:10.1109/10.58593 PMID:2227969

Dash, D. P., & Kolekar, M. H. (2017, September). Epileptic seizure detection based on EEG signal analysis using hierarchy based Hidden Markov Model. In *International Conference on Advances in Computing, Communications and Informatics (ICACCI)*, (pp. 1114-1120). IEEE. 10.1109/ICACCI.2017.8125991

de Chazal, P., & Reilly, R. B. (2006). A patient-adapting heartbeat classifier using ECG morphology and heartbeat interval features. *IEEE Transactions on Biomedical Engineering*, *53*(12), 2535–2543. doi:10.1109/TBME.2006.883802 PMID:17153211

de Oliveira, L. S., Andreão, R. V., & Sarcinelli-Filho, M. (2011, August). Premature ventricular beat classification using a dynamic Bayesian network. In *Annual International Conference of Engineering in Medicine and Biology Society, EMBC*, (pp. 4984-4987). IEEE. 10.1109/IEMBS.2011.6091235

Dong, X., Wang, C., & Si, W. (2017). ECG beat classification via deterministic learning. *Neurocomputing*, *240*, 1–12. doi:10.1016/j.neucom.2017.02.056

Fancott, T., & Wong, D. H. (1980). A minicomputer system for direct high speed analysis of cardiac arrhythmia in 24 h ambulatory ECG tape recordings. *IEEE Transactions on Biomedical Engineering*, *BME-27*(12), 685–693. doi:10.1109/TBME.1980.326593 PMID:7461643

Franc, V., & Hlavác, V. (2002). Multi-class support vector machine. In *International Conference on Pattern Recognition* (Vol. 2, pp. 236-239). IEEE. 10.1109/ICPR.2002.1048282

Ge, D., Srinivasan, N., & Krishnan, S. M. (2002). Cardiac arrhythmia classification using autoregressive modeling. *Biomedical Engineering Online*, *1*(1), 5. doi:10.1186/1475-925X-1-5 PMID:12473180

Gutiérrez-Gnecchi, J. A., Morfin-Magana, R., Lorias-Espinoza, D., del Carmen Tellez-Anguiano, A., Reyes-Archundia, E., Méndez-Patiño, A., & Castañeda-Miranda, R. (2017). DSP-based arrhythmia classification using wavelet transform and probabilistic neural network. *Biomedical Signal Processing and Control*, *32*, 44–56. doi:10.1016/j.bspc.2016.10.005

Hadhoud, M. M., Eladawy, M. I., & Farag, A. (2006, November). Computer aided diagnosis of cardiac arrhythmias. In *International Conference on Computer Engineering and Systems*, (pp. 262-265). IEEE.

Huikuri, H. V., Castellanos, A., & Myerburg, R. J. (2001). Sudden death due to cardiac arrhythmias. *The New England Journal of Medicine*, *345*(20), 1473–1482. doi:10.1056/NEJMra000650 PMID:11794197

Jha, C. K., & Kolekar, M. H. (2015, December). Performance analysis of ECG data compression using wavelet based hybrid transform method. In *International Conference on Microwave, Optical and Communication Engineering (ICMOCE)* (pp. 138-141). IEEE. 10.1109/ICMOCE.2015.7489709

Jha, C. K., & Kolekar, M. H. (2016, January). Efficient ECG data compression and transmission algorithm for telemedicine. In *International Conference on Communication Systems and Networks (COMSNETS)* (pp. 1-6). IEEE. 10.1109/COMSNETS.2016.7439988

Jha, C. K., & Kolekar, M. H. (2017). ECG data compression algorithm for tele-monitoring of cardiac patients. *International Journal of Telemedicine and Clinical Practices*, *2*(1), 31–41. doi:10.1504/IJTMCP.2017.082106

Jha, C. K., & Kolekar, M. H. (2018). Electrocardiogram data compression using DCT based discrete orthogonal Stockwell transform. *Biomedical Signal Processing and Control*, *46*, 174–181. doi:10.1016/j.bspc.2018.06.009

Jha, C. K., & Kolekar, M. H. (2018). Classification and Compression of ECG Signal for Holter Device. In *Biomedical Signal and Image Processing in Patient Care* (pp. 46–63). IGI Global. doi:10.4018/978-1-5225-2829-6.ch004

Khalaf, A. F., Owis, M. I., & Yassine, I. A. (2015). A novel technique for cardiac arrhythmia classification using spectral correlation and support vector machines. *Expert Systems with Applications*, *42*(21), 8361–8368. doi:10.1016/j.eswa.2015.06.046

Kolekar, M. H. (2011). Bayesian belief network based broadcast sports video indexing. *Multimedia Tools and Applications*, *54*(1), 27–54. doi:10.100711042-010-0544-9

Kolekar, M. H., & Dash, D. P. (2015). A nonlinear feature based epileptic seizure detection using least square support vector machine classifier. In IEEE Region 10 Conference TENCON (pp. 1-6). IEEE.

Kolekar, M. H., & Sengupta, S. (2015). Bayesian network-based customized highlight generation for broadcast soccer videos. *IEEE Transactions on Broadcasting*, *61*(2), 195–209. doi:10.1109/TBC.2015.2424011

Kutlu, Y., & Kuntalp, D. (2012). Feature extraction for ECG heartbeats using higher order statistics of WPD coefficients. *Computer Methods and Programs in Biomedicine*, *105*(3), 257–267. doi:10.1016/j.cmpb.2011.10.002 PMID:22055998

Li, P., Wang, Y., He, J., Wang, L., Tian, Y., Zhou, T. S., ... Li, J. S. (2017). High-performance personalized heartbeat classification model for long-term ECG signal. *IEEE Transactions on Biomedical Engineering*, *64*(1), 78–86. doi:10.1109/10.650355 PMID:27046844

Liang, W., Zhang, Y., Tan, J., & Li, Y. (2014). A novel approach to ECG classification based upon two-layered HMMs in body sensor networks. *Sensors (Basel)*, *14*(4), 5994–6011. doi:10.3390140405994 PMID:24681668

Lin, L. C., Yeh, Y. C., & Chu, T. Y. (2014). Feature Selection Algorithm for ECG Signals and Its Application on Heartbeat Case Determining. *International Journal of Fuzzy Systems*, *16*(4).

Linh, T. H., Osowski, S., & Stodolski, M. (2003). On-line heart beat recognition using Hermite polynomials and neuro-fuzzy network. *IEEE Transactions on Instrumentation and Measurement*, *52*(4), 1224–1231. doi:10.1109/TIM.2003.816841

Mar, T., Zaunseder, S., Martínez, J. P., Llamedo, M., & Poll, R. (2011). Optimization of ECG classification by means of feature selection. *IEEE Transactions on Biomedical Engineering*, *58*(8), 2168–2177. doi:10.1109/TBME.2011.2113395 PMID:21317067

Martis, R. J., Acharya, U. R., Mandana, K. M., Ray, A. K., & Chakraborty, C. (2013). Cardiac decision making using higher order spectra. *Biomedical Signal Processing and Control*, *8*(2), 193–203. doi:10.1016/j.bspc.2012.08.004

Martis, R. J., Acharya, U. R., & Min, L. C. (2013). ECG beat classification using PCA, LDA, ICA and discrete wavelet transform. *Biomedical Signal Processing and Control*, *8*(5), 437–448. doi:10.1016/j.bspc.2013.01.005

Martis, R. J., Chakraborty, C., & Ray, A. K. (2009). A two-stage mechanism for registration and classification of ECG using Gaussian mixture model. *Pattern Recognition*, *42*(11), 2979–2988. doi:10.1016/j.patcog.2009.02.008

Martis, R. J., Krishnan, M. M. R., Chakraborty, C., Pal, S., Sarkar, D., Mandana, K. M., & Ray, A. K. (2012). Automated screening of arrhythmia using wavelet based machine learning techniques. *Journal of Medical Systems*, *36*(2), 677–688. doi:10.100710916-010-9535-7 PMID:20703662

Melgani, F., & Bazi, Y. (2008). Classification of electrocardiogram signals with support vector machines and particle swarm optimization. *IEEE Transactions on Information Technology in Biomedicine*, *12*(5), 667–677. doi:10.1109/TITB.2008.923147 PMID:18779082

Mert, A., Kılıç, N., & Akan, A. (2014). Evaluation of bagging ensemble method with time-domain feature extraction for diagnosing of arrhythmia beats. *Neural Computing & Applications*, *24*(2), 317–326. doi:10.100700521-012-1232-7

Moody, G. B., & Mark, R. G. (2001). The impact of the MIT-BIH arrhythmia database. *IEEE Engineering in Medicine and Biology Magazine*, *20*(3), 45–50. doi:10.1109/51.932724 PMID:11446209

Motinath, V. A., Jha, C. K., & Kolekar, M. H. (2016). A novel ECG data compression algorithm using best mother wavelet selection. In *International Conference on Advances in Computing, Communications and Informatics (ICACCI)* (pp. 682-686). IEEE. 10.1109/ICACCI.2016.7732125

Pal, S., & Mitra, M. (2010). Detection of ECG characteristic points using multiresolution wavelet analysis based selective coefficient method. *Measurement*, *43*(2), 255–261. doi:10.1016/j.measurement.2009.10.004

Pan, J., & Tompkins, W. J. (1985). A real-time QRS detection algorithm. *IEEE Transactions on Biomedical Engineering*, *32*(3), 230–236. doi:10.1109/TBME.1985.325532 PMID:3997178

Raj, S., & Ray, K. C. (2017). ECG signal analysis using DCT-based DOST and PSO optimized SVM. *IEEE Transactions on Instrumentation and Measurement*, *66*(3), 470–478. doi:10.1109/TIM.2016.2642758

Sahoo, S., Kanungo, B., Behera, S., & Sabut, S. (2017). Multiresolution wavelet transform based feature extraction and ECG classification to detect cardiac abnormalities. *Measurement*, *108*, 55–66. doi:10.1016/j.measurement.2017.05.022

Shadmand, S., & Mashoufi, B. (2016). A new personalized ECG signal classification algorithm using block-based neural network and particle swarm optimization. *Biomedical Signal Processing and Control*, *25*, 12–23. doi:10.1016/j.bspc.2015.10.008

Thomas, M., Das, M. K., & Ari, S. (2015). Automatic ECG arrhythmia classification using dual tree complex wavelet based features. *AEÜ. International Journal of Electronics and Communications*, *69*(4), 715–721. doi:10.1016/j.aeue.2014.12.013

Übeyli, E. D. (2007). ECG beats classification using multiclass support vector machines with error correcting output codes. *Digital Signal Processing*, *17*(3), 675–684. doi:10.1016/j.dsp.2006.11.009

Weston, J., & Watkins, C. (1998). *Multi-class support vector machines*. Technical Report CSD-TR-98-04, Department of Computer Science, Royal Holloway, University of London.

Yeh, Y. C., Wang, W. J., & Chiou, C. W. (2009). Cardiac arrhythmia diagnosis method using linear discriminant analysis on ECG signals. *Measurement*, *42*(5), 778–789. doi:10.1016/j.measurement.2009.01.004

Zadeh, A. E., Khazaee, A., & Ranaee, V. (2010). Classification of the electrocardiogram signals using supervised classifiers and efficient features. *Computer Methods and Programs in Biomedicine, 99*(2), 179-194.

Zhu, J., He, L., & Gao, Z. (2014). Feature extraction from a novel ECG model for arrhythmia diagnosis. *Bio-Medical Materials and Engineering*, *24*(6), 2883–2891. PMID:25226994

Chapter 5
Melanoma Image Classification Based on Multivariate Parametric Statistical Tests of Hypothesis

K. Seetharaman
Annamalai University, India

ABSTRACT

This chapter proposes a novel method, based on the multivariate parametric statistical tests of hypotheses, which classifies the normal skin lesion images and the various stages of the melanoma images. The melanoma images are categorized into two classes, such as initial stage and advanced stage, based on the degree of aggressiveness of the cancer. The region of interest is identified and segmented from the input skin melanoma image. The features, such as HSV color, shape, and texture, are extracted from the region of interest. The features are treated as a feature space, which is assumed to be a multivariate normal random field. The proposed statistical tests are employed to identify and classify the melanoma images. The proposed method yields an average correct classification up to 91.55% for the normal skin lesion versus the initial and the advanced stages of the melanoma images, up to 91.39% for initial stage melanoma versus the normal skin lesion and the advanced stages melanoma, and up to 92.27% for the advanced stage melanoma versus the normal skin lesion and the initial stage melanoma. The proposed method yields better results.

INTRODUCTION

The advances in computer vision system have exponentially increased the applications of image processing methods in many fields. Particularly, the medical imaging system, such as ultrasonography, computed tomography (CT), magnetic resonance (MR) imaging system, cancer analysis and classification, and nuclear medicine, those are used to assist doctors in diagnosis, treatment, and research. Nowadays, many corporate-based healthcare organizations use Robotics for complicated surgery with the assist of

DOI: 10.4018/978-1-5225-7796-6.ch005

a specialized surgeon in the respective domain. In order to make the computerized analysis of medical image processing systems as an effective and efficient tool, a proper image classification method is required. The classification refers to assigning a physical object or incident into one of a set of predefined categories. The classification plays a noteworthy role in disease classification, like cancer identification, segmentation and classification, brain disease classification, CT liver image classification, X-ray image segmentation, gene classification, etc. The medical image classification is more sensitive, because they could vary with a minute feature or signature. This chapter concentrates on melanoma image classification, based on a multivariate parametric statistical methods. It is observed from the literature that the existing methods identify or classify whether a skin image is melanoma or not. Though, clinically the melanoma has been categorized into four groups, based on the degree of aggressiveness of the cancerous, the existing methods classify only two groups, that is, whether the skin image is melanoma or not. This motivated to develop this chapter to classify a three different category of melanoma images, namely (i) normal dermoscopic images; (ii) initial stage melanoma; (iii) advanced stage melanoma. The proposed classification method is developed based on the statistical tests of hypothesis, such as the test for equality of covariance and the test for equality of mean vector. The test for equality of covariance compares the covariance of two groups, whereas the test for equality of mean vector compares the mean vectors of the two groups.

BACKGROUND

Despite there are a number of methods available for medical image classification, some methods require high computational complexity for feature extraction and classification (Li & Shen, 2018; Lee et al., 2018; Ma et al., 2017), for instance the method which comprises of deep learning, deep convolutional learning while some other methods follow a lot of procedures for feature extraction (Lee et al., 2018; Ma et al., 2017; Silveria et al., 2009). The medical image classification comprises of image acquisition, preprocessing, feature extraction, classification, and performance evaluation. The pre-processing is a course of actions that is executed on raw image data, in order to achieve a best recital of a data set. It has a significant impact on the performance of the classification algorithm. Data pre-processing phase, in medical image processing, comprises of image cropping, filtering, segmentation, gradient operations and scaling. Feature extraction engages feature estimation and feature selection methods. A considerable number of texture feature extraction methods available in the literature, such as Gabor, Haralick's, and wavelet histogram, and so on; each of them describes some aspects of image contents. Therefore, feature extraction is a process of analyzing objects and images, which extracts the most prominent features that corresponds to various classes of objects. Therefore, it is worth to state that improving the feature extraction process will improve the performance of a described classification algorithm.

The X-ray medical images play a noteworthy role in clinical diagnosis of the diseases. It has turned the attention of the computer vision community to the medical image analysis such as classification, segmentation, compression, and retrieval. Pourghassem and Ghassemian (2008) have proposed a hierarchical medical image classification, based on a perfect set of various shape and texture features; and a tessellation-based spectral feature as well as a directional histogram has been proposed. They have adopted a merging scheme, which applies three measures -- *accuracy*, *miss-classified ratio*, and *dissimilarity* – to detect the overlapping classes. The accuracy and miss-classified ratio realizes a supervised classification technique, and the last one realizes an unsupervised clustering technique. This method is evaluated with a database, which consists of 9100 medical X-ray images of 40 classes. It provides accuracy rate of 90.83% on 25 merged classes in the first level. If the correct class is considered within the best three matches, this value will increase to 97.9%. In the past two decades, due to its precision, computed tomography (CT) is used to image the liver and diagnose its diseases. The computer-assisted methods facilitate the extraction of organ shapes from medical images, and helps to diagnose disease entities. Chen et al. (1998) have proposed an automatic diagnostic system for CT-liver image classification, based on a modified probabilistic neural network (PNN) [MPNN] classifier which includes the Kohonen self-organizing algorithm to reduce the number of training patterns, and normalized fractional Brownian (NFB) feature bitmap. They have adopted a texture feature-based classification system to discriminate two types of liver tumors, *hepotoma* and *hemageoma*. Gletsos et al. (2003) proposed a method, based on feed-forward neural networks (NN), which identifies regions of interest (ROI)from non-enhanced CT images of normal liver, hepatic cysts, hemangiomas, and hepatocellular carcinomas. The features are extracted from the spatial gray-level co-occurrence matrices obtained from the ROIs. The NN method classifies the images in three stages: (i) classifies into normal or pathological liver regions; (ii) characterizes the pathological liver regions as *cyst* or *other disease*; (iii) classifies other disease into hemangioma or hepatocellular carcinoma. They have adopted three feature selection techniques to each individual NN: (i) sequential forward selection; (ii) sequential floating forward selection; (iii) a genetic algorithm for feature selection. They have reported that the genetic algorithm results in lower dimensional feature vectors and improved classification performance. Rajendran and Madheswaran (2010) proposed a method based on image mining with association rule and hybrid classifier for classification of brain tumor in the CT scan brain images. Tsai et al. (2004) have proposed a system with *fuzzy logic* for classification of ECG images, based on the triangle and trapezoid, and Gaussian-distributed membership functions (GDMF). It discriminates myocardial heart disease from echocardiographic images; detects and classify clustered micro-calcifications from mammograms. The shapes of the GDMF are optimized using the Genetic-algorithm. Castro et al. (2016) proposed a method, which classifies the density of the enlarged Perivascular spaces (PVS) in the basal ganglia (BG), based on texture description of structural brain MRI. The texture of the BG region is described by means of first order statistics, such as mean, median, standard deviation, minimum and maximum, quartile deviation, and the features derived from the co-occurrence matrix, both types of features computed from the original image and the coefficients yielded by the discrete wavelet transform and local binary patterns. Rasku et al. (2007) have investigated whether hidden Markov models can be used to recognize and classify balance signals extracted from two subject groups, the healthy and patients suffering from otoneurological vertiginous diseases; they have reported that these models with 7–15 states were able to recognize the healthy subjects from the patients with the accuracy between 70% and 90% although their balance measurements were visually very similar and difficult to separate two groups.

The literature reveals that the texture component plays a significant role in medical image analyses, such as classification, segmentation, compression, edge detection, and the retrieval, because most of the medical images are constituted with the texture properties; and the texture properties establish a spatial relationship among the pixels. This chapter concerns with the melanoma versus non-melanoma (normal) image classification; and the melanoma images are categorized into initial stage melanoma and advanced stage melanoma.

Causes of Skin Cancer and Its Risks

Normally, the skin cells develop in a controlled and proper way, that is, the healthy and fresh cells move the older cells towards the skin's surface, where they die and eventually fall off. But, when some cells damage the DNA, the fresh cells may begin to grow out of the control and can eventually form a mass of cancerous cells.

The ultraviolet (UV) ray is one of the factors that causes the melanoma. Sunlight is a main source of UV rays. The Tanning beds and sun lamps are other sources of the UV rays. The skin cancer develops to grow itself, while the UV rays affect the DNA of genes that control skin cell growth. If a close relative, such as parent, child or sibling, have had melanoma, then there is a greater possibility of developing melanoma..

The risk of melanoma seems to be increasing with the people under the age of 40, especially for the women (Fritz, 2013; Castroa, 2016). Observing the warning signs of skin cancer could help to ensure the cancerous changes that are detected and treated before the cancer has spread to other parts of the body. The melanoma skin cancer can be cured successfully, if it is detected in the early stage.

Types of Skin Cancer

The skin cancer begins in the cells that make up the outer layer (epidermis) of your skin. One type of skin cancer called *basal cell carcinoma* begins in the basal cells, which make skin cells that continuously push older cells toward the skin surface. As new cells move upward, they become flattened squamous cells, where a skin cancer called *squamous cell carcinoma* can occur. The *Melanoma*, another type of skin cancer, which arises in the pigment cells known as melanocytes.

MAIN FOCUS OF THE CHAPTER

Clinically, melanoma has been categorized as four stages, based on the prognostics of the experts in the concerned domain (dermatology and cancer) about the anatomic structure of the melanoma. The melanoma is characterized, based on their attributes such as *tumour* (T), *node* (N), and *metastasis* (M). The problem of melanoma image classification is still a challenging problem, because identification of the melanoma and feature extraction are too difficult. The TNM staging method could facilitate the researchers for effective classification or identification of the melanoma images, provided the four stages of the melanoma images and the normal skin lesion image of a person, who has been affected by the melanoma, are available. But, in practice, it is too difficult to get the normal skin lesion and four stages of the melanoma images of a person (Winston W Tan, 2018). Therefore, this chapter takes account of the features, such as color, shape, and texture, for melanoma classification. In this chapter, the melanoma images are categorized into two groups: (i) initial stage and (ii) advanced stage; the stage-2, stage-3, and stage-4 are grouped and coined as advanced stage; and the normal skin lesion image as an another group. This chapter takes account of the statistical methods, such as test for equality of covariances, and the test for equality of mean vectors, for effective identification of the melanoma and classification of the dermoscopic images into three classes. An overview of the proposed method is illustrated in Figure 1.

Figure 1. Overview of the proposed method

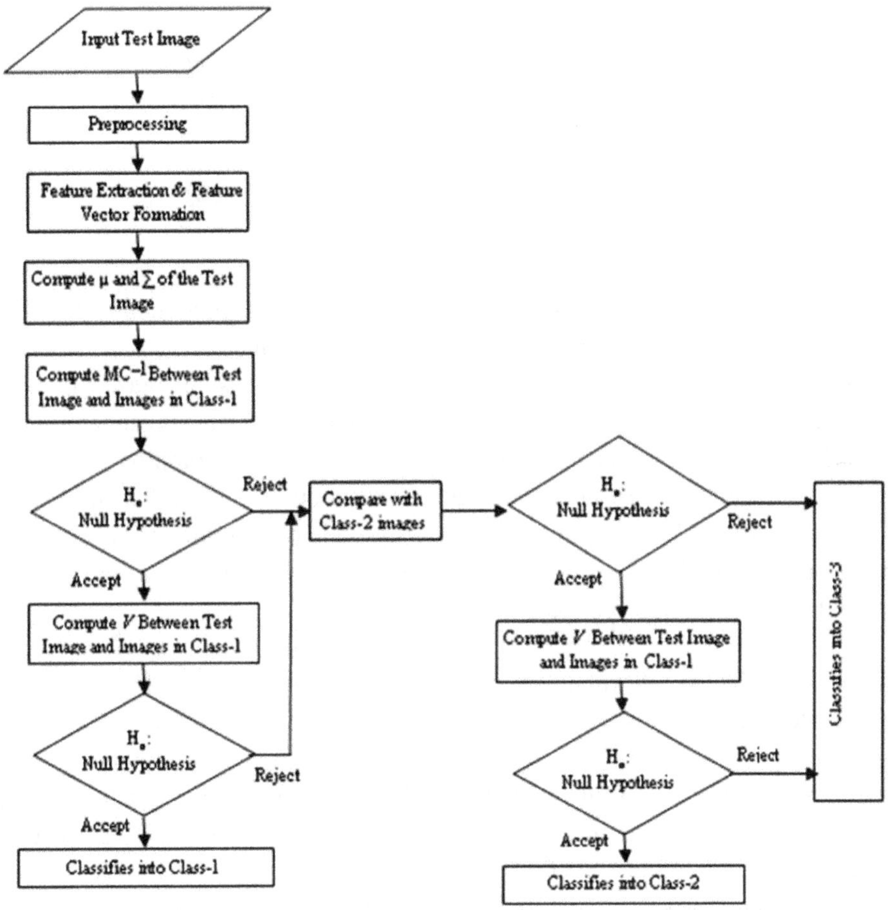

CHARACTERISTICS OF MELANOMA

This chapter takes account of the nature and structure or layout of the melanoma skin cancer, that is, the color (C) features, shape (Asymmetry, Border, Diameter) feature, Evolution (E), and texture orientation features. Generally, the terminology of ABCDE characteristics used in the context of melanoma skin cancer.

- **Color:** Usually, the color of a normal lesion is uniform with a single color. If there is a change in the single color, that is, the single color changes to different colors, like shades of brown, tan or black, red, white, and blue, it means the beginning stage of the melanoma. For a sample, the normal and the melanoma images have been presented in Figures 2 and 3.
- **Shape:** On the malignant stage, the shape of the mole or lesion changes to contour shape from round; symmetry to asymmetry; border may change from smooth round to rough contour; diameter could vary. For a sample, the normal mole and the evolution of the melanoma skin cancer is shown in Figure 2. The changes of the shape can be characterized as follows.
    - **Asymmetry:** The shape of one half does not match the other half.

Figure 2. Stages of evolution of cancer images

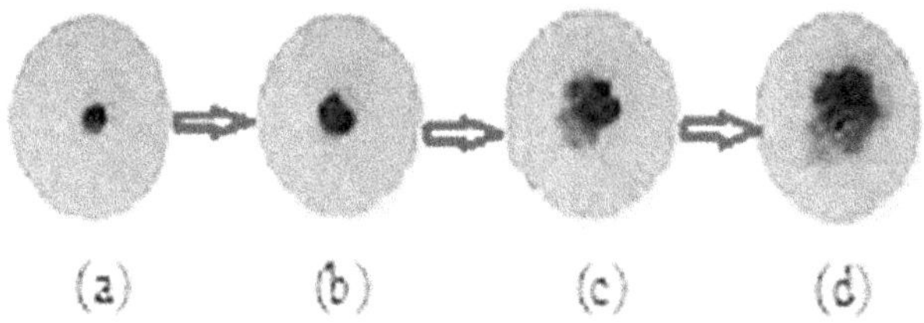

- ◦ **Border:** There exist irregular border; the edges are often ragged, notched, or blurred in outline. The pigment may spread into the neighboring regions.
- ◦ **Diameter:** The size of the malignant has changed, that is, increased than the previous. Melanomas can be tiny, but most of them are larger than 6 millimeters or about 1/4 inch.
- ◦ **Evolution:** The mole has changed over the past few weeks or months.
- **Texture:** The surface of the lesion may change from smooth to rough, that is, the skin on the surface may break down and look scraped. It may become hard or lumpy. The surface may ooze or bleed. Sometimes the melanoma is itchy, tender, or painful. The surface of the melanoma could be characterized in terms of texture properties.

The image in Figure 2(a) is a normal lesion with round shape and a single color; image in Figure 2(b) begins to change of color and shape; image in Figure 2(c) uneven borders; image in Figure 2(d) is in asymmetrical shape.

It is observed from Figure 3 that the attributes of the malignant images, such as color, shape, and texture layout play a significant role in the evolution of the malignant skin cancer. Thus, this chapter takes account of the color, shape, and texture features for various stages of the melanoma classification. Since the features play a noteworthy role in the medical image classification, it is important to identify and extract appropriate features.

Figure 3. (a): Normal lesion; (b): smaller than 6 mm; (c): single color; (d): borders are even; (e): symmetry; (f) changes in color, shape and other attributes; (g) larger than 6 mm; (h): more than one color; (i): uneven border; (j): asymmetry

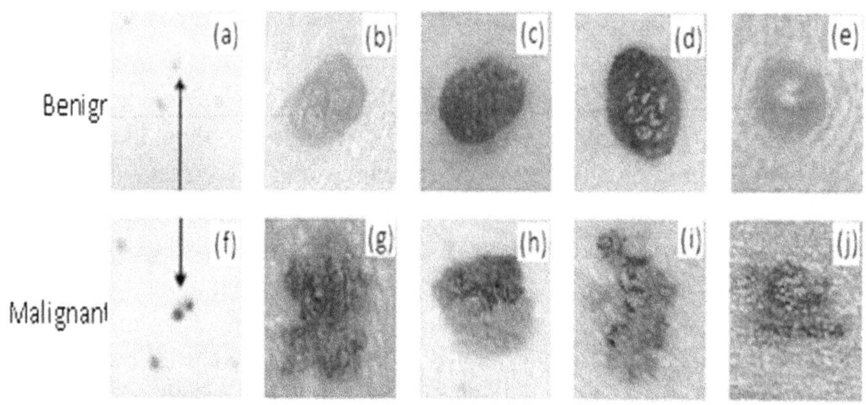

FEATURE EXTRACTION

Color Feature

The given melanoma skin cancer image is converted to the HSV (hue, saturation, and value) color space, because HSV color space is more effective than the other color spaces for feature extraction. The H represents the hue of the color, which ranges from 0° to 360°; S denotes the saturation, which denotes the amount of color mixed with white and its value ranges from 0 to 1; V represents the intensity value of the pixel, which ranges from 0 to 255. The conversion of the RGB color image to the HSV color is briefed below.

$$H = 60^\circ \times H^c$$

where,

$$H^c = \begin{cases} \frac{G' - B'}{C} \bmod 6, & \text{if V = R'} \\ \frac{B' - R'}{C} + 2, & \text{if V = G'} \\ \frac{R' - G'}{C} + 4, & \text{if V = B'} \end{cases}$$

$$R' = \frac{R}{255};$$

$$G' = \frac{G}{255};$$

$$B' = \frac{B}{255}$$

$$\mathrm{V = max(R, G, B);} \quad \mathrm{m = min(R, G, B); C = V - m}$$

$$S = \begin{cases} 0, & \text{if V=0} \\ \frac{C}{V}, & \text{otherwise} \end{cases}$$

Shape Feature

The boundary of the given input melanoma image is identified, based on the edge detection method proposed by Seetharaman & Krishnamoorthy (2007). The boundary could be round shape, if it is a benign lesion or a normal mole; the boundary is contour, if it is a melanoma. In order to extract the shape features, the region of interest (RoI) of the melanoma image is segmented. A pixel is arbitrarily selected from the boundary of the RoI; the distance is computed, in terms of pixel, between the arbitrarily selected pixel and the pixel in straight opposite direction, and a straight line is drawn between the pixels in straight opposite direction of the boundary of the RoI. A midpoint (pixel)of the straight line is computed, based on the expression in Equation (1); and the location of the midpoint pixel is stored with *midx(i) and midy(i)*, {i = 1, 2, …, 36}; i is the index of the number of midpoint pixels.

$$\text{midpoint}=\frac{\text{number of pixels between two boundary pixels}}{2} \tag{1}$$

Likewise, 12 midpoint pixels are computed; the column and row indices of the midpoint pixel are stored with *row_index(i)* and *col_index(i)*. An average of the *row_index* and the *col_index* are computed for the 12 midpoint pixels using the expressions in Equations. (2) and (3). The average of the *row_index* and c*ol_index* is fixed as a centre of the contour shape. The centre of the contour, *cont_cent(r_loc_average, c_loc_average),* is computed as follows.

$$r\_loc\_average = \frac{\sum_{i=1}^{24} row\_index(i)}{12} \tag{2}$$

$$c\_loc\_average = \frac{\sum_{i=1}^{24} col\_index(i)}{12} \tag{3}$$

The maximum distance from the centre of the contour to a pixel in its boundary is identified, which is fixed as a radius; and a circle is drawn, based on the radius with origin, $circle(x_o, y_o, r_o)$. The centre of the contour is moved to the origin of the circle, which is illustrated in Figure 3. A twenty four feature points are selected each at 15° angular distance, which are treated as shape features.

Texture Feature

The surface of the lesion image is smooth and fine. The texture surface changes to a rough surface with a broken skin layout, while the benign lesion grows towards the melanoma. Therefore, the texture features play a significant role in differentiating the melanoma from normal skin lesion and identifying the stages of the melanoma. The autocorrelation function (ρ) plays a noteworthy role in characterizing the texture (Seetharaman & Palanivel, 2013). Thus, this paper takes into the account of autocorrelation for characterizing the melanoma images in terms of texture properties.

The degree of aggressiveness of the melanoma is measured based on the surface of the melanoma. The surface of the melanoma is characterized by the first order autocorrelation. In order to compute the autocorrelation, the RoI is subjected to the experiment with overlapping windows of size 3×3. The autocorrelation function expressed in (5) is employed to compute the autocorrelation between the center pixel of the window and its neighboring pixels. The expression in (4) is rewritten as in (5) for a computational purpose. The neighboring pixels to the center pixel of the window are formed as a one dimensional vector for computational simplicity.

$$\rho_k = \frac{E(f_t - \mu)E(f_{t+k} - \mu)}{\sigma^2} \tag{4}$$

where, f_t represents the pixel intensity value; μ represents mean intensity value; σ^2 represents variation among the pixel intensity values; k is the *lag* variable, which denotes the order of the autocorrelation. In this case the order is one.

$$\rho_k = \frac{E(f_c - \mu)E(f_k - \mu)}{\sigma^2} \tag{5}$$

In Equation (5), f_c and f_k represent the centre and its neighboring pixels respectively.

The autocorrelation values are treated as one of the features, which effectively characterizes the surface of the melanoma images, in terms of texture properties. The surface properties play a noteworthy role in identifying the stages of the melanoma.

Figure 4. Shape feature extraction

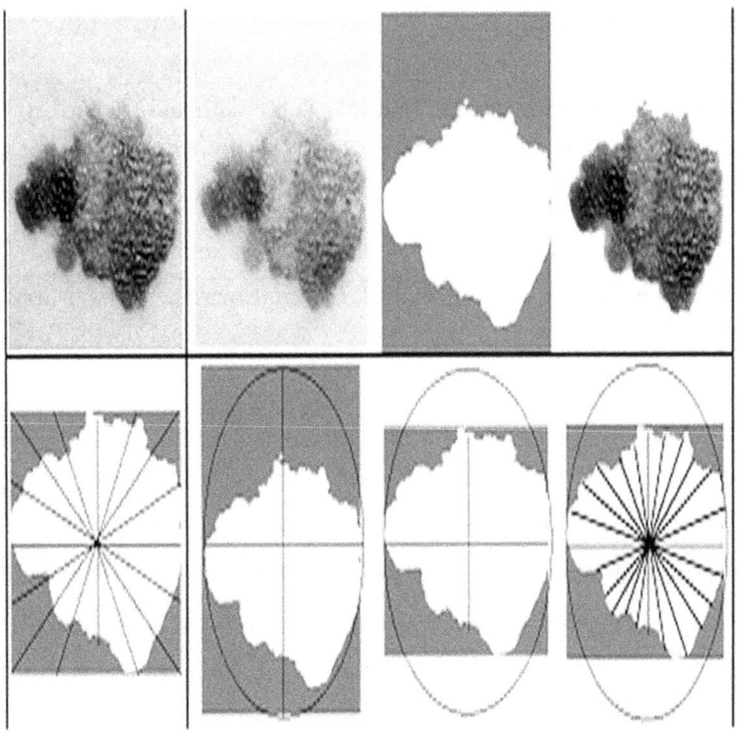

Feature Vector Formation

The extracted color, shape, and texture features are formed as a bag-of-features (BoF) as follows. The color melanoma image is converted to the HSV color space, because the HSV color model is more effective than the RGB color model. The shape features are extracted, based on the shape, that is, symmetry or asymmetry; the border features, that is, whether the border of the melanoma is round or contour shape; diameter of the shape, that is, almost the diameter of the normal mole or benign lesion is same in all directions, whereas it differs in the case of malignant melanoma images. A twenty four feature points along the boundary are selected, and the distances between the center and the boundary points are computed that represent the size and shape of the melanoma image. The surface of the melanoma is characterized by autocorrelation function, and that are treated as a texture feature.

$$FV = (H, S, V, \text{shape, texture}) \tag{6}$$

CLASSIFICATION METHODS

In order to identify whether a melanoma image is cancerous or not, a test for equality of covariance and a test for equality of mean vector are applied. If the outcome of the test indicates the symptom of the melanoma, further it is classified into the initial stage, and the advanced stage. The task of classification is the identification of a group of pixels, or a region of interest in the image that are cohesive to be clustered from other types of pixels, or a region of interest in the image and assigns each possible cohesive group of pixel or regions of interest to a known stage of the melanoma.

Basis of the Proposed Test Statistic

Let X be a random variable that represents the intensity value with additive noise of a pixel at location (k, l) in a color melanoma image. The pixel $f(k,l) \in \Re^3$ is a linear combination of three colors, such as red, green, and blue, that is, $f(k, l) = \left[r(k, l),\ g(k, l),\ b(k, l)\right]^T$, where T represents the transformation of the vector. The mean intensity value of each color is represented by μ_r, μ_g and ¼$_b$ respectively, and the covariance matrix is denoted by Σ. The multivariate normal density function of the melanoma image, $F(k, l)$, is given by

$$F(k,l) = \frac{1}{\left(\sqrt{2\Pi}\right)^3 |\Sigma|} \exp\left(-\tfrac{1}{2}(x-\mu)^T \Sigma^{-1} (x-\mu)\right) \tag{7}$$

The density function mentioned in Eq (7) can be denoted as $n\left(x : \mu, \Sigma\right)$ and the distribution law as $N\left(\mu,\ \Sigma\right)$. The i-th diagonal element of the covariance matrix, Σ, is the variance, σ_{ii}, of the i-th component of $F(k, l)$. The mean vector of each color of the pixels in the image is

$$\mu = \mathrm{E}\left(\mathrm{X}\right) = \mathrm{E}\begin{bmatrix} x_r \\ x_g \\ x_b \end{bmatrix} = \begin{bmatrix} \mu_r \\ \mu_g \\ \mu_b \end{bmatrix} \tag{8}$$

and the covariance matrix is

$$\Sigma = \begin{bmatrix} \sigma_{rr} & \sigma_{rg}\rho & \sigma_{rb}\rho \\ \sigma_{gr}\rho & \sigma_{gg} & \sigma_{gb}\rho \\ \sigma_{br}\rho & \sigma_{bg}\rho & \sigma_{bb} \end{bmatrix} = \begin{bmatrix} \sigma_r^2 & \sigma_{rg}\rho & \sigma_{rb}\rho \\ \sigma_{gr}\rho & \sigma_g^2 & \sigma_{gb}\rho \\ \sigma_{br}\rho & \sigma_{bg}\rho & \sigma_b^2 \end{bmatrix} \tag{9}$$

where, σ_r^2, σ_g^2 and σ_b^2 are the variations among the intensity values of red, green, and blue colors respectively; σ_{rg} represents the interaction between the red and green colors; similarly, σ_{rb} and σ_{gb} represent the interaction between the corresponding colors; ρ represents correlation or interrelation between the corresponding color pixels. The covariance matrix $\pounds$ is symmetric and positive definite.

Test for Equality of Covariance

First, let us discuss the problem of generalized case, that is, q-populations, and p-components in each population. Let $x_{(\alpha)}^{(g)}, \alpha = 1,\ 2,\ \ldots, N_g;\ \ \mathrm{g} = 1,\ 2,\ \ldots,\ \mathrm{q}$ be an observation from the g-th population, $N(\text{¼}^{(g)},\ \pounds_g)$. The hypothesis,

$$\begin{aligned} H_0 &: \pounds_1 = \pounds_2 = \ldots = \pounds_q \\ H_a &: \pounds_1 \neq \pounds_2 \neq \ldots \neq \pounds_q \end{aligned} \tag{10}$$

the equality of covariance matrices of q-populations with p-components of multivariate normal populations can be tested against the alternative of general positive definite matrices by a modified generalized likelihood-ratio test statistic. The generalized likelihood function for the above said observations is

$$\mathrm{L} = \prod_{\mathrm{g}=1}^{\mathrm{q}} \frac{1}{(\sqrt{2\tilde{A}})^{\mathrm{pN_g}} \left(\sqrt{|\pounds_{\mathrm{g}}|}\right)^{\mathrm{N_g}}} \exp\left[-\frac{1}{2}\sum_{\pm=1}^{\mathrm{N_g}} (\mathrm{x}_{\pm}^{(\mathrm{g})} - \text{¼}^{(\mathrm{g})})^{\mathrm{T}} \pounds_{\mathrm{g}}^{-1} (\mathrm{x}_{\pm}^{(\mathrm{g})} - \text{¼}^{(\mathrm{g})})\right] \tag{11}$$

The covariance matrix, Σ_g, is positive definite and $\Sigma_1 = \Sigma_2 = \ldots = \Sigma_q$, and $\mu^{(g)}$ is any vector in the parameter space, Ω. The maximum likelihood estimates of $\mu^{(g)}$ and Σ_g in Ω are given by

$$\hat{\mu}_{\Omega}^{(g)} = \bar{x}^{(g)},\ \Sigma_{\Omega}^{g} = \frac{1}{N_g} A_g,\ \mathrm{g} = 1,2\ldots,\mathrm{q} \tag{12}$$

where,

$$A_g = \sum_{g,\alpha} (x_\alpha^g - \overline{x}^{(g)})^T (x_\alpha^g - \overline{x}^{(g)})$$

is a sum of squares of cross products of variation about the mean of the components in a sample, which is drawn from the multivariate normal population.

The maximum likelihood estimates of $\mu^{(g)}$ in Ω are given by Equation (9), $\hat{\mu}_\Omega^{(g)} = \overline{x}^{(g)}$, since the maximizing values of $\mu^{(g)}$ are the same regardless of $\sum_g$. The function is to be maximized with respect to $\sum_1 = \ldots = \sum_q = \sum$, say,

$$\frac{1}{(\sqrt{2\pi})^{pN} \left(\sqrt{|\sum_g|}\right)^N} \exp\left[-\frac{1}{2}\sum_{g=1}^{q}\sum_{\alpha=1}^{N_g} (x_\alpha^{(g)} - \mu^{(g)})^T \ \Sigma^{-1}(x_\alpha^{(g)} - \mu^{(g)})\right] \tag{13}$$

By the following Lemma [32], the maximizing value of $\sum$ is

$$\hat{\Sigma}_\varpi = \frac{1}{N} A \tag{14}$$

Lemma: If D is positive definite of order p, the maximum of $f(g) = N \ \log|G| - \mathrm{tr}(G^{-1})D$ with respect to positive definite matrices G exists, occurs at $G = (1/N)D$, and has the value $f[(1/N)D] = pN \ \log N - N \ \log|D - pN|$

Let A_g be the unbiased estimate of $\sum_g$, based on n_g degrees of freedom, where $n_g = N_g - 1$ to the usual case of a random sample of N_g observation vectors from the g-th population. When H_0 is true,

$$A = \frac{1}{\sum n_g} \sum_{g=1}^{q} n_g A_g \tag{15}$$

is the pooled estimate of the common covariance matrix. The test statistic

$$MC^{-1} = \left(\sum n_g \ln|A| - \sum_{g=1}^{q} n_g \ln A_g\right) C^{-1} \tag{16}$$

is approximately distributed with chi-square variate with degrees of freedom $1/2\,(q-1)p(p+1)$ (Anderson, 2003), where

$$C^{-1} = 1 - \frac{2p^2 + 3p - 1}{6(p+1)(q-1)}\left(\sum_{g=1}^{q}\frac{1}{n_g} - \frac{1}{\sum n_g}\right) \tag{17}$$

The objective of this chapter is to classify the normal lesion image and the malignant melanoma image (q = 2), and each population consists of three components (p = 5), namely color features, such as H, S, and V, shape, and texture features. Here, the aim is to test the hypothesis that the test image is affected by malignant or not, that is,the null hypothesis $H_0 : \Sigma_t = \Sigma_{mm}$, where Σ_t and Σ_{mm} represent the covariance matrices of the test image and the malignant melanoma image. The pooled estimate of the common covariance matrix A can be computed as follows.

$$A = \left(\frac{1}{(N_1 - 1) + (N_2 - 1)}\right)\left[(N_1 - 1)A_1 + (N_2 - 1)A_2\right] \tag{18}$$

The test statistic for the case of the two populations is given by

$$M = \left(\left[(N_1 - 1) + (N_2 - 1)\right] \ln|A|\right) - \left(\left[(N_1 - 1)\ln(A_1) + (N_2 - 1)\ln|A_2|\right]\right) \tag{19}$$

If $MC^{-1} \leq \chi_\nu^2(\alpha)$, then the hypothesis is accepted, that is, the test image belongs to the class of malignant image. Otherwise, that is, $MC^{-1} > \chi_\nu^2(\alpha)$, the hypothesis is rejected, that is, the test image does not belong to the class of melanoma image, where, $\nu = 1/2\,(q-1)p(p+1)$, and α is the level of significance.

Test for Equality of Mean Vectors

As discussed in the preceding section, if the covariance of the test image and the class of melanoma images pass the covariance test, then it proceeds to test the equality mean vector of the test image and the class of malignant melanoma image with the assumption of equal variances. After observing the outcome of the two tests, it is concluded that whether the two images fall in the same class or not. To achieve this, the test for equality of mean vectors is performed on the images. Let $x_{(\alpha)}^{(g)}$, $\alpha = 1,2,\ldots,N_g$; g = 1,2,...,q, be an observation from the g-th population, $N(\mu^{(g)}, \Sigma_g)$. The aim of this section is to test the hypothesis

$$\begin{aligned} H_0 &: \mu^{(1)} = \mu^{(2)} = \ldots = \mu^{(g)} \quad \text{Null hypothesis} \\ H_1 &: \mu^{(1)} \neq \mu^{(2)} \neq \ldots \neq \mu^{(g)} \quad \text{Alternate hypothesis} \end{aligned} \tag{20}$$

The proposed test statistic

$$V = \left|N \hat{\Sigma}_\Omega\right| \Big/ \left|N \hat{\Sigma}_\varpi\right| \tag{21}$$

is distributed as a chi-squared variate with degrees of freedom $\nu = 1/2(q-1)p(p+1)$ (Anderson, 2003), where,

$$N\hat{\Sigma}_\Omega = \sum_{g,,\alpha} x_\alpha^{(g)} x_\alpha^{(g)T} - \sum_g N_g \bar{x}^{(g)} \bar{x}^{(g)'T} \quad (22)$$

$$N\hat{\Sigma}_\Omega = \sum_{g,a} \left(x_a^{(g)} - \bar{x}^{(g)} \right) \left(x_a^{(g)} - \bar{x}^{(g)} \right)^T \quad (23)$$

$$N\hat{\Sigma}_\varpi = \sum_{g,\alpha} \left(x_\alpha^{(g)} - \bar{x} \right) \left(x_\alpha^{(g)} - \bar{x} \right)^T \quad (24)$$

where, $\bar{x}_\alpha^{(g)} = \frac{1}{N_g} \sum_{\alpha=1}^{N_g} x_\alpha^{(g)}$, $\bar{x} = \frac{1}{N} \sum_{g,\alpha} x_\alpha^{(g)}$, and $N = N_1 + N_2 + \ldots + N_q$. The $\hat{\Sigma}_\varpi$ is an estimate of the Σ when $\mu^{(1)} = \mu^{(2)} = \ldots = \mu^{(g)}$, and $\hat{\Sigma}_\Omega$ is a weighted average of the estimate of the Σ.

In the proposed work, there are only two populations (q=2) and each consists of five components (p= 5). Hence, Eqsuations (23) and (24) can be re-written as in Equation (25).

$$N\hat{\Sigma}_\Omega = \sum_{\alpha=1}^{N} \left(x_\alpha^{(1)} - \bar{x}^{(1)} \right) \left(x_\alpha^{(1)} - \bar{x}^{(1)} \right)^T + \sum_{\alpha=1}^{N} \left(x_\alpha^{(2)} - \bar{x}^{(2)} \right) \left(x_\alpha^{(2)} - \bar{x}^{(2)} \right)^T \quad (25)$$

If $V < \chi_\nu^2(\alpha)$, then the hypothesis is accepted, that is, the test image falls in the class of malignant melanoma image; otherwise, that is, $V > \chi_\nu^2(\alpha)$, then the hypothesis is rejected, it means that the images fall in different classes.

If the test image and the class of the melanoma images pass the aforementioned two tests, such as test for equality of covariance and test for equality of mean vectors, at the 25% level of significance, then the test image is classified in the class of the melanoma image.

FEATURE DATABASE CONSTRUCTION

In order to implement the theoretical concepts discussed in the previous sections, 1419 dermoscopic images were collected from various health care centres and downloaded from the Internet. They have been categorized into three classes: (i) class – 1, normal skin lesion images; (ii) class – 2, initial stage of the skin melanoma images; (iii) class – 3, advanced stage of the skin melanoma images. The 1419 dermoscopic images comprise of 509 normal skin lesion images, 302 initial stage melanoma images, and 608 advanced stage melanoma images.

The features, such as color, shape, and texture, are extracted as in Equation (6) from the images collected; and they are treated as a feature space. The feature space is assumed to be a multivariate normal random field. The mean vector, covariance matrix, and the number of samples, N, of each image are computed, and they are stored as a feature database. The principal and upper diagonal elements are stored in the feature database because the covariance matrix is a symmetric; by which half of the storage space could be reduced.

PERFORMANCE EVALUATION

The performance of the proposed statistical tests of hypothesis-based method was evaluated, based on the Lachenbruch's holdout procedure (Lachenbruch & Mickey, 1968). The correct classification and misclassification rates were measured by applying the Lachenbruch's holdout procedures expressed in Equations (26) and (27) respectively. Let n_{iC}^{H} and n_{iM}^{H} be the number of correctly classified and the misclassfied observations of the i-th group respectively, where i = 1,2, ...p; and n_i represents the number of observations belong to the i-th group, then an estimate of the expected actual correct classification rate E(ACR), and the estimate of the expected actual misclassification rate E(AER) are as follows; and the notation $\hat{E}$ denotes the estimate of the AER and ACR. Since this chapter deals only with three categories of the melanoma images, p is fixed to 3.

$$\hat{E}(AER) = \frac{\sum_{i=1}^{p} n_{iM}^{H}}{\sum_{i=1}^{p} n_i} \times 100 \tag{26}$$

$$\hat{E}(ACR) = \frac{\sum_{i=1}^{p} n_{iC}^{H}}{\sum_{i=1}^{p} n_i} \times 100 \tag{27}$$

IMPLEMENTATION

A test image is given as input to the proposed classification method, which extracts the color, shape, and texture features that are formed as a feature vector as in Equation (6), which is treated as a feature space, and is assumed to be a multivariate normal random field. The mean vector, covariance matrix, and the number of samples, N, are computed from the test image. First, the covariance of the test image is compared with the covariance of the class-1 images stored in the feature database by applying the expression in Equation (16). If the images pass the test for equality of covariance, then proceeds to the test for equality of the mean vector; otherwise, it is assumed that the test image falls in other classes. If the test image pass both the tests (mean and covariance tests), then it is classified into the class-1 images; otherwise, it is assumed that the test image falls in other classes. Similarly, the test image is compared to the class-2 and class-3 images. The significance (probability) values of the three tests (test image versus normal; test image versus initial; test image versus advanced) are compared, and the minimum of the them (significance probability) is selected. Now, the test image is classified into the class, which has minimum significance probability value.

The mean vector, covariance matrix, and the number of samples, N, are computed from the given input test image. The statistic MC^{-1} is computed, based on the expression in Equation (16), for the mean vector, covariance matrix, and the number of samples, N, of the test image and the features of the class-1 images stored in the feature database. The computed statistic, MC^{-1}, is compared to the critical values, $\chi_{\nu}^{2}(\alpha)$ at different significance levels as listed in Tables 1 – 3. After performing the null hypothesis test on trial basis at different significance levels from 1% to 40%, the average significance level is fixed at 25% for the class-1 images. If the computed MC^{-1} value is less than or equal to the critical value, $\chi_{\nu}^{2}(\alpha)$, at the significant level, $\alpha = 0.25$, then the null hypothesis is accepted. Furthermore, the test for equality of mean vectors is conducted for the same dataset. If the computed test statistic value, *V* expressed in Equation (21), is less than or equals to the critical value $\chi_{\nu}^{2}(\alpha)$ at the level of significance, 25%, then the null hypothesis is accepted. If the test image passes both the tests (test for equality of covariances and test for equality of mean vectors), then it is inferred that the test image falls in class-1 images, that is, the test image falls in the category of normal skin lesion images; otherwise, it is inferred that the test image falls in other classes. Similarly, the test image is compared with other categories, that is, class-2 and class-3 images at the level of significance, 25%.

While fixing the level of significance at higher level, that is, at 30% and above, there is a possibility of the image belongs to other clasess (class-2 and class-3) falls in the class-1. In this context, the test image could be categorized into the class, which has the minimum significant probability value for the acceptance of the null hypothesis test for the two classes. The outcome of the classification results is tabulated in the Tables 1 – 3, and the average correct classification and misclassification are tabulated in Table 4.

Table 1. Rate of classification for normal skin lesion versus other classes

Significance level (α)	Normal Skin Lesion (%)	Initial Stage Melanoma (%)	Advanced Stage Melanoma (%)
1%	72.53	17.48	09.99
5%	78.61	13.35	08.04
10%	86.85	08.07	05.08
15%	90.88	05.61	04.51
20%	95.16	03.23	01.61
25%	99.86	00.14	00.00
30%	100.00	00.00	00.00
35%	100.00	00.00	00.00
40%	100.00	00.00	00.00

Table 2. Rate of classification for initial stage melanoma versus other classes

Significance level (α)	Initial Stage Melanoma (%)	Normal Skin Lesion (%)	Advanced Stage Melanoma (%)
1%	69.65	17.48	12.87
5%	78.53	11.43	10.04
10%	86.62	08.24	05.14
15%	91.33	04.86	03.81
20%	96.66	02.13	01.21
25%	99.96	00.04	00.00
30%	100.00	00.00	00.00
35%	100.00	00.00	00.00
40%	100.00	00.00	00.00

Table 3. Rate of classification for advanced stage melanoma versus other classes

Significance level (α)	Advanced Stage Melanoma (%)	Normal Skin Lesion (%)	Initial Stage Melanoma (%)
1%	71.23	15.42	13.35
5%	77.63	11.36	11.01
10%	83.38	07.49	09.13
15%	88.66	05.15	06.19
20%	95.82	01.62	02.56
25%	99.16	00.47	00.37
30%	100.00	00.00	00.00
35%	100.00	00.00	00.00
40%	100.00	00.00	00.00

The classification results of the normal skin lesion image verses other categories of the melanoma, such as initial and advanced stage images, are tabulated in Table-1 reveal that the test statistics classify the melanoma images 100% correctly at the higher significance level, that is, at 30% and above; but, at the same time, the proposed test statistic classifies the other categories of the melanoma images into the normal melanoma images. At the lower significant level, that is, at 15% and below, the test statistic results with mixed classification rates among the three categories of the melanoma images, whereas the test statistic yields a correct classification rate at the level of significance from 25% to 30%. The range of the level of significance, from 25% to 30%, is identified after conducting a rigorous experiment on a trial and error basis.

Similarly, the same classification study is conducted with the initial stage melanoma versus normal skin lesion images and the advanced melanoma images, for which the test statistic yields almost 100% correct classification at the level of significance, from 25% to 30%. The proposed statistic gives mixed classification results at the lower significance level, at 15% and below. But, the test statistic correctly classifies the initial stage melanoma images at the higher level of significance, but mis-classify the normal skin lesion and the advanced stage melanoma images into the class of initial stage melanoma images. The obtained classification results are presented in Table 2.

Table 4. Average correct classification and misclassification in percent

	Predicted membership						
		Normal Skin Lesion	Initial Stage Melanoma	Advanced Stage Melanoma	Correct Classification (%)	Mis-classification (%)	
Actual membership	Normal Skin Lesion	456	27	16	91.55	8.45	
	Initial Stage Melanoma	11	276	15	91.39	8.61	
	Advanced Stage Melanoma	19	28	561	92.27	7.73	

It is observed from the results tabulated in Table 3, the proposed test statistic yields nearer to 100% or 100% correct classification at the level of significance from 25% to 30% for the classification of advanced melanoma images versus initial stage melanoma images and normal skin lesion images. The proposed statistic gives a mixed classification result at the lower level of significance, at 15% and below. But, the test statistic gives a correct classification of the advanced stage melanoma images at the higher level of significance, whereas the statistic mis-classifies the normal skin lesion images and initial stage melanoma images into the class of advanced stage melanoma images.

Figure 5. Correct classification: Normal versus initial and advanced stages; initial versus normal and advanced stages; advanced versus normal and initial

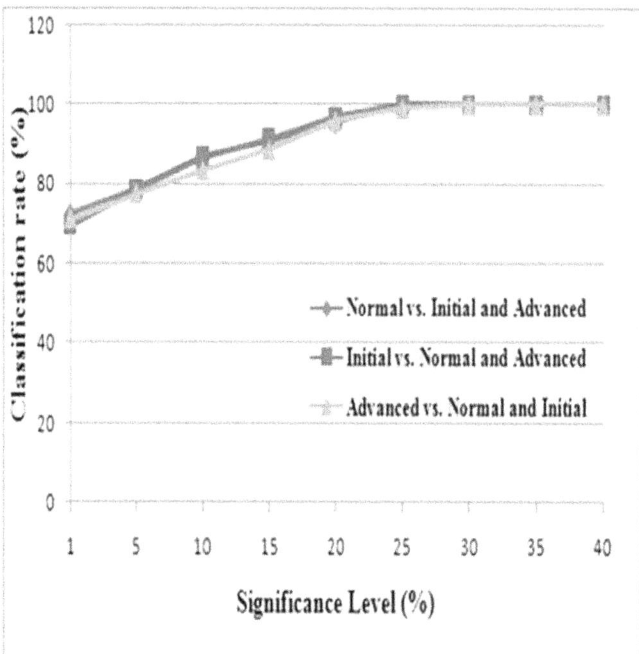

Furthermore, an actual correct classification and misclassification rates are computed using the expressions in Eqs. (26) and (27), based on the results obtained and that has been presented in Table 4. The proposed test statistic gives a correct classification up to 91.55% of the normal skin lesion images; 91.39% for the initial stage melanoma images; and 92.27% for advanced stage melanoma images. The correct classification of the proposed method is graphically represented in Figure 4.

FUTURE RESEARCH DIRECTION

The melanoma image classification is a challenging problem with the use of features, such as color, shape, and texture, available in the present context. Though, the proposed test statistic method effectively classifies the melanoma images with the color, shape, and texture features, it could yield better classification results, if the TNM-based (Tumor, Node, and Metastatis) staging system adopted. The TNM-based grouping method is fully based on the anatomic stage/prognostic groups clinical data. It is also a challenging problem of feature extraction in the clinical environment. If the TNM-based feature extraction for the melanoma is possible, the proposed test statistic is more effective and efficient for melanoma image identification and classification. Due to the difficulties of extracting features at each stage, that is, stage-1, stage-2, stage-3, stage-4, and the normal skin lesion, the proposed method considered only the three groups, such as normal skin lesion, initial stage melanoma, and advanced stage melanoma. But, still the existing methods deal only with two groups, that is, normal skin lesion and melanoma image.

CONCLUSION

This chapter was developed based on the multivariate parametric statistical tests of hypothesis, such as a test for equality of the mean vector and a test for the equality of covariance, for skin cancer melanoma image classification. This chapter categories the melanoma images into three groups, such as normal skin lesion, initial stage melanoma, and advanced stage melanoma. This chapter compares and classifies each category of images individually, that is, normal versus initial and advanced stages; initial stage versus normal and advanced stages; advanced stage versus normal and initial stages. The proposed statistical test-based method gives an average correct classification up to 91.55% for normal skin lesion versus initial and advanced stage melanoma; up to 91.39% for the initial stage melanoma versus the normal skin lesion image and the advanced stage melanoma; up to 92.27% for advanced stage melanoma versus the normal skin lesion and the initial stage melanoma. The advantages of the proposed method are that it classifies three groups of skin melanoma images, whereas the existing methods classify or identify whether the images is affected by melanoma or not; and it consumes less computational time for feature extraction and classification. The proposed method gives better results.

REFERENCES

Anderson, T. W. (2003). *An introduction to multivariate statistical analysis* (3rd ed.). John Wiley & Sons, Inc.

Carlson. (2018). *National Comprehensive Cancer Network Clinical Practice Guidelines in Oncology (NCCN Guidelines)*. Retrieved from http://www.nccn.org

Castroa, V. G., Hernandeza, M. V., Armitageb, P. A., & Wardlawa, J. M. (2016). Texture-based classification for the automatic rating of the perivascular spaces in brain MRI. *Procedia Computer Science*, *90*, 9–14. doi:10.1016/j.procs.2016.07.003

Chen, E. L., Chung, P. C., Chen, C. L., Tsai, H.-M., & Chang, C.-I. (1998). An Automatic Diagnostic System for CT Liver Image Classification. *IEEE Transactions on Biomedical Engineering*, *45*(6), 783–794. doi:10.1109/10.678613 PMID:9609943

Fritz, A., Percy, C., Jack, A., Shanmugaratnam, K., Sobin, L., Parkin, D. M., & Whelan, S. (2013). *WHO International Classification of Diseases for Oncology* (3rd ed.). ICD-O. Retrieved from www.who.int/classifications/icd/adaptations/oncology/

Gletsos, M., Mougiakakou, S. G., Matsopoulos, G. K., Nikita, K. S., Nikita, A. S., & Kelekis, D. (2003). A Computer-Aided Diagnostic System to Characterize CT Focal Liver Lesions: Design and Optimization of a Neural Network Classifier. *IEEE Transactions on Information Technology in Biomedicine*, *7*(3), 153–162. doi:10.1109/TITB.2003.813793 PMID:14518728

Kaur, R., Albano, P. P., Cole, J. G., Hagerty, J., LeAnder, R. W., Moss, R. H., & Stoecker, W. V. (2015). Real-time supervised detection of pink areas in dermoscopic images of melanoma: Importance of color shades, texture and location. *Skin Research and Technology*, *21*(4), 466–473. doi:10.1111rt.12216 PMID:25809473

Lachenbruch, P. A., & Mickey, M. R. (1968). Estimation of Error Rate in Discriminant Analysis. *Technometrics*, *10*(1), 1–10. doi:10.1080/00401706.1968.10490530

Lee, H. D., Mendesb, A. I., Spolaôra, N., Olivaa, J. T., Parmezana, A. R. S., Wua, F. C., & Fonseca-Pintob, R. (2018). Dermoscopic Assisted Diagnosis in Melanoma: Reviewing Results, Optimizing Methodologies and Quantifying Empirical Guidelines. *Knowledge-Based Systems*, *158*, 9–24. doi:10.1016/j.knosys.2018.05.016

Li, Y., & Shen, L. (2018). Skin Lesion Analysis towards Melanoma Detection Using Deep Learning Network. *Sensors (Basel)*, *18*(556), 2–16. PMID:29439500

Ma, M., Manuel, J., & Tavares, R. S. (2017). Effective features to classify skin lesions in dermoscopic images. *Expert Systems with Applications*, *84*, 92–101. doi:10.1016/j.eswa.2017.05.003

Pourghassem, H., & Ghassemian, H. (2008). Content-based medical image classification using a new hierarchical merging scheme. *Computerized Medical Imaging and Graphics*, *32*(8), 651–661. doi:10.1016/j.compmedimag.2008.07.006 PMID:18789648

Rajendran, P., & Madheswaran, M. (2010). Hybrid Medical Image Classification Using Association Rule Mining with Decision Tree Algorithm. *Journal of Computers*, *2*(1), 127–136.

Rasku, J., Juhola, M., Toppila, E., & Pyykko, I. (2007). Recognition of balance signals between healthy subjects and otoneurological patients with hidden Markov models. *Biomedical Signal Processing and Control*, *2*(1), 1–8. doi:10.1016/j.bspc.2006.12.005

Seetharaman, K., & Krishnamoorthi, R. (2007). A Statistical Framework Based on A Family of Full Range Autoregressive Models for Edge Extraction. *Pattern Recognition Letters*, *28*(7), 759–770. doi:10.1016/j.patrec.2006.11.003

Seetharaman, K., & Palanivel, N. (2013). Texture Characterization, Representation, Description and Classification Based on a Family of Full Range Gaussian Markov Random Field Model. *International Journal of Image and Data Fusion*, *4*(4), 342–362. doi:10.1080/19479832.2013.804007

Silveira, M., Nascimento, J. C., Marques, J. S., Marçal, A. R. S., Mendonça, T., Yamauchi, S., ... Rozeira, J. (2009). Comparison of Segmentation Methods for Melanoma Diagnosis in Dermoscopy Images. *IEEE Journal of Selected Topics in Signal Processing*, *3*(1), 35–45. doi:10.1109/JSTSP.2008.2011119

Tsai, D.-Y., Lee, Y., Sekiya, M., & Ohkubo, M. (2004). Medical image classification using genetic algorithm based fuzzy-logic approach. *Journal of Electronic Imaging*, *13*(4), 780–788. doi:10.1117/1.1786607

Winston, W. T. (2018). *TNM Classification for Malignant Melanoma: TNM Classification for Malignant Melanoma*. Retrieved from https://emedicine.medscape.com/article/2007147-overview

Section 2
Analysis of Healthcare

Chapter 6

Improvement of Variant Adaptable LSTM Trained With Metaheuristic Algorithms for Healthcare Analysis

Tarik A. Rashid
University of Kurdistan Hewler, Iraq & Salahaddin University – Erbil, Iraq

Mohammad K. Hassan
University of Kurdistan Hewler, Iraq

Mokhtar Mohammadi
University of Human Development, Iraq

Kym Fraser
University of Kurdistan Hewler, Iraq

ABSTRACT

Recently, the population of the world has increased along with health problems. Diabetes mellitus disease as an example causes issues to the health of many patients globally. The task of this chapter is to develop a dynamic and intelligent decision support system for patients with different diseases, and it aims at examining machine-learning techniques supported by optimization techniques. Artificial neural networks have been used in healthcare for several decades. Most research works utilize multilayer layer perceptron (MLP) trained with back propagation (BP) learning algorithm to achieve diabetes mellitus classification. Nonetheless, MLP has some drawbacks, such as, convergence, which can be slow; local minima can affect the training process. It is hard to scale and cannot be used with time series data sets. To overcome these drawbacks, long short-term memory (LSTM) is suggested, which is a more advanced form of recurrent neural networks. In this chapter, adaptable LSTM trained with two optimizing algorithms instead of the back propagation learning algorithm is presented. The optimization algorithms are biogeography-based optimization (BBO) and genetic algorithm (GA). Dataset is collected locally and another benchmark dataset is used as well. Finally, the datasets fed into adaptable models; LSTM with BBO (LSTMBBO) and LSTM with GA (LSTMGA) for classification purposes. The experimental and testing results are compared and they are promising. This system helps physicians and doctors to provide proper health treatment for patients with diabetes mellitus. Details of source code and implementation of our system can be obtained in the following link "https://github.com/hamakamal/LSTM."

DOI: 10.4018/978-1-5225-7796-6.ch006

INTRODUCTION

Many pieces of research have been carried out to provide the prediction, detection, and classifications for many diseases. According to international diabetes federation, the number of people suffered from diabetes mellitus has increased lately to 225 million people worldwide (Pradhan, Ranjit & Sahu, 2011). Providing the system that can help doctors and patients with diabetes to predict this disease is a big step toward solving many problems in an early stage. This chapter aims to use machine learnings optimization algorithms to enhance doctor's decisions. Artificial neural networks (ANN) considered as the most popular one among all. ANN can have different algorithms for training (Peretto, 1992). There are many classes of neural networks, which classified according to their learning algorithms. Most research works used the multilayer perceptron feed-forwarded trained with back propagation algorithm or its variants to achieve diabetes mellitus classification. In this chapter work, an MLP is used, as it is a class of feed-forward artificial neural network. MLP consists of three layers, where each neuron uses a nonlinear activation function except for neurons at the input layer. However, training multilayer perceptron is slow in terms of convergence and falling easily into local minima (Park, 2006). Thus, recurrent neural networks are used to overcome these problems and obtaining more accuracy in the result. Recurrent neural networks consist of feedback connection so that the activations can flow round in a loop and recurrent neural networks have many forms in terms of architecture. One type of recurrent neural network consists of a standard multilayer perceptron plus loop and capable of having some sort of memory. Recurrent neural networks can memorize relevant events over time and also can deal with arbitrary input data, not just static input data only which makes recurrent networks in principle more powerful than multilayer perceptron (Shanker, 1996). Standard recurrent neural network algorithms for learning to store information over time take too long and lack of long-term dependency. To overcome these problems in standard recurrent neural networks, LSTM proposed which is a more advanced form of recurrent neural networks and a particular type of a recurrent neural network in which they are capable of learning long-term dependencies or avoiding long-term dependency problem (Hochreiter, 2001; Schmidhuber et al., 2007; Schmidhuber, 1997). LSTM unit contains a cell, an input gate, an output gate, and a forget gate. Each of the three gates can be thought of as a conventional artificial neuron, as in a multilayer neural network. LSTM is very useful and more accurate than a standard recurrent neural network, which is why big companies like Apple and Microsoft have used it (Zifan & Gharibzadeh, 2006). As for optimization techniques, two algorithms are used in this work to optimize LSTM. BBO used as the main algorithm, which is an evolutionary algorithm, and GA used as the second. Datasets collected locally and another dataset used for evaluations purposes.

This chapter organized as follows: Section 2 describes the background and previous research works. Details and types of diabetes presented in section 3. Section 4 provides details about ANN in general. Details about classifiers presented in section 5. In section 6, optimizers explained. Details about the methodology, process of data collection, simulation and results presented in section 7, and finally, the conclusion and future works presented in section 8.

BACKGROUND

Diabetes mellitus is a most separated disease in world nowadays. In the past most research works are just focusing identifying the types of diabetes, but these identification is not enough to solve the problem because there is a problem of prediction of glucose rate in the blood also finding relationship between chronic diseases for example eyes infection, kidneys failure, and heart problems. The main problem is there is no strong intelligent system that can reduces the gape produced by normal system for diagnosing patient with diabetes diseases.Machine learning can help doctors to detect the diabetes disease earlier. Patients and physicians can benefit from the prediction's results as early detection reduces patient's health risk. There are various artificial intelligence techniques for diabetes detection. For these techniques to provide better results, they need to learn from data sets (Negrato, Cobas & Gomes, 2012). Techniques used in this area are Support Vector Machine, Fuzzy C-means, Principal Component Analysis, Navies Bayes Classifier, Decision Trees, and Artificial Neural Networks. An artificial neural network is a technique that works like or similar to human brain and inspired by the way biological nervous systems works in processing the information. It has capabilities to learn from input data and predict the output data or results by configuring it for a specific application, such as, pattern recognition or data classification (Andrej, 2011). Artificial neural networks are used in diabetes detection for feature extraction when combined with powerful algorithm. However, for training the network, it takes large effort.

Apart from what mentioned above, many researchers have used ANN in diagnosing diabetes mellitus as in (Gregory & Nejhdeh, 1998), which proposed a model for diagnosing diabetes mellitus. Supervised and unsupervised used as learning algorithms. Support Vector Machine used for processing the inputs. Real-time dataset taken as input based on the physical conditions. Their system proved that ANN for diagnosing diabetes gave better results than other techniques. (Khaled, Osama & Tim, 2002) have diagnosed diabetes by trying to predict the glucose levels in the near future based on the current level. They used the ANN for predicting the diabetes. Time series dataset on diabetic blood glucose patients recorded for about one month. They used feature extraction on time series dataset and trained ANN using this knowledge to predict the blood glucose levels of a diabetic patient with a good accuracy. Rajeeb, Vaibhav, Gagan, and Barnali (2008) have used BP algorithm with ANN to predict diabetes mellitus. They used binary classification to predict diabetes and the person to be diabetic falls under category 1 and not diabetic falls under category 0. Supervised multilayer feed-forward network with BP learning algorithm used for accomplishing this classification, which is the basic architecture of ANN. The inputs to the system are Fasting Blood Sugar test result, Post Plasma Blood Sugar test, age, sex, Random Blood Sugar test result, and their occupation (Zachary & Lipton, 2017). The system achieved Classification accuracy of 92.5they proposed Recurrent Neural Networks using Long Short-Term Memory to diagnose diabetes. They establish the effectiveness of a simple LSTM network for modelling clinical data.

Diabetes Mellitus

Diabetes mellitus (DM) is a disease in which the level blood glucose is higher than a normal person is. The patient who diagnosed with diabetes will lose the ability to produce insulin. The main role of insulin is to lower blood sugar in the body by different mechanisms (Shanker, 1996). Genetic or environmental factors can cause diabetes mellitus. DM can be divided into two major types, type 1diabetes (T1D) and type 2diabetes (T2D). There is still much to be discovered and clarified. The processes of diagnosing and evaluating of appropriate treatment in diabetes can establish a significant basis toward the medical handling of the disease. The two main DM types are described as follows:

Figure 1. Type 1 diabetes
(Negrato, Cobas & Gomes, 2012)

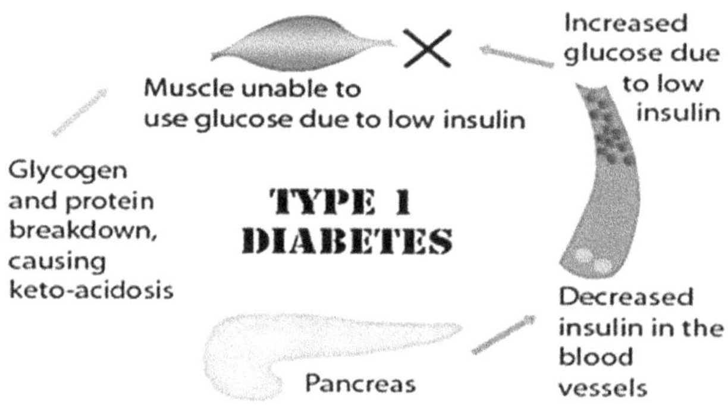

Type 1 Diabetes

Type 1 diabetes is a chronic disease that occurs when the pancreas releases the small amount of insulin or does not make insulin at all. Several factors can affect or cause type I diabetes, including genetics and infection with certain viruses. Type 1diabetes mostly occurs in childhood, but adults are also vulnerable to this disease (Negrato, Cobas & Gomes, 2012) as shown in Figure 1.

Type 2 Diabetes

Type 2 diabetes is another type of diabetes in which the body produces insulin, but not enough. Unfortunately, there is no cure for this disease, but there are significant components of the treatment of diabetes, which can enhance it like Diet, Exercise, Oral hypoglycemic therapy, and Insulin Therapy (Wang, 2005) as shown in Figure 2.

Figure 2. Type 2 diabetes
(Negrato, Cobas & Gomes, 2012)

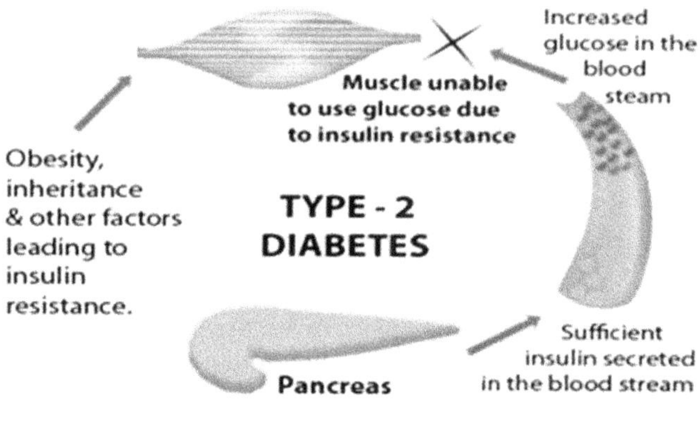

Figure 3. Biological and artificial neuron
(Nagai, 2000)

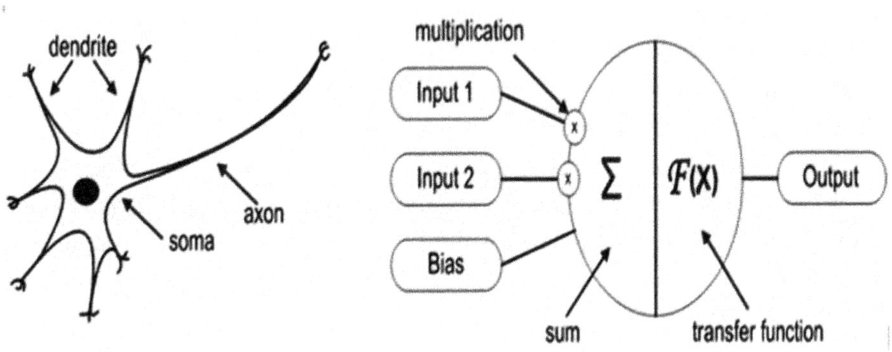

Artificial Neural Networks

The history of neural networks begins in the early 1940's were Warren McCulloch and Walter Pitts introduced models of neurological networks based on neurons. They proposed an application to recognize special patterns by neural networks. An Artificial Neural Network is a model in which simulates the functionalities of biological neural networks (Aggarwal & Song, 1997). For ANN to extract features in datasets, first it must go through learning processes. Deep learning neural networks can extract different features in datasets. There are three major learning techniques; they are supervised learning, unsupervised learning, and reinforcement learning (Nikolic, 2015). There are many types of neural networks with different use cases and levels of complexity. The basic type of neural network is a feed forward neural network. A more advanced one is the recurrent neural network. There are also convolutional neural networks, Hopfield networks, and many others (Sietsma & Dow, 1991). Artificial neuron is a building block for artificial neural network. The design and functionalities of artificial neuron are inspired by biological neuron (Nagai, 2000). In artificial neuron, the information comes in by inputs. Artificial neuron then sums the weighted inputs, bias, and processes the sum with a transfer function. At the exit, the information comes out via outputs. Figure 3 shows a biological neuron and an artificial neuron.

Mathematical description of artificial and biological neurons shown in the below equation (Meyer, Scheich, 1997):

$$y_{(x)} = F\left(\sum_{i=0}^{m} W_i\left(k\right).X_i\left(k\right) + b\right) \tag{1}$$

here $X_i(k)$ is input value in discrete time k where I start from 0 to m, $W_i(k)$ is weight value in discrete time k where i start from 0 to m, b is bias, F is a transfer function, and $Y_{(x)}$ is output value in discrete time k.

Classifiers

In this section, multi-layer perceptron and long short-term memory neural networks are described:

Multi-Layer Perceptron

The simplest type of neural network is Feed-Forward where information goes from input to hidden then to output in one direction (Fukushima, K. 2013). There is feed-forward artificial neural network with single perceptron and more advanced feed forward artificial neural network is called multi-layer feed-forward, which used for analytical description. In many applications, these networks apply a sigmoid function as an activation function. Back propagation is a learning technique, which is used mostly by multi-layer networks, but in this work, Biogeography-Based Optimization (BBO) and Genetic Algorithm (GA) are used to update the weight and biased values. The output with the correct answer is fed back through the network in order to reduce the value of the error function. The activation function of MLP is shown in the below equation:

$$y_i = (1 + e^{-x})^{-1} \tag{2}$$

here, y_i is the output of the ith neuron and $x$is the weighted sum of the input connections.

Long Short Term Memory

Long Short Term Memory is an improvement type of the recurrent artificial neural networks topologies and proposed by Sepp Hochreiter and Jurgen Schmidhuber in the late 90s. LSTM is different from basic recurrent artificial neural networks in which it can learn from its experience to process, classify and predict time series data with very long time lags, which means that LSTM is capable of remembering value for any length of time (Mohs, Wescourt & Atkinson, 1973). This makes LSTM outperform other recurrent artificial neural networks. The architecture of LSTM consists of chained together modules and information can pass in between. The difference comes from the cells internally. Each unit or cell in

Figure 4. LSTM artificial neural networks

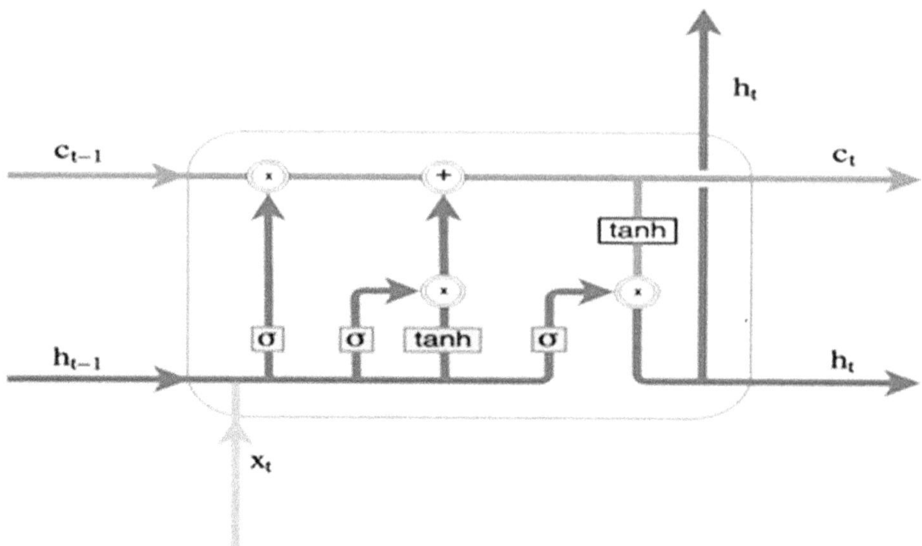

LSTM sends its state and a hidden state to the next cell, and every cell contains four interacting neural network layers instead of a single one. These four layers form three "gates" in which together they give LSTM capability of remembering value for long time and control when the input is important enough remembering it, when to forget it, and when to output the value (Sudharsan, Peeples & Shomali, 2014). The structure of LSTM is shown in Figure 4.

It is vital to decide about the information, which will be disposed from the cell state. This can be decided by the forget gate, which uses a sigmoid function as expressed below (Christopher, 2015):

$$f_t = \sigma\left(h_{t-1} \cdot U_f + x_t \cdot W_f + b_f\right) \tag{3}$$

where f_t represent the forget layer, σ signifies sigmoid activation function at f_t, U_f. signifies weight link to previously hidden states, W_f represents weight link to the input patterns, and b_f represents the biases at f_t. In addition, it is so significant to regulate new information, which can be saved in the cell state. This step is done via two parts: The input gate layer i_t that decides about the values, which are going to be modernized and temporary cell state layer $\tilde{C}_t$. that produces values of a new candidate in a vector, which can be added to the state (see equations 4 and 5):

$$i_t = \sigma\left(h_{t-1} \cdot U_i + x_t \cdot W_i + b_i\right) \tag{4}$$

Now, i_t, represents the input layer, σ signifies sigmoid activation function at i_t, U_i characterizes weight link to the previous hidden states, W_f represents weight link to the input patterns, and b_i represents the biases at i_t.

$$\tilde{C}_t = \tanh\left(h_{t-1} \cdot U_c + x_t \cdot W_c + b_c\right) \tag{5}$$

Here, $\tilde{C}_t$. is the temporary state layer, σ represents the sigmoid function at $\tilde{C}_t$., $\tilde{C}_t$ is the weight link to the previously hidden states, W_C. presents link connection to the input patterns, and b_C is the biases at . $\tilde{C}_t$.

Following, the new cell state is update using the old cell state as expressed below:

$$C_t = i_t * \tilde{C}_t + C_{t-1} * f_t \tag{6}$$

Thus, the output layer gate o_t is expressed as below:

$$o_t = \sigma\left(h_{t-1} \cdot U_o + x_t \cdot W_o + b_o\right) \tag{7}$$

here o_t represents the output layer, σ represents the sigmoid function at o_t, U_o is the weightlink to previous hidden states, W_0, represents weight link to the input patterns, and b_0 represents the biases at o_t. .Finally, the LSTM output is expressed as follows:

$$h_t = \tanh\left(C_t\right) * o_t \tag{8}$$

Optimizers

Nature has inspired many researchers in many ways to think about their working mechanisms. Because of that, many algorithms are inspired by nature. Based on those mechanisms, many algorithms are developed, such as, particle swarm optimization and biogeography based optimization algorithms (Islam & Murase, 2001). In the most generic term, the main source of inspiration is nature. Therefore, almost all new algorithms can be referred to as nature-inspired. Two optimizers are used in this work, these are:

Biogeography-Based Optimization Algorithm

Biogeography-Based Optimization Algorithm is a new population-based evolutionary algorithm (EA) that was introduced by Dan Simon in 2008 and is based on island biogeography (Meyer & Scheich, 1997). Each island has its own features as simple biotas. Good biotic and abiotic factors in BBO affect the richness of species on any island yet, if the island has many good features, then it will attract more species and good solutions. BBO consists of two operators: migration operator and mutation operator. Each island in BBO represents one solution, if the island has lots of good biotic, the living, such as, diversity of prey, trees, shrubs, meadow, and abiotic non-living like a distance of isolation, wind, temperature, humidity, water, and area factors means that it's a good solution. The purpose of the migration process is to use high ISI islands as a source of modification to share their features with low ISI islands. A mutation is a random event. In nature, the mutation process could happen on one feature or multiple features. Most observed mutations are harmful, like predators from other islands, tsunamis, volcanos, diseases or earthquakes, which are not directed to be useful.

Genetic Algorithm

A Genetic algorithm is one of the search techniques that used in term of calculating to find out true of estimated solutions for optimization and search problems. A Genetic algorithm could be considered as an international search heuristics and those algorithms are a particular class of evolutionary algorithms that use technique inspired by evolutionary biology, such as, inheritance, mutation, selection, and crossover (Mantzaris, Anastassopoulos & Adamopoulos, 2011). The basic components common to almost all genetic algorithms are:

1. A fitness function
2. A population
3. Reproduce chromosome Selection
4. Crossover to produce the next generation of chromosomes
5. Random mutation

The fitness function is the function that the procedure is trying to enhance and it is one of the most essential portions of the process. The term chromosome refers to a numerical value or values that represent a candidate solution to the problem that the genetic algorithm is trying to solve. Each candidate solution is encoded as an array of parameter values, a process that is also found in other optimization algorithms (García, Ortiz & Martínez, 2006). Chosen chromosomes are to create two offspring. The mutation operator randomly flips individual bits in the new chromosomes (turning a 0 into a 1 and vice versa). Naturally, mutation happens with a very low probability, such as, 0.001. Some algorithms implement the mutation operator before the selection and crossover operators; this is a matter of preference. At first glance, the mutation operator may seem unnecessary. In fact, it plays an important role, even if it is secondary to those of selection and crossover. Selection and crossover maintain the genetic information of fitter chromosomes, but these chromosomes are only fitter relative to the current generation.

Methodology

The main steps undertaken to implement the system explained in the methodology. The system is separated into two different neural networks. In the beginning, the MLP is applied to two Data sets (Cancer and Diabetes). BBO and GA optimizations algorithms update the weights and biases. Second, the LSTM applied to the same data sets and the same optimizations algorithms are used to update the weights. The results between two networks and algorithms are compared based on the accuracy rate of results.

Data Collection

In this work, two datasets are used. First, the Wisconsin Breast Cancer datasets from the UCI Machine Learning Repository is used as first data set. The number of attributes that included in the dataset is 32. The attributes are: ID, Diagnosis, and 30 real-valued input feature. This dataset is available at the University of California, Irvine UCI, fetched from UCI Web Portal and downloaded from UCI repository (Mangasarian & Wolberg, 1990b; Mangasarian & Wolberg, 1990b).Second, diabetes dataset for (501 patients) from the local Clinic for DM patients has been collected through different processes like testing and interviewing (Rashid & Abdulla, 2018). 26 variables have been collected for DM patients. Two types of records obtained; the first type is those variables that have units such as Weight (kg), Height (cm), and S.BP (mg/dl). The second type is those variables that logically recorded as 0 or 1. These logically variables are related to some symptoms that DM patients might have felt them, such as, Polyuria, Weakness, Numbness, and Coma. A brief description of these datasets presented in Table 1.

Design and Implementations

Firstly, feed forward MLP network has been successfully applied in diagnosing diabetes as the main object as well as for diagnosing cancer. Secondly, LSTM is applied to overcome long-term decency. Two data sets are used one for Cancer and other one for diabetes. The biogeography based optimization algorithm and Genetic algorithm are used as optimizations methods. The design of this system with

Table 1. Data sets description

Dataset	No. of Attribute	No. of Instance	No. of Classes
Cancer (WDBC)	32	569	2
Diabetes	26	501	2

Figure 5. MLP with optimizer's implementation design

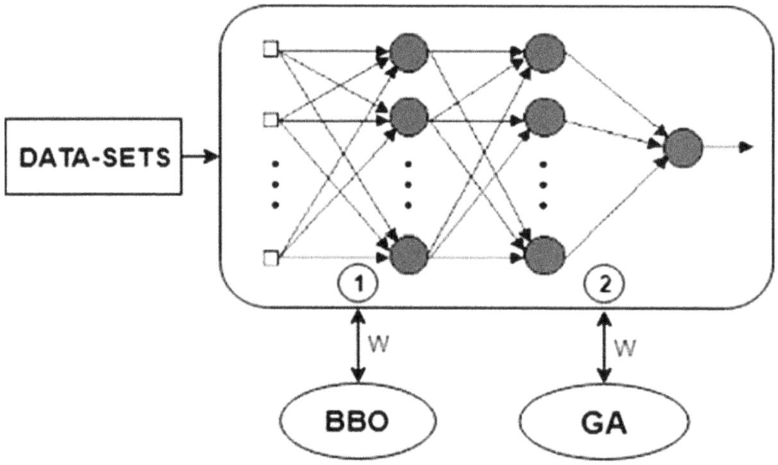

MLP neural networks as well as two optimizations (BBO and GA) and two datasets (Diabetes and Cancer) are shown in Figure 5. Thus, the two models of MLP with BBO and GA are created and labeled as MLPBBO and MLPGA.

The design of this system with LSTM neural networks as well as two optimizations (BBO and GA) and two datasets (Diabetes and Cancer) are shown in Figure 6. Thus, the two models of LSTM with BBO and GA are created and labeled as LSTMBBO and LSTMGA.

The data sets are fed to the networks MLPGA, MLPBBO, LSTMGA and LSTMBBO, then weights and biases are updated to get better accuracy results and less error rate. The results for each data set with different networks and algorithms are differentiated and separated.

Figure 6. LSTM with optimizer's implementation design

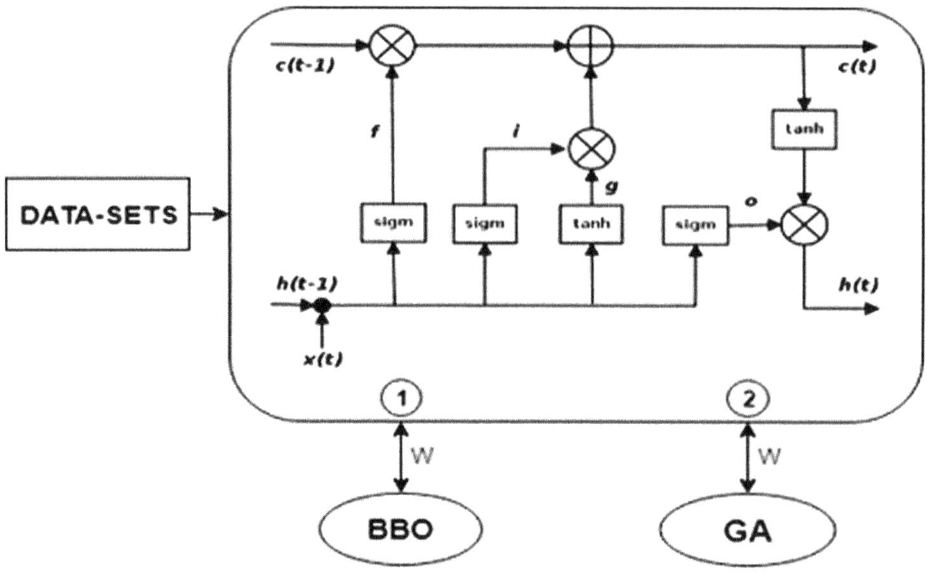

Table 2. Prediction class

Actual Class	Predicted Class	
	Class 1	**Class 0**
Class 1	TP	FN
Class 0	FP	TN

This section demonstrates the main test scenarios that have been conducted. The overall results and tests are further discussed and analyzed. Two test cases carried out, the first test case for MLPGA and MLPBBO neural networks is implemented and second one for the LSTMGA and LSTMBBO artificial neural networks is implemented. As we have explained in data collection that two datasets are used, diabetes and cancer. The two networks and algorithms are tested for all datasets. Results are presented in each stage of the algorithms and networks. For presenting the data, experimental and graphical methodologies are utilized. Confusion matrix is a visualization tool, which is used to show the relationships between outcomes and predicted classes. The accuracy and AUC are based on the confusion matrix.

When making a binary prediction, there are 4 types of outcomes needs to be considered:

1. Consider predicting 0 while the class is actually 0: this is called a True Negative
2. Consider predicting 0 while the class is actually 1: this is called a False Negative
3. Consider predicting 1 while we should have the class is actually 0: this is called a False Positive
4. Consider predicting 1 while we should have the class is actually 1: this is called a True Positive

To get the confusion matrix, we go over all the predictions made by the model see Table 2, and count how many times each of those 4 types of outcomes occurs:

The Accuracy of the system is calculated based on the Equation (9):

$$Accurecy = \frac{TP + TN}{TP + FN + FP + TN} \tag{9}$$

The AUC is an abbreviation for area under the curve. It is used in classification analysis in order to determine which of the used models predicts the classes best. An example of its application is ROC curves. Here, the true positive rates are plotted against false positive rates (Hand, 2009).

The AUC of the system is calculated based on Specify and Sensitivity see equation (10) and (11):

$$Specifity = \frac{TN}{TN + FP} \tag{10}$$

$$Sensivity = \frac{TP}{FN + TP} \tag{11}$$

There are six measuring parameters in this work to measure the performance of networks: True Positive (TP), True Negative (TN), False Positive (FP), False Negative (FN), AUC, and the accuracy rate. The test and results are divided in to two parts: the first part MLPBBO and MLPGA are used on Diabetes data sets. The second part LSTMBBO and LSTMGA are used on two datasets, Diabetes and Cancer. Figures and tables present the test results.

Fitness Function for LSTMBBO to Update the Weights

The pseudocde of fitness function for LSTMBBO to update the weights is presented below:

```
Pseudocode
[
Function FitnessFunctionLSTM(weights) {
Map: = map Vector for LSTM (weights),
Result assigned to LSTM Classify ([Best,MinCost] = BBO(dim,net,inputs,targets))
Return [error rate [result, label]]
 ]
Calculation the optimum solution of BBO
Pseudocode
[
Result BBO assigned to BBO (fitness Function, optimType= [OPTIONS, MinCost,
AvgCost, InitFunction, CostFunction, FeasibleFunction,
MaxParValue, MinParValue, Population] = Init (DisplayFlag, ProblemFunction, Ra
ndSeed,net,inputs,targets,dim)
Optwieghts BBO assigned to resuiltBBO
Print [fitnessFunction[resultsBBO]]
Returen[resuiltBBO]
]
```

Figure 7. Accuracy for MLPBBO and MLPGA on diabetes data set

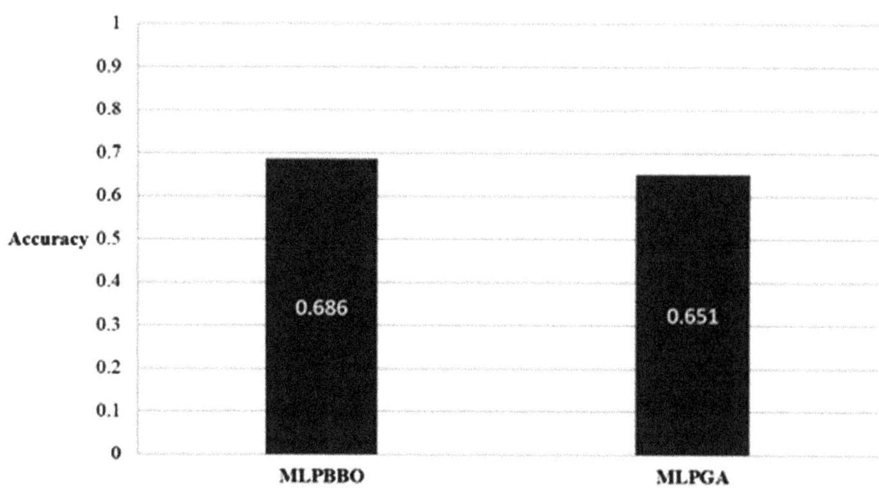

Figure 8. AUC parameters for MLPBBO on diabetes dataset

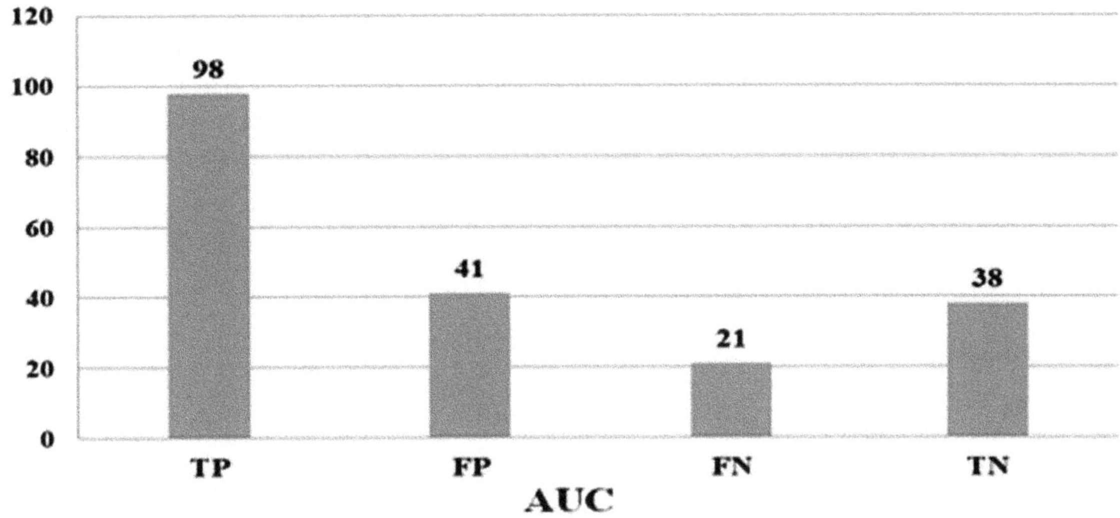

Table 3. MLPs iteration and population detail on diabetes dataset

Algorithms trained on Diabetes	Iteration	Population
MLPBBO	30	500
MLPGA	30	500

Test Results for MLP Neural Networks

The test results are described in the tables and figures below. The MLPBBO and MLPGA neural networks with 30 iterations and 500 populations are implemented on Diabetes data sets as shown in Table 3.

The accuracy rate, which is calculated based on the Equation (9) shown in Figure 7 for MLPBBO and MLPGA for diabetes data set.

The MLPBBO performs better then MLPGA as shown in Figure 7, the MLPBBO scores higher accuracy rate 0.68% while MLPGA is 0.65. The parameters True Positive (TP), True Negative (TN), False Positive (FP), and False Negative (FN), for MLPBBO and MLPGA networks are shown in Figures 8 and 9 respectively were the accuracy and AUC are calculated based on these parameters.

Table 4. MLPBBO and MLPGA classification results

Algorithms	Dataset	Accuracy	AUC	TP	FP	FN	TN
MLPBBO	Diabetes	0.68	0.72	98	41	21	38
MLPGA	Diabetes	0.65	0.69	80	38	17	25

The AUC rate is calculated based on the on the Specify and Sensitivity for MLPBBO is shown in figure 10.

The AUC rate is calculated based on the on the Specify and Sensitivity for MLPGA is shown in figure 11.

The classification results are shown in Table 4. It can be seen from the table, MLPBBO performs better than MLPGA. MLPBBO has higher accuracy and AUC rate with lower error rate, while MLPGA has lower accuracy and AUC rate and higher error rate.

Figure 9. AUC parameters for MLPGA on diabetes dataset

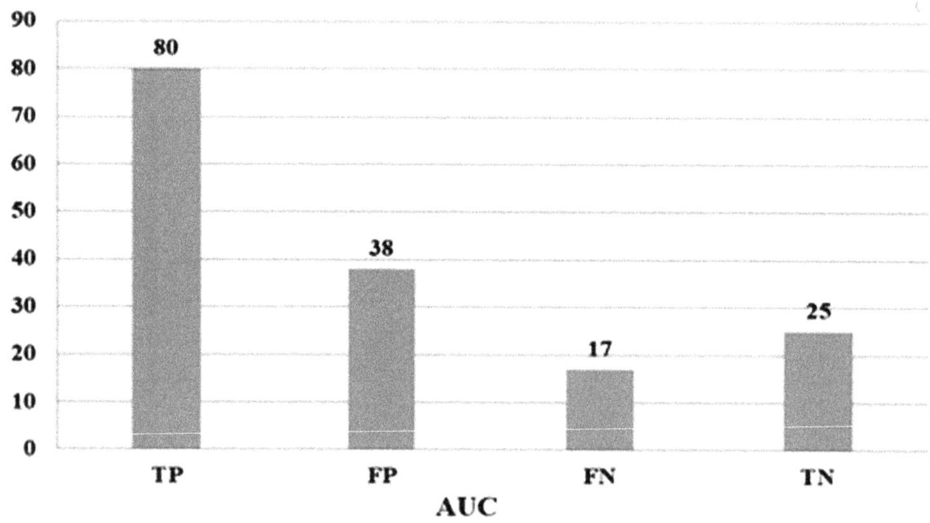

Figure 10. AUC for MLPBBO on diabetes dataset

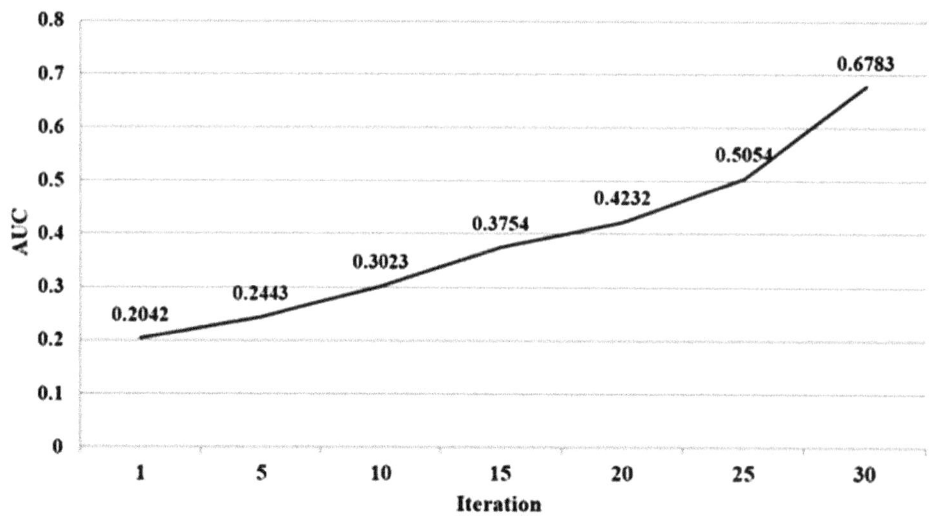

Figure 11. AUC for MLPGA on diabetes dataset

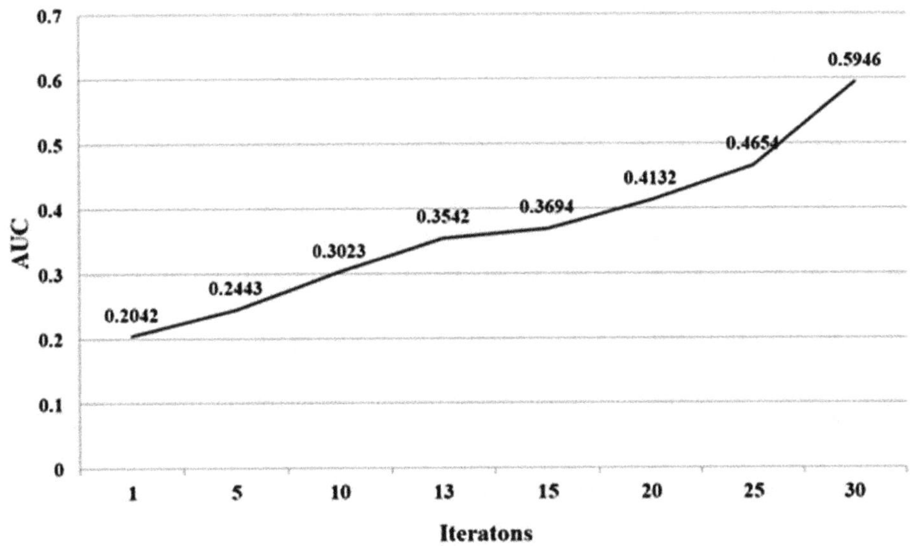

Test Results for LSTM Networks

The test results are described in the tables and figures below. The LSTMBBO and LSTMGA neural networks with 30 iterations and 500 populations are implemented on Diabetes data sets as shown in Table 5.

The accuracy rate, which is calculated based on the Equation (9) shown in Figure 14 for LSTMBBO for Cancer data set, LSTMGA for Cancer data set, LSTMBBO for Diabetes data set and LSTMGA for Diabetes data set. As we can see that LSTMBBO for Cancer data set scores the highest accuracy, which is 0.96, while LSTMBBO for Diabetes data set scores 0.77. At the time, LSTMGA on cancer data set scores 0.95 and for diabetes data set scores 0.72, which is lower than the results or the accuracy of LSTMBBO on the same data sets. That result proves that LSTMBBO performs better than LSTMGA.

The parameters True Positive (TP), True Negative (TN), False Positive (FP), False Negative (FN), for LSTMBBO optimizer for Cancer and Diabetes is shown in Figure 13.

The parameters True Positive (TP), True Negative (TN), False Positive (FP), and False Negative (FN) for LSTM with GA optimizer for Cancer and Diabetes are shown in Figure 14. The accuracy and AUC are calculated based on these parameters.

The parameters from Figure 13 shows that the TP rate for LSTM with BBO is higher than the TP from GA and TN from LSTMBBO also is higher than the LSTMGA, which proves that LSTMBBO performs better than LSTMGA while comparing them which each other. The AUC rate is calculated

Table 5. LSTMBBO and LSTMGA Iteration and population details on diabetes and cancer datasets

Algorithms trained on Cancer and Diabetes	Iteration	Population
LSTMBBO	30	500
LSTMGA	30	500

Figure 12. Accuracy for LSTMBBO and LSTMGA on cancer and diabetes datasets

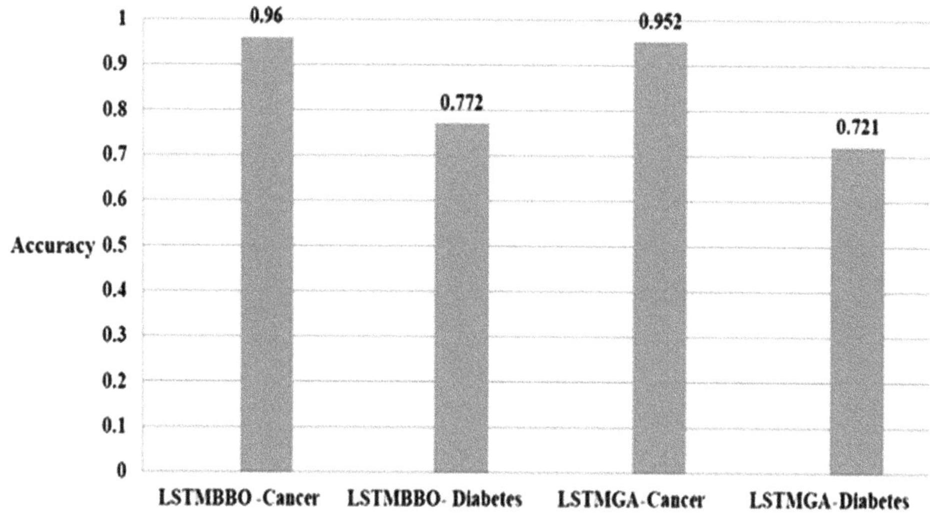

Figure 13. AUC parameters for LSTMBBO on diabetes and cancer dataset

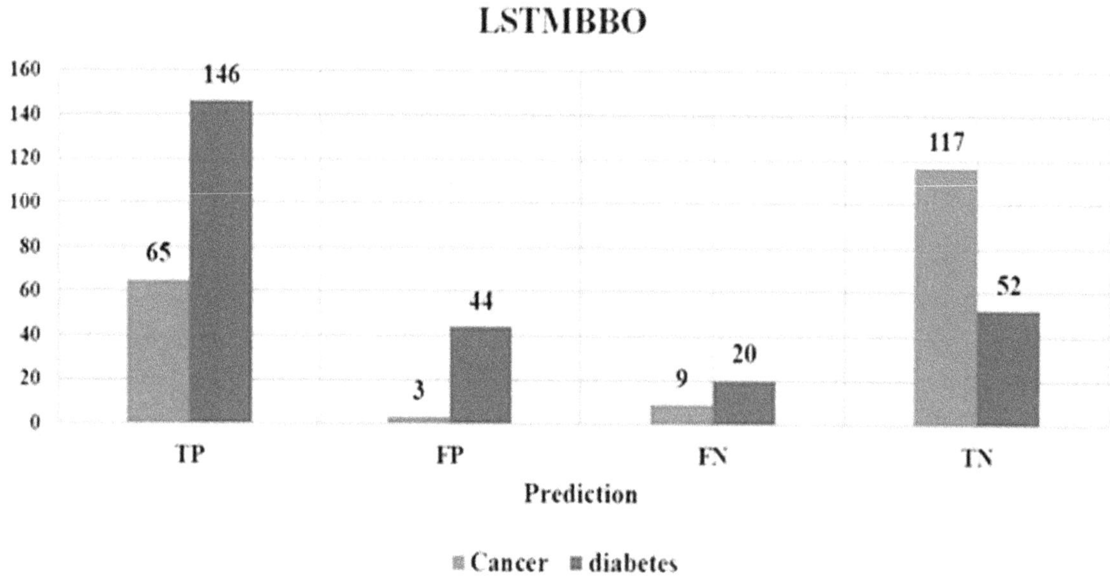

based on the on the Specify and Sensitivity for LSTMBBO for Cancer and Diabetes as well the AUC rate for LSTMGA for Cancer and Diabetes are shown in the figure below.

Figure 15 shows that LSTMBBO for cancer AUC rate is 0.991 while LSTMBBO for Diabetes data set is 0.837. LSTMGA for Cancer 0.972 and LSTMGA for Diabetes are 0.721. These results again proving that LSTMBBO performs better than LSTMGA while comparing their AUC results as shown in Table 6.

Figure 14. AUC parameters for LSTMGA-diabetes and cancer

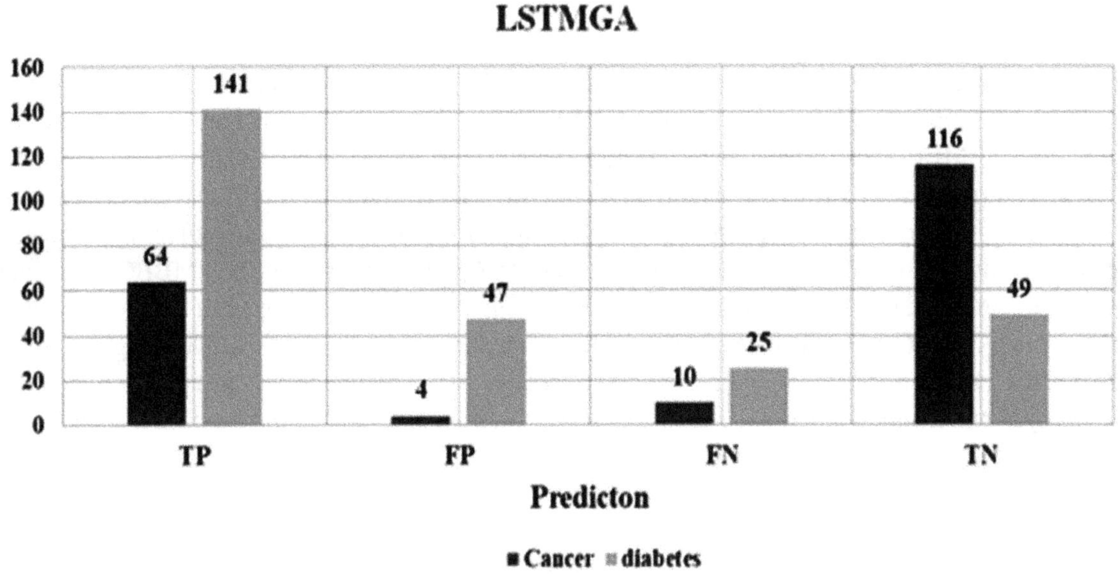

Figure 15. AUC result for LSTMBBO and LSTMGA

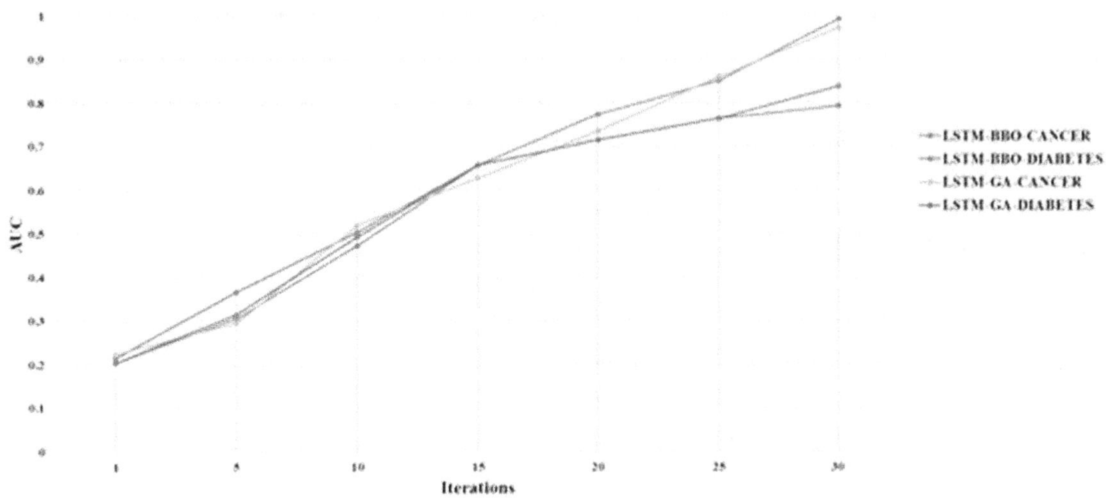

Table 6. Classification results for LSTMBBO and LSTMGA

Algorithms	Dataset	Accuracy	AUC	TP	FP	FN	TN
LSTMBBO	Cancer	0.960	0.99	65	3	9	117
LSTMBBO	Diabetes	0.772	0.83	146	44	20	52
LSTMGA	Cancer	0.952	0.97	64	4	10	116
LSTMGA	Diabetes	0.721	0.79	141	47	25	49

Discussion

The results prove that our proposed methods produce promising results. As shown in Table 5 the accuracy rate for LSTMBBO for cancer data set is 0.96 while the same network with the same data set for LSTMGA accuracy is 0.95. This proves that LSTMBBO performs better than LSTMGA does as well as for LSTMBBO for diabetes data set produces better result than LSTMGA with the same data set. If we compare LSTM with MLP neural networks, we can see significant differences between them from performance and accuracy perspective. LSTMBBO for diabetes data set scores 0.77 accuracy rates higher than MLPBBO with same data set which 0.68 with less error but LSTMBBO takes more time for processing data. The AUC for LSTMBBO is 0.99 for cancer dataset while LSTMGA is 0.97 with the same dataset and for diabetes data set is less. The parameters TP true positive is higher than FP false positive as well as TN true negative is higher than FN false negative for all data sets, which proves that this system with all data sets and classifiers scores promising accuracy and produces a good result.

CONCLUSION

This chapter has proposed problems of MLP and recurrent neural network architectures and proposed LSTM architecture as an alternative to MLP recurrent neural network to deal with problems of learning speed and accuracy due to long-term dependencies. This chapter uses two different optimizers based on Nature Inspired Algorithms, such as, Biogeography based optimization and Genetic algorithm to train LSTM neural networks. Two data sets were used to examine all models, one for Cancer and other one for Diabetes. Same parameters were used for all models. The developed neural network was applied to diagnose the diabetes and Cancer by classifying patients into Diabetic or not diabetic as well as for cancer based on a number of content related features. First, metaheuristic algorithm BBO for training the feed forward neural network with multilayer MLP was used, and Genetic algorithm GA was used to train same network with diabetes data set. The same algorithms were used to train LSTM neural networks with two data sets for Cancer and Diabetes. The developed approach was evaluated and compared with other neural networks trained by Biogeography based optimizations and Genetic Algorithms. After that, the two optimizers were compared based on their accuracy results. The experiments have shown that LSTM in the term of network has better quality results than MLP networks. The experiments showed that LSTM with BBO performed better than LSTM with GA in the term of optimizers; BBO had better result and accuracy. The accuracy for LSTM with BBO was 0.96 while the accuracy for LSTM with GA was 0.95. In the term of the network performance, LSTM produced 0.83 accuracy result with diabetes while MLP produces 0.77 with same data sets. Finally, this chapter has provided a new method for detecting diabetes patients with higher accuracy result by applying LSTM to overcome the problems with MLP and standard RNN with two types of optimization algorithms and two different datasets in the health care field.

The future work for this chapter will include the verification of the BBO and GA algorithm on other types of neural networks and investigating the effectiveness of LSTM and algorithms with larger datasets. Prediction different diseases and diabetes with different data sets and time series data sets using LSTM neural networks could also be considered. Using different algorithms with LSTM such as Harmony Search and Krill heard is also can be one of the important future works.

ACKNOWLEDGMENT

The authors would like to thank University of Kurdistan Hewler (UKH) for their continuous effort and support.

If there is only one funding agency:

This research work is supported by the UKH [UKH 10].

REFERENCES

Aggarwal, R., & Song, Y. (1997). Artificial neural networks in power systems. Part 1: General introduction to neural computing. *Power Engineering Journal, 11*(3), 129–134. doi:10.1049/pe:19970306

Andrej, K., Janez, B., & Kos, A. (2011). Introduction to the Artificial Neural Networks. *Methodological Advances and Biomedical Applications*.

Christopher, O. (2015). *Understanding LSTM Networks*. Retrieved from https://colah.github.io/posts/2015-08-Understanding-LSTMs/

Fukushima, K. (2013). Artificial vision by multi-layered neural networks: Neocognitron and its advances. *Neural Networks, 37*, 103–119. doi:10.1016/j.neunet.2012.09.016 PMID:23098752

García, N., Ortiz, D., & Martínez, C. (2006). An alternative approach for neural network evolution with a genetic algorithm: Crossover by combinatorial optimization. *Neural Networks, 19*(4), 514–528. doi:10.1016/j.neunet.2005.08.014 PMID:16343847

Gregory, H., & Nejhdeh, G. (1998). A self-organizing estimator for hypoglycaemia monitoring in diabetic patients. *20th annual international conference of IEEE engineering in medicine and biology society, 20*(3), 23-29.

Hand, D. (2009). Measuring classifier performance: A coherent alternative to the area under the ROC curve. *Machine Learning, 77*(1), 103–123. doi:10.100710994-009-5119-5

Hochreiter, S., Bengio, Y., Frasconi, P., & Schmidhuber, J. (2001). Gradient flow in recurrent nets: the difficulty of learning long-term dependencies. In S. C. Kremer & J. F. Kolen (Eds.), *A Field Guide to Dynamical Recurrent Neural Networks*. IEEE Press.

Islam, M., & Murase, K. (2001). A new algorithm to design compact two-hidden-layer artificial neural networks. *Neural Networks, 14*(9), 1265–1278. doi:10.1016/S0893-6080(01)00075-2 PMID:11718425

Khaled, E., Osama, B., & Tim, R. (2002). Predicting blood glucose levels in diabetes using feature extraction and artificial neural networks. *International Conference on Information and Communication Technologies*, 18-27.

Mangasarian, O. L., & Wolberg, W. H. (1990a). Cancer diagnosis via linear programming. *SIAM News, 23*(5).

Mangasarian, O. L., & Wolberg, W. H. (1990b). Multisurface method of pattern separation for medical diagnosis applied to breast cytology. *Proceedings of the National Academy of Sciences of the United States of America*, *87*(23), 9193–9196. doi:10.1073/pnas.87.23.9193 PMID:2251264

Mantzaris, D., Anastassopoulos, G., & Adamopoulos, A. (2011). Genetic algorithm pruning of probabilistic neural networks in medical disease estimation. *Neural Networks*, *24*(8), 831–835. doi:10.1016/j.neunet.2011.06.003 PMID:21723704

Meyer, U., & Scheich, H. (1997). Artificial implementation of auditory neurons: A comparison of biologically motivated models and a new transfer function oriented model. *Biological Cybernetics*, *77*(2), 123–130. doi:10.1007004220050373 PMID:9323861

Mohs, R., Wescourt, K., & Atkinson, R. (1973). Effects of short-term memory contents on short-and long-term memory searches. *Memory & Cognition*, *1*(4), 443–448. doi:10.3758/BF03208906 PMID:24214639

Nagai, T. (2000). Artificial neural networks estimate the contribution of taste neurons to coding. *Physiology & Behavior*, *69*(1-2), 107–113. doi:10.1016/S0031-9384(00)00194-3 PMID:10854922

Negrato, C., Cobas, R., & Gomes, M. (2012). Temporal changes in the diagnosis of type 1 diabetes by diabetic ketoacidosis in Brazil: A nationwide survey. *Diabetic Medicine*, *29*(9), 1142–1147. doi:10.1111/j.1464-5491.2012.03590.x PMID:22269058

Nikolic, K. (2015). Stochastic Search Algorithms for Identification, Optimization, and Training of Artificial Neural Networks. *Advances in Artificial Neural Systems*, *2015*, 1–16. doi:10.1155/2015/931379

Park, H. (2006). Part 2: Multilayer perceptron and natural gradient learning. *New Generation Computing*, *24*(1), 79–95. doi:10.1007/BF03037294

Peretto, P. (1992). *An Introduction to the Modeling of Neural Networks*. Cambridge, UK: Cambridge University Press. doi:10.1017/CBO9780511622793

Pradhan, M., Ranjit, & Sahu, K. (2011). Predict the onset of diabetes disease using Artificial Neural Network (ANN). *International Journal of Computer Science & Emerging Technologies, 2*.

Rajeeb, D., Vaibhav, B., Gagan, G., & Barnali, D. (2008). *Application of artificial neural network technique for diagnosing diabetes mellitus. In IEEE Region 10 Colloquium and the Third ICIIS* (pp. 18–23). Kharagpur: IEEE.

Rashid, T. A., & Abdulla, S. A. (2018). A Hybrid of Artificial Bee Colony, Genetic Algorithm, and Neural Network for Diabetic Mellitus Diagnosing. *ARO-The Scientific Journal of Koya University, 6*(1), 55-64. doi:10.14500/aro.10368

Sasakawa, T., Hu, J., & Hirasawa, K. (2007). A brainlike learning system with supervised, unsupervised, and reinforcement learning. *Electrical Engineering in Japan*, *162*(1), 32–39. doi:10.1002/eej.20600

Schmidhuber, J. (1997). Discovering neural nets with low Kolmogorov complexity and high generalization capability. *Neural Networks*, *10*(5), 857–873. doi:10.1016/S0893-6080(96)00127-X PMID:12662875

Schmidhuber, J., Wierstra, D., Gagliolo, M., & Gomez, F. (2007). Training Recurrent Networks by Evolino. *Neural Computation, 19*(3), 757-779.

Shanker, M. (1996). Using Neural Networks to Predict the Onset of Diabetes Mellitus. *Journal of Chemical Information and Computer Sciences*, *36*(1), 35–41. doi:10.1021/ci950063e PMID:8576289

Sietsma, J., & Dow, R. (1991). Creating artificial neural networks that generalize. *Neural Networks*, *4*(1), 67–79. doi:10.1016/0893-6080(91)90033-2

Singh, S., & Sachdeva, G. (2012). Yagi-Uda Antenna Design Optimization for Maximum Gain using different BBO Migration Variants. *International Journal of Computers and Applications*, *58*(5), 14–18. doi:10.5120/9278-3471

Sudharsan, B., Peeples, M., & Shomali, M. (2014). Hypoglycemia Prediction Using Machine Learning Models for Patients With Type 2 Diabetes. *Journal of Diabetes Science and Technology*, *9*(1), 86–90. doi:10.1177/1932296814554260 PMID:25316712

Wang, M. (2005). Extension Neural Network-Type 2 and Its Applications. *IEEE Transactions on Neural Networks*, *16*(6), 1352–1361. doi:10.1109/TNN.2005.853334 PMID:16342480

William, H. W. (1995). General Surgery Dept. University of Wisconsin, Clinical Sciences Center.

Zachary, C., & Lipton, D. (2017). *Learning to Diagnose with LSTM Recurrent Neural Networks.* Cornell University Library.

Zifan, A., & Gharibzadeh, S. (2006). The chaotic nature of temper in humans: A long short-term memory recurrent neural network model. *Medical Hypotheses*, *67*(3), 658–661. doi:10.1016/j.mehy.2006.02.032 PMID:16624500

Chapter 7
Medical Image Segmentation and Analysis

Ramgopal Kashyap
Amity University – Chhattisgarh, India

ABSTRACT

An improved energy-based technique with a Lattice Boltzmann method organizes with the neighborhood and global energy terms, local term propels to pull the frame and constrain it to protest limit, decides noteworthy points of interest not confined to, snappy planning, automation, invariance of exact medical image segmentation, and analysis. Consequently, the worldwide vitality fitting term drives the advancement of the frame at a division of the question limit. The worldwide vitality term relies upon the worldwide division computation, which can better catch drive information of pictures than mixture area-based dynamic shape technique. Both neighborhood and worldwide terms are ordinarily acclimatized to construct a level set strategy to divide pictures with exactness. The level set technique with Boltzmann system uses neighborhood mean, a quality which engages it as far as possible. The proposed chapter gathers gainful purposes of intrigue not stuck just using expedient process, computerization, and right helpful picture partitions.

INTRODUCTION

The programmed division is extremely a testing assignment it's as yet an unsolved issue for most medicinal applications because of wide assortment associated with picture modalities, encoding parameters, and natural fluctuation. The manual division is repetitive and each now and again not appropriate in the clinical schedule. Therefore, self-loader division techniques which require end client collaboration utilized as a part of occasions where programmed calculations fall flat. A wide assortment of self-loader division strategies exists that will generally be grouped into voxel-based techniques, where the end client attracts seed things to characterize fore and foundation voxels and surface-based strategies, where decent protest is reproduced relying upon forms or subject models (Drapikowski & Domagała, 2014). Picture division can without much of a stretch continue on three different ways, physically, intelligent, self-loader and programmed. The division is the route toward allotting a photo into semantically

DOI: 10.4018/978-1-5225-7796-6.ch007

interpretable regions. The inspiration driving division is to weaken the photo into parts that are critical concerning a particular application. Picture division is usually used to discover articles and points of confinement like lines twist in pictures. The result of picture division is a course of action of territories that all in all cover the entire picture, or a game plan of structures removed from the photo. Each one of the pixels in a locale is near concerning any trademark or handled property, for instance, shading, power, or surface. Coterminous regions are on a very basic level phenomenal with respect to a comparative trademark. Division subdivides a photo into its constituent areas or things. That is, it sections a photo into indisputable locale that are planned to relate immovably with things or features of eagerness for the photo. Division can similarly be seen as a methodology of gathering together pixels that have practically identical characteristics. The level to which the subdivision is passed on depends upon the issue being comprehended. That is, the division should stop when the objects of eagerness for an application have been separated. There is no explanation behind passing on division past the level of detail required to recognize those parts. The methodology divides picture pixels into non-covering areas with the ultimate objective that: Each zone is homogeneous i.e. uniform similar to the pixel characteristics, for instance, constrain, shading, range, or surface.

Segmentation Concept

To understand the concept using mathematical representation here{Ri} is a segmentation of an entire image R if:

1. R=j=1nRj the union of all regions covers entire R
2. Ri∩RjFor all i and j, i≠j there is no overlap of the regions
3. P (Ri) for i = 1, 2... n, P is the intelligent consistency predicate characterized over the focuses in set Ri
4. 4. P (Ri∪Rj)=false, for i and j and Ri and Rj are neighboring districts.
5. Ri is an associated area, I = 1, 2... n All pixels must be relegated to areas. Every pixel must have a place with a solitary locale as it were. Every area must be uniform. Any combined match of nearby districts must be non-uniform. Every district must be an associated set of pixels.

A few Predicate Examples

1. P(R) =True, if |g(x1, y1) – g(x2, y2)|<=ε for all(x1, y1), (x2, y2) in R
2. P(R) =True, if T1<=g(x, y) <=T2 for all (x, y) in R where T1and T2are thresholds that define the region.
3. P(R) = True if |f (j,k)-f(m,n)|≤ Δ and false otherwise

Where (j,k) and (m, n) are the coordinates of neighboring pixels in region R. This predicate expresses that an area R is uniform if (and just if) any two neighboring pixels contrast in dim level of no more than Δ.

4. P(R) = True if |f(j,k)-μR|≤ Δand false otherwise

Where f (j, k) is the gray-level of a pixel with coordinates (j, k) and μR is the mean gray level of all pixels in R. All pixels must be doled out to locales. Every pixel must have a place with a solitary locale as it were. Every locale must be uniform any blended combine of nearby locales must be non-uniform and every locale must be an associated set of pixels.

Classifications of Segmentation

Manual Segmentation

The pixels on a similar force cluster could physically be discussed; however, obviously, this is an exceptionally tedious strategy on the occasion the picture is huge. A superior decision is dependably to check the forms of the articles. This may be done discretely through the console, giving higher precision, yet little speed or it might be finished with the specific mouse with higher speed yet less exactness. The manual procedures all have in like manner the measure of time spent in following the things, and HR are exceptionally expensive. Following calculations can likewise use geometrical figures like ovals to close the limits of the items. This has been completed a lot of therapeutic reasons, however, the approximations may not be great (Siegel, 2014). Intelligent division of restorative pictures has been explored by Olabarriaga and Smeulders. As to division errands, both self-loader and intuitive alludes to calculations that require some type of client input. From the perspective, intelligent division (Olabarriaga & Smeulders, 2001) differs from the self-loader division from the part of the individual and therefore from the algorithmic necessities, particularly concerning the calculation times in addition to the interface utilized with respect to the human-PC communication.

In qualification to self-loader division, an intuitive division puts the individual into a basic part all through the division undertaking. At the point when it's in self-loader divisions the individual information is commonly helpful for reinstatement of some programmed calculation, in intuitive division, the division is normally an iterative procedure where brief answers are created from each client contribution to display the client a chief criticism on the impact produced by the calculation in light of the present parameters got from the info information. This enables the individual to assess the impact and to specifically respond to it. As a final product, an intuitive division calculation must be sufficiently quick to permit such a constant recommendation (Naegel & Passat, 2014). An outstanding illustration, only for this class of division calculations in 2D will be the live-wire calculation. Other than the as of now examined necessities, the procedure associated with intelligent division also postures prerequisites for the perception of cutting-edge novice comes about and for the human PC communication, that happens to be both fundamental to have a natural and productive utilization of an intuitive division strategy.

Automatic Segmentation

The completely programmed division will be hard to execute because of high intricacy and variety of pictures. Most calculations need to have exactly from the earlier data to execute the division, and for a way to be programmed, this from the earlier data must be accessible to the specific PC. They required from the earlier data could, for example, be clamor level and the likelihood of the articles having a selective dissemination (Huang & Pun, 2015).

Table 1. Difference between semi-automatic and interactive segmentation method

Criteria	Semi-Automatic	Interactive
Division process	Fire and overlook	Iterative
Role of client	Instatement and parameterization	Controlling and adjusting
Manipulation/Input	Direct or aberrant	Indirect
Execution prerequisites	Direct	Quick (constant reaction)

Semiautomatic Segmentation

Self-loader division consolidates the utilization of both manual and programmed division by giving some underlying data in regards to the structures; to continue with customized strategies. Intuitive picture divisions attempt to locate the "brilliant way" between completely programmed picture division and completely manual client drawing (Ryba & Zelezny, 2015). They all endeavor to adjust between the client's capacity to determine to start insights and the PC's capacity to naturally entire them. Dynamic forms strategies permit the client to draw an underlying shape that must be either completely typified by a protestor to completely encase the thing. The "in or potentially out" decision was made in the specific execution since all clients have to a great degree "swell terms inciting speed" that is pre-intended to be either positive or maybe negative (Panin & Knoll, 2006). Drawing the hidden shape can be viewed as giving "free bits of knowledge" on the count. If an individual needs to offer specific shape guides he has no possibility to get toward doing accordingly Table 1 is demonstrating the distinction between self-loader and intuitive division.

Motivation

In medicinal imaging research, the division is by and large the first step which permits later quantitative measurements, conclusion, and fixes arranging, and displaying in regards to anatomical structures. Medicinal imaging advancements, similar to CT, MRI notwithstanding PET, have been generally given to different restorative strategies. Contrasted with ordinary restorative determination, they highlight a non-obtrusive yet great approach to research the interior structures and activities of human figures. With the assistance of such innovation, specialists can obtain multi-dimensional data like 2-D cuts, 3-D volumetric pictures on the locale of intrigue, which encourages the general execution of both subjective notwithstanding quantitative examination. This examination supplies significant data for finding and in addition careful arranging subsequently may soothe the agonies to the patients to some degree. Therapeutic picture division is normally the initial step of most examination systems effectively expressed. It is additionally a significant advance that decides a last consequence of the full application since different examination completely depends upon the information out of this progression. For example, to assemble a type of 3-D volumetric model from various medicinal pictures, division in 2-D pictures should be as exact as is conceivable; something else, the measure of the recreated model will presumably not be right, and representation of this model will potentially (Kashyap & Tiwari, 2018). A resulting restorative control and examination step sometimes incorporate measurement, enlistment, creation, and PC supported the finding. Return for capital invested every so often incorporate mind, bone houses, vessels, delicate tissues, and so forth. Therapeutic picture division assumes a critical part for instance, in the use of cardiovascular conclusion, offered the division with respect to cardiovascular tissues all through continuous cuts, volumetric models of the heart and circulatory system can be remade by just displaying the blood flow inside, specialists can pinpoint one's heart issue and measure the hazard quantitatively (Kashyap & Gautam, 2017). Perception with respect to the heart can furthermore help specialists in making evaluations. The division with the different organs or tissues is imperative to restorative choice makings, such since infection classification notwithstanding ailment hazard examination. The division comes about to give the establishment notwithstanding essential for center around the partition, highlight expulsion, and quantitative rating. Moreover, contemporary therapeutic imaging methods like CT, MRI, and PET frequently have a lot of pictures which create medicinal imaging research a dull and battle. In this way, it is important to create unsupervised picture examination techniques all through medicinal pictures. Aside from this intelligent approach with quick preparing is additionally required for handling restorative pictures. The work can be roused by the prerequisite to offer unsupervised, right and strong picture division techniques all through routine clinical circumstance.

Challenges in Medical Image Segmentation

As of late, different medicinal picture division approaches have been and numerous significant changes have been gotten. Be that as it may, because of weaknesses in medicinal services imaging frameworks, restorative pictures can contain distinctive assortments of ancient rarities. These ancient rarities can influence the item information and perplex the pathology. A few ancient rarities can be alleviated by the attractive imaging innovation and some require post control. In clinical research, the normal wonders made are clamor, power inhomogeneity, and fractional volume impacts that happen to be considered as the open issues in restorative picture division (Kashyap & Gautam, 2015). There are various systems to section a photograph into areas which may be homogeneous. Not every one of the strategies is appropriate for therapeutic picture examination as a result of many-sided quality and mistake. There's no standard picture division method that may deliver palatable outcomes for all imaging applications like mind MRI, cerebrum disease analysis et cetera. Ideal determination of highlights, tissues components are thought of as principle confinements for mind picture division. Exact division in abundance of the full field of view is interference (Ahirwar, 2013). Administrator heading and manual thresholding are by and large different hindrances to portion cerebrum picture. Amid the division treatment confirmation of advantages is another reason for trouble

Picture division will be the issue of expelling frontal area objects from the foundation in a picture. It is among the most key issues in PC vision and has intrigued numerous inquiries about consistently. As the simple use in PCs increment over the long haul, solid picture division is required in more application, in the mechanical, restorative and furthermore individual fields. Completely programmed division keeps on being an open issue due to a wide assortment of conceivable articles' blend, thus evidently the utilization of human "clues" is unavoidable. Intelligent picture division gives in this manner turn out to be increasingly well known among inquiring about these days (Dimitriou & Delopoulos, 2013). The objective of the intelligent division has removed the object(s) from the foundation in an exact way, utilizing client information in a way that requires negligible discussion and insignificant answer time. This proposition will unquestionably begin by portraying general procedures to arrange division approaches, proceeds with a careful overview of existing form-based intelligent picture division systems, and ends by presenting a radical new consolidated altering and furthermore division apparatus (Gao, Kikinis, Bouix, Shenton & Tannenbaum, 2012). Picture division is a vital issue with picture examination alongside picture understanding. It is additionally a basic issue of PC vision and example acknowledgment. The Active Contour Models (ACM) are the best strategies in picture division and the basic thought of ACM is to advance a bend as illustrated by some specific imperatives to extricate the required protest. These common dynamic shape models are ordered as an edge based and district-based the two kinds have their extraordinary paybacks and negatives, and the decision between them to use in applications is dictated by the distinctive attributes with the pictures (Aitfares, Bouyakhf, Herbulot, Regragui & Devy, 2013). The model forms an edge based capacity utilizing picture edge realities, which can produce the shape on the protest limits (Feng, Li, Gao, Yan & Xue, 2016). The edge-based capacity in accordance with the picture slope can investigate the correct impediments, for the pictures with extreme clamor or perhaps a powerless edge. Then again, a district-based model uses measurable data to build up a locale, ceasing capacity which could stop the form of advancement between particular areas (Zhao, Liang, Wu & Ding, 2017). Contrasted with the edge-based model this model can improve the situation for pictures with obscured closes. The district based model isn't touchy to the introduction of the level set capacity and can perceive the question's limitations (Zhang, Wen, Xu & Meng, 2016). Locale based models are favored for picture division since they give change over the edge based model in a couple of perspectives, it has constraints. The normal area-based models which are in parallel pictures with the supposition that each and every picture locale can be homogeneous, don't work splendidly for pictures with force inhomogeneity and it is touchy to the primer form and the developing bend might be caught into provincial minima (Li, Jiang, Shi & Li, 2015).In the expansion, the Chan-Vese (CV) strategy isn't reasonable for speedy preparing on the grounds that, in every emphasis, the standard powers inside and past shape should wind up being figured, which enhances the calculation time. The exemplary district based models which are in the parallel pictures, don't work successfully if the objective picture contains power inhomogeneous locales in it (Kashyap & Piersson, 2018a). The neighborhood parallels fitted demonstrates by implanting close-by picture data and can fragment pictures with power inhomogeneity which is significantly more precise rather than arranged systems. The basic thought is to present the Gaussian part work, in spite of the fact that it partitions well the pictures with power inhomogeneity. It got high computational time unpredictability (Zhuang, Dierckx & Zaidi, 2016). Subsequently, the division process takes a critical time contrasted with old division systems. Zhang a functioning form strategy roused by local image fitting (LIF) vitality, which gives same division, comes about and contains less time multifaceted nature contrasted with LBF model (Li, He, Chunli & Hongjie, 2017).

Noise

Commotion is frequently atypical marvel inside therapeutic pictures in the greater part of the imaging systems using x-beam or gamma photons, most by far of picture clamor is produced by the arbitrary qualities on the photons circulated inside the picture, this is by and large assigned quantum sound. Extreme commotion can undoubtedly significantly influence the sharpness of the pictures it can cover and moderate up the deceivability of specific highlights inside the picture, in this manner affect the division impacts. Some prominent techniques for general answers for clamor evacuation strategies in PC vision are recorded inside Table 1. These sorts of strategies can productively lessen clamor, however various despite everything them have space for development. For instance, the anisotropic nonlinear dispersion filtering is normally ground-breaking in limiting clamor inhomogeneous places and diminishing the diffusivity in the edges of a picture, be that as it may, the cycle measure of the anisotropic dispersion demonstrate is obscure.

Figure 1. Left image: MRI image with noise, right image: Improved MRI image

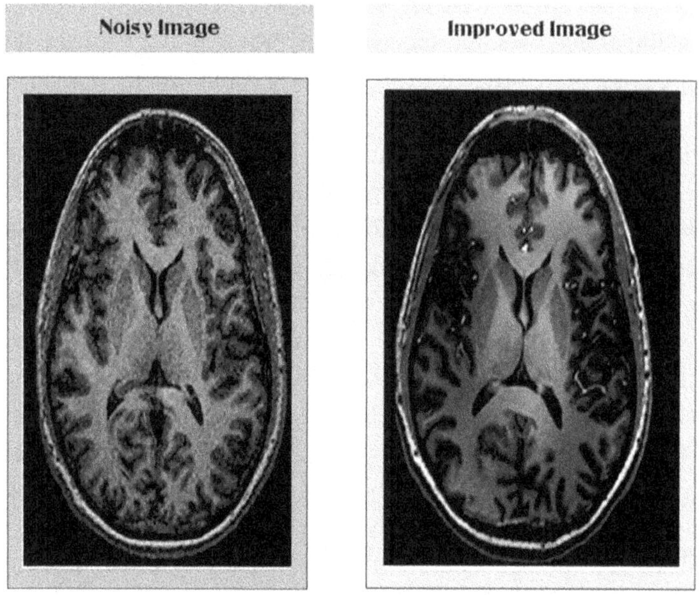

The value regarding pixels is updated using the weighted average with the samples where the actual neighborhood is similar to the neighborhood with the current pixel. On the off chance that the cycle number is generally huge, the edge will be significantly obscured. On the off chance that the emphasis number is typically little, the commotion will be held. In this manner, the anisotropic dissemination model could be enhanced by routinely assessing the time number. Therapeutic pictures tend to endure much significantly more clamor than reasonable pictures to do the character of the securing gadgets. This clearly postures awesome inconveniences to any photo division strategy (Kashyap & Piersson, 2018b). So clamor can diminish and numerous gadgets raise the part volume that is, for the most part, they normal procurement with a thick cut. This (among different reasons) realizes obscuring the edges between the articles, which settle on choices, hard for programmed gear (Cui & Fan, 2018). Figure 1 demonstrates a case of MRI with clamor and without having a commotion, the expulsion of clamor is critical for restorative picture division.

Intensity Inhomogeneity

Force inhomogeneity is perceived as a smooth spatially differing perform which adjusts the quality inside initially homogeneous districts. The regular pattern of thickness inhomogeneity inside MRI is caused by the inclination field. The Bias field flag is regularly a low recurrence and furthermore smooth flag that will degenerate MR pictures, particularly those made by old MRI gadgets. Picture handling calculations like division, surface examination or even classification that use dim level costs of picture pixels wouldn't create attractive impacts. A pre-preparing step can be right for the inclination field sign before submitting hurtful MRI pictures for such calculations. Figure 2 demonstrates a case of MR picture with and without the predisposition field. Contrasted and the ordinary

Figure 2. Presence of intensity inhomogeneity in medical images

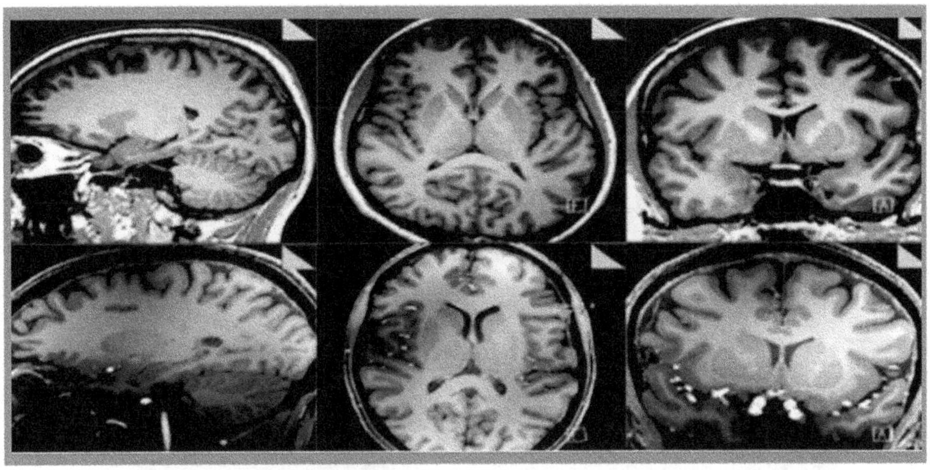

MR picture, the center segment of the thickness inhomogeneity picture is darker contrasted with the encompassing regions that are regularly misclassified as an extra piece of tissue. Subsequently, the added substance predisposition field should be evacuated as an approach to enhance the division precision (Caponetti, Castellano & Corsini, 2017) some current intensity inhomogeneity is recorded inside Figure 2.

SIGNIFICANCE OF THIS CHAPTER

The utilization of PC supported conclusion strategies to enhance how much restorative treatment has turned into an interesting issue all through medicinal imaging notwithstanding indicative radiology examination. A few division strategies happen to be in this particular theory. The requirement for this postulation is reflected inside after angles. Medicinal pictures regularly consolidate unwanted ancient rarities, including commotion, thickness all through homogeneity and incomplete volume impacts. In spite of the fact that a considerable measure of division techniques in which, the precision and vigor of the division come about typically are not tasteful, when managing restorative pictures having significant commotion, feeble edges, and inhomogeneity, notwithstanding incomplete volume results. Some division procedures still have a region for development. Also, the examination of helpful pictures can be a bleak and complex errand just in light of the way that it usually incorporates a considerable measure of data. Thusly, more correct, overwhelming and unsupervised division philosophies than existing frameworks should be. The prior learning, for instance, surface, territory, appearance, and estimate, et cetera inside remedial picture examination can essentially streamline the division errand. Some clinical data in the remedial space may very well be brought into the particular division figuring, like the general anatomical kind of the inquiry, the particular characteristics of different imaging gear, the assignment of dull level estimations of the assorted tissues, and the spatial geometric nostalgic association between different tissues.

Figure 3. Segmentation results of GOGAC method for microarray images

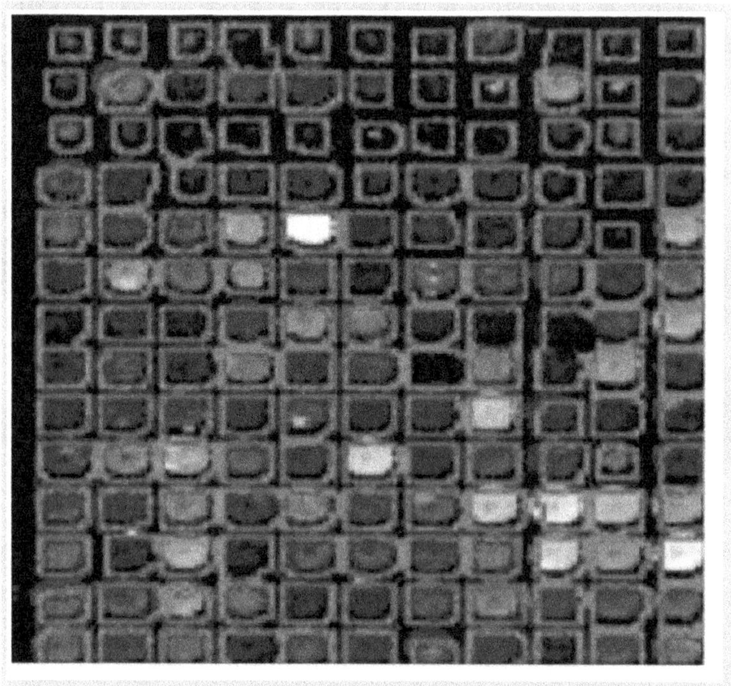

Aims and Objectives

Correct Segmentation

Picture division perseveres with incorrect results, various procedures have been made for overhaul comes to fruition, yet a couple of systems put aside such a lot of time for estimation and some methodology gives over divided comes to fruition. The Globally Optimal Geodesic Active Contour (GAC) is one if the best procedure in light of imperativeness, yet it stuck in neighborhood minima and gives erroneous results. Here microarray pictures have pulled in much thought because of the disappointment of making precisely isolated spots (Waoo, Kashyap & Jaiswal, 2010). Figure 3 shows the real division result picture obtained while using the GAC. In the occasion that divided result will be erroneous and it will be given for help examination of the photo, by then no doubt it will give wrong results since it will impact the whole method like information extraction, examination, estimation, and evaluation (Jones, Xie & Essa, 2014). The point is to improve and precise outcome with the goal that the right investigation must be produced through division.

Interactive Segmentation

Intelligent picture division includes little client communication to incorporate client expectation for the division procedure and is likewise a functioning exploration zone these days since it can do agreeable division comes about that is unattainable by the real best in class programmed picture division calculations. This proposal considers the indistinguishable issue of in what capacity can intelligently portion a type of forefront questions out from its encompassing capabilities. The objective ought to be to build up an astute picture division strategy with instruments that let clients to intelligently division with a little measure of natural communications. Here the issue with conventional strategies is each time, the technique gives diverse outcome as a result of the introduction of form area is extraordinary and it gives wrong investigation result. The other target is to build up a successful division strategy which is autonomous from the choice; it will diminish the many-sided quality of the techniques (Jones, Xie & Essa, 2014). A decent intelligent picture division strategy requests are: (1) given a reasonable client input, the calculation should deliver instinctive division that reflects anybody purpose; (2) the calculation ought to be proficient all together that it can give immediate visual criticism.

Fast Segmentation

Picture division will be the front phase of various works in impression handling, for example, protest arrange pressure in light of these sorts of necessities, a great impression division calculation must have the accompanying around three focal points: (1) rapidly quick, (2) great condition availability, and (3) great condition coordinating. The spot developing technique gives great division comes about, yet the quickness is moderate. The k-implies and the watershed techniques are quick, however, needs enhancements by correlation; the strategy can accomplish the objectives related to high productivity and additionally better execution too. The outcome related with k-implies is divided and in addition pack, the sectioning result will squander an exorbitant measure of an asset for all of us to record these limits. The strategy exploits inside the k-implies and these watershed techniques inside the framework unwavering quality period (Peng, Zhu & Wang, 2016). In any case, should state the trustworthiness is more regrettable contrasted with the locale developing technique. The picture fragmenting calculation as the front-organize preparing related with picture pressure and that is the quick quickness, the great appearance network of sectioning result, and the great condition coordinating.

Positron Emission Tomography

PET is regularly an imaging methodology about diagnosing and finding the phases of different sorts of growth, including lung, mind, and neck, heart and cerebrum this is the atomic medication picture determination strategy that makes a three-dimensional realistic or picture with respect to utilitarian process procedures.

In any case, the patient could be infused with isotope tracer the irregular tissues assimilate the tracer for the higher rate in correlation with ordinary tissues, creating tracer focus higher in unhealthy tissue. Next, the positron outflow happens in the occasion the proton-rich isotope (Unstable Father or mother Nucleus) rots. A Proton rots with a Neutron, a Positron or a Neutrino. In the wake of voyaging a shorter separation (3-5mm), the positron offered experiences an electron from the encompassing condition. Next both the particles converge and additionally "destroy" 1 an alternate, emanating γ beams in inverse ways every which can be gotten because of γ camera. At last, the PC recreates the radioactivity into the 3D image of body or zone alongside past ordinary tracer take-up the PET image is given in Figure 4 like alternate sweeps, may PET outputs quantify cell level metabolic changes happening in an organ or tissue. This gives PET leverage over different advancements in deciding if sores frameworks are considerate or may be harmful, disposing of the need for careful biopsies on the off chance that PET outputs more

Figure 4. Demonstrates the PET framework

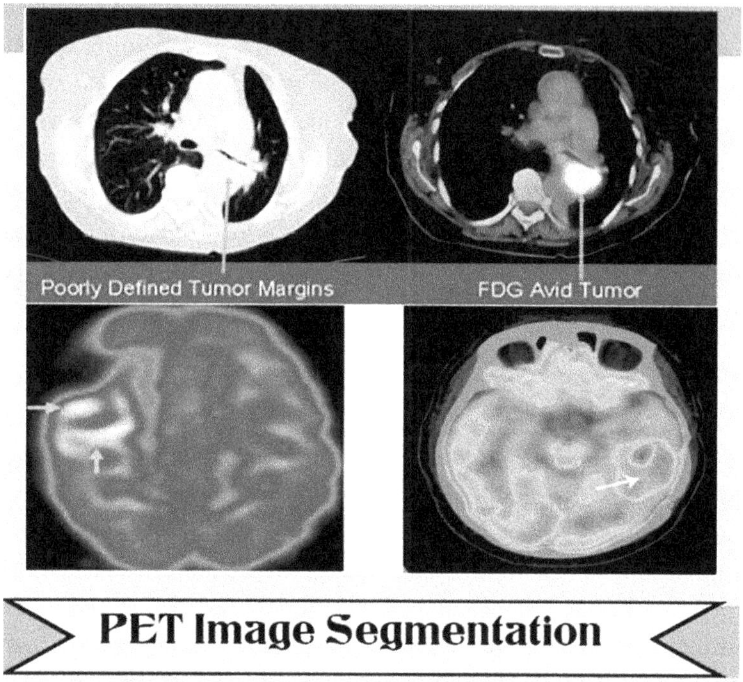

often than not are negative (Wilson, Coleman & Turkington, 2011). In supplement, PET can analyze ailments at their soonest organizes, since infection forms regularly center on practical changes in the cell level. CTs or MRIs, generally, can't perceive alterations until the point that infirmities begin to cause changes in the structure of internal organs or tissues. A PET compass is routinely used close by a MRI or possibly a CT yield to show a whole three-dimensional perspective of the organ and the zone of infection inside that organ. Nowadays, mix of PET and MRI as for treatment masterminding has become noteworthy thought.

Energy-Based Image Segmentation Method

A champion among the most predominant essentialness based model which has been viably used as a piece of twofold phase division with the supposition that each photo region is verifiably homogeneous. Regardless, the CV shows does not work splendidly for the images with constrain inhomogeneity. These and Chan extended their work to utilize multiphase level set abilities to address various territories. These models are known as the piecewise consistent (PC) models (Ogorodnikov, Sereseva and Kargapolova, 2016). Regardless, both the CV and the PC models have the disservice depicted beforehand. In order to divide pictures with drive inhomogeneities, Vese and Chan and Tsai two near models, which are called piecewise smooth (PS) model. In any case, these strategies are computationally inefficient. The LBF (local binary fitting) model, which uses the nearby picture data as imperatives, can well section objects with force inhomogeneities. Besides, LBF display has preferred execution over PC and PS models in division precision and computational proficiency. A novel ACM demonstrate that can be utilized to fragment pictures with power inhomogeneities it uses the neighborhood picture data to build a LIF vitality

Figure 5. Stages of image analysis process

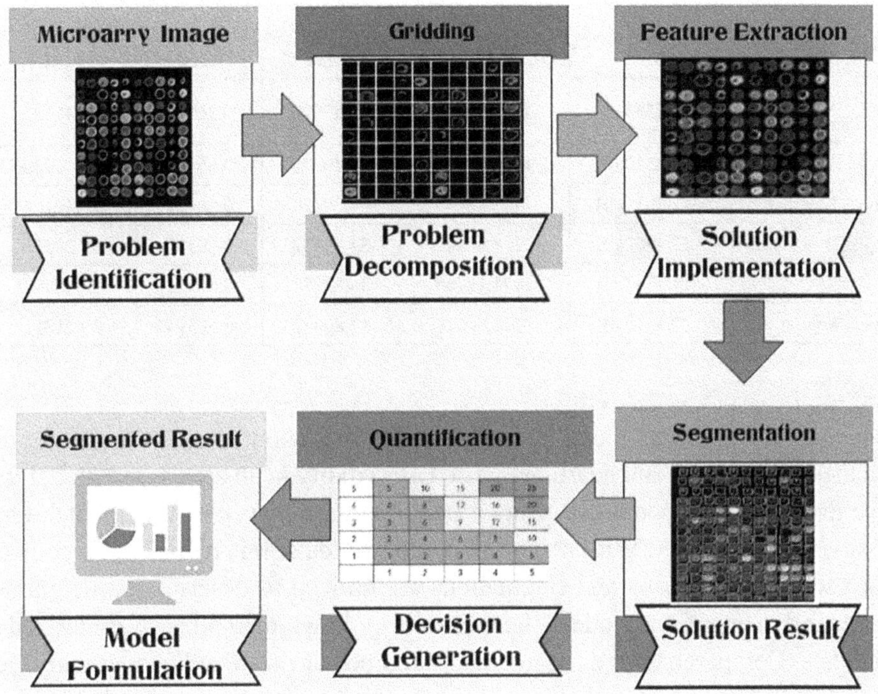

work (Miao, Huang, Zhou, Wang & Liu, 2018), which can be seen as a requirement of the contrasts between the fitting picture and the first picture. Moreover, a novel strategy is utilized to regularize the level set capacity by utilizing Gaussian bit sifting. Also, re-introduction isn't required in the strategy. The intricacy investigation and exploratory outcomes demonstrate that the strategy is more effective than the LBF display while yielding comparative outcomes. The LBF demonstrate by installing the nearby picture data can portion pictures with power inhomogeneities and is significantly more productive and exact than the PS method. The fundamental thought is to present a portion work in this work, a novel dynamic shape demonstrate driven by the LIF vitality utilitarian has less computational intricacy than the LBF vitality practical (Juneja & Kashyap, 2016). A novel level set technique in light of Gaussian separating was utilized to execute the variational plan, and the test comes about uncovered that it isn't just vigorous to keep the vitality work that ascertains the qualities and stuck in nearby minima yet in addition equipped for moving the level set capacity normal. An analysis showed that the enhanced technique can accomplish fulfilling division comes about as the LBF display, yet it is considerably more effective. It ought to be called attention to that the Gaussian regularizing level set method (Feng & Jiang, 2010) can be effortlessly reached out to unadulterated PDE driven LSM, stages of microarray image analysis process is given in Figure 5.

The novel dynamic shape display inside a variational level set recipe for impression division and target confinement. They consolidate LIF term and in addition a worldwide impression fitting term to drive the shape development. This composes can effectively portion pictures alongside force inhomogeneity utilizing the shape beginning anyplace in the impression. This compose is executed by level set technique, which can dispose of the prerequisite associated with the statement. The test comes about showed that model has preferable execution over the CV model and LIF display. They affirmed its adequacy in dif-

Table 2. Image error measurement comparison of method with geodesic dynamic contour, globally optimal geodesic active contour, local binary fitting model, local region model, and local intensity fitting model

S.N.	Method	PSNR	MSE	RMSE	UIQI	MAE	SNR
1.	Geodesic Active Contour	+17.6535 dB	1124.92733	33.53994	0.56134	29.42330	-8.66585 dB
2.	LBF	+17.4329 dB	1183.54933	34.40275	0.56484	29.41930	-8.65918 dB
3.	Proposed Method	+17.4611 dB	1175.88649	34.29120	0.58922	29.19164	-8.59064 dB
4.	LIF	+17.4502 dB	1178.84548	34.33432	0.60389	29.28552	-8.60989 dB
5.	GOGAC	+17.4787 dB	1171.12769	34.22174	0.57231	29.48097	-8.65585 dB
6.	Local Region	+17.3310 dB	1211.65018	34.80877	0.56594	29.21311	-8.62334 dB

ferent engineered pictures and real pictures, and the test comes about method its points of interest with respect to exactness, capability, and heartiness. The LBF vitality in an area based model for more exact and productive division. The model draws upon neighborhood power implies, which empowers it to adapt to intensity inhomogeneity. With neighborhood power data, this model can recoup protest limits precisely both nearby force means and fluctuations are utilized to describe the neighborhood power conveyance in their dynamic form models, the local energy-based method is characterized observationally in their models. Comparable types of neighborhood power mean and changes are Mumford Shah model. The intuitive Segmentation utilizing an irregular walker will be more probable in achieving the seed with the last advances, and in this way, it may maintain a strategic distance from division spillage and contracting inclination. It displays the best strength to seed amount, yet minimal vigor to seed position contrasted and the diagram cuts and arbitrary walker calculations, yet every one of these techniques is tedious and a portion of the strategies is not ideal for the precise division of the medicinal pictures. The enhanced GOGAC division comes about were tried on pictures from the microarray database by Stanford University. Here utilized the human fringe blood mononuclear cell pictures. The fragmented outcomes are hearty on account of right division, especially for those spots whose pixels are outside the divided locale and, here found these outcomes are extremely powerful for precise picture examination.

PSNR esteem for the technique is higher than every one of the strategies in the underneath table acknowledge geodesic dynamic shape strategy and the lower estimation of the MSE and RMSE indicates less blunder and the estimations of UIQI and MAE has demonstrated that the strategy is better. Pearson connection coefficient fortifies the relationship between pixels that is higher than the all analyzed technique as found in Table 2 (Kashyap & Gautam, 2017).

The approach conquers the issues of off-base division and intensity inhomogeneity with the current strategies (Ali, Rada & Badshah, 2018) the method can't require more client connection; the approach is roused by a natural vision for the enhanced division for restorative pictures. The trial comes about it has been watched that general execution is superior to the traditional level set methods to deal with manage power inhomogeneity and diminishes time, vigorous and amend result within the sight of clamor and pitifully communicated spots and pictures. The procedure shows a marked separation workability to discard the need related with re-presentation and regularization are fruitful under the noteworthy power inhomogeneity issue and contains better results which have a use other technique. It utilizes each edge and the spot information to section a photo into no covering spot and in perspective of thought to stop the bend. It is associated with new region subordinate SPF reason that uses the particular picture neighborhood information gained while using the LBF imperativeness method by displaying this SPF work (Li, He, Chunli & Hongjie, 2017) in perspective of adjacent picture fitting (LIF). This orchestrated approach will section pictures close by inhomogeneity and MR pictures to exhibit the relentless quality, practicality, and intensity of the estimation. Locale based ACM is decisive balances the signs from the weight drive inside and past the form and handles pictures with various powers inside the forefront. In addition, it can be vigorous to part clamor and gives high productivity alongside quick meeting. This model is ordinarily hearty to shape will stop the improvement close, maybe keeping in mind the end goal to frail sides. Inside offered strategy, the specific advance with the form introduction that moves as indicated by the interior and outer energies in the picture and moves shape (Eun, Jung & Park, 2017). This exploration work the picture utilizes the usefulness and advances toward areas to remove the protest limits utilizing picture data like edge, edges and power estimation of the picture. In this part, the force estimation of the pictures assumes critical part during the time spent precise outcome for that group mid esteem is computed for the introduction of the shape. To move the specific level set inwards, numerous individuals figure the indoor sub locale, including zero level, needs utilizing $\phi > 0$. This SDF fulfills the attractive property $|\nabla I| = 1$. The activity useful (ϕ) hard circles the zero phases set toward completed limits (Jiang, Feng & Gao, 2011). Keeping ϕ pre-customized and limiting the power E with respect to $c1$ and $c2$, it disposes of the need of introduction that is computationally extremely expensive. Regularization utilizing Gaussian bit gives better smoothing outcomes with no vitality spillage when contrasted with the zone smoothing alongside the acknowledgment.

The adjusted SPF work consolidates another SPF usefulness, which utilizes veil term keeping in mind the end goal to authorize level set up development. It characterizes the signs in the weight powers and district of enthusiasm for the request to form contracts when clear of articles and extends when in the question. This gives without parameter division encompassing, requiring negligible purchaser intercession. Clearly depend worldwide mean inside and far from the shape as inside the C-V display simply isn't adequate to level power conveyances demonstrated the pictures to develop to be sectioned have frontal areas seen as more mind-boggling toughness disseminations. To beat this test, here presented the correct worldwide middle or maybe a worldwide mean inside vitality term for being limited (Ali, Badshah, Chen, Khan & Zikria, 2017). The model may overcome the restriction around the C-V demonstrate in regards to the symmetry on this power syndication, which isn't exactly in almost all genuine pictures. Specific Binary alongside Gaussian choice regularized sum set uses what's so incredible about both GAC chooses C-V plan (Kashyap, Gautam & Tiwari, 2018). In the real substitution of edge halting usefulness, an area based signed pressure function (SPF) has moved toward becoming created and this SPF work to control the particular bearing of movement. Inverse signs about the limits on the thing in this performance make the necessities to skilled to grow when it is inside the real limit and therapists when it's outside the genuine limit.

Comparison Regard to Effectiveness and Accuracy

In this part, examination between the real technique with a few division approaches the first was dynamic forms without edges in regards to picture division, the second one wound up being Active contour as per the local Gaussian dispersion displayed, the third one wound up being Active contour driven by neighborhood picture fitting vitality in addition to the last one was a level set strategy within the sight of force inhomogeneities exhibited. Figure 6 demonstrates the outcomes for segmentation of started from

Figure 6. Contour initialization and regularization using energy-based method

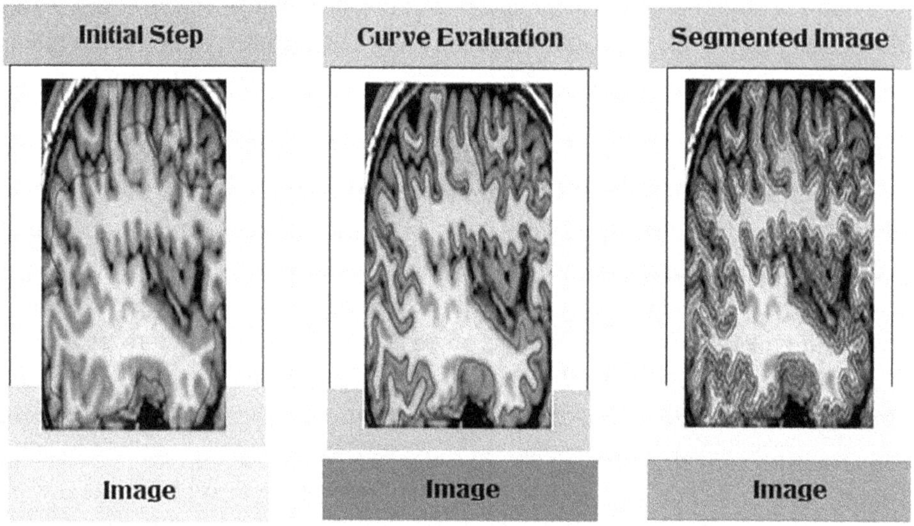

contour initialization and curve evaluation from that point on bend movement steps are exhibited not long after adequate advanced, got an area of intrigue and the approach can be uncovered.

Comparison in Terms of Speed and Accuracy

In this part, the examination of the system with CV methodology, Improved CV, neighborhood picture fitting essentialness; a level set technique with inclination revision. Each one of the CPU time is open in Table 4. For quality and precision, it very well may be seen how the methodology gives better result stood out from Chan Vese, updated Chan Vese, local image fitting imperativeness system, and level set procedure control inhomogeneities whatever the shape and the circumstance of the basic twist. The resulting changes with the entire basic frame and you should run the figuring so you can pick the best result; along these lines, this strategy can't be used, made arrangements for exact and authentic division, CV show uses territory information and considered as a champion among the most used models for division (Chen, Huang & Chen, 2013). One of the various discernible parts of the CV shows is which

Table 3. Comparison of method with improved CV and LBF method

	Time Elapsed 40 Iterations (Time in Seconds)		
Images	**Improved CV**	**LBF**	**Proposed Method**
Brain Image	42.2570	42.9964	6.95209
Test Image	276.0517	433.7730	5.36582
Vessel Image	30.1480	42.6795	3.43219
MRI Image	128.7563	173.875	3.15436
ART Image	73.05454	115.525	14.53183

it performs well for the photos having feathery without closes. In any case, being an obstruction, your CV technique Table 3 is demonstrating a correlation among CV and LBF strategy constantly accept picture having power homogeneity, the area picture fitting methodology gives the best possible result.

It is required to run the specific calculation more than once so as to pick the most helpful outcome; in this manner, these strategies can't be utilized in regards to exact alongside appropriate division, CV method utilizes spot data alongside considered among the most utilized models with respect to the division. Among the noticeable properties of the CV method in which it performs well for the pictures alongside fluffy or without parameters, However, the specific CV demonstrate dependably assumes the specific picture alongside power homogeneity, nearby impression fitting procedure gives the suitable outcome yet the technique is speedier, comparison of global energy-based method with local energy-based methods are given in Figure 7.

Energy Based Method With Lattice Boltzmann Method

The issue of intelligent picture division is the common utilization of little frontal area or foundation seeds from clients to extricate the forefront district. One noteworthy issue with current calculations for intelligent division utilizing their preference of the bounding box which covers the protest which is to be sectioned. The strategy will make client characterized jumping boxes with outside vitality that assess the division comes about. To process the fit box to the ground-truth frontal area and marginally enlarge it by 5% of the aggregate pixels in the all headings and to take it as the bouncing box alongside vitality and grow this jumping box as indicated by the required vitality in the ways and in the wake of performing crash and gushing the jumping box will give exact outcome, choice of the question won't subject to the positioning client will get same outcomes from choosing anyplace in the picture this is the signature accomplishment of the technique (Izham, Fukui & Morinishi, 2014). This is for intuitive catching of pictures and better division comes about and an intelligent caught picture for quick preparing that is done through utilizing computational liquid progression systems for therapeutic picture division with a few

Figure 7. Comparisons between the methods using local energy and global energy

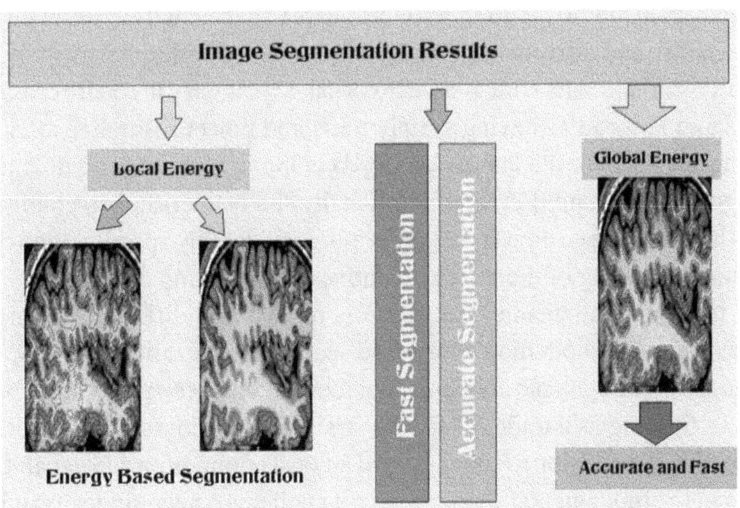

Figure 8. Energy-based method using partial differential equation for energy minimization

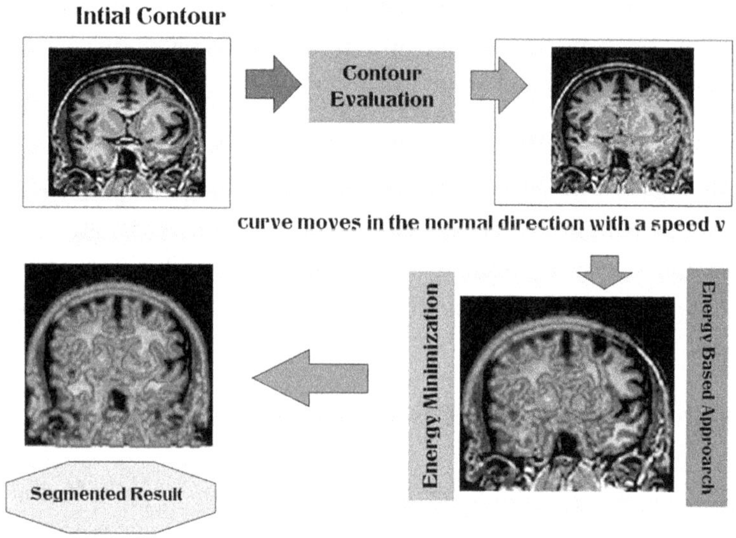

alterations Figure 8 is showing accurate segmentation process by an energy-based method with energy minimization that uses partial differential equation.

The cross-segment Boltzmann technique has been made from the help of quantifiable mechanics as a nice choice numerical methodology for showing physical ponders in fluid streams. Rather than the standard numerical plans, for instance, restricted qualification system and unpleasant segment method use normally noticeable conditions for planning. The essential room starts stacked with particles while the second room starts empty from the physical point of view, the Boltzmann strategy can be interposed as an amplifying focal point for fluid mechanics while a telescope for sub-nuclear movement and it has been successfully associated for the coupling of sub-nuclear components in the tiny world and fluid stream in the clearly unmistakable. The fundamental idea behind cross segment gas automata is that moment interchanges of fake particles living on the minute network can provoke the relating distinguishable conditions to delineate comparative fluid streams. In the midst of the correspondence, which is containing crash and expansion or spouting with cross area speeds, lattice symmetry accept a key part in saving mass and vitality and also ensuring the jaunty power security.

The foremost lattice gas automata with 4-cover rotational symmetry in square cross segment was made by Hardy, de Pazzis and Pomeau achieving simply mass and power insurance after that the hexagonal symmetry was satisfactory to save the dapper vitality keeping in mind the end goal to recuperate spread condition, reaction scattering condition, and additionally the Navier-Stokes conditions (Amrouche & Rejaiba, 2015) and the two-arrange nine speed show it is considerably speedier than the standard models with linearization and unraveling of the effect executive in Boltzmann condition .

The noteworthy test with Boltzmann system is it is particularly difficult to achieve higher than the second demand of exactness for both momentary and spatial discretization plus, because there are more allotment limits than the hydrodynamic elements to screen, it can't keep up a vital separation from the for the most part genuine figuring as a trade off for the straightforwardness. In the procedure, a cushioned outside power is affecting the division to snappy, solid against commotion and capable whatever the position or the condition of the fundamental shape it can get challenges unequivocally. It has, first the upside of the fuzzy c means (FCM) which controls the propelling curve through the cooperation level of the

Figure 9. The velocity vector of the model with two dimensional vectors

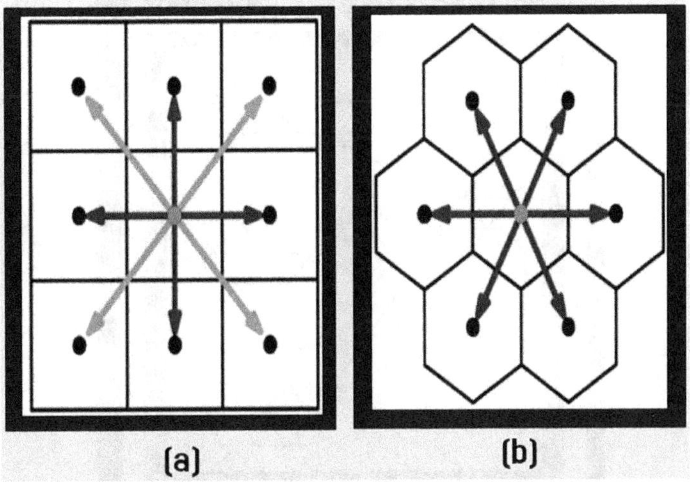

present pixel, second, the advantages of the imperativeness based procedure is that it is self-sufficient of topological contrast fit as a fiddle, size, and presentation of the dissent and, third, the purposes of intrigue are it extraordinarily sensible for parallel programming as a result of its neighborhood and unequivocal nature. The peculiarity of the methodology lies first in the treatment of division. Here made two moves up to the customary system: "iterative estimation" and "perfect breaking point condition" that decreases the customer relationship for a given nature of result and brisk division. Incidental points of confinement recommend that an atom which leaves the system at one edge will restore the structure at the opposite edge with hard restricts, the direct of a fluid got in a box is reproduced, while with infrequent cutoff points, it is the lead of a fluid in an irregular system which is mirrored. It is regularly possible to join as far as possible, for instance by having hard vertical breaking points on opposite sides and infrequent cutoff points on the other two. Power can be reenacted in the method self-assertively changing some particle speed toward the power with a given probability. Each one of these rules known, it is possible to play out a proliferation. The plainly visible energy can be found by a comparable normal of the hubs' force. The cross-section vectors in the display are c1 = (1, 0), c2 = (1/2, $\sqrt{3}/2$), c3 = (−1/2, $\sqrt{3}/2$), c4 = (−1, 0), c5 = (−1/2, −$\sqrt{3}/2$) and c6 = (1/2, −$\sqrt{3}/2$) these are appeared in Figure 9.

A hexagonal framework grants two possible goals for a head-on crash which protect both mass and power, sketched out in Figure 9. This is novel in connection to the HPP show, where there is only a solitary possible assurance, which is to occur, is picked aimlessly for each effect, with make back the initial investment with probability. In light of this stochastic part in the model, it isn't any longer totally deterministic and does not have adequate vitality reversal property of the 4 speed. As indicated, it very well may be resolved that the technique gives a direct according to the incompressible Navier-Stokes conditions. From the determination, one can demonstrate that the kinematic thickness of the framework must be

$$\text{V}= \frac{\Delta x^2}{\Delta t}\left(\frac{1}{2\rho\left(1-\rho\frac{\rho}{6}\right)^3}-\frac{1}{8}\right) \tag{1}$$

Figure 10. The head-on collision rule for the model

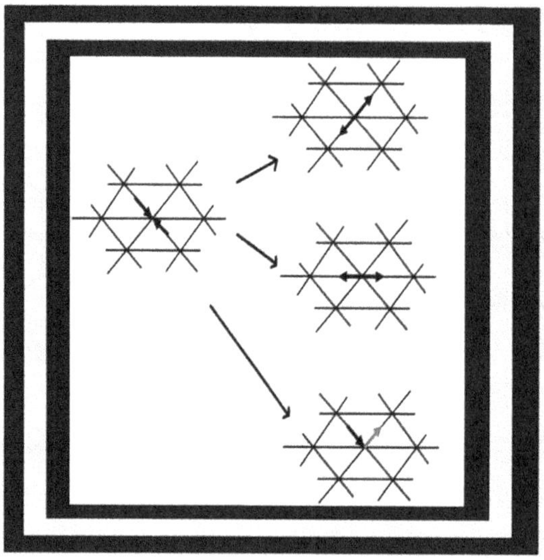

where ρ is the balance thickness of the gas, this can be found as the normal molecule thickness of the whole framework. To see from this condition the consistency can turn out to be discretionarily huge in the breaking points $\rho \to 0$ and $\rho \to 6$, showing no particles in the framework and a most extreme number of particles in the framework, separately. The insignificant consistency for the model is discovered when $\rho = 3/2$.

Assortments exist in the display the extra crashes are presented the show is basically the Lattice Boltzmann method and dynamic shape demonstrate (Beneš & Kučera, 2015) with a difference in the cross section and the impact rules. Along these lines, it holds every one of the benefits of the customary model, for example, little storage room requests, correct flow, and parallelism. It expels the most basic inconvenience, that of the inalienable anisotropy of the customary model, giving a conduct predictable with the incompressible Navier-Stokes conditions given in Figure 10. The issue of factual clamor remains

Figure 11. The method of collision handling

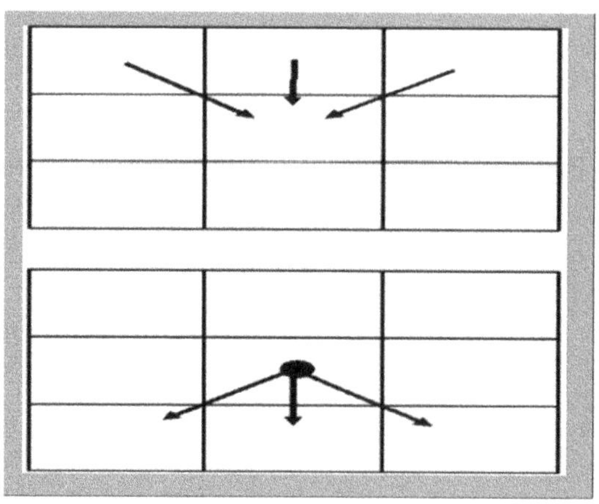

Figure 12. The computational node and boundary calculation

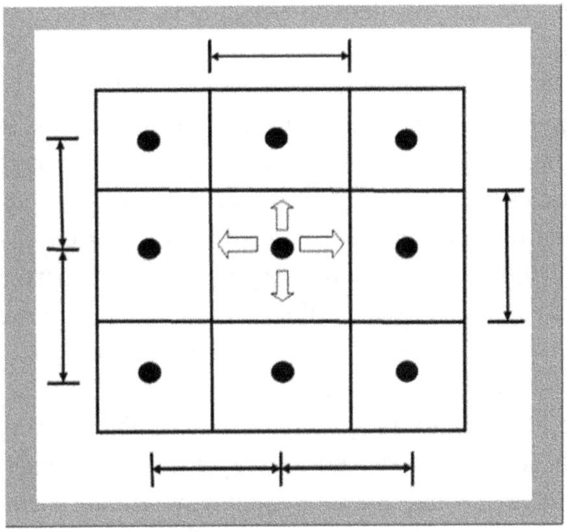

this is a general issue when endeavoring to recuperate naturally visible amounts from minute extension reenactments, as the infinitesimal framework is liable to arbitrary changes that vanish in as far as possible. Then again, if the subject of intrigue is concentrating such changes in genuine frameworks; this measurable commotion is a coveted property.

An essential property the technique holds from its cross-section gas progenitors is a region in each progression given over, every hub is refreshed independently from the others on account of this parallelism can accomplish and the strategy can use the same number of processors as there are hubs in the lattice. Nothing has been said yet in regards to the issue of beginning conditions and collision handling criteria is given in Figure 11. Constrained volume system subdivided space into little control volumes that are known as cells through the cross section and the system depicts the cutoff points of the control volumes while the computational center at the point of convergence of the control volume and the important insurance is satisfied accurately completed the control volume. The net change through the control volume restrain is the total of the integrals over the four control volume faces (six out o 3D). The control volumes don't cover and the estimation of the integrand isn't open at the control volume faces and is directed by contribution.

The Periodic edges go about as if they are related with the opposite edge of the structure. If the left and right edges of a system are infrequent, a particle spread which streams left at the left edge of the structure will return at the right edge, heading left. In a 2D structure, the left, right cutoff points or conceivably the best base breaking points can be irregular.

Figure 12 demonstrates the computational hub and limit condition, neighboring center points across over discontinuous breaking points. An incidental farthest point regularly induces that the structure is discontinuous. This can be needed in circumstances where a discontinuous lead is inspected, for instance, the spread of a plane sound wave in a channel, where the length of the structure makes back the initial investment with the wavelength (Krithivasan, Wahal & Ansumali, 2014). The other fundamental cross-segment Boltzmann confine is the hard divider, which reflects particles back and guarantees a non-slip condition with zero speed at the divider. There are two minor takeoffs from this method, the on-network or full-way ricochet back system and the mid-structure or halfway weave back procedure. In these two procedures, certain center points in the system are separate as dividers and are appropriately not a bit of the fluid.

The particle dispersals in divider centers are not easygoing towards balance and don't go about according to the cross segment Boltzmann headway condition. The on-system strategy is the less demanding of the two procedures. In the accident adventure of the cycle, where the fluid center points are easygoing, each one of particles' headings is pivoted with the objective that the particles are sent back toward the way they started from. The accident step is balanced for the divider center points; be that as it may, the spilling step is unaltered. In the mid-organize strategy, particles which are set to stream into a divider center point are reflected instead of spilled. Here, the spouting development is changed while the effect step proceeds as previously. In both skip back procedures, the reasonable position of the divider is completely the divider center points and the fluid centers close-by it. This can be seen, for instance by taking a gander at the mid-arrange system is somewhat more difficult to execute than the on-network procedure, yet the mid-structure methodology gives a better exactness that is the inspiration than use mid-cross section dividers amid the time spent a system are incidental, an atom flow which streams left at the left edge of the structure will return at the right edge, heading left (Wang, Shu and Yang, 2016). In a 2D structure, the left-right points of confinement, and also the best base breaking points, can be intermittent and hard divider the method which reflects particles back and guarantees a non-slip condition with zero speed at the divider. There are two minor takeoffs from this methodology, the on-lattice or full-course ricochet back strategy and the mid-system or halfway skip back procedure. In these two strategies, certain centers in the system are separate as dividers and are in this way not a

Figure 13. Lattice Boltzmann method eliminating partial differential equation for fast segmentation

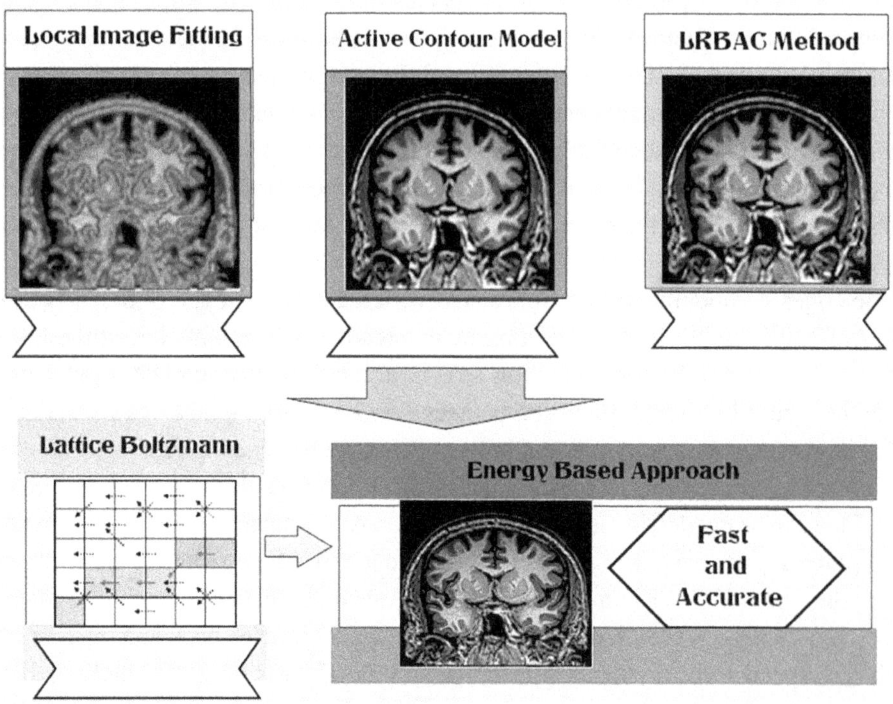

bit of the fluid. The particle allotments in divider center points are not easygoing towards balance and don't go about according to the lattice Boltzmann improvement condition. The on-organize procedure is the less unpredictable of the two techniques. In the accident advance of the cycle, where the fluid center points are easygoing, each one of particles' headings is pivoted with the objective that the particles are sent back toward the way they began from. The accident step is changed for the divider center points, yet the spouting development is unaltered. In the mid-arrange system, particles which are set to stream into a divider center point are reflected as opposed to spouted. Here, the spilling step is balanced while the accident step proceeds as previously. In both ricochet back systems, the intense position of the divider is altogether the divider centers and the fluid centers bordering it Figure 13 is demonstrating the technique with the cross section Boltzmann strategy for quick division of pictures.

This is physically appropriate in light of the fact that solid dividers have a satisfactory disagreeableness to keep any smooth development parallel to the divider. Furthermore, the uttermost cells that delimit the space are separate as breaking point cells with the weave back condition. In the midst of their revive, these telephones still anticipate that entrance will cells that are outside of the territory, which is the implied spirit cells. To avoid one of a kind treatment for those cells another layer of point of confinement cells is put around the region (Wang, Shu & Yang, 2016). Regardless, the additional layer of farthest point cells are not set up in a framework Boltzmann step, they simply exist to avoid a special treatment for as far as possible cells. In this way, all the LBM figurings can be adequately enlivened on the GPU; body forces can be added to the LBM as an outside commitment to control the stream direct.

EXAMINATIONS AND RESULT ANALYSIS

The trail fragment is depicted in two areas; the underlying section shows the precision and the comfort of the methodology by differentiating it and the regular imperativeness based techniques the second part epitomizes the limit of the procedure with respect to speed and capability. In the use of the methodology, the estimation of the feathery parameter is set to three, and Convection coefficient is kept at 0.08. Every one of the techniques has been executed utilizing Matlab R2014b introduced on a PC Pentium(R) Dual-Core CPU E5500 processor with a clock speed of 2.80 GHz and 2 GB of RAM.

Examination in Terms of Effectiveness and Accuracy

In this part, examination of the technique with four division strategies is given. The first was dynamic shapes without edges presented by T. Chan and L. Vese et al. (Kang, Kim, Lee, Shin & Shin, 2014) for picture division, the second one was presented by Kaihua Zhang et al. (Zhang, Song & Zhang, 2010), the third one was presented by Li et al. (Li, Zeng, Xu, Chen & Yan, 2016) and the last one was presented by Chunming Li, et al. (Wang, Zhang, He, Chang & Yang, 2015).To analyze that the technique gives the best division comes about it gives cease and effective question limit. The technique by Chen et al. Furthermore, the strategy by Li et al. both are not succeeding in light of the fact that because of the feeble edges distinguishing proof. The strategy by Huihui Song et al invest more energy in the emphasizes, moreover, the subsequent forms show numerous discontinuities The technique by Li et al. gives over divided outcomes and takes additional time; it is hence less strong than the strategy, and besides, the nature of the division utilizing the technique is powerful to commotion and gives the best outcomes.

Table 4. Pearson correlation coefficient comparison of the method with geodesic active contour, globally optimal geodesic active contour, local binary fitting model, local region model, and local intensity fitting model

S.N.	Method	Pearson Correlation Coefficient	
		Original Image vs Noisy Image	Original Image vs Original Image
1	Local Intensity Fitting	30051.00372	34981.00000
2	Geodesic Active Contour	29633.67067	34981.00000
3	Local Binary Fitting	29735.21324	34981.00000
4	GOGAC	29769.78693	34981.00000
5	Local Region Model	29843.18299	34981.00000
6	Proposed Method	30192.33511	34981.00000

Comparison in Terms of Speed and Efficiency

In this part, connection of the system with the outstanding CV method, improved CV, close-by picture fitting methodology, upgraded level set procedure with inclination amendment and the technique. All the CPU times are appeared in Table 3. Concerning and precision, it tends to be seen that the methodology gives ideal result over the Chan Vese, upgraded Chan Vese, adjacent picture fitting essentialness procedure and level set system, whatever the shape and the circumstance of the hidden frame the result

Figure 14. Demonstrates the segmentation results of medical MRI and CT images of the human body (a) Using the active contour method. (b) Shows the segmentation result using Boltzmann method

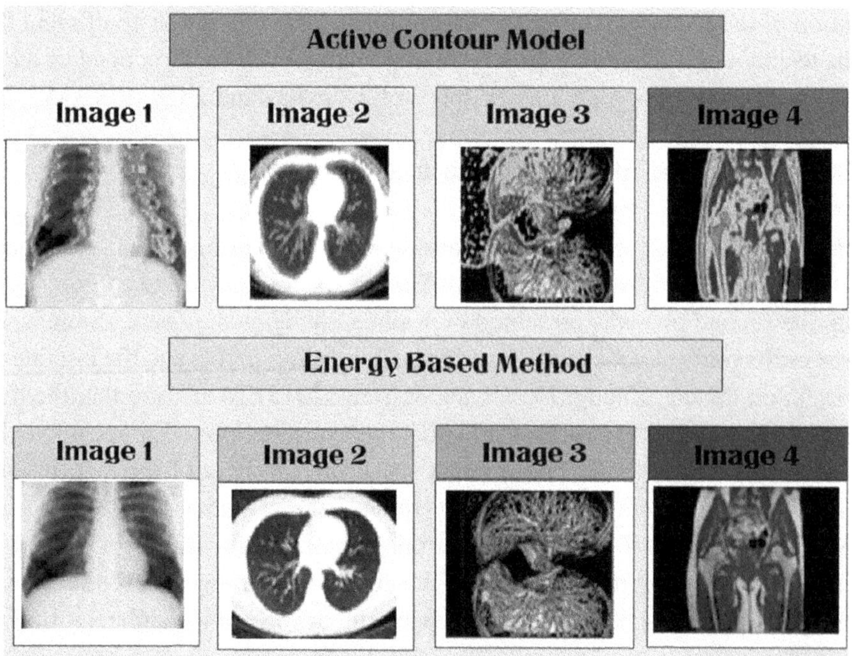

changes with the fundamental shape and one should run the figuring a couple of times remembering the ultimate objective to pick the best result. Thusly, these systems can't be used for the correct and genuine division, C-V technique uses area information and considered as a champion among the most comprehensively used models for the division. One of the prominent purposes of enthusiasm of the C-V show is that it performs well on the photos with cushioned or even without edges. Regardless, as a requirement, the C-V model constantly expect the photo with control homogeneity, the area picture fitting aftereffects of the customary vitality based strategy is given in Figure 14.

Here the impression of the technique gives the most astounding division comes to fruition; whatever the shape and the region of the hidden frame and the resultant structures are smooth and reliable. Figure 14 exhibits the area picture fitting procedure where starting from position impacts the last delayed consequence of division incorrect result downs the accuracy of the strategy.

CONCLUSION

Reinitializing the particular level set ability to some checked partition work all through the headway used for keeping up stable advancement and being sure appealing results. From the practical viewpoint, the restoration procedure is every now and again rather convoluted and costly. The locale based LSM with a balanced stamped partition ability to take out the need related with restoration and regularization work commendably under the high power inhomogeneity issue and has better results in connection with various procedures. It utilizes both edge and the spot information to segment a photo into no covering spot and in light of controlling the propelling curve in through investment degree in the present pixel being inside or outside the dynamic shape. This is executed through stamped weight work that uses the adjacent information in the photo. The procedure will area imaging with drive inhomogeneity and put on MR pictures to exhibit the reliability, feasibility, and generosity in the figuring. The best approach to manage naturally area the closer view dissent of excitement from a photo is to remark on a bouncing box that covers the bleeding edge question. By then, a matched naming is performed to achieve a refined division. The framework Boltzmann system thusly is another and promising other alternative to the standard Navier– Stokes solvers in the region of Computational Fluid Dynamics (CFD). Because of the gigantic necessity for memory and preparing time most CFD issues can't be lit up on a singular PC deficient time, thusly the solvers must be parallelized. In perspective of the comprehended parallelism of the methodology, this ensures a better than average quickens. Numerical reenactment of the PDEs for the most part requires high-drive count and broad use of computational resources.

To discretize the PDEs that incites clarifying a sparse straight structure. The parallelisms of PC counts are winding up continuously fundamental today, as the latest years' example in processors was to put a greater number of CPUs on each processor as opposed to drastically improving the speed of each CPU. Additionally, the ascent of all around helpful plans getting ready units, which can be looked tremendously parallel processors, offers to invigorate new open entryways for a speedy check of parallelizable issues. This is a term for issues which are particularly simple to parallelize, and where the quicken in the check is about straight with the quantity of processor focuses used. The reason behind the cross area Boltzmann's essential parallelization is that assignments on the system are close-by, with the objective that each center can be invigorated self-sufficiently of others. It should not bewilder that the lattice Boltzmann procedure gives direct, according to the wave condition, and that it very well may be used to imitate acoustics. Everything considered, the compressible Navier-Stokes condition can be repeated using the cross area Boltzmann methodology and the wave condition can be gotten from compressible Navier-Stokes. Clearly, for unadulterated wave condition diversions, there will probably be all the more intense numerical methodologies. The cross-area Boltzmann technique's quality is being a full Navier Stokes solver, which suggests that it very well may be used to reenact non-straight acoustics in complex streams.

REFERENCES

Ahirwar, A. (2013). Study of Techniques used for Medical Image Segmentation and Computation of Statistical Test for Region Classification of Brain MRI. *International Journal Of Information Technology And Computer Science*, *5*(5), 44–53. doi:10.5815/ijitcs.2013.05.06

Aitfares, W., Bouyakhf, E., Herbulot, A., Regragui, F., & Devy, M. (2013). Hybrid region and interest points-based active contour for object tracking. *Applied Mathematical Sciences*, *7*, 5879–5899. doi:10.12988/ams.2013.38483

Ali, H., Badshah, N., Chen, K., Khan, G., & Zikria, N. (2017). Multiphase segmentation based on new signed pressure force functions and one level set function. *Turkish Journal of Electrical Engineering and Computer Sciences*, *25*, 2943–2955. doi:10.3906/elk-1606-260

Ali, H., Rada, L., & Badshah, N. (2018). Image Segmentation for Intensity Inhomogeneity in Presence of High Noise. *IEEE Transactions on Image Processing*, *27*(8), 3729–3738. doi:10.1109/TIP.2018.2825101 PMID:29698205

Amrouche, C., & Rejaiba, A. (2015). Navier-Stokes equations with Navier boundary condition. *Mathematical Methods in the Applied Sciences*, *39*(17), 5091–5112. doi:10.1002/mma.3338

Beneš, M., & Kučera, P. (2015). Solutions to the Navier-Stokes equations with mixed boundary conditions in two-dimensional bounded domains. *Mathematische Nachrichten*, *289*(2-3), 194–212. doi:10.1002/mana.201400046

Caponetti, L., Castellano, G., & Corsini, V. (2017). MR Brain Image Segmentation: A Framework to Compare Different Clustering Techniques. *Information*, *8*(4), 138. doi:10.3390/info8040138

Chen, Y., Huang, M., & Chen, S. (2013). Automatic Color Segmentation by Colormap and Edge Detection by Chan Vese Method for Tongue Image. *Journal of Applied Sciences (Faisalabad)*, *13*(18), 3676–3683. doi:10.3923/jas.2013.3676.3683

Cui, Z., & Fan, Q. (2018). A "Nonconvex+Nonconvex" approach for image restoration with impulse noise removal. *Applied Mathematical Modelling*, *62*, 254–271. doi:10.1016/j.apm.2018.05.035

Dimitriou, N., & Delopoulos, A. (2013). Motion-based segmentation of objects using overlapping temporal windows. *Image and Vision Computing*, *31*(9), 593–602. doi:10.1016/j.imavis.2013.06.005

Drapikowski, P., & Domagała, Z. (2014). Semi-Automatic Segmentation of Ct/Mri Images Based on Active Contour Method for 3D Reconstruction of Abdominal Aortic Aneurysms. *Image Processing & Communications*, *19*(1), 13–19. doi:10.1515/ipc-2015-0002

Eun, S., Jung, E., & Park, D. (2017). Effective Brain Contour Segmentation based on Active Contour Model. *Journal Of Next-Generation Convergence Information Services Technology*, *6*(2), 75–88. doi:10.29056/jncist.2017.12.07

Feng, W., Li, Y., Gao, S., Yan, Y., & Xue, J. (2016). A Novel Flame Edge Detection Algorithm via A Novel Active Contour Model. *International Journal Of Hybrid Information Technology*, *9*(9), 275–282. doi:10.14257/ijhit.2016.9.9.26

Feng, R., & Jiang, H. (2010). Edge Based Level Set with Gaussian Filtering Regularized and its Application in Liver Segmentation. *Advanced Materials Research, 121-122*, 222-227. Retrieved from www.scientific.net/amr.121-122.222

Gao, Y., Kikinis, R., Bouix, S., Shenton, M., & Tannenbaum, A. (2012). A 3D interactive multi-object segmentation tool using local robust statistics driven active contours. *Medical Image Analysis*, *16*(6), 1216–1227. doi:10.1016/j.media.2012.06.002 PMID:22831773

Huang, G., & Pun, C. (2015). Robust Interactive Segmentation Using Color Histogram and Contourlet Transform. *International Journal Of Computer Theory And Engineering*, *7*(6), 489–494. doi:10.7763/IJCTE.2015.V7.1007

Izham, M., Fukui, T., & Morinishi, K. (2014). Simulation of three-dimensional homogeneous isotropic turbulence using the moment-based lattice Boltzmann method and LES-lattice Boltzmann method. *Journal of Fluid Science and Technology, 9*(4). doi:10.1299/jfst.2014jfst0064

Jiang, H., Feng, R., & Gao, X. (2011). Level set based on signed pressure force function and its application in liver image segmentation. *Wuhan University Journal of Natural Sciences*, *16*(3), 265–270. doi:10.100711859-011-0748-5

Jones, J., Xie, X., & Essa, E. (2014). Combining region-based and imprecise boundary-based cues for interactive medical image segmentation. *International Journal for Numerical Methods in Biomedical Engineering*, *30*(12), 1649–1666. doi:10.1002/cnm.2693 PMID:25377853

Juneja, P., & Kashyap, R. (2016). Optimal approach for CT image segmentation using improved energy based method. *International Journal of Control Theory and Applications*, *9*(41), 599–608.

Kang, H., Kim, B., Lee, J., Shin, J., & Shin, Y. (2014). Automatic left and right heart segmentation using power watershed and active contour model without edge. *Biomedical Engineering Letters*, *4*(4), 355–361. doi:10.100713534-014-0164-9

Kashyap, R., & Gautam, P. (2015). Modified region based segmentation of medical images. *International Conference on Communication Networks (ICCN)*, 209–216. 10.1109/ICCN.2015.41

Kashyap, R., & Gautam, P. (2017). 'Fast Medical Image Segmentation Using Energy-Based Method', Biometrics. *Concepts, Methodologies, Tools, and Applications*, *3*(1), 1017–1042. doi:10.4018/978-1-5225-0983-7.ch040

Kashyap, R., Gautam, P., & Tiwari, V. (2018). Management and Monitoring Patterns and Future Scope. In Handbook of Research on Pattern Engineering System Development for Big Data Analytics. IGI Global. doi:10.4018/978-1-5225-3870-7.ch014

Kashyap, R., & Piersson, A. (2018a). *Impact of Big Data on Security. In Handbook of Research on Network Forensics and Analysis Techniques* (pp. 283–299). IGI Global. doi:10.4018/978-1-5225-4100-4.ch015

Kashyap, R., & Piersson, A. (2018b). Big Data Challenges and Solutions in the Medical Industries. In Handbook of Research on Pattern Engineering System Development for Big Data Analytics. IGI Global. doi:10.4018/978-1-5225-3870-7.ch001

Kashyap, R., & Tiwari, V. (2018). Active contours using global models for medical image segmentation. *International Journal of Computational Systems Engineering*, *4*(2/3), 195. doi:10.1504/IJCSYSE.2018.091404

Krithivasan, S., Wahal, S., & Ansumali, S. (2014). Diffused bounce-back condition and refill algorithm for the lattice Boltzmann method. *Physical Review. E*, *89*(3), 033313. doi:10.1103/PhysRevE.89.033313 PMID:24730973

Li, D., He, Q., Chunli, L., & Hongjie, Y. (2017). Local Binary Fitting Segmentation by Cooperative Quantum Particle Optimization. *TELKOMNIKA*, *15*(1), 531. doi:10.12928/telkomnika.v15i1.3159

Li, D., He, Q., Chunli, L., & Hongjie, Y. (2017). Local Binary Fitting Segmentation by Cooperative Quantum Particle Optimization. *TELKOMNIKA*, *15*(1), 531. doi:10.12928/telkomnika.v15i1.3159

Li, X., Jiang, D., Shi, Y., & Li, W. (2015). Segmentation of MR image using local and global region based geodesic model. *Biomedical Engineering Online*, *14*(1), 8. doi:10.1186/1475-925X-14-8 PMID:25971306

Li, Z., Zeng, L., Xu, Y., Chen, J., & Yan, B. (2016). Level set method for image segmentation based on local variance and improved intensity inhomogeneity model. *IET Image Processing*, *10*(12), 1007–1016. doi:10.1049/iet-ipr.2016.0352

Miao, J., Huang, T., Zhou, X., Wang, Y., & Liu, J. (2018). Image segmentation based on an active contour model of partial image restoration with local cosine fitting energy. *Information Sciences*, *447*, 52–71. doi:10.1016/j.ins.2018.02.007

Naegel, B., & Passat, N. (2014). Interactive Segmentation Based on Component-trees. *Image Processing On Line*, *4*, 89–97. doi:10.5201/ipol.2014.71

Ogorodnikov, V., Sereseva, O., & Kargapolova, N. (2016). Stochastic models of piecewise-constant and piecewise-linear non-Gaussian processes based on Poisson flows. *Russian Journal of Numerical Analysis and Mathematical Modelling*, *31*(3). doi:10.1515/rnam-2016-0018

Olabarriaga, S., & Smeulders, A. (2001). Interaction in the segmentation of medical images: A survey. *Medical Image Analysis*, *5*(2), 127–142. doi:10.1016/S1361-8415(00)00041-4 PMID:11516707

Panin, G., & Knoll, A. (2006). Fully Automatic Real-Time 3D Object Tracking using Active Contour and Appearance Models. *Journal of Multimedia*, *1*(7). doi:10.4304/jmm.1.7.62-70

Peng, Y., Zhu, Y., & Wang, Y. (2016). A fast medical image segmentation method of based on initial contour forecast segmentation model. *International Journal Of Computing Science And Mathematics*, *7*(3), 212. doi:10.1504/IJCSM.2016.077863

Ryba, T., & Zelezny, M. (2015). An automatic image segmentation algorithm involving shortest path basins. *Pattern Recognition and Image Analysis*, *25*(1), 89–95. doi:10.1134/S1054661815010162

Siegel, C. (2014). Re: Fully Automated Prostate Segmentation on MRI: Comparison with Manual Segmentation Methods and Specimen Volumes. *The Journal of Urology*, *192*(3), 767. doi:10.1016/j.juro.2014.06.025

Utyuzh, O., Wilk, G., & Wodarczyk, Z. (2007). Numerical symmetrization of state of identical particles. *Brazilian Journal of Physics*, *37*(2c). doi:10.1590/S0103-97332007000500007

Wang, L., Zhang, H., He, K., Chang, Y., & Yang, X. (2015). Active Contours Driven by Multi-Feature Gaussian Distribution Fitting Energy with Application to Vessel Segmentation. *PLoS One*, *10*(11), e0143105. doi:10.1371/journal.pone.0143105 PMID:26571031

Wang, Y., Shu, C., & Yang, L. (2016). Boundary condition-enforced immersed boundary-lattice Boltzmann flux solver for thermal flows with Neumann boundary conditions. *Journal of Computational Physics*, *306*, 237–252. doi:10.1016/j.jcp.2015.11.046

Waoo, N., Kashyap, R., & Jaiswal, A. (2010). DNA nano array analysis using hierarchical quality threshold clustering. *2010 2nd IEEE International Conference on Information Management and Engineering*, 81–85.

Wilson, J., Coleman, R., & Turkington, T. (2011). Variable-time positron emission tomography leg protocol to equalize noise for positron emission tomography/computed tomography acquisitions. *Nuclear Medicine Communications*, *32*(9), 868–872. doi:10.1097/MNM.0b013e328347f1a3 PMID:21799371

Zhang, K., Song, H., & Zhang, L. (2010). Active contours driven by local image fitting energy. *Pattern Recognition*, *43*(4), 1199–1206. doi:10.1016/j.patcog.2009.10.010

Zhang, X., Wen, X., Xu, H., & Meng, Q. (2016). Synthetic aperture radar image segmentation based on edge-region active contour model. *Journal of Applied Remote Sensing*, *10*(3), 036014. doi:10.1117/1.JRS.10.036014

Zhao, F., Liang, H., Wu, X., & Ding, D. (2017). Region-based Active Contour Segmentation Model with Local Discriminant Criterion. *International Journal Of Security And Its Applications*, *11*(7), 73–86. doi:10.14257/ijsia.2017.11.7.06

Zhuang, M., Dierckx, R., & Zaidi, H. (2016). Generic and robust method for automatic segmentation of PET images using an active contour model. *Medical Physics*, *43*(8Part1), 4483–4494. doi:10.1118/1.4954844 PMID:27487865

KEY TERMS AND DEFINITIONS

CFD: Computational fluid dynamics is a branch of liquid mechanics that utilizations numerical investigation and information structures to take care of and break down issues that include liquid streams. PCs are utilized to play out the counts required to mimic the collaboration of fluids and gases with surfaces characterized by limit conditions. With rapid supercomputers, better arrangements can be accomplished. Continuous research yields programming that enhances the exactness and speed of complex reenactment situations, for example, transonic or turbulent streams. Beginning trial approval of such programming is performed utilizing a breeze burrow with the last approval coming in full-scale testing (e.g., flight tests).

LSM: Level set method are a calculated system for utilizing level sets as an instrument for numerical investigation of surfaces and shapes. The benefit of the level-set model is that one can perform numerical calculations including bends and surfaces on a settled cartesian framework without having to parameterize these articles. This is known as the Eulerian approach also. The level-set strategy makes it simple to take after shapes that change topology, for instance, when a shape parts in two, creates gaps, or the invert of these activities. All these make the level-set technique an extraordinary apparatus for demonstrating time-shifting items, similar to swelling of an airbag, or a drop of oil skimming in water.

Chapter 8
Heart Disease Diagnosis:
A Machine Learning Approach

Siddhartha Kumar Arjaria
Rajkiya Engineering College Banda, India

Abhishek Singh Rathore
Independent Researcher, India

ABSTRACT

In the modern era of information technology, machine learning algorithms are used in different domains for boosting the quality of decision making. The correct decision making about the disease diagnosis is one of the applications where these approaches are applied successfully for assisting the doctors. Correct and timely diagnosis of disease is the primary requirement of effective treatment. Today, one of the most leading causes of death is heart disease. This chapter deals with the application of different machine learning algorithms for effective heart disease diagnosis. Diagnosis through the machine learning algorithms involves the three major steps, data preprocessing, feature selection, and classification. The chapter covers the experimental study of performance of SVM, ANN, logistic regression, random forest, KNN, AdaBoost, Naive Bayes, decision tree, SGD, CN2 rule inducer approaches.

INTRODUCTION

In the recent time the medical field shows tremendous improvement in diagnosis and treatment of diseases. The timely and accurately diagnosis of any disease is helpful for effective treatment. Traditionally, the examination the signs and symptoms of the patient physically by a doctor is the most common way to diagnose the disease. Wrong diagnosis, causes the high treatment cost and the risk of life. In order to improve the accuracy of disease diagnosis, nowadays in the medical field, machine learning techniques are being used. The main data mining task involves in disease diagnosis is classification; for this many algorithms have been proposed by the researchers. Presently heart disease is considered to be one of the most fatal disease in both men and women. In year 2012, World Health Organization (WHO) claims that heart disease is the reason of more than 31% global death. In the present work we will explore various machine learning methods being used for heart disease diagnosis. Few of them are Artificial Neural

DOI: 10.4018/978-1-5225-7796-6.ch008

Network, Support vector Machine, Random Forest, Logistic Regression, K-Nearest Neighbor approach (KNN), Ada Boost, and Naive Bayes, Decision tree, SGD and CN2 rule inducer.

Heart

The heart is considered to be most important organ of the body. A healthy heart is important for healthy life the heart has four chambers that are separated by valves and divided into two halves (Figure 1, Human Heart Diagram, n.d.). There are two chambers in each half. One chamber is known as atrium and other one is ventricle. The role of the atrium is blood collection, and the role of the ventricles is to push blood out of the heart. The role of right half of the heart is pushing oxygen-poor blood to the lungs in which blood cells can gain more oxygen. Then from lungs this newly oxygen rich blood moves into the left atrium and the left ventricle. The role of the left ventricle is to push this oxygen-rich blood to the different organs of the body. For the healthy body the proper functioning of the heart is very important.

The life style along with other factors causes the malfunction of the heart and thus leads towards the heart or cardiac disease. Heart attack or stroke or cardiac attack is the most commonly used term for heart disease. There are many reasons for heart attack but high risk people share some common set of factors. These factors are summarized in Table 1.

Figure 1.

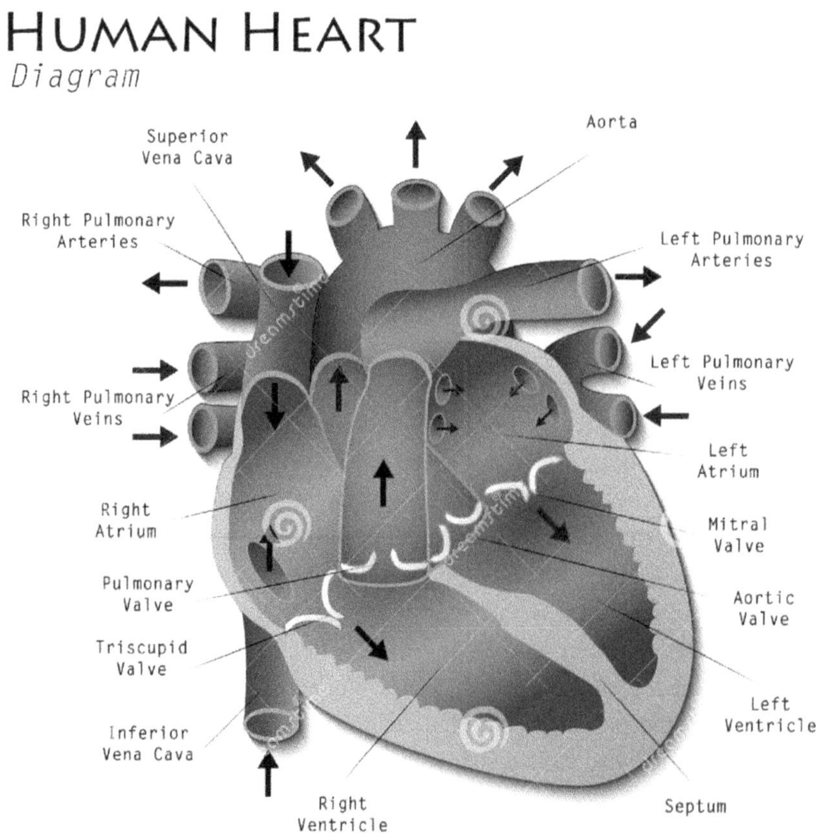

Table 1. Common factors showing a high risk of heart attack

S.No	Attribute Name	Type	Role	Values
1	Age(In Years)	Numeric	Feature	
2	Sex	Categorical	Feature	{ Male; female}
3	CP(Chest Pain)	Categorical	Feature	{Asymptomatic ; Atypical angina, Non-anginal ; Typical angina}
4	Rest SBP (resting blood pressure)	Numeric	Feature	
5	Chol (Cholesterol)	Numeric	Feature	
6	Fasting Blood Sugar>120	Categorical	Feature	{True; False}
7	Rest ECG	Categorical	Feature	{Normal; ST-T wave abnormality ; Left ventricular hypertrophy }
8	Maximum heart rate	Numeric	Feature	
9	Exang(Exercise induced angina)	Categorical	Feature	{1 = Yes; 0 = No}.
10	ST by exercise	Numeric	Feature	
11	Slope(The slope of ST segment)	Categorical	Feature	{Up sloping; Flat; Down sloping.}
12	major vessels colored	Numeric	Feature	
13	Thal	Categorical	Feature	{Normal; Fixed defect; Reversible defect}
14	Diameter narrowing	Categorical	Target	{0;1}

The objective of the chapter is to study the performance of SVM, ANN, Logistic regression, Random Forest, KNN, Ada Boost, Naive Bayes, Decision Tree, SGD, CN2 rule inducer approaches. The experiments have been performed on publicly available benchmark UCI Statlog (Heart) dataset (Dua & Karra Taniskidou, 2017). The remainder of the chapter is organized as follows. Section 2 includes the work done in this area. Section 3 summarizes the widely used classification techniques and the performance of those algorithms are listed in section 4. Later future recommendation and conclusion is provided.

BACKGROUND

With the emergence of digital pathology labs, various computing techniques are used for disease diagnosis. Data mining techniques are widely used for categorization and prediction (Awang & Palaniappan, 2007) of medical problems. For healthcare prediction, association rule mining contributed significantly (Ordonez, et al., 2001; Deepika, 2011; Durairaj & Meena, 2011). Less relevant or irrelevant rules are significantly removed in association rule mining (Ordonez C, 2006). Principal Component Analysis (PCA) is applied to binary regression model; that works on the presumed dependent variables showing the presence or absence of disease (Jilani, Yasin, Yasin, & Ardil, 2009). Evolution classifier is applied with PCA to generate classifier rules from electronic medical records (Luukka & Lampinen, 2010). C4.5 is used for decision tree for heart disease risk assessment (Karaolis, Moutiris, Hadjipanayi, & Pattichis, 2010).

A web-based intelligent system applied hybrid approach using naïve-Bayes, neural network and decision tree to find out disease patterns from age, sex, blood pressure and sugar level to predict the chances of having heart disease (Palaniappan & Awang, 2008). Prediction of cardiovascular risk, the Levenberg - Marquardt algorithm is employed in two-layer neural network (Fidele, Cheeneebash, Gopaul, & Goorah, 2009). To predict disease; MAFIA algorithm is applied to find hidden patterns, which are then used by Multilayer Perceptron to train the weights of a neural network (Patil & Kumaraswamy, 2009).

Artificial intelligence, especially Bayesian inference techniques are applied to Sphygmogram signals and hemodynamic analysis are used to diagnose cardiovascular disease, but the uncertainties are bottlenecked. A multi-stage Bayesian Inference Net with fuzzy rules applied to overcome those bottlenecks (Sekar & Dong, 2014). Bayesian classifier is applied on features extracted by linear discriminant analysis of heart rate variability measures (Asyali, 2003). Distribution-free Bayes optimal classifier for synthetic dataset provides better worst case accuracy. It eliminates equality constraints on a hyper - plane by minimizing on upper bounds in worst case settings (Huang, Yang, King, Lyu, & Chan, 2004).

A hybrid two phase fuzzy inference engine improves decision making uncertainty and information's vagueness by considering evidential parameters (Khatibi & Montazer, 2010). A multi-stage fuzzy rule-based decision system populates the decision tree from demographic and historical data (Tsipouras, et al., 2008). The parameters are automatically optimized from an annotated dataset. Another decision support system based on Rough Set Theory, generates rules and fuzzified them from discretizing the attributes (Setiawan, Venkatachalam, & Hani, 2009). Dempster–Shafer evidence theory based fuzzy inference engine is applied over the hybrid method of PROCAM and FRS guidelines for the prediction(Vahid & Gholam, 2010).

Particle Swarm Optimization is employed with Mamdani Fuzzy Inference for heart disease diagnosis (Muthukarupan & Erib, 2012). A Neuro-fuzzy network (Ayat & Khosravanian, 2014) and rough set based clustering (Kumar & Arasu, 2017) fuzzy based expert systems are proposed for improved accuracy of heart disease diagnosis. Another clinical decision system identifies suitable attributes with deviations and employs weighted fuzzy rules & decision tree rules to predict risk of heart disease (Anooj, 2011). The Shannon entropy is used to reduce dimensions of features extracted through discrete wavelet transform. Adaptive Neuro-fuzzy inference classifier is used to diagnose the heart disease (Uguz, 2012).

Deep learning techniques, especially Convolutional Neural Networks (CNN) are currently used on cardiac images. The deep convolutional neural network is applied on endomyocardial biopsy images to predict cardiac disease (Nirschl, et al., 2018). A deep survival analysis is applied to electronic health record (HER) data to predict risk of coronary heart disease. Since EHR is high-dimensional, basic conditional models are unable to handle missing covariates, Bayesian framework is employed with deep survival analysis (Rangnath, Perotte, Elhadad, & Blei, 2016). A 3D convolutional network exploits 3D-HOL layer to identify defective heart structures. A deeply-supervised pathway is employed to accelerate learning. It uses additional companion loss that learns more discriminate features rapidly (Li, Zhang, Shi, & Wang, 2016). An 11-layer CNN is picks up features from ECG signals. Max-pooling is used for dimension reduction after each convolution with minimum information loss (Acharya, et al., 2018).

In recent years, of adaptive network based fuzzy inference system (ANIFS) is widely used in different medical diagnostic systems. A hybrid optimization model of ANIFS classifier (for continuous values) and linear discriminant analysis is developed for prediction purpose (Yang, Kim, Kang, & Lee, 2014). Another model applied multiple kernel learning with ANIFS based deep learning for heart disease diagnosis (Manogaran, Varatharajan, & Priyan, 2018). However, the model considersa limited number of parameters for classification.

Long-term and short-term physiological time-series information of patients are also used by different authors for prediction. Hidden Markov model (Krogh, 1994), mismatch tree-based kernels (Eskin

& Pevzner, 2002), dynamic time wrapping (Pazzani & Ratanamahatana, 2005) techniques are used for learning parameters. Symbolic mismatch, a parameter-less technique identifies high-risk patients in long-term time-series (Syed & Guttag, 2011).

A patch-based interactive algorithm applied to uniformly slice segments of MRI images. At each iteration, short-axis plane of MRI images is segmented manually to automatically define the remaining volume of image using patch-based segmentation (Pace D.F., 2015). Rotation Forest based classification algorithm is used for heart disease prediction (Ozcift & Gulten, 2011).

Genetic Algorithm based feature selection method is employed to extract more relevant features for better prediction (Yen, Zheng, Jiang, Peng, & Xaio, 2008; Tan, Teoh, Yu, & Goh, 2009). Genetic Algorithm is applied to determine features from short-term heart rate variability measures. A KNN classifier is used to evaluate the performance of feature selection (Isler & Kantalp, 2007). While another work applied SVM with Genetic Algorithms for feature selection (Gokulnath & Shantharajah, 2018). Apriori, Predictive Apriori and Teritus methods are used for feature selection (Nahar, Imam, Tickle, & Chen, 2013). Radial Basis Function transforms features into kernel space. F-Score values are used to extract relevant features from this feature space (Polat & Gunes, 2009). Fisher score and forward/reverse feature selection algorithms are proposed with the Mathew correlation coefficient score for selection of feature subset. A kernel-based SVM is used for disease diagnosis (Saqlain, et al., 2018).

Particle swarm optimization and support vector machine are combined to assess risk of having the disease from ultrasound images (Raghavendra, et al., 2017). Heart rate variability signals are-decomposed non-linearly into different mono-component functions classes. PNN and SVM are applied to classify different classes (Acharya, et al., 2017).Different feature extraction and classification algorithms have been applied in heart disease prediction and identification with better accuracy. The objective of this study is to compare different machine learning algorithms for heart disease prediction.

MAIN FOCUS OF THE CHAPTER

For applying the data mining techniques effectively, feature selection is an important task. Data mining tasks when applied on relevant features, it will produce the accurate result in minimum time. The feature selection algorithms identifies the significant feature set by providing the score to different features. Many feature selection algorithms are being used by researchers. Information gain (IG) is one of the feature selection algorithms that measures how much “information” a feature provides about the class. Features that partition the data into classes accurately will give maximal information. Unrelated features will give a little or no information. In other words, IG measures the reduction in entropy.

The Table 2 shows the ranking of features on the basis of information gain. The Table 1 shows thal as the most informative feature. In the experiment, these features are applied on different classifiers and judged the performance of the classifier algorithm on the basis of different measures e.g. the accuracy, precision, recall and F1 measures.

Once features are extracted, different supervised and unsupervised learning algorithms are applied to predict diseases accurately. Classification is the process to create a model for finding the appropriate classes for the unknown data samples. Classification model is constructed using the supervised learning approach, first train the model and then test it with unknown data samples. Several Classification techniques are used for disease diagnosis. In this section, few of classification algorithms are employed, that are used in experimental study of the chapter.

Table 2. Features identified based on information gain

S.No	Features	Information Gain
1	Thal	0.2080
2	Chest Pain	0.2050
3	Major Vessels Colored	0.1797
4	ST By Exercise	0.1453
5	ExercIndAng	0.1391
6	Max HR	0.1230
7	Slope Peak Exc ST	0.1124
8	Age	0.0578
9	Gender	0.0572
10	Rest ECG	0.0241
11	Cholesterol	0.0161
12	Rest SBP	0.0149
13	Fasting Blood Sugar > 120	0.0004

Feed-Forward Back Propagation Neural Network

Feed-forward back propagation neural network (Figure 2, Determining the Appropriate Amount of Anesthetic Gas Using DWT and EMD Combined with Neural Network - Scientific Figure on ResearchGate., n.d.) is used as a classifier for heart disease diagnosis. An ANN is a popular machine learning approach that simulates the behavior of the human brain to some degree. It mimics the "learning" and "generalization" abilities of the human brain to solve the highly nonlinear complex classification problem of the real world. An artificial neural network (ANN) is a computational model that have of highly interconnecting processing elements (neurons) operating in parallel. A neuron is a mathematical unit which calculates the weighted sum of its inputs and the output of the network produced with the support of each neuron.

Figure 2.

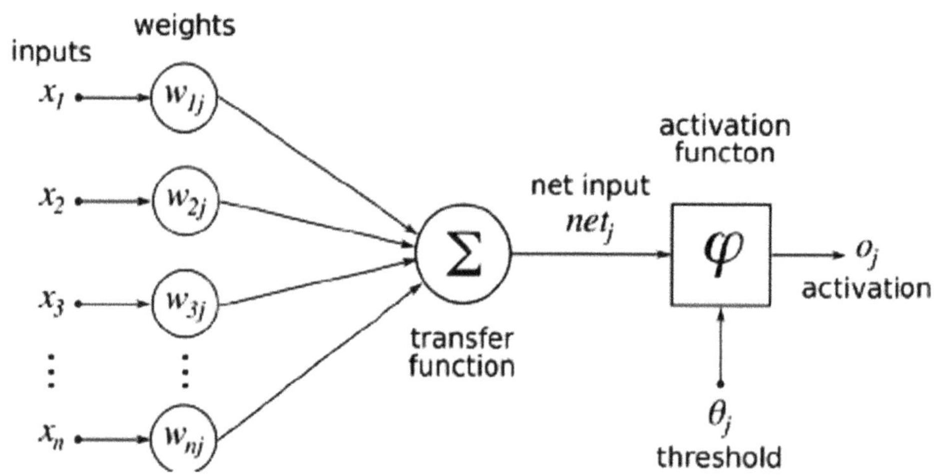

Training data set: (x_i, y_i) $1 \leq i \leq N$
x_i is a vector corresponding to an input sample data having P input attribute $1 \leq P \leq 13$
y_i is a target variable with a class label of either 1 or 0

Neural networks are organized in layers. Each layer in the network is the group of neurons. Feed forward neural network has an input layer as first layer, an output layer as last layer and one or more hidden layers in between. Each neuron in a layer is connected with each neuron in the next layer through a weighted connection w. The interconnection link between the layers is assigned with the initial random weights. During the training phase of Neural Network the input training samples along with output is applied to the network. This attached output is desired output. The input layer is responsible for receiving the inputs and to transmit it to the next layer. The hidden layer takes the weighted sum of input sent by the input layer and mathematically processes it using the appropriate activation function. Now, hidden units direct the output towards the neurons in the next layer for further processing. There can be one or more hidden layer so next layer can be either hidden layer or output layer. This process continues till the network produces the output. This output is known as the current output. The squared error between the desired output and the current output is calculated. This is given by:

$$E = \frac{1}{2}\sum_{j}\left(t_{pj} - o_{pj}\right)^2 \tag{1}$$

where, t_{pj} is a desired output and o_{pj} is a current output

In order to minimize the error E the weights are modified in the backyard pass from output towards the input and modified the weights of each layer by a proportion δ of the overall error E. After the weights modification the training samples are presented again to the network and the same process continues iteratively, until there is error reaches up to the desired minimum value.

After each iteration the squared error between the actual output and the desired output is calculated and employs gradient descent to minimize the sum of squared error by propagating the error signals in backward direction and thus weights are adjusted for the multilayer neural network. Figure 3 shows the architecture of artificial neural network. The neural network is first trained and then tested. The performance of classifier is tested on different number of features.

Bayesian Classifier

It is a simple and efficient statistical classification method to predict the class membership probabilities. It works on the principle of Bayes theorem and estimates the posterior probability. Naïve Bayesian classifier assumes attribute independence. In this approach, symptoms of a patient using the features are observed and then find the probability of disease.

It is a statistical method for classification that adopts the supervised learning approach.It is a probabilistic model that determines the probabilities of the output class of the testing instance by applying the Bayes theorem.

Given training data X, posterior probability of a hypothesis H, Conditional probability $P(H|X)$, follows the Bayes theorem

Figure 3.

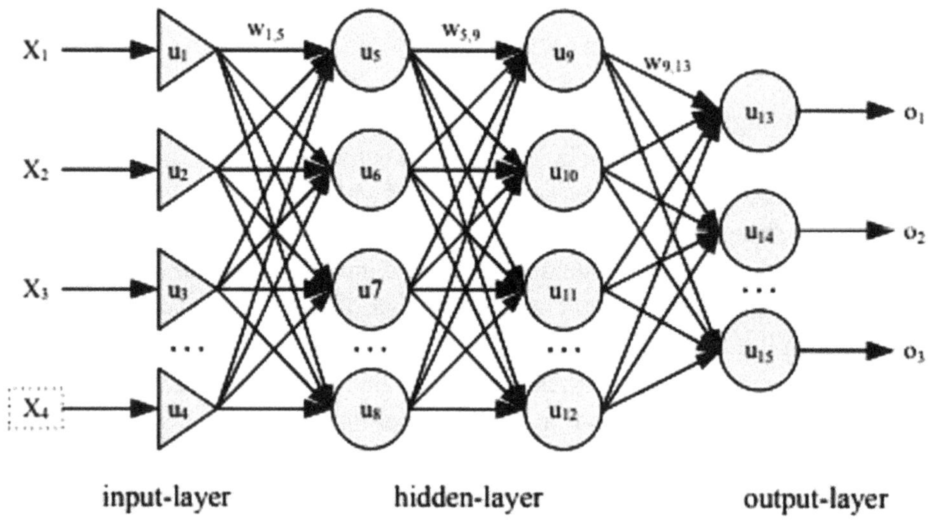

$$P(H|X) = P(X|H)P(H)/P(X) \tag{2}$$

Each data sample is denoted by a *P* dimensional feature vector, $X = (A_1, A_2 ..... A_P)$. There are *m* classes, $C_1, C_2 ...... C_m$. Class of unknown data sample *X* will decided by Posterior probability. Sample *X* belongs to the class that have highest posterior probability, conditioned if and only if:

$$P(C_i/X) > P(C_j/X) \text{ for all } 1 < = j < = m \text{ and } j != I \tag{3}$$

Class C_i for which $P(C_i/X)$ is maximized is known as the maximum posteriori hypothesis. As *P(X)* is constant for all classes, only $P(X|C_i)P(C_i)$ need be maximized. That is, the naive probability assigns an unknown sample *X* to the class C_i.

The class prior probabilities $P(C_i)$ may be estimated by $P(C_i) = n_i/n$,

where, n_i is the number of training samples of class C_i, and *n* is the total number of training samples.

K-Nearest Neighbor (KNN) Classifier

KNN simple and straightforward data mining techniques work on the principle of majority of votes. The KNN algorithm also known as case based reasoning, example based reasoning and lazy learner, etc. KNN stores all the cases and then find the class of new instances by finding the similarity measure. Similarity measure is calculated by finding the distance. The distance is calculated using one of the following measures n Euclidean Distance, Minkowski Distance, Mahalanobis Distance.

If the first instance is $(a_1, a_2, a_3 ... a_n)$ and the second instance is $(b_1, b_2, b_3, ...b_n)$, the distance between them is calculated by the following formula for Euclidean Distance:

$$\sqrt{\sum_{i=1}^{n}\left(a_i - b_i\right)^2}$$

To find the class of new instance x_q

Step 1: Find the K training instances which are closest x_q instance
Step 2: Pick the K instances nearest to x_q by finding the distance
Step 3: Return the class of x_q as the class that appears maximally among the K instances.

Random Forest

Random forest is a group or ensemble of Classification and Regression Trees (CART). The method combines the idea of "bagging" with the random selection of features to construct a collection of decision trees. Random Forest has mainly two properties, first it is not sensitive to noise in the dataset and secondly the problem of over fitting is not a matter of concern in it. Random forest consists several trees and each tree is trained separately. Random forest has been built by combining the predictions of these trees. Construction of random forest needs to make choices about the type of predictor used for each leaf, splitting method applied at leafs and method of infusing the randomness in the tree.Parameters like selection of Base classifier, a number of attribute used in base classifier, selection of split measure at each node of tree, number of passes required is needed to determine the result

Training data set: (x_i, y_i) $1 \leq i \leq N$

where, x_i is a vector corresponding to an input sample data having P input attribute $1 \leq P \leq 13$and y_i is a target variable with a class label of either 1 or 0.

The number of training data set contains be N number of training samples with aP number of attributes. At a node of tree the m out of P number of input features are used in the decision making. Select N training samples from this tree by picking them with replacement from available N training samples, i.e. select the bootstrap sample and remaining samples are used for the error estimation of this tree. For each node of the tree, randomly choose m out of P features in the decision making at that node. Now on the basis of these m features calculate the best split. Each tree is grown-up fully without pruning. For predicting the class label of new sample, it is pushed down the tree and it is assigned with the class label of the training sample of that terminal node where it ends up. This process is iterated over all trees in the ensemble and average vote of all trees is calculated for predicting the output.

Logistic Regression

Logistic Regression is a popular classification method that uses the probabilistic statistics of the data. Logistic regression is similar to linear regression. In it, unlike linear regression a binary output y is predicted by combining the Input values (x) linearly using weights. In other words, we can say that it predicts the probability of an outcome by fitting data to a logistic function.Logistic regression is a statistical method suitable where the outcome depends on one or more independent variables.It essentially uses the logistic function or sigmoid function. This function takes any real-valued number and map it into a value between 0 and 1, but never exactly at those limits.

$$z= b_0+ b_1x_1 + b_2 x_2+ b_3 x_3 + . . + b_nx_n$$

where b_0: bias or intercept term and $b_1,b_2,b_3,...b_n$ are the coefficient for the input value $x_1,x_2,x_{3.....}x_n$. and predicted output

$$y = 1/\left(\left(1 + e^{\wedge}\left(-z\right)\right)\right) \quad (4)$$

Logistic regression works in two phases, training and testing phase. In the training phase, to learn the model the samples from the datasets is taken. Learning ends with the best values of b_0, $b_1,b_2,b_3,...b_n$. To judge the performance of the model the response of model is tested on unknown samples in testing phase.

Decision Tree

The decision tree is a predictive model that maps observations of sample to sample's target value. The goal is to make a decision tree model is to predict the target variable value on the basis of input variables. In tree each interior node denotes an input variable and the edges to child nodes for all the values of that input variable. Each leaf node denotes a value of the target variable. To find the target value for the given set of input value we have to explore the path from the root node to a leaf node. By exploring the path from the root node to leaf node the decision tree approach generates if –then classification rules. Learning of this tree can be done by splitting the source set into subsets on the basis of an attribute value test. For each derived subset the process is repeated in a recursive manner. This is also known as recursive partitioning. This process carries on until no further expansion in the tree. This recursion terminates if all instances for a particular node belongs to the same class or if there is no remaining attributes on which the instances cannot be partitioned further. There is only one rule for every sample in the tree.

Data comes in records of the form:$(x, y) = (x_1, x_2, x_3, ...,x_k, y)$

where, y is dependent or the target variable. The input variables, x_1, x_2, x_3 etc. are the input attributes. In the decision tree, each internal nodes have a decision function of one or more attributes. Some popular Decision tree methods are CART, CHAID, ID3and C4.5. The construction of C4.5 decision tree applies information theory or entropy concept to find the information gain of every attribute and in turn decide the attributes location in decision tree.

AdaBoost

The adaptive Boosting algorithm, also known as Ada-boost is ensemble classifier. Ensemble classifier forms the strong classifier by combining many weak classifiers. In this algorithm weak classifiers are added iteratively and thus form well-correlated true classifier. Each weak classifier is trained using a random subset of the overall training set, random subset is not actually 100% random. It creates a strong classifier using a set of weak classifiers. If considering the weak classifier alone; it may produce the poor classification result. But multiple weak classifiers are combined and assign the appropriate weight in final voting; we can achieve good performance in terms of good classification accuracy for overall classifier. The weak classifiers correlated to the actual classifier in a very weak manner. Strong ensemble learning classifier is created by using the adaptive Boosting algorithm.

Boosting Ensemble Method

It builds a model using the training data and then form the second model to correct the errors from the first model. The models are added iteratively until a maximum number of models are added or the training set is predicted perfectly.

Each instance in the training dataset is provided with a weight. The initial weight assignment of training sample x_i is set to: weight $(x_i) = 1/n$, where n is the number of training instances.

These weighted samples are used to prepare a weak classifier. These weak classifiers are used only for binary classification problems. The classifier makes a binary decision and outputs +1 or -1 value.

For the trained model the rate of misclassification is calculated and it is given by:

$$misclassification\ rate{:}\ error = (correctly\ classified\ samples - n) / n \tag{5}$$

Again, this is modified for assign the weights of training instances:

$$error = sum(w(i) * terror(i)) / sum(w) \tag{6}$$

where, w is the weight for training instance i and terror is the prediction error for training instance i which is 1 if misclassified and -1 if correctly classified.

To provide the weight for the prediction made by the trained model, stage value is calculated as:

$$stage = ln((1\text{-}error) / error) \tag{7}$$

In final prediction stage, weight provides more weight for more accurate models. The training weights are updated in such a way so that more weights are assigned to incorrectly predict training instances, and vice-versa.

The weight updating of one training instance (w) is given by:

$$w = w * exp(stage * terror) \tag{8}$$

where, w is the weight for a specific training instance terror is the error the weak classifier made predicting the output variable for the training instance, evaluated as:

$$terror = 0\ if(y == p),\ otherwise\ 1 \tag{9}$$

where, y is the output variable for the training instance and p is the prediction from the weak learner.

This has the effect of not changing the weight if the training instance, was classified correctly and making the weight slightly larger if the weak learner misclassified the instance. Weak classifiers are added iteratively and trained using the weighted training data until a predefined number of weak classifier have been considered or there is improvement can be made on the training dataset.

Support Vector Machine (SVM)

It is another most widely used classifier that will work on the principle of approximate implementation of the method of structural risk minimization. SVM (Figure 4, (Eliot, 2018) is known as the maximum margin classifier as its aim is to minimize the empirical classification error and maximize the geometric margin. SVMs can do non-linear classification by mapping their inputs into high-dimensional feature spaces. It first maps the input vectors into a decision value, and then using the significant threshold value it performs the classification. This kernel trick builds the classifier without explicitly any information of feature space. In SVM the data samples are represented as points in space, and they are mapped in such a way that the data samples belong to different class are separated by a gap that is as wide as possible.

Training data set: $(x_i y_i)\ 1 \leq i \leq N$

where, x_i is a vector corresponding to an input sample data having P input attribute $1 \leq P \leq 13$ and y_i is a target variable with a class label of either 1 or -1.

Pattern denoted by the subset $y_i = +1$ and the pattern denoted by the subset $y_i = -1$ are linearly separable. The equation of separating hyper plane is

$$w^T x + b = 0 \tag{10}$$

where, x is input vector, w is an adjustable weight vector, and b is a bias. The weight vector w will indicate the perpendicular direction to separating hyper plane. For the weight vector w and a bias b, margin of separation ρ is defined as the separation between the separating hyper plane and the closest data point.

Figure 4.

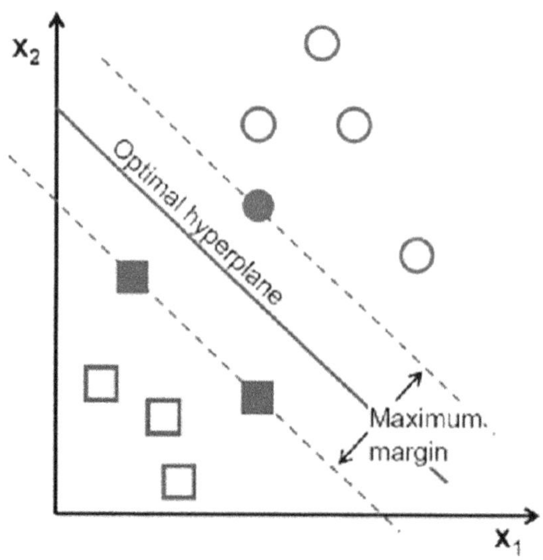

Thus, it will give the geometric construction of an optimal hyper plane for a two- dimensional input space. When the training data set is linearly separable,then these hyper planes are selected in such a way that there are no points between them. The distance between the hyper planes will be 2/ | ρ |. Maximize the distance between the hyper plane is done by minimizing | ρ |, we need to ensure for all i

$$w^T x_i + b \geq 0 \; for \; yi = +1$$

and

$$w^T x_i + b < 0 \; for \; yi = -1 \tag{11}$$

SOLUTIONS AND RECOMMENDATIONS

Widely used standard classification algorithms are evaluated to suggest recommendations. To evaluate the performance of learning algorithms the UCI Statlog (Heart) dataset (Dua & Karra Taniskidou, 2017) is used. The dataset contains the 303 records and each there are 13 out of 76 features are utilized in this study (refer to Table 3**).** 10-fold cross validation is applied to the data for classification task. The performance of SVM, ANN, Logistic regression, Random Forest, KNN, Adaboost, Naive Bayes, Decision Tree, SGD, CN2 rule inducer approaches are evaluated on all 13 features (refer Table 4, Table 5, Table 6, Table 7, and Table 8).

The comparison between different classifier are shown in Table 4- 8Different classifiers are applied, and classification results suggest that Naïve Bayes classifier performs better than other classifier. The basic reason behind the success of Naïve Bayes classifier (NBC) is that degree of class overlapping is small in used dataset. Another reason is that wrapped features extracted by information gain, provide optimized features and thus NBC outperforms in current context. NBC assumes all the features independent, whereas other classifiers tries to find certain interactions between features. Recent studies also suggest that NBC has better resilience to missing data than the graphical models based classifiers (Shi & Liu, 2011). Since the classification is based relative comparison, NBC even not providing exact probabilities, it surprisingly works well than others algorithms for classification by find relative probabilities with faster estimations.

Model size of NBC is small and constant with used dataset and thus do not try to overfit the data like remaining classifier does. Simply it picks best features and beats other classifier in the current domain. NBC is generative in nature, it will perform better with scalability measure.

FUTURE RESEARCH DIRECTIONS

From the study it can be concluded that a substantial amount of research work on heart disease diagnosis can be found. Since the accuracy of the classifier depends on most relevant features. This first important thing is to identify suitable and evidential attributes. Information gain based feature extraction technique is applied in this study. Topic model based dimension reduction and information extraction techniques

Table 3. The glimpses of data, there are 303 instances and each have attributes

S. No.	Diameter narrowing	Age	Gender	Chest Pain	Rest SBP	Cholesterol	fasting blood sugar > 120	rest ECG	max HR	exercindang	ST by exercise	Slope Peak Exc ST	Major Vessels Colored	Thal
1	0	63	male	typical ang	145	233	1	left vent hypertrophy	150	0	2.3	downsloping	0	fixed defect
2	1	67	male	asymptomatic	160	286	0	left vent hypertrophy	108	1	1.5	flat	3	normal
3	1	67	male	asymptomatic	120	229	0	left vent hypertrophy	129	1	2.6	flat	2	reversable defect
4	0	37	male	non-anginal	130	250	0	normal	187	0	3.5	downsloping	0	normal
5	0	41	female	atypical ang	130	204	0	left vent hypertrophy	172	0	1.4	upsloping	0	normal
6	0	56	male	atypical ang	120	236	0	normal	178	0	0.8	upsloping	0	normal
7	1	62	female	asymptomatic	140	268	0	left vent hypertrophy	160	0	3.6	downsloping	2	normal
8	0	57	female	asymptomatic	120	354	0	normal	163	1	0.6	upsloping	0	normal
9	1	63	male	asymptomatic	130	254	0	left vent hypertrophy	147	0	1.4	flat	1	reversable defect
10	1	53	male	asymptomatic	140	203	1	left vent hypertrophy	155	1	3.1	downsloping	0	reversable defect
11	0	57	male	asymptomatic	140	192	0	normal	148	0	0.4	flat	0	fixed defect
12	0	56	female	atypical ang	140	294	0	left vent hypertrophy	153	0	1.3	flat	0	normal
13	1	56	male	non-anginal	130	256	1	left vent hypertrophy	142	1	0.6	flat	1	fixed defect
14	0	44	male	atypical ang	120	263	0	normal	173	0	0.0	upsloping	0	reversable defect
15	0	52	male	non-anginal	172	199	1	normal	162	0	0.5	upsloping	0	reversable defect
16	0	57	male	non-anginal	150	168	0	normal	174	0	1.6	upsloping	0	normal
17	1	48	male	atypical ang	110	229	0	normal	168	0	1.0	downsloping	0	reversable defect
18	0	54	male	asymptomatic	140	239	0	normal	160	0	1.2	upsloping	0	normal
19	0	48	female	non-anginal	130	275	0	normal	139	0	0.2	upsloping	0	normal
20	0	49	male	atypical ang	130	266	0	normal	171	0	0.6	upsloping	0	normal
21	0	64	male	typical ang	110	211	0	left vent hypertrophy	144	1	1.8	flat	0	normal
22	0	58	female	typical ang	150	283	1	left vent hypertrophy	162	0	1.0	upsloping	0	normal

can be used for more relevant features. Another issue with classifiers is the stability of the classifier. Most of classifier works better on best/average case, therefore lots of efforts are needed in worst case settings.

Most of the classifiers works on image data only. The genetic code of patient are still not explored of future heart disease predictions. Deep learning models can be applied on genetic codes but number of epochs are still problem for creating learning models. The new system must be proposes the solution for challenges of the present system for early diagnosis of the disease.

Table 4. Accuracy on different features

S.No	Method	13	12	11	10	9	8	7	6	5	4	3	2	1
1	**Neural Network**	0.86	0.84	0.85	0.86	0.87	0.83	0.82	0.80	0.80	0.79	0.8	0.78	0.59
2	**SVM**	0.88	0.88	0.89	0.89	0.89	0.88	0.88	0.88	0.88	0.88	0.79	0.69	0.58
3	**Random Forest**	0.88	0.88	0.89	0.89	0.89	0.87	0.87	0.87	0.87	0.87	0.86	0.80	0.71
4	**Logistic Regression**	0.90	0.90	0.90	0.90	0.90	0.90	0.90	0.90	0.89	0.89	0.87	0.78	0.60
5	**kNN**	0.68	0.68	0.67	0.71	0.70	0.71	0.81	0.80	0.85	0.85	0.86	0.71	0.76
6	**AdaBoost**	0.74	0.74	0.73	0.76	0.78	0.76	0.77	0.79	0.81	0.78	0.84	0.78	0.60
7	**Naive Bayes**	0.91	0.91	0.91	0.91	0.91	0.90	0.90	0.90	0.90	0.90	0.88	0.80	0.61
8	**DecisionTree**	0.69	0.70	0.71	0.74	0.74	0.71	0.72	0.73	0.78	0.80	0.85	0.79	0.61
9	**SGD**	0.50	0.50	0.50	0.50	0.50	0.50	0.50	0.50	0.50	0.50	0.50	0.50	0.50
10	**CN2 rule inducer**	0.78	0.81	0.81	0.83	0.79	0.81	0.81	0.82	0.84	0.83	0.85	0.81	0.60

Table 5. CA on different features

S.No	Method	13	12	11	10	9	8	7	6	5	4	3	2	1
1	**Neural Network**	0.79	0.76	0.79	0.80	0.80	0.78	0.78	0.77	0.77	0.75	0.83	0.73	0.76
2	**SVM**	0.83	0.82	0.83	0.82	0.84	0.84	0.83	0.83	0.82	0.83	0.81	0.74	0.76
3	**Random Forest**	0.80	0.80	0.80	0.80	0.82	0.79	0.80	0.81	0.79	0.79	0.82	0.74	0.76
4	**Logistic Regression**	0.84	0.85	0.85	0.85	0.84	0.85	0.85	0.83	0.83	0.83	0.84	0.72	0.76
5	**kNN**	0.65	0.65	0.65	0.68	0.69	0.70	0.77	0.76	0.80	0.81	0.81	0.58	0.75
6	**AdaBoost**	0.74	0.74	0.73	0.76	0.78	0.77	0.77	0.80	0.77	0.74	0.82	0.73	0.76
7	**Naive Bayes**	0.83	0.84	0.83	0.83	0.83	0.82	0.84	0.83	0.84	0.81	0.85	0.73	0.76
8	**Decision Tree**	0.73	0.74	0.75	0.77	0.76	0.73	0.73	0.74	0.76	0.77	0.84	0.74	0.76
9	**SGD**	0.84	0.84	0.83	0.85	0.85	0.84	0.84	0.84	0.84	0.83	0.82	0.75	0.76
10	**CN2 rule inducer**	0.73	0.73	0.74	0.74	0.71	0.70	0.73	0.73	0.76	0.75	0.82	0.74	0.76

Table 6. F1 measure on different features

S.No	Method	13	12	11	10	9	8	7	6	5	4	3	2	1
1	**Neural Network**	0.77	0.73	0.77	0.79	0.79	0.76	0.76	0.74	0.75	0.73	0.80	0.66	0.74
2	**SVM**	0.82	0.80	0.81	0.80	0.82	0.81	0.80	0.81	0.80	0.80	0.78	0.68	0.74
3	**Random Forest**	0.78	0.77	0.78	0.77	0.80	0.76	0.78	0.79	0.77	0.77	0.80	0.68	0.74
4	**Logistic Regression**	0.82	0.83	0.82	0.82	0.82	0.83	0.83	0.81	0.81	0.81	0.82	0.66	0.74
5	**kNN**	0.60	0.60	0.61	0.65	0.66	0.67	0.73	0.71	0.77	0.78	0.78	0.58	0.72
6	**AdaBoost**	0.72	0.72	0.71	0.74	0.76	0.75	0.75	0.77	0.74	0.70	0.79	0.66	0.74
7	**Naive Bayes**	0.82	0.82	0.81	0.81	0.81	0.80	0.82	0.81	0.82	0.79	0.83	0.67	0.74
8	**DecisionTree**	0.71	0.71	0.72	0.73	0.73	0.69	0.70	0.70	0.72	0.74	0.81	0.68	0.74
9	**SGD**	0.81	0.81	0.81	0.82	0.83	0.81	0.82	0.82	0.81	0.80	0.79	0.72	0.74
10	**CN2 rule inducer**	0.71	0.69	0.71	0.71	0.69	0.68	0.70	0.71	0.73	0.71	0.79	0.68	0.74

Table 7. Precision on different features

S.No	Method	13	12	11	10	9	8	7	6	5	4	3	2	1
1	**Neural Network**	0.75	0.76	0.78	0.77	0.78	0.75	0.76	0.76	0.74	0.73	0.83	0.76	0.74
2	**SVM**	0.82	0.82	0.84	0.82	0.86	0.85	0.84	0.86	0.84	0.86	0.85	0.79	0.74
3	**Random Forest**	0.81	0.79	0.79	0.81	0.82	0.79	0.80	0.80	0.78	0.79	0.82	0.77	0.74
4	**Logistic Regression**	0.85	0.87	0.86	0.86	0.85	0.87	0.87	0.84	0.84	0.84	0.84	0.73	0.74
5	**kNN**	0.63	0.64	0.63	0.65	0.67	0.67	0.80	0.78	0.81	0.82	0.81	0.53	0.74
6	**AdaBoost**	0.72	0.72	0.71	0.74	0.76	0.74	0.74	0.79	0.76	0.73	0.83	0.76	0.74
7	**Naive Bayes**	0.82	0.83	0.83	0.82	0.82	0.80	0.83	0.84	0.85	0.81	0.87	0.75	0.75
8	**DecisionTree**	0.70	0.71	0.73	0.77	0.75	0.72	0.73	0.73	0.75	0.77	0.87	0.79	0.75
9	**SGD**	0.86	0.86	0.84	0.86	0.87	0.86	0.85	0.88	0.86	0.85	0.84	0.74	0.74
10	**CN2 rule inducer**	0.71	0.72	0.73	0.72	0.69	0.67	0.71	0.71	0.76	0.75	0.84	0.79	0.75

Table 8. Recall on different features

S.No	Method	13	12	11	10	9	8	7	6	5	4	3	2	1
1	**Neural Network**	0.80	0.71	0.76	0.81	0.80	0.77	0.76	0.73	0.76	0.73	0.78	0.59	0.73
2	**SVM**	0.81	0.78	0.78	0.78	0.78	0.78	0.77	0.76	0.76	0.74	0.72	0.59	0.73
3	**Random Forest**	0.75	0.76	0.76	0.73	0.78	0.73	0.76	0.78	0.76	0.74	0.78	0.61	0.73
4	**Logistic Regression**	0.80	0.80	0.79	0.79	0.79	0.79	0.79	0.77	0.78	0.77	0.79	0.60	0.73
5	**kNN**	0.57	0.57	0.60	0.66	0.66	0.67	0.67	0.66	0.74	0.74	0.76	0.65	0.71
6	**AdaBoost**	0.71	0.71	0.71	0.73	0.76	0.75	0.76	0.76	0.71	0.68	0.76	0.59	0.73
7	**Naive Bayes**	0.81	0.81	0.80	0.80	0.80	0.80	0.81	0.78	0.78	0.77	0.80	0.60	0.73
8	**DecisionTree**	0.71	0.72	0.71	0.71	0.72	0.66	0.67	0.68	0.70	0.71	0.76	0.59	0.73
9	**SGD**	0.76	0.76	0.78	0.79	0.79	0.76	0.78	0.76	0.76	0.76	0.75	0.70	0.73
10	**CN2 rule inducer**	0.71	0.66	0.69	0.71	0.68	0.69	0.70	0.70	0.70	0.67	0.73	0.59	0.73

After identifying heart disease, next work will be personalized medicine recommendation. This medicine management system will include not only the symptoms but also the genetic signatures and biomedical parameters too. These additional parameters will identify the state of the disease. Therefore, Personalization is the future.

CONCLUSION

Nowadays, heart disease is one of the most chronic diseases faced by the human race. Early diagnosis can help in prevention of such chronic disease. With the emergence of digital pathology, artificial intelligence and machine learning contributes a lot. It provides essential power of intelligent computing to diagnose disease early. Various machine learning and data mining algorithms are studied in this chapter and performance of the algorithms are evaluated on the UCI Statlog dataset. This chapter summarized and evaluated the performance of the common and widely used classification techniques for heart disease diagnosis. Information gain based feature selection technique combined with various classifiers to get better prediction.

REFERENCES

Acharya, U. R., Fujita, H., Oh, S. L., Hagiwara, Y., Tan, J. H., Adam, M., & Tan, R. S. (2018). Deep convolutional neural network for the automated diagnosis of congestive heart failure using ECG signals. *Applied Intelligence*, 1–12.

Acharya, U. R., Fujita, H., Sudarshan, V. K., Oh, S. L., Muhmmand, A., Koh, J. E., ... Tan, R. S. (2017). Application of empirical mode decomposition (EMD) for automated identification of congestive heart failure using heart rate signals. *Neural Computing & Applications*, *28*(10), 3073–3094. doi:10.100700521-016-2612-1

Anooj, P. K. (2011). Clinical decision support system: Risk level prediction of heart disease using weighted fuzzy rules and decision tree rules. *Central European Journal of Computer Science*, *1*(4), 482–498.

Asyali, M. H. (2003). Discrimination power of long-term heart rate variability measures. *Proceedings of the 25th Annual International Conference of the IEEE Engineering in Medicine and Biology Society* (pp. 200-203). Cancun, Mexico: IEEE. 10.1109/IEMBS.2003.1279568

Awang, R., & Palaniappan, S. (2007). Web based Heart Disease Decision Support System using Data Mining Classification Modeling techniques. In iiWAS, (pp. 177-187). Jakarta: Academic Press.

Ayat, S., & Khosravanian, A. (2014). Identification and classification of Coronary Artery disease patients using Neuro-Fuzzy Inference system. *Journal of Mathematics and Computer Science*, *13*(02), 136–141. doi:10.22436/jmcs.013.02.05

Deepika, N. (2011). Association Rule for Classification of Heart Attack Patients. *IJAEST*, *11*(2), 253–257.

Determining the Appropriate Amount of Anesthetic Gas Using DWT and EMD Combined with Neural Network - Scientific Figure on ResearchGate. (n.d.). Retrieved June 2018, 15, from ResearchGate: https://www.researchgate.net/Artificial-neuron-model-43_fig2_275965841

Dua, D., & Karra Taniskidou, E. (2017). *Statlog (Heart) Data Set.* Retrieved from UCI Machine Learning Repository: http://archive.ics.uci.edu/ml/datasets/Statlog+%28Heart%29

Durairaj, M., & Meena, K. (2011). A Hybrid Prediction System using Rough Sets and Artificial Neural Network. *International Journal of Innovative Technology and Creative Engineering*, *1*(7), 16–23.

Eliot, L. (2018, Jan 19). *Support Vector Machines (SVM) for AI Self-Driving Cars.* Retrieved from AITrends: https://aitrends.com/ai-insider/support-vector-machines-svm-ai-self-driving-cars/

Eskin, E., & Pevzner, P. A. (2002). Finding composite regulatory patterns in DNA sequences. *Bioinformatics (Oxford, England), 18*(Suppl 1), 354–363. doi:10.1093/bioinformatics/18.suppl_1.S354 PMID:12169566

Fidele, B., Cheeneebash, J., Gopaul, A., & Goorah, S. S. (2009). Artificial neural network as a clinical decision-supporting tool to predict cardiovascular disease. *Trends in Applied Sciences Research, 4*(1), 36–46. doi:10.3923/tasr.2009.36.46

Gokulnath, C. B., & Shantharajah, S. P. (2018). An optimized feature selection based on genetic approach and support vector machine for heart disease. *Cluster Computing*, 1–11.

Huang, K., Yang, H., King, I., Lyu, M. R., & Chan, L. (2004). The Minimum Error Minimax Probability Machine. *Journal of Machine Learning Research, 5*, 1253–1286.

Human Heart Diagram. (n.d.). Retrieved May 21, 2018, from Dreamstime: https://www.dreamstime.com/stock-illustration-human-heart-diagram-illustration-image55185229

Isler, Y., & Kantalp, M. (2007). Combining classical HRV indices with wavelet entropy measures improves to performance in diagnosing congestive heart failure. *Computers in Biology and Medicine, 37*(10), 1502–1510. doi:10.1016/j.compbiomed.2007.01.012 PMID:17359959

Jilani, T. A., Yasin, H., Yasin, M., & Ardil, C. (2009). Acute coronary syndrome prediction using data mining techniques-an application. *World Academy of Science, Engineering and Technology, 59*(4), 295–299.

Karaolis, M. A., Moutiris, J. A., Hadjipanayi, D., & Pattichis, C. P. (2010). Assessment of the Risk Factors of Coronary Heart Events Based on Data Mining With Decision Trees. *IEEE Transactions on Information Technology in Biomedicine, 14*(3), 559–566. doi:10.1109/TITB.2009.2038906 PMID:20071264

Khatibi, V., & Montazer, G. A. (2010). A fuzzy-evidential hybrid inference engine for coronary heart disease risk assessment. *Expert Systems with Applications, 37*(12), 8536–8542. doi:10.1016/j.eswa.2010.05.022

Krogh, A. (1994). Hidden Markov models for labeled sequences. In *International Conference on Pattern Recognition* (pp. 140-144). Jerusalem: The IEEE Computer Society. 10.1109/ICPR.1994.576891

Kumar, S., & Arasu, G. T. (2017). Rough set theory and fuzzy logic based warehousing of heterogeneous clinical databases. *International Journal of Uncertainty, Fuzziness and Knowledge-based Systems, 25*(3), 385–408. doi:10.1142/S0218488517500167

Li, J., Zhang, R., Shi, L., & Wang, D. (2016). Automatic Whole-Heart Segmentation in Congenital Heart Disease Using Deeply-Supervised 3D FCN. In First International Workshops, RAMBO 2016 and HVSMR 2016.10129 (pp. 111-118). Athens: Reconstruction, Segmentation, and Analysis of Medical Images: LNCS.

Luukka, P., & Lampinen, J. (2010). A Classification method based on principal component analysis and differential evolution algorithm applied for prediction diagnosis from clinical EMR heart data sets. In Y. Tenne & C. K. Goh (Eds.), *Computational Intelligence in Optimization. Adaptation, Learning, and Optimization* (pp. 263–283). Springer. doi:10.1007/978-3-642-12775-5_11

Manogaran, G., Varatharajan, R., & Priyan, M. K. (2018). Hybrid Recommendation System for Heart Disease Diagnosis based on Multiple Kernel Learning with Adaptive Neuro-Fuzzy Inference System. *Multimedia Tools and Applications*, *77*(4), 4379–4399. doi:10.100711042-017-5515-y

Muthukarupan, S., & Erib, M. J. (2012). A hybrid PSO based fuzzy expert system for the diagnosis of Coronary heart system. *Expert Systems with Applications*, *39*, 11657–11665. doi:10.1016/j.eswa.2012.04.036

Nahar, J., Imam, T., Tickle, K. S., & Chen, Y.-P. P. (2013). Association rule mining to detect factors which contribute to heart disease in males and females. *Expert Systems with Applications*, *40*(4), 1086–1093. doi:10.1016/j.eswa.2012.08.028

Nirschl, J. J., Janowczyk, A., Peyster, E. G., Frank, R., Margulies, K. B., Feldman, M. D., & Madabhushi, A. (2018). A deep-learning classifier identifies patients with clinical heart failure using whole-slide images of H&E tissue. *PLoS One*, *13*(4), e0192726. doi:10.1371/journal.pone.0192726 PMID:29614076

Ordonez, C. (2006). Association rule discovery with the train and test approach for heart disease prediction. *IEEE Transactions on Information Technology in Biomedicine*, *10*(2), 334–343. doi:10.1109/TITB.2006.864475 PMID:16617622

Ordonez, C., Omincenski, E., de Braal, L., Santana, C. A., Ezquerra, N., Taboada, J. A., ... Garcia, E. V. (2001). Mining Constraint Association Rules to Predict Heart Disease. In *IEEE International Conference of Data Mining* (pp. 433-440). San Jose, CA: IEEE.

Ozcift, A., & Gulten, A. (2011). Classifier ensemble construction with rotation forest to improve medical diagnosis performance of machine learning algorithms. *Computer Methods and Programs in Biomedicine*, *104*(3), 443–451. doi:10.1016/j.cmpb.2011.03.018 PMID:21531475

Pace, D. F. D. A. (2015). Interactive Whole-Heart Segmentation in Congenital Heart Disease. In MICCAI 2015.9351 (pp. 80-88). Munich, Germany: LNCS Springer.

Palaniappan, S., & Awang, R. (2008). Intelligent heart disease prediction system using data mining techniques. *International Journal of Computer Science and Network Security*, *8*(8), 108–115.

Patil, S. B., & Kumaraswamy, Y. S. (2009). Intelligent and effective heart attack prediction system using data mining and artificial neural network. *European Journal of Scientific Research*, *31*(4), 642–656.

Pazzani, M. J., & Ratanamahatana, C. A. (2005). Exact indexing of dynamic time warping. *Knowledge and Information Systems*, *7*(3), 358–386. doi:10.100710115-004-0154-9

Polat, K., & Gunes, S. (2009). A new feature selection method on classification of medical datasets: Kernel F-score feature selection. *Expert Systems with Applications*, *36*(7), 10367–10373. doi:10.1016/j.eswa.2009.01.041

Raghavendra, U., Acharya, U. R., Gudigar, A., Shetty, R., Krishnananda, N., Pai, U., ... Nayak, C. (2017). Automated screening of congestive heart failure using variational mode decomposition and texture features extracted from ultrasound images. *Neural Computing & Applications*, *28*(10), 2869–2878. doi:10.100700521-017-2839-5

Rangnath, R., Perotte, A., Elhadad, N., & Blei, D. (2016). Deep Survival Analysis. In *Proceedings of the 1st Machine Learning in Health Care*, (pp. 101-114). Los Angeles, CA: Academic Press.

Saqlain, S. M., Sher, M., Shah, F. A., Khan, I., Ashraf, M. U., Awais, M., & Ghani, A. (2018). Fisher score and Matthews correlation coefficient-based feature subset selection for heart disease diagnosis using support vector machines. *Knowledge and Information Systems*, 1–29.

Sekar, B. D., & Dong, M. (2014). Function Formula Oriented Construction of Bayesian Inference Nets for Diagnosis of Cardiovascular Disease. *BioMed Research International*. PMID:25247174

Setiawan, N. A., Venkatachalam, P. A., & Hani, A. F. (2009). Diagnosis of coronary artery disease using artificial intelligence based decision support system. In *International Conference on Man-Machine Systems*, (pp. 1-5). Batu Ferringhi, Penang: Academic Press.

Shi, H., & Liu, Y. (2011). Naïve Bayes vs. Support Vector Machine: Resilience to Missing Data. In *International Conference on Artificial Intelligence and Computational Intelligence* (pp. 680-687). Chengdu, China: LNCS, Springer. 10.1007/978-3-642-23887-1_86

Syed, Z., & Guttag, J. (2011). Unsupervised Similarity-Based Risk Stratification for Cardiovascular Events Using Long-Term Time-Series Data. *Journal of Machine Learning Research*, *12*, 999–1024.

Tan, K. C., Teoh, E. J., Yu, Q., & Goh, K. C. (2009). A hybrid evolutionary algorithm for attribute selection in data mining. *Expert Systems with Applications*, *36*(4), 8616–8630. doi:10.1016/j.eswa.2008.10.013

Tsipouras, M. G., Exarchos, T. P., Fotiadis, D. I., Kotsia, A. P., Vakalis, K. V., Naka, K. K., & Michalis, L. K. (2008). Automated Diagnosis of Coronary Artery Disease Based on Data Mining and Fuzzy Modeling. *IEEE Transactions on Information Technology in Biomedicine*, *12*(4), 447–458. doi:10.1109/TITB.2007.907985 PMID:18632325

Uguz, H. (2012). Adaptive neuro-fuzzy inference system for diagnosis of the heart valve diseases using wavelet transform with entropy. *Neural Computing & Applications*, *21*(7), 1617–1628. doi:10.100700521-011-0610-x

Vahid, K., & Gholam, A. M. (2010). A fuzzy-evidential hybrid inference engine for coronary heart disease risk assessment. *Expert Systems with Applications*, *37*(12), 8536–8542. doi:10.1016/j.eswa.2010.05.022

Yang, J.-G., Kim, J. K., Kang, U. G., & Lee, Y. H. (2014). Coronary heart disease optimization system on adaptive-network-based fuzzy inference system and linear discriminant analysis (ANFIS–LDA). *Personal and Ubiquitous Computing*, *18*(6), 1351–1362. doi:10.100700779-013-0737-0

Yen, H., Zheng, J., Jiang, Y., Peng, C., & Xaio, S. (2008). Selecting critical clinical features for heart diseases diagnosis with a real-coded genetic algorithm. *Applied Soft Computing*, *8*(2), 1105–1111. doi:10.1016/j.asoc.2007.05.017

ADDITIONAL READING

Navab, N., Hornegger, J., Well, W. M., & Frangi, A. F. (Eds.). (2015). *Medical Image Computing and Computer-Assisted Intervention*. Springer.

Zuluaga, M. A., Bhatia, K., Kainz, B., Moghari, M. H., & Pace, D. F. (Eds.). (2016). *Reconstruction, Segmentation, and Analysis of Medical Images*. Springer.

KEY TERMS AND DEFINITIONS

Accuracy: In classification, it one of the metric to evaluate the classification model and defined as: Accuracy=(Number of correct predictions)/(Total number of predictions).

Classification: It is task of classifying the data into predefined number of classes. It is a supervised approach. The tagged data is used to create classification model that will be used for classification on unknown data.

Deep Learning: It is class of one machine learning algorithms that can be supervised, unsupervised, or semi-supervised. It uses multiple layers of processing units for feature extraction and transformation.

Deep Survival Analysis: In context of electronic health records, it is hierarchical generative approach to analyze the survival time of the patient.

F1-Measure: For uneven class distributions, accuracy does not work well, F1-measure, another evaluation metric is used. It is harmonic average works better even if false positives and false negatives are different.

Particle Swarm Optimization: It is an optimization method that iteratively tries to improve solution based on certain measures.

Sphygmogram Signals: Used to measure blood pressure.

Chapter 9
Real-Time Cardio Monitoring and Characterization of Diseases Introducing Statistical and Spectrogram Analysis

Soumyendu Bhattacharjee
Maulana Abul Kalam Azad University of Technology, India

Subham Ghosh
JIS College of Engineering, India

Biswarup Neogi
JIS College of Engineering, India

ABSTRACT

This chapter provides significant theoretical and systematic frameworks and the latest empirical research towards the development of an automated cardiovascular disorder diagnostic system with the classifier. This research proposes an accurate non-invasive model of the cardiovascular diseases diagnostic system. This model of diagnostic system support superior mobility with continuous real-time monitoring facility. This monitoring system will uncover a new dimension towards cardiovascular research. A physician will able to monitor several heart patients remotely with this device. Also, they can prescribe proper medicine remotely to the patient in an emergency. The system also has a provision to alert the patient by predicting the specific type of cardiovascular disorder accurately. An automated cardiovascular disorder diagnostic system development focuses towards the prime objective. Another objective is the adoption of modern classification technique for detecting cardiovascular disorders with high accuracy.

INTRODUCTION

The cardiovascular disorder has now been a massive problem throughout the world. According to the W.H.O. (World Health Organization) The cardiovascular diseases were responsible for an estimated 17.7 million deaths globally in 2015, representing around 31% of all global deaths (World Health Organization

DOI: 10.4018/978-1-5225-7796-6.ch009

[WHO], 2017). The malfunction of human heart and disorder in the blood circulation system including arteries and vain are responsible for the cardiovascular disorder. Several important factors are responsible for cardiovascular disorder including taking a heavy amount of medicine, unbalanced and unhealthy lifestyles like drinking excessive alcohol, smoking, and excessive consumption of high-caloric food like red meat, egg, and high blood pressure, obesity, diabetes, mental stress. These risk factors severely reduce functional activity of heart and blood circulation system. The abnormal functionality of heart pumping and blood circulation system is the main cause of several fatal diseases like mitral stenosis, rheumatic heart disease, mitral valve regurgitation, and aortic regurgitation, myocardial infarction, tricuspid regurgitation, aortic stenosis, asthma, tricuspid stenosis, ischemic heart disease with including the deadly heart attack. As a result, the scientists are looking forward to taking advantage of further development related to cardiovascular disorders. The effect of advancement in engineering in our society; a vast change has taken place in medical science. Now the conceptual development of an automated cardiovascular disorder diagnostic system has been proposed for detecting several cardiovascular diseases with the high level of accuracy. The diseases we are dealing with here are Myocardial Syndrome, Myocardial Infarction, Heart Attack, and Sinus Syndrome.

Myocardial infarction (MI) is the irreversible death (necrosis) of heart muscle secondary to prolonged lack of oxygen supply (ischemia). Patients with typical MI may have the prodromal symptoms in the days preceding the event such as Fatigue, Chest discomfort, Malaise.

Acute myocardial infarction is a life-threatening cardiovascular problem that occurs when blood flow to the heart muscle is abruptly cut off. That is a serious cause of permanent tissue damage. This life-threatening condition generally occurred due to the blockage in one or more of the coronary arteries in the cardiac system.

Sick sinus syndrome also is known as sinus node disease or sinus node dysfunction is the name for a collection of heart rhythm problems (arrhythmias) in which the sinus node the heart's natural pacemaker doesn't work accurately. The sinus node is an area of specific cells in the upper right chamber of the heart that controls the rhythm of the heart. Normally, the sinus node of the heart produces a steady pace of regular electrical impulses. In sick sinus syndrome, these signals are abnormally paced. It is relatively uncommon, but the risk of developing sick sinus syndrome increases with age.

A heart attack appears if the flow of oxygen-rich blood to a segment of heart muscle abruptly becomes blocked and the heart can't get oxygen. If blood flow isn't restored quickly, the section of heart muscle begins to die.

A view of the heart's activity, which generated during the cardiac cycle, is provided by the view of electrocardiogram (ECG). The condition human cardiovascular system can be depicted through the detailed analysis of ECG signal graph. Here in this scenario, two different types of classification models are introduced in the segment of cardio-diagnostic system for efficiently detecting a specific type of heart disease.

THE ECG signal analysis and simulation in terms of spectrogram representation is the essential element in this study for diagnosing various cardiovascular disease. The spectrogram analysis of the human heart ECG signal for detecting the abnormalities of the cardiovascular system has been studied. The spectrum of the signal frequencies is visually represented by spectrogram analysis with the variation of time and frequency. The innovative spectrogram analysis model of ECG signal has been proposed for visual detection of various fatal heart problem like myocardial infarction, myocardial syndrome, sick sinus syndrome, heart attack. Along with this, the generalized study of heart ECG signal has been observed. An electrocardiogram abbreviated as EKG or ECG is a test that measures the electrical activity of the heartbeat. A typical ECG tracing is a repeating cycle of three electrical entities: a P wave (atrial depolarization), a QRS complex (ventricular depolarization) and a T wave (ventricular repolarization). The study of spectrogram in this chapter is a major field of work. A spectrogram is a visual representation of the spectrum of frequencies in a sound or other signal as they vary with time and frequency. The frequency also varies in accordance with the various conditions of the heart.

Now accumulating analysis this various state of the heart, a new algorithm has developed which may guide the scientists to achieve their goals towards the development of continues heart monitoring model. This heart monitoring model introduces diseases diagnostic model for heart by accepting the modern classifiers.

BACKGROUND ANALYSIS

Study on Human Heart: In 2014 a ventricular assist device was patented that connected with electrodes and responsible for smooth blood flow (Choi & Min, 2014). The motor, pump, and blood circulation can be demonstrated with the aid of time extension with maximum price $\tau = 1$ sec. The goal is to accomplish a step response with much less than 5% consistent country error and less than 10% overshoot. Moreover, to graph a controller the use of a PID controller (Ghosal, Darbar, Neogi, Das, & Tibarewala, 2012). An efficient heart rate control algorithm was designed by testing various control system methods. Some pacemaker controlling mechanisms including Zeigler-Nichols based PID controller were analyzed to find out best-suited heart bit controller. It was assumed that the pacemaker control system is the example of negative feedback based closed loop control system. The neural network based PID control system is best for controlling of heart bit for the pacemaker (Castro & Malathi, 2018). A Fuzzy logic based PID control algorithm was developed and simulated by Zhao et al. in 2014. The fuzzy PID controller has some advantages including system robustness and advanced control precision compared with conventional PID controller. Many heart rate controllers have been analyzing for optimum performance. In 2016 fractional-order PID controller was designed that almost outperformed all other control mechanisms like fuzzy logic controller, traditional PID controller in terms of stability, rise time, stability, settling time. This Ziegler-Nichols tuning based control system has less than 2% overshoot problem, and that is essential for the stability of heart pacemaker control (Arunachalam, Kapa, Mulpuru, Friedman & Tolkacheva, 2016). O.H. Frazier tested a battery powered Electric Ventricular Assist Device that allows a patient to maintain their daily life activity. The low-speed torque motor pumps the blood efficiently to maintain a proper heartbeat (Frazier, 1994).

The diagnostic system for ECG rhythm monitoring (Hamilton & Tompkins, 1986) was based on syntactic approaches. A given frame of the signal is first approximated piecewise linearly into a set of line segments that are completely specified in terms of their length and slope values. In paper (Ghaffari, Golbayani & Ghasemi, 2008) MIT-BIH Arrhythmia Database has been used for the detecting the performance of real-time QRS detection algorithms for the selection of QRS detectors. In an article (Hai-Ying & Kun-Mean, 2008) ECG detection has been performed using continuous wavelet transform (CWT). Wavelet transforms are applied to decompose the signal into a set of coefficients that describe the signal frequency content at given times. Article (Portet, Hernandez & Carrault, 2005) proposes an embedded real-time QRS detection algorithm system. In an article (Zeraatkar & Kermani, 2010) the QRS detection algorithm is based on the Empirical Mode Decomposition (EMD). Empirical mode decomposition can decompose the signal into a series of intrinsic mode function (IMFs). The QRS detector (Meissimilly,

Rodriguez, Rodriguez, Gonzalez & Caiiizares, 2003) is based on the Hamilton- Tompkins algorithm. The preprocessor stage enhances the QRS complex by reducing the contribution of the non-correlated noise. In paper (Whan Lee, Seop Kim, Lee, Lee & Lee, 2002) the algorithm is used for the characteristics of reconstructed phase portraits by delay coordinate mapping utilizing lag rotundity for real-time detection of QRS complexes in ECG signals. The method (Zhengzhong, Fanxue & Xu, 2011) consists of combining the differential threshold method and the amplitude detection method utilized for localization of R-waves. Article (Pueyo, Sörnmo & Pablo Laguna, 2008) presents a Hilbert transform method for extraction of the fetal heart rate. The method may be applied to signals derived from a single channel or an array of channels. In this paper (Chatterjee, Gupta, Bera & Mitra, 2011) an FPGA implementation of Real Time QRS Detection is presented.

Cardiovascular Disorder Diagnosis System is a rising trend in medicinal and engineering trade. A pacemaker is a small device, positioned in the chest or abdomen, that generates electrical pulses to prompt the heartbeat in a normal rate to resume the regular lifestyle of a person by providing relief from fatigue and fainting caused due to the irregular rhythm of the heart (Bhattacharjee, et.al., 2013; Cohn et.al., 2000). For generating and implementing the heart equation depending on various diseases with different ages of human, control theory approach is implemented (Cook & Shaper, 1988). Clinical implications and diagnosis system for heart failure are defined (Cohn et al. & Cowie et al., 2000; Garg et al., 2005) and discussed the effects of the computerised decision support systems for heart disease patients. In 2007, Polat et al. represented an automatic heart disease detection system using fuzzy resource allocation system with machine learning mechanism (Haider, 2008). Mann et al. (2011) designed a system that can detect, diagnose and treat cardiovascular disease. (Nagendra et al., 2006) discussed a technique for improving the condition of chronic diseases through biomedical signal monitoring. ECG signal analysis with polynomial function and curve fitting for data analysis is a modern trend (Kleiger, Miller, Bigger, & A.J., 1987). Mathematical modelling with polynomial equation analysis for an ECG generator is discussed (Kovács, 2012) by extracting the features of the signal. A virtual health management technique for patients related to various cardiovascular diseases is depicted by Lehto et al. (Lehto, Oinas-Kukkonen, Pätiälä, & Saarelma, 2013).

Study On Diseases Classification: In 2013, the World Health Organization and the World Heart Federation reported that more than 17 million people died from cardiovascular diseases (CVD) and around 3 million of these deaths happened beforehand the age of 60 (Sony, Ansari, Sharma & Sony, 2011). Yet, 90% of those deaths were expected to be avoidable, if patients have correctly been spotted and classify in early and improving their daily routines (Choi & Min, 2014). CVD passing away are caused by high blood pressure of about 13%, while tobacco effects in 9%, diabetes 6%, lack of workout 6% and obesity 5% in the United States. Worldwide health issues are credited to cardiovascular diseases by 30%. All over the world, 12.3 million (25.8%) of people pretentious by CVD in the earlier years has been increased by 17.3 million that is approx. 31.5% till now. It has been estimated that CVD death rate of 272 per 100 000 populations in India is higher than the overall average of 235 per 100 000 populations. Premature mortality in terms of years of life lost because of CVD in India increased by 59%, from 23.2 million to 37 million (Saktheeswari & Adalarasu, 2017).

The different types of CVD are coronary artery disease, heart attack, arrhythmia, heart failure, congenital heart defects, cardiomyopathy and peripheral artery disease. The different tools used for diagnosing of CVD are Electrocardiography (ECG), Phonocardiography, Echocardiography, Halter monitoring, coronary angiography, intravascular ultrasound, Cardio visor. In other source, Cardiovascular disease (CVD) includes coronary artery diseases (CAD) such as angina and myocardial infarction that are commonly

Figure 1. An ECG signal: (a) Generated by simulation (b) obtained in clinic

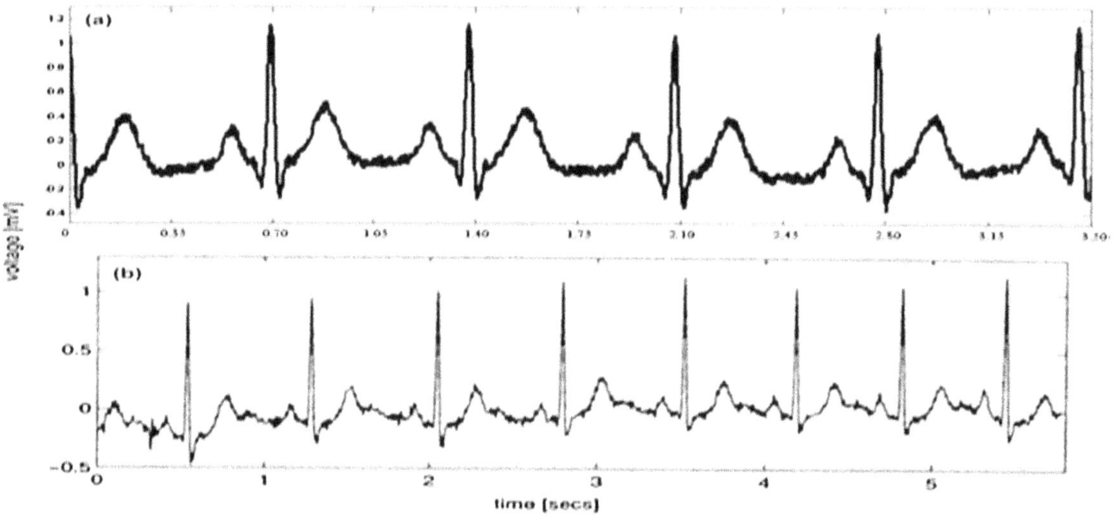

known as a heart attack. Other CVDs include stroke, heart failure, hypertensive heart disease, rheumatic heart disease, cardiomyopathy, heart arrhythmia, congenital heart disease, valvar heart disease,, aortic aneurysms, peripheral artery disease, thromboembolic disease, and venous thrombosis. The initial recognition of irregular heart conditions is the most important to classify heart issues and avoid unexpected cardiac death. The patients with similar heart conditions almost have similar electrocardiogram (ECG) signals. Electrocardiogram (ECG) is an essential tool at the present time for analyzing the Cardiovascular Diseases (CVD). The study on the ECG signal gives us a comprehensive data on the patient's cardiac health status. ECG is a simple and specific analytical test for imposing rhythms of heart.

Two classifiers are built to classify ECG signals according to the parameter deviations. In 1972 the preliminary model of the ECG signal was described by Zeeman (Zeeman, 1972), however the effects of the parasympathetic and sympathetic nervous system are not measured. A new model for ECG signal is proposed in Yatollahi et.al. (2005), where a novel consideration conferring to the deeds of the parasympathetic and sympathetic nervous system is mentioned and applied in the Zeeman model. Through these predict heart condition of clinically obtained ECGs more indeed with these classifiers.

Moreover, another discussable point is in maximum cases cardiac arrhythmias which are also one of the most common causes of death and as a result, their accurate detection has been of great interest in biomedical studies, actually don't show any consistent changes in ECG signal, therefore a Halter monitor is needed. Halter monitor is an ECG recorded over a longer period of time (i.e. longer than thirty minutes), which helps the detection of dysrhythmias that may happen briefly and unpredictably throughout that period.

The ECG signal is generated through MATLAB by applying the parameters from (Vafaie, Ataei, & Koofigar, 2014) and explained in Figure 1(a).The real ECG signal which has physiognomies analogous to the simulated ECG is demonstrated in Figure 1(b) to compare real ECG and ECG signal generated by simulating.

ECG signals based numerous methods have been suggested for ischemic beat classification, which assesses the ST segment changes and the T-wave variations with different approaches (Goletsis, Papaloukas, Fotiadis, Likas, & Michalis, 2004). Their appraisal progression is based upon parametric modeling

(Papaloukas, Fotiadis, Likas, & Michalis, n.d.), wavelet transform (Papaloukas, Fotiadis, Likas, Liavas, & Michalis, 2001), set of rules and artificial neural networks (Mahmoodabadi, Ahmadian, & Abolhasani, 2005). Although these methods have achieved acceptable results, enhancements can be made.

Mahmoodabadi et al (2005) suggested an approach for ECG highlight extraction comprising of Daubechies Wavelets transform. These component extraction systems for electrocardiogram (ECG) depended on the multi-resolution wavelet transform. The ECG signals decided for preparing were obtained from Modified Lead II (MLII). The scaling capacity of the wavelet filter is further personally like the shape of the ECG signal which is achieved for better identification. The foremost step of their approach was to diagnose the ECG signal by evacuating the identical wavelet coefficients at higher scales. At that point, QRS complexes are recognized and every one complex is used to trace the peaks of the individual waves, including onsets and offset of the P and T waves which are available in one cardiac cycle. Proposed approach uncovered that ECG include extraction achieved sensitivity of 99.18% and a positive predictively of 98% (Mahmoodabadi, Ahmadian, & Abolhasani, 2005).

Zhao et al (2005) utilized wavelet transform and support vector machines (SVM) for highlight extraction. The order of the system here the system is characterized using three segments including information preprocessing, highlight extraction and classification of ECG signs. The feature vector of ECG information is accomplished by consolidating two distinctive feature extraction techniques. The wavelet transform extricates the coefficient of the transform as the components of every ECG section. Autoregressive displaying (AR) gives the transient structures of ECG waveforms are support vector machine (SVM) characterizes diverse ECG heartbeat. The general exactness of the proposed approach by PC simulation result 99.68%. (Qibin Zhao, & Liqing Zhan)

Sani Saminu et al (2014) proposed wavelet Feature Extraction for ECG Beat Classification. The R-T interval specimens are calculated using discrete wavelet transform (DWT) and mean, median, standard deviation, maximum, minimum, energy and entropy which are considered as the measurable parameters of wavelet coefficients are used as a time-frequency domain feature. The hybrid technique which is proposed in this work has been tested by classifying the ECG beats into three conditions, for example, ordinary, right bundle branch block (Rbbb) and paced beat utilizing the signal from Massachusetts Institute of Technology Beth Israel Hospital (MIT-BIH) arrhythmia database and prepared utilizing Matlab 2013 condition. Neural system back propagation calculation has been used for the order of ECG signal as a result of its straightforwardness. R-T interim components which are proportional gives normal precision of 98.22%, the proposed half and half technique gives a promising outcome with normal exactness of 99.84% by utilizing computational many sided quality with reduced classifier (Sani Saminu, Nalan Özkurt and Ibrahim & Abdullahi Karaye, 2005).

Sreelakshmi T G and Seethal Paul (2015) proposed a precise ECG highlight extraction strategy for distinguishing various cardiovascular diseases. Here the target of their work is creating techniques to analyse and distinguish little transforms in ECG waves and complexes that show cardiovascular disease and disorders. Different cardiovascular disorders like arrhythmia, sinus tachycardia, third degree atrioventricular block, right package branch block, left package branch block, sinus bradycardia, expanded cardiomyopathy, Artial Fibrillation, Flutter, Supraventricular Tachycardia (SVT) and myocardial localized necrosis by utilizing wavelet transform. Wavelet transform is an effective strategy for highlight extraction and can be used alongside neural system structures to build efficient model for diagnosis of bio signals. (Sreelakshmi & Seethal Paul, 2015)

In other way, Data mining techniques plays an important role for predicting or diagnosing diseases with good accuracy and avoid in traditional healthcare environments, diagnosis of a disease depends on doctor's decision for identifying it as the most likely cause depending on a person's symptoms. However, this leads to unwanted errors that resulting on more medical costs and affecting the quality of service provided to patients (Power, Sharda & Burstein, 2015).Surveys such as have been discussed the impact and power of data mining techniques in predicting systems.

MAIN FOCUS OF THE CHAPTER

Issues, Controversies, Problems

To enlargement of the resource of people died from cardiovascular diseases that usually know as a heart attack. It can classify through numerous satiation. In these chapter discussions will spotlighted over the basic four heart attacks, those are Ischemic heart disease, Six-sinus syndrome, myocardial Infraction and myocardial syndrome.

A heart attack which also called Myocardial Infarction usually occurs when a blood clot blocks blood flow to the heart. Deprived of blood, soft tissue loses oxygen and dies. Symptoms include tightness or pain in the chest, neck, back or arms, as well as weakness, wooziness, anomalous heartbeat and nervousness. Women are more likely to have atypical symptoms than men. Treatment ranges from lifestyle changes and cardiac rehabilitation to medication, stents and bypass surgery.

To verify by some of reporting of Apollo Hospitals and others resource that majority of heart attack happen over 60 ages.

Further to noticeable issue is Coronary artery disease (CAD) which is also known as atherosclerotic heart disease and ischemic heart disease. To more closely the usual cause is the build-up of plaque. This causes coronary arteries to narrow, limiting blood flow to the heart. Coronary artery disease can range from no symptoms, to chest pain, to a heart attack. Treatments include lifestyle changes, medication, angioplasty and surgery.

Figure 2. Development of ischemic heart disease
(Shaw, Bugiardini & Merz, 2009)

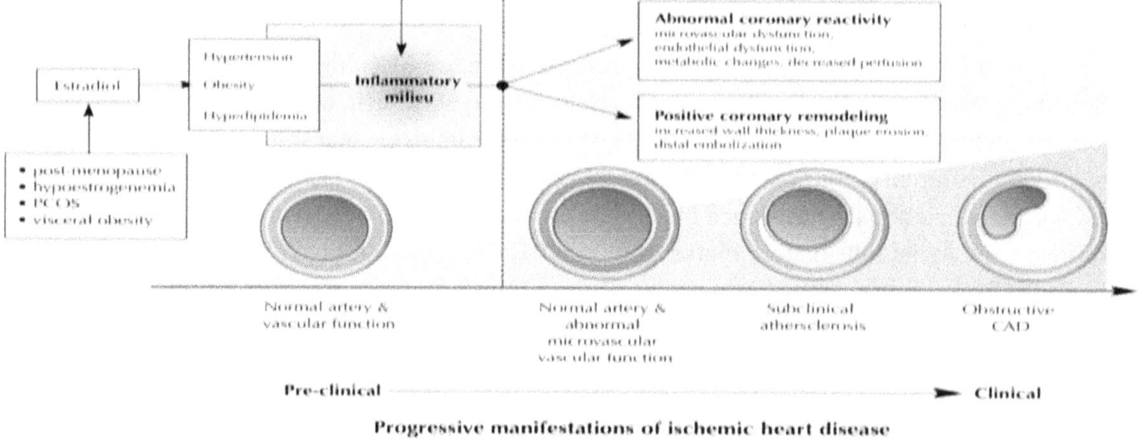

Figure 3. Cardiac problem regarding to sick-sinus syndrome
(Jensen, Gronroos, Chen, Folsom, Heckbert & Alonso, 2014)

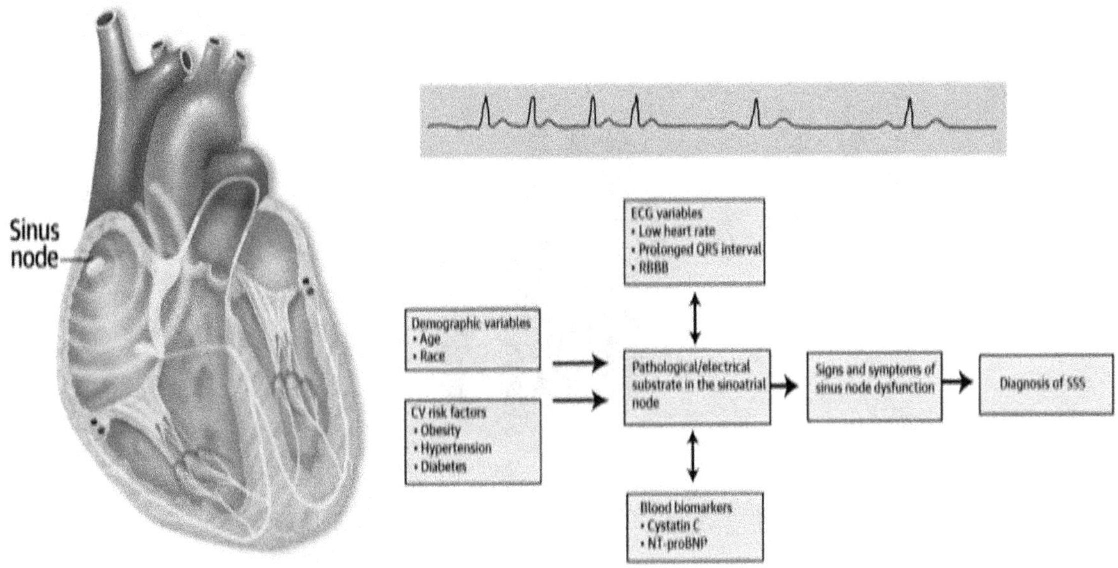

Moreover, coronary artery disease can range from no symptoms, to chest pain, to a heart attack. Although can have no symptoms, but people may experience like pain in the chest, gastrointestinal happen indigestion or nausea, the whole body will wooziness or sweating and also common symptoms like other heart attack is fast heart rate or shortness of breath.

To study sick-sinus syndrome (SSS) is very interesting to count heart beats and Complications are to facing in result of many abnormal heart rhythms or arrhythmias including sinus arrest, sinus node blocks to exit, sinus bradycardia, and other types of bradycardia. Sick sinus syndrome may also be associated

Figure 4. ECG signal variation in sick-sinus
(Keller & Lemberg, 2007)

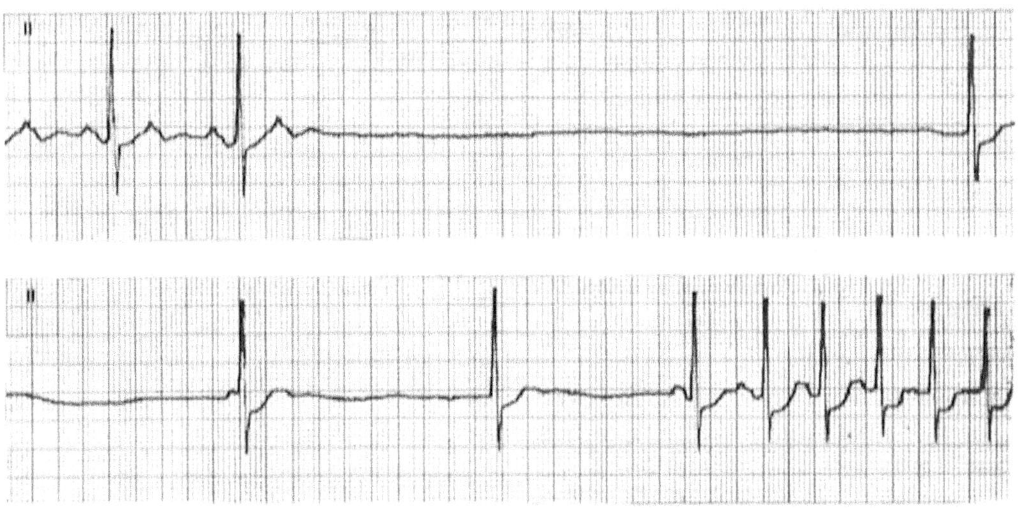

Figure 5. Representation of acute coronary syndrome
(Luscher & Templin, 2016)

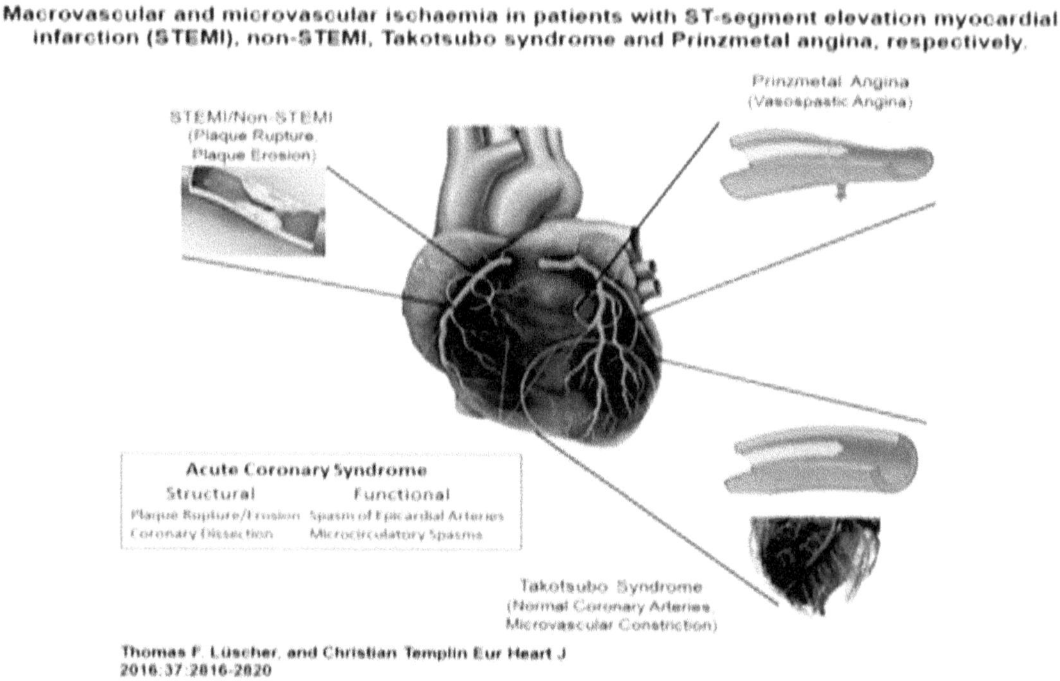

with tachycardia's (fast heart rate) such as atrial tachycardia (PAT) and atrial fibrillation. Tachycardia's that occur with sick sinus syndrome are characterized by a long pause after the tachycardia. Sick sinus syndrome is also associated with azygos continuation of interrupted inferior vena cava.

Disorders that cause scarring, degeneration, or damage to the sinoatrial node can cause sick sinus syndrome, including sarcoidosis, amyloidosis, hemochromatosis, Chagas disease, and cardiomyopathies. Abnormal heart rhythms are often caused or worsened by medications such as digoxin, calcium channel blockers, beta-blockers, sympatholytic medications, and anti-arrhythmic.

In last myocardial syndrome or popularly known as acute coronary syndrome is a condition brought on by a sudden reduction or blockage of blood flow to the heart. Myocardial syndrome atheroma rupture is most commonly found 60% when compared to atheroma erosion (30%), thus causes the formation of thrombus which block the coronary arteries.

Symptoms may include heart attack-like chest pressure, chest pressure while resting or doing light activity or sudden heart stoppage. People are also experience that pain in the chest, arm or jaw with held on that Pain circumstances happen in the chest at rest or with exertion also. Shortness of breath or shortness of breath on exercise and chest pressure or sweating is also common effect.

All of these conditions are treatable if diagnosed quickly. Treatment may include medication, such as blood thinners, clot busters or beta blockers. Surgery may be required. But most effective preventions are to avoid smoking, scheming high blood pressure and high blood cholesterol, maintain the diabetes, care for non-physical inactivity, monitoring overweight or obese and also to take care of if there was a family history of chest pain, heart disease or stroke.

METHODOLOGY

Comparative Analysis

In this graph shows the result of Heart Attack result with comparison between heart attack line graphs against normal heart beats. Here heart beats are representing along with x-axis and the time parameter are in with y-axis. In this graph shows two different color to diffract each from another where black represent normal heart and the other one heart attack by ochre. In normal heart beats are the sampled with ECG signal and it is obtained from continuous ECG signal acquired in experimental surroundings with two known parameters, and heart attack is the signal, generated by simulating. Both the normal heart beats and heart attack are plotted in the same frequency in this line graph.

Among these line graph noticeable that each one-time interval 50 beats gap have shown a useful notch which differ to approachable condition of heart beats. In normal heart beats shows three pick point in total but one has very sharp point notch and other two are avoidable notch. To compare with heart attack there, have five in total with a fatty healthy notch which represent a big time interval condition, not to a normal one.

The shape and size of the different notch on this ECG signal parameter which is concern that the patient might have a blocked artery in the heart. A blocked heart artery can cause a heart attack, which is a medical emergency requiring immediate treatment by an interventional cardiologist.

In this graph shows the result of Ischemic heart disease result with comparison between Ischemic heart disease line graphs against normal heart beats. Here heart beats are representing along with x-axis and the time parameter are in with y-axis. In this graph shows two different color to diffract each from another where black represent normal heart and the other one ischemic heart disease by sky-blue. In normal heart beats are the sampled with ECG signal and it is obtained from continuous ECG signal

Figure 6. Normal heart with heart attack

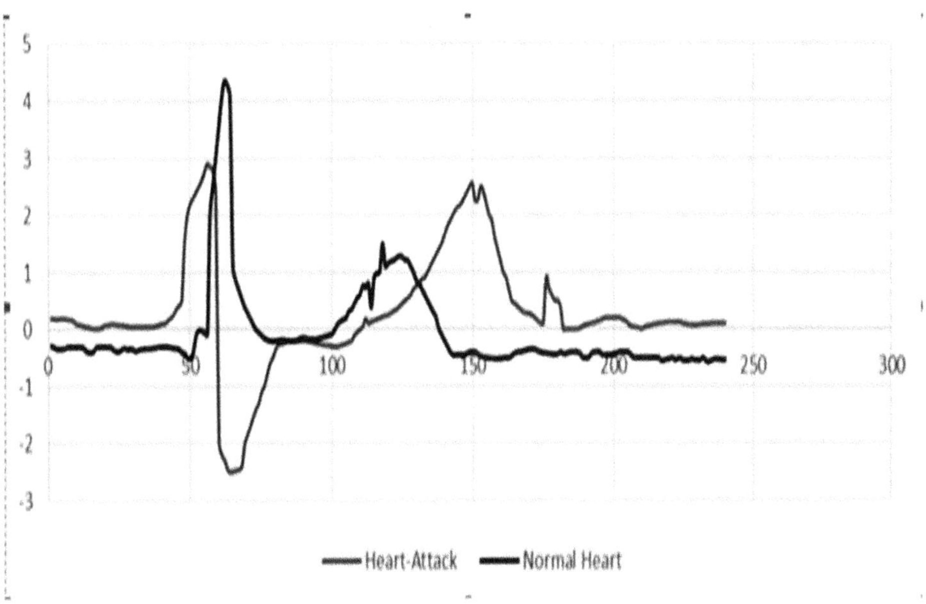

Figure 7. Ischemic heart disease

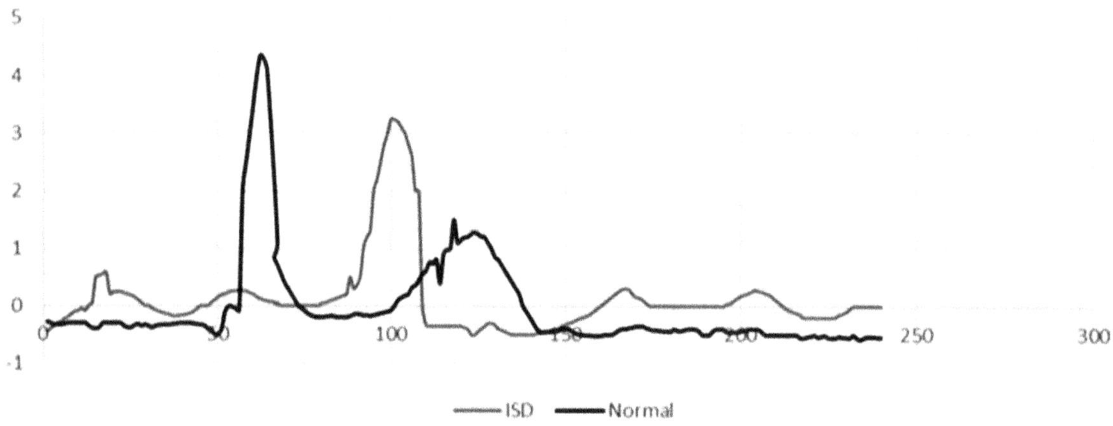

picked up in experimental backgrounds with two known variable parameters, and ischemic heart disease is the signal, generated by pretending. Both the normal heart beats and ischemic heart disease are plotted in the same frequency in this line graph.

Among these line graph noticeable that each one-time interval 50 beats gap have shown a useful notch which differ to approachable condition of heart beats. In normal heart beats shows three pick point in total but one has very sharp point notch and other two are avoidable notch. To compare with ischemic heart disease there, have five in total with a too healthy notch which represent a big time interval condition, not to a normal one with last two notch ware plotted by a non-response time interlude.

Figure 8. Six-sinus syndrome

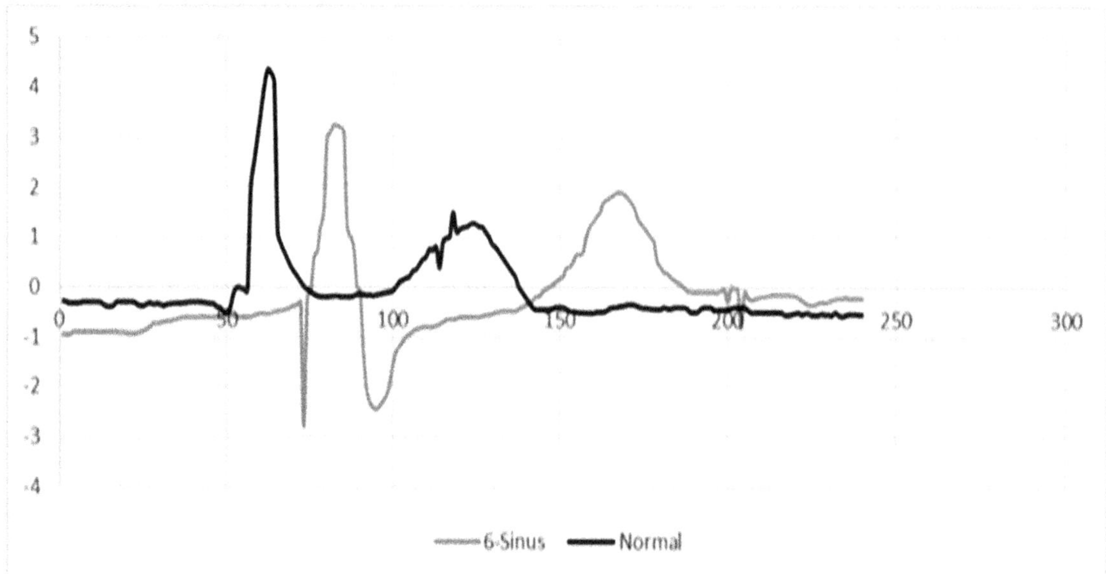

Figure 9. Myocardial infraction

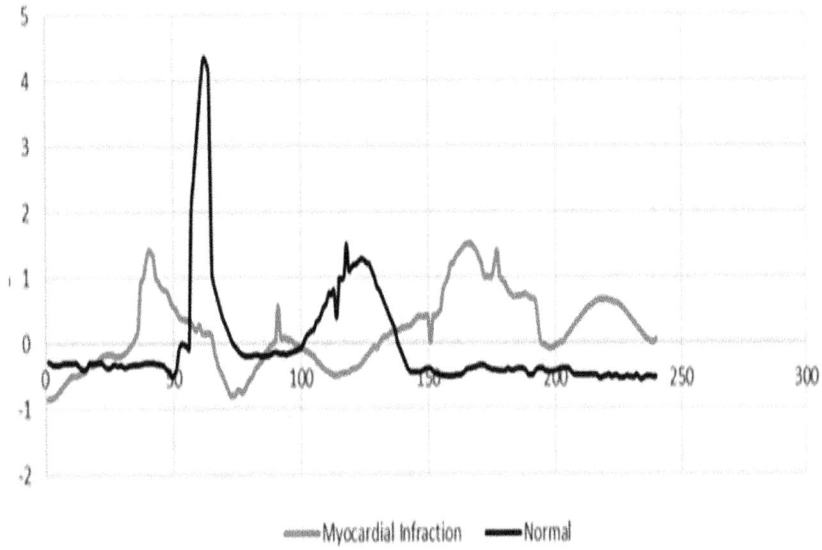

Also here again the shape and size of the altered notch on this ECG signal bound which is distress that the patient might have a blocked blood vessel in the heart. A blocked heart artery can cause a heart attack, which is a medical emergency requiring immediate treatment by an interventional cardiologist.

In this line graph demonstrations, the outcome of Six-sinus syndrome result with appraisal among Six-sinus syndrome line graphs against normal heart beats. Here heart beats are representing along with x-axis and the time parameter are in with y-axis. In this graph shows two different color to diffract each from another where black represent normal heart and the other one six-sinus syndrome by sab-green. In normal heart beats are the sampled with ECG signal and it is obtained from continuous ECG signal acquired in experimental surroundings with two known parameters, and heart attack is the signal, generated by simulating. Both the normal heart beats and heart attack are plotted in the same frequency in this line graph.

Among these line graph noticeable that each one-time interval 50 beats gap have shown a useful notch which differ to approachable condition of heart beats. In normal heart beats shows three pick point in total but one has very sharp point notch and other two are avoidable notch. To compare with Six-sinus syndrome there have six in total with a fatty healthy notch which represent a big time interval condition, not to a normal one.

The shape and size of the altered notch on this ECG signal parameter which is concern that the patient might have a blocked artery in the heart. A blocked heart artery can cause a Six-sinus syndrome, which is a medical emergency requiring instantaneous cure by an interventional cardiologist.

In this graph shows the result of myocardial Infraction result with comparison between myocardial Infraction line graphs against normal heart beats. Here heart beats are representing along with x-axis and the time parameter are in with y-axis. In this graph shows two different color to diffract each from another where black represent normal heart and the other one myocardial Infraction by red. In normal heart beats are the sampled with ECG signal and it is obtained from continuous ECG signal acquired in experimental surroundings with two known parameters, and myocardial Infraction is the signal,

Figure 10. Myocardial syndrome

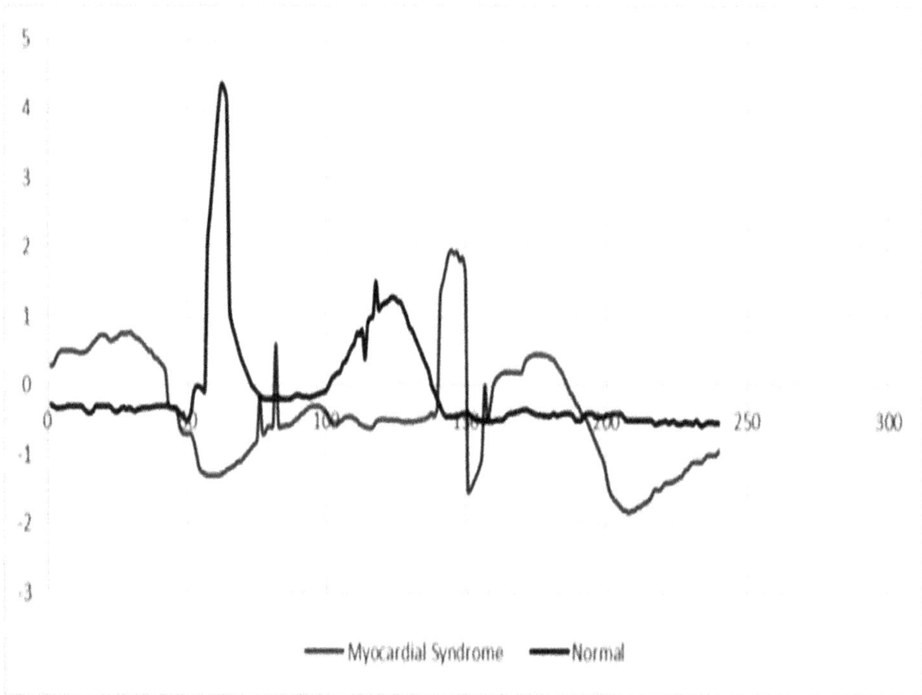

generated by simulating. Both the normal heart beats and myocardial Infraction are plotted in the same frequency in this line graph.

Among these line graph noticeable that each one-time interval 50 beats gap have shown a useful notch which differ to amenable situation of heart beats. In normal heart beats shows three pick point in total but one has very sharp point notch and other two are avoidable notch. To compare with myocardial Infraction there, have many notch in total with a low and healthy which represent a big time interim state, not to an average individual.

Moreover, the shape and size of the different notch on this ECG signal parameter which is anxiety that the patient might have a blocked artery in the heart. A blocked heart artery can cause a myocardial Infraction that is a medical emergency requiring immediate treatment by an interventional cardiologist.

In this graph portrayed the result of myocardial syndrome result with comparison between myocardial syndrome line graphs against normal heart beats. Here heart beats are representing along with x-axis and the time parameter are in with y-axis. In this graph shows two different color to diffract each from another where black represent normal heart and the other one myocardial syndrome by ink-blue. In normal heart beats are the sampled with ECG signal and it is obtained from continuous ECG signal acquired in experimental surroundings with two known parameters, and myocardial syndrome is the signal, generated by simulating. Both the normal heart beats and myocardial syndrome are intrigued in the same rate of recurrence in this line graph.

Surrounded by these lines graph noticeable that each one-time interval 50 beats gap have shown a useful notch which differ to approachable condition of heart beats. In normal heart beats shows three pick point in total but one has identical shrill point nick and other two are not inevitable indentation. To

Figure 11. Normal heart signal with its spectrogram

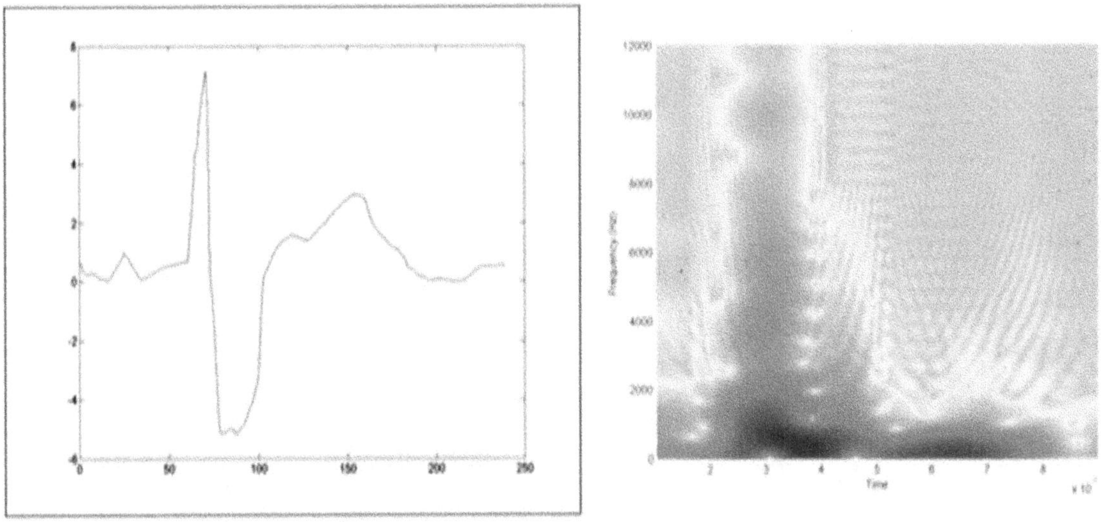

equate with myocardial syndrome there, have four in total with a greasy vigorous notch which represent a big time interval condition, not to a normal one. The shape and size of the different notch on this ECG signal parameter which is anxiety that the patient might have a blocked artery in the heart. A blocked heart artery can cause a heart attack, which is a medical emergency requiring immediate treatment by an interventional cardiologist.

Spectrogram Analysis

Aim for the chapter stands to a point of data interpretation through spectrogram. Below is the normal heart wave with its spectrogram following various heart diseases and their spectrogram respectively. Following are the diseases discussed in the research study. At the initiation of the spectrogram of the normal cardiac response, it is observed, from 0 to 1mS, the frequency of moderate level components remains present, representing the P wave characteristics, containing about 8 kHz of frequency. From 1mS to 2mS, time interval represents Q wave depolarization effect leaving the low amount of low components. The 2mS to 4mS time interval contains the high amount of high-frequency components representing the high P wave.

Rest of the time intervals represent the presence of frequency of low-frequency components depicting the normal heart rhythm.

Myocardial Infarction

Myocardial infarction (MI) is the irreversible death (necrosis) of heart muscle secondary to prolonged lack of oxygen supply (ischemia). Patients with typical MI may have the prodromal symptoms in the days preceding the event such as Fatigue, Chest discomfort, Malaise. (Hai-Ying & Kun-Mean, 2008) Spectrogram for the myocardial infarction depicting the abnormalities, starting with the elevated P wave in 0mS to 2mS time interval containing around 10kh of the frequency with reddish yellow plots in the

Figure 12. Myocardial infarction waveform and spectrogram

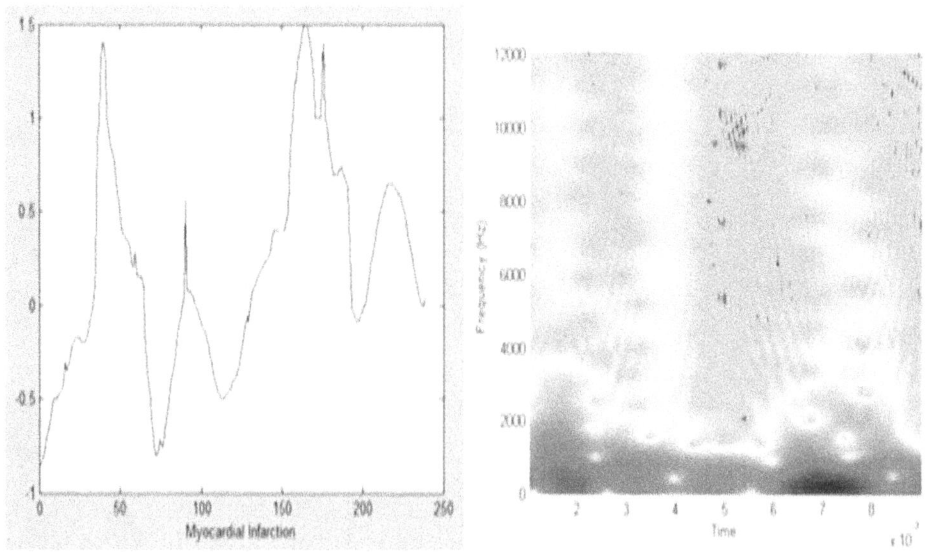

beginning and ending with greenish yellow plots. In the time interval of 2mS to 3mS greenish yellow plots are present with around 5kh of frequency denoting slight depolarization. The main abnormality can be observed by the next time interval of 3.5mS to 4.5mS a high spectral density is presently stated as ST elevation representing high repolarization with 12kh of frequency.

This drastic change in the atrial section causes the disease. And for the next time intervals, it is almost the repetition of the previous states. For time interval 4.5mS to 6mS blue and greenish plots are present and for rest, the moderate elevation is observable with 10 KHz of frequency representing the diseased states of the cardiac muscles.

Myocardial Syndrome

The spectrogram analysis reveals the operation of the human heart through the variation of signals in different time intervals. At the first time interval of 0 to 1mS, the spectral density of the frequencies are almost absent. In the time interval of 1mS to 2.5mS, the moderate-high frequencies of yellow colored plots with a frequency around 10kh is present and this is followed by the 3mS to 4mS time interval again moderate to high-frequency plots remain present denoting spectral power density on the higher side with almost 12kh frequency plots. These are the abnormalities from a normal heart in which these two elevations remain absent to the most extent. And the same phenomenon repeats itself having an absence of initial P wave in the time interval of 4mS to 5mS and elevations with high and moderate frequencies of 12kh frequencies in the time interval of 5mS to 7mS.And the rest are low frequencies present in the last phases of the timescale.

Sick Sinus Syndrome

Sick sinus syndrome also known as sinus node disease or sinus node dysfunction is the name for a group of heart rhythm problems (arrhythmias) in which the sinus node the heart's natural pacemaker doesn't

Figure 13. Myocardian syndrome waveform and spectrogram

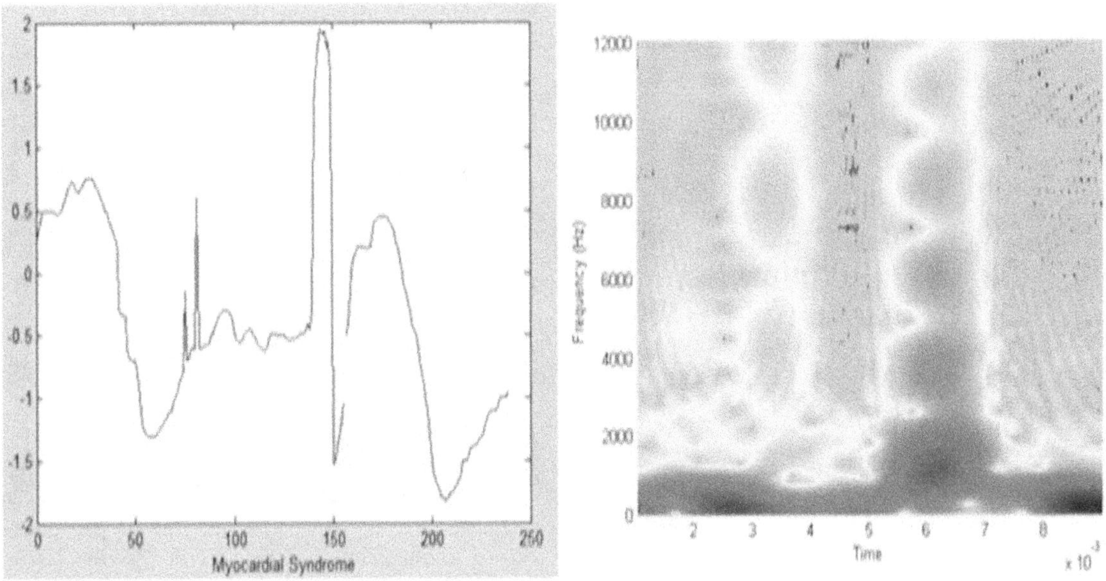

work properly. The sinus node is an area of specialized cells in the upper right chamber of the heart that controls the rhythm of the heart. Normally, the sinus node produces a steady pace of regular electrical impulses. In sick sinus syndrome, these signals are abnormally paced. It is relatively uncommon, but the risk of developing sick sinus syndrome increases with age (Portet, Hernandez & Carrault, 2005). Spectrogram of sinus syndrome reveals blue plots on both sides of the highly elevated spectrum containing high frequency. At the initial phase of the spectrogram from 0mS to 2.5mS, the waves are absent denoting low or null frequency with the blue and slightly yellow colored plots which are an abnormal variation of the normal condition. From 2.5mS to 4.5mS time interval the frequency elevations containing high-frequency plots of around 12kh represented by the red and high yellow plots.

In the later phase, the repetition of the absence of the moderate frequencies in the time interval of 5mS to 6mS containing around 1kh frequency, represented by blue or greenish blue plots, which should have been a bit high in a normal heart. In the time interval of 6mS to 7mS, the presence of low to moderate frequencies denote the repetition of the previous phenomenon of absence of the initial P wave containing few KHz of frequencies for the greenish-yellow plots. And lastly, the time intervals 8mS to 9mS the only elevation of the R wave with high moderate frequencies with the yellow colored plots represent the abnormalities from the normal heart.

Heart Attack

A heart attack happens when the flow of oxygen-rich blood to a section of heart muscle suddenly becomes blocked and the heart can't get oxygen. If blood flow isn't restored quickly, the section of heart muscle begins to die (Hamilton & Tompkins, 1986). Spectrogram of general heart attack if schematized, it is observable that, in the initial stages the absence of the frequencies of the P wave is there in a small aspect which is denoted by the greenish-yellow plots in the 0mS to 1mS time interval containing slight

Figure 14. Sick sinus syndrome waveform and spectrogram

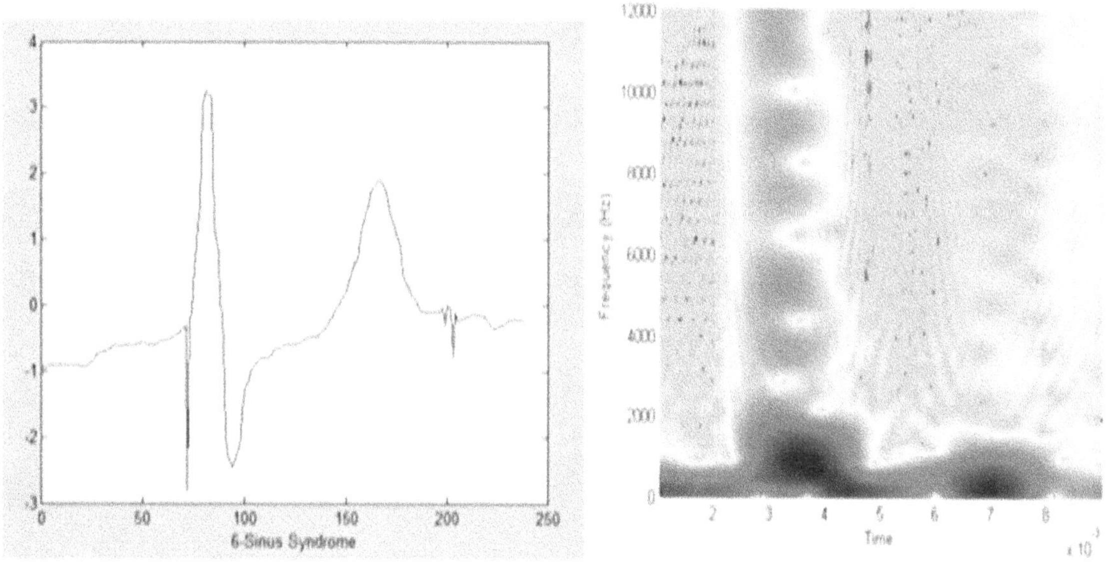

depolarization of the cardiac muscles for few KHz of frequency. Then for the 2mS to 3.5mS time interval, contains high-frequency spectral density shown by the yellow and red plots with 12kh of frequency by the scale representing huge depolarization of the muscles. For the time interval of 3.5mS to 5.5mS the repolarization of the cardiac muscles tends to operate on a high scale with the greenish yellow plots having low to moderate frequency range.

Figure 15. Heart attack waveform and spectrogram

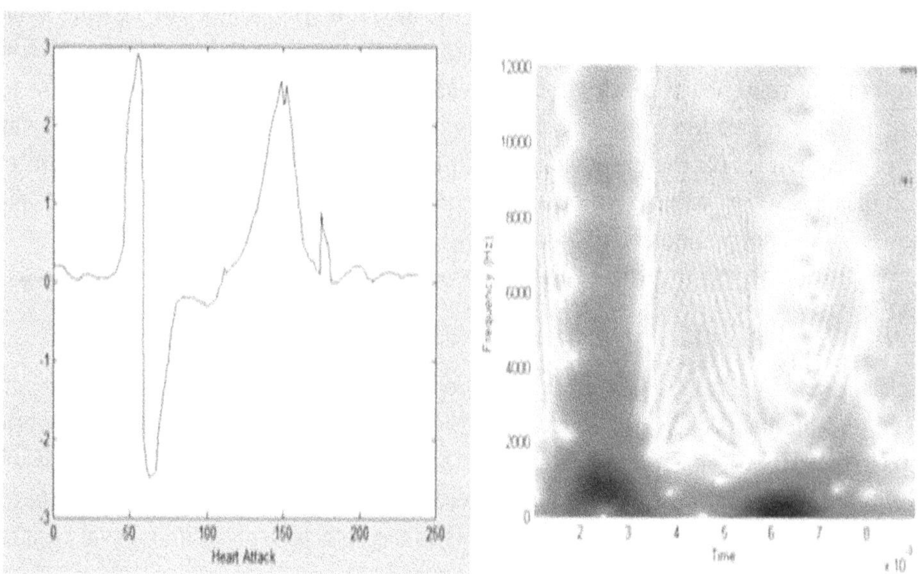

In the next time interval of 5.5mS to 6.5mS, the continued repolarization takes place denoted by reddish yellow plots having moderate to high frequency an elevated plot appears with almost 10kh of frequency creating the main abnormality of the cardiac muscles, increasing conductance afterwards and resulting heart attack.

TABULAR REPRESENTATION OF SPECTRAL COMPARATIVE STUDY

To start with this section, the above data are taken into account. The table depicts the contrasting review of the different diseases with the spectrogram analysis of the same in comparison to the normal heart signal(spectrogram). The differences of the different diseased signals with that to normal heart are described in Table 1.

RESULT ANALYSIS

Mathematical Algorithm for Detecting Heart Condition

The analytical study based upon the mathematical approach has been described here. The ECG signal has been analyzed for detecting the health condition of human by some mathematical deduction. An algorithm based on some mathematical deduction is presented here. The proposed algorithm uses coefficient of variation of ECG signal defined by the pattern variation of the entire ECG graph. The coefficient of variation (CV) can be explored as the relative variability of the signal curve. Mathematically the coefficient of variation (CV) is expressed as the ratio of standard deviation of a series of variable numerical data and the mean value of the same serial data.

Table 1. Frequency spectrum comparisons table for heart diseases

Time Intervals	Myocardial Infarction	Myocardial Syndrome	Sick Sinus Syndrome	Heart Atack
1-2mS	Less spectrum presence in P wave	Lesser impulse of P wave	Absence of P wave	Absence of P wave
2-3mS	Absence of spectrum	Absence of required spectrum	No change	Quicker appearance of spectrum
3-4mS	Absence of required spectrum	Less spectrum presence	Lesser impulse	No change
4-5mS	Absence of impulse	Absence of spectrum	Lesser amount of spectrum	Absence of impulse
5-6mS	Absence of impulse	Presence of higher impulse	Absence of impulse	Absence of impulse
6-7mS	No change	Presence of greater spectrum	No change	No change
7-8ms	Presence of elevated impulse	Absence of impulse	No change	Presence of higher spectrum
8-9mS	No change	No change	Presence of elevated spectrum	No change

The coefficient of variation (CV) = $\frac{\sigma}{\mu}$ (1)

The σ depicts standard deviation of a numerical data series. And the mean value of the data series is represented as μ.

The standard deviation is the calculation of the dispersion of a series of numerical data from its mean. Mathematically it is expressed as =

$$\sqrt{\frac{\sum \left|y-\mu\right|^{2}}{X}} \quad (1(a))$$

The ∑ shows "sum of", y is a value in the numerical data series, μ represents the mean of the numerical data series, and X is the number of data points in the data series.

The mean value of an entire numerical data series is also calculated as summing up all of the given numerical data in the data series and dividing by the number of data pointes in the same data series.

Mathematically it is expressed as =

$$\frac{\sum a}{x} \quad (1(b))$$

The ∑ shows "sum of", a depicts all values in the numerical data series, and x is the number of data points in the data series.

The proposed model algorithm is highly capable for differentiating multiple cardio-vascular syndrome. The health status of the heart can be identified using the coefficient of variation. The -21.0 valued coefficient of variation is expressed as healthy heart of a person. The sick-sinus syndrome and Myocardial Syndrome have been exploited by using coefficient value of -4.6 and -2.24 respectively. Although the deadly Myocardial Infarction shows the coefficient of variation (CV) value +2.5 by analyzing the ECG graph. Then the most fatal the heart attack can be analyzed mathematically through coefficient of variation (CV).

The 3.5 value of coefficient of variation (CV) represent the ECG graph of a heart attack patient.

Table 2. Co-efficient variation of heart condition

Heart Condition	Co-Efficient of Variation =(Standard Deviation / Mean)
Normal Heart	-21.0 (approx.)
Heart Attack	3.5 (approx.)
Sick sinus syndrome	-4.6 (approx.)
Myocardial Syndrome	-2.24 (approx.)
Myocardial Infarction	2.5 (approx.)

FUTURE RESEARCH DIRECTIONS

The proposed model based approach leads to identify and characterize some cardiovascular problem and attempt to recover from the health problem. The analytical research on the human heart and current available technology on the human cardiovascular system will initiate to develop an IoT based cardiovascular diagnostic system with automatic cure system through some software simulation using real-time ECG signal data and various realistic control analogy of human heart system.

The generated mathematical equation-based model of various states of heart using analysis of ECG signal after the simulation will drive to the further development for hardware designing and modelling implementing. A circuitry model based approach will be conducted for developing the prosthetic heart driving circuit utilizing VLSI circuitry analysis through accumulating the idea of mathematical model and ECG signal analysis. In the near future, a wireless body worn healthcare device will be developed for automatic detection and cure without using any traditional medicine with real-time IOT based monitoring.

In addition to the device will communicate with a preferred medical person in the emergency situation through the body mounted device if any problem arises. In the near feature an IOT based cardiac health monitoring system will be developed based on the proposed classification using human heart ECG signal. The device will aware the patient, doctor and other people before the arrival of critical condition by analyzing the ECG signal. This early detection of cardiac problem will help the patient to cure quickly and accurately.

CONCLUSION

A generalized method for observing of the abnormalities of cardiac muscles than the normal condition, a newer different aspect needed to be developed to appear in comparatively detailed, easier and a very precise description of the normal and diseased states. The envelope and spectrogram analysis of the behavior of cardiac muscles fulfil the requirement that represents a more favorable result as a description in time and frequency of normal and diseased states.

This method of representing would include further observable phenomenon to clarify the reasons of specific diseased states from the separate spectrograms. The analysis will also prove to be much easier to observe diseased states to any common man. A mathematical algorithm based systematic structure has presented for detecting the disorder of cardiac muscle. The resultant coefficient of variation has already been estimated and stored for some heart problem.

The diagnostic model able to predicts proper disease by comparing between static databases and calculated coefficient of variation of ECG signal. It is also capable of providing medical enrichment denoting broader aspects to describe, analyze and appear as a result in a detailed and easier manner. Quite similarly much more diseases can be inspected through this manner. Adding to this context a quantitative study can also be done on the variable diseases and their spectrogram study which incurs minimal data requirement and effortless study. In the near the future, a model based approach towards the recovering from the cardiovascular problem without using any medicine will be developed based on the diagnostic approach.

REFERENCES

Arunachalam, S. P., Kapa, S., Mulpuru, S.K., Friedman, P.A., & Tolkacheva, E.G. (2016). Intelligent fractional-order pid (fopid) heart rate controller for cardiac pacemaker. In *Healthcare Innovation Point-Of- Care Technologies Conference (HI-POCT), 2016 IEEE*. IEEE.

Bhattacharjee, S., Mazumder, A., Das, Z., Kumar, L., Shree, K., & Neogi, B. (2013). Study on cardio-vascular diseases with compression of generalized ECG signal to support biomedical advancement. *International Journal of Advanced Research in Electrical. Electronics and Instrumentation Engineering*, *2*(10), 5213–5219.

Castro, V. J. F., & Malathi, R. (2018). Design of advanced control strategies for cardiovascular system. *Materials Today: Proceedings*, *5*(1), 1960–1966. doi:10.1016/j.matpr.2017.11.299

Chatterjee, H. K., Gupta, R., Bera, J. N., & Mitra, M. (2011). An FPGA implementation of Real Time QRS Detection. *International Conference on Computer and Communication Technology*, 274-279. 10.1109/ICCCT.2011.6075114

Choi, S. W., & Min, B. G. (2014). *Ventricular assist device cannula and ventricular assist device including the same*. US Patent 8,771,165.

Cohn, J. N., Ferrari, R., & Sharpe, N. (2000). Cardiac remodelling – concepts and clinical implications: A consensus paper from an international forum on cardiac remodeling. *Journal of the American College of Cardiology*, *35*(3), 569–582. doi:10.1016/S0735-1097(99)00630-0 PMID:10716457

Cook, D. G., & Shaper, A. G. (1988). Breathlessness, lung function and the risk of heart attack. *European Heart Journal*, *9*(11), 1215–1222. doi:10.1093/oxfordjournals.eurheartj.a062432 PMID:3234413

Cowie, M. R., Wood, D. A., Coats, A. J. S., Thompson, S. G., Suresh, V., Poole-Wilson, P. A., & Sutton, G. C. (2000). Survival of patients with a new diagnosis of heart failure: A population based study. *Heart (British Cardiac Society)*, *83*(5), 505–510. doi:10.1136/heart.83.5.505 PMID:10768897

Dubey, A., Patel, R., & Choure, K. (2014). An efficient data mining and ant colony optimization technique (DMACO) for heart disease prediction. *International Journal of Advanced Technology and Engineering Exploration.*, *1*(1), 1–6.

Frazier, O. (1994). First use of an untethered, vented electric left ventricular assist device for long-term support. *Circulation*, *89*(6), 2908–2914. doi:10.1161/01.CIR.89.6.2908 PMID:8205707

Garg, A. X., Adhikari, N. K., McDonald, H., Rosas-Arellano, M. P., Devereaux, P. J., Beyene, J., & Haynes, R. B. (2005). Effects of computerized clinical decision support systems on practitioner performance and patient outcomes: A systematic review. *Journal of the American Medical Association*, *293*(10), 1223–1238. doi:10.1001/jama.293.10.1223 PMID:15755945

Ghaffari, A., Golbayani, H., & Ghasemi, M. (2008). A new mathematical based QRS detector using continuous wavelet transform. Computers and Electrical Engineering, 34, 81–91.

Ghosal, G., Darbar, R., Neogi, B., Das, A., & Tibarewala, D. N. (2012). Application of swarm intelligence computation techniques in pid controller tuning: A review. In *Proceedings of the International Conference on Information Systems Design and Intelligent Applications 2012 (INDIA 2012)*. Springer.

Goletsis, Y., Papaloukas, C., Fotiadis, D. I., Likas, A., & Michalis, L. (2004). Automated ischemic beat classification using genetic algorithm and multicriteria decision analysis. *IEEE Transactions on Biomedical Engineering, 51*(10), 1717–1725. doi:10.1109/TBME.2004.828033 PMID:15490819

Guendouzi, F., & Attari, M. (2013). Polynomial modeling of the ECG signals. *IEEE 2013 International Conference on Computer Medical Applications (ICCMA)*, 1–5. 10.1109/ICCMA.2013.6506177

Hai-Ying, Z., & Kun-Mean, H. (2008). Embedded Real-Time QRS Detection Algorithm for Pervasive Cardiac Care System. *ICSP2008 Proceedings*, 2150- 2153.

Haider, S. (2008). *U.S. Patent Application 12/192,216*. U.S. Patent and Trademark Office.

Hamilton, P. S., & Tompkins, W. J. (1986). Quantitative Investigation of QRS Detection Rules Using the MIT/BIH Arrhythmia Database. *IEEE Transactions on Biomedical Engineering, BME-33*(12), 1157–1165. doi:10.1109/TBME.1986.325695 PMID:3817849

Jensen, P. N., Gronroos, N. N., Chen, L. Y., Folsom, A. R., Heckbert, S. R., & Alonso, A. (2014). Incidence of and risk factors for sick sinus syndrome in the general population. *Journal of the American College of Cardiology, 64*(6), 531–538. doi:10.1016/j.jacc.2014.03.056 PMID:25104519

Jokic, S., Delic, V., Peric, Z., Krco, S., & Sakac, D. (2011). Efficient ECG modeling using polynomial functions. *Elektronika ir Elektrotechnika, 110*(4), 121–124. doi:10.5755/j01.eee.110.4.304

Keller, K. B., & Lemberg, L. (2006). The sick sinus syndrome. *American Journal of Critical Care, 15*(2), 226–229. PMID:16501143

Keller, K. B., & Lemberg, L. (2007). Iatrogenic sick sinus syndrome. *American Journal of Critical Care, 16*(3), 294–297. PMID:17460324

Kleiger, R. E., Miller, J. P., Bigger, J. T. Jr, & Moss, A. J. (1987). Decreased heart rate variability and its association with increased mortality after acute myocardial infarction. *The American Journal of Cardiology, 59*(4), 256–262. doi:10.1016/0002-9149(87)90795-8 PMID:3812275

Kovács, P. (2012). ECG signal generator based on geometrical features. *Annales Universitatis Scientarium Budapestinensis de Rolando Eötvös Nominatae Sectio Mathematica, 37*, 247–260.

Lehto, T., Oinas-Kukkonen, H., Pätiälä, T., & Saarelma, O. (2013). Virtual health coaching for consumers: A persuasive systems design perspective. *International Journal of Networking and Virtual Organisations, 13*(1), 24–41. doi:10.1504/IJNVO.2013.058440

Lüscher, T. F., & Templin, C. (2016). Is takotsubo syndrome a microvascular acute coronary syndrome? Towards a new definition. *European Heart Journal, 37*(37), 2816–2820. doi:10.1093/eurheartj/ehw057 PMID:26966148

Mahmoodabadi, S. Z., Ahmadian, A., & Abolhasani, M. D. (2005). ECGFeature Extraction using Daubechies Wavelets. *2005 IEEE Engineering in Medicine and Biology 27th Annual Conference*.

Meissimilly, G., Rodriguez, J., Rodriguez, G., Gonzalez, R., & Caiiizares, M. (2003). Microcontroller-Based Real-Time QRS Detector for Ambulatory Monitoring. *Proceedings of the 25 Annual International Conference of the IEEE EMBS*, 2881-2884. 10.1109/IEMBS.2003.1280520

Papadimitriou, S., Mavroudi, S., Vladutu, L., & Bezerianos, A. (2001, May). Ischemia detection with a self-organizing map supplemented by supervised learning. *IEEE Transactions on Neural Networks*, *12*(3), 503–515. doi:10.1109/72.925554 PMID:18249884

Papaloukas, C., Fotiadis, D. I., Likas, A., Liavas, A. P., & Michalis, L. K. (2001). A knowledge-based technique for automated detection of ischemic episodes in long duration electrocardiograms. *Medical & Biological Engineering & Computing*, *39*(1), 105–112. doi:10.1007/BF02345273 PMID:11214261

Papaloukas, C., Fotiadis, D. I., Likas, A., & Michalis, L. K. (2002). An expert system for ischemia detection based on parametric modeling and artificial neural networks. *Processings of the European Medical Biological Engineering Conference.*

Papaloukas, C., Fotiadis, D. I., Likas, A., & Michalis, L. K. (2002). An ischemia detection method based on artificial neural networks. *Artificial Intelligence in Medicine*, *24*(2), 167–178. doi:10.1016/S0933-3657(01)00100-2 PMID:11830369

Pitas, I., Strintzis, M. G., Grippas, S., & Xerostylides, C. (1983). Machine classification of ischemic electrocardiograms. Presented at the *IEEE Mediterranean Electrotechnical Conf.*, Athens, Greece.

Portet, F., Hernandez, A. I., & Carrault, G. (2005). Evaluation of realtime QRS detection algorithms in variable contexts. *Medical & Biological Engineering & Computing*, *43*(3), 379–385. doi:10.1007/BF02345816 PMID:16035227

Power, D. J., Sharda, R., & Burstein, F. (2013). Decision support systems. John Wiley & Sons, Ltd.

Pueyo, E., Sörnmo, L., & Laguna, P. (2008). QRS Slopes for Detection and Characterization of Myocardial Ischemia. *IEEE Transactions on Biomedical Engineering*, *55*(2), 468–477. doi:10.1109/TBME.2007.902228 PMID:18269981

Sadh, A. S., & Shukla, N. (2013). Association rules Optimization: A survey. *International Journal of Advanced Computer Research*, *3*(9), 111–115.

Saktheeswari, R., & Adalarasu, K. (2017). Survey on signal processing techniques for diagnoising cardiovascular diseases. *2017 International Conference on Innovations in Information, Embedded and Communication Systems (ICIIECS).* 10.1109/ICIIECS.2017.8276116

Saminu, S., Özkurt, N., & Karaye, I. A. (2008). Wavelet Feature Extraction for ECG Beat Classification. *2014 IEEE 6th International Conference on Adaptive Science & Technology (ICAST).*

Shaw, L. J., Bugiardini, R., & Merz, C. N. B. (2009). Women and ischemic heart disease: Evolving knowledge. *Journal of the American College of Cardiology*, *54*(17), 1561–1575. doi:10.1016/j.jacc.2009.04.098 PMID:19833255

Sony, J., Ansari, U., Sharma, D., & Sony, S. (2011). "Predictive data mining for medical diagnosis: an overview of heart disease prediction" International Journal of Computer Science and Engineering, vol. 3. Ahmad, P., Qamar, S. & Rizvi, S.Q.A. (2015) Techniques of data mining in healthcare: A review. *International Journal of Computers and Applications*, *120*(15).

Sreelakshmi, T.G., & Paul, S. (2015). *An Accurate ECG Feature Extraction Method for Detecting Multiple Cardiovascular Diseases*. Retrieved from: http://www.ijiset.com/v1s9/IJISET_V1_I9_08.pdf

Vafaie, M. H., Ataei, M., & Koofigar, H. R. (2014). Heart diseases prediction based on ECG signals' classification using agenetic-fuzzy system and dynamical model of ECG signals. *Biomedical Signal Processing and Control*, *14*, 291–296. doi:10.1016/j.bspc.2014.08.010

Whan Lee, J., Kim, S. K., Lee, B., Lee, B., & Lee, M. H. (2002). A Real Time QRS Detection Using DelayCoordinate Mapping for the Microcontroller Implementation. *Annals of Biomedical Engineering*, *30*(9), 1140–1151. doi:10.1114/1.1523030 PMID:12502225

World Health Organization. (2017). *Cardiovascular diseases (CVDs)*. Retrieved October 17 May 2017, from http://www.who.int/news-room/fact-sheets/detail/cardiovascular-diseases-(cvds)

Yang, G., Xie, L., Mäntysalo, M., Zhou, X., Pang, Z., Da Xu, L., ... Zheng, L. R. (2014). A health-IoT platform based on the integration of intelligent packaging, unobtrusive bio-sensor, and intelligent medicine box. *IEEE Transactions on Industrial Informatics*, *10*(4), 2180–2191. doi:10.1109/TII.2014.2307795

Yatollahi, A. A., Jafarnia Dabanloo, N., McLemon, D., Johari Majd, V., & Zhang, H. (2005). A comprehensive model using modified Zeeman model for generating ECG sig-nals. *Iran. J. Electr. Electron. Eng.*, *1*, 88–93.

Zeeman, E. C. (1972). *Differential Equations for the Heartbeat and Nerve Impulse*. Coventry, UK: Math-ematics Institute, University of Warwick.

Zeraatkar, E., & Kermani, S. (2010) Improving QRS Detection for Artifacts Reduction. *Proceedings of the 17th Iranian Conference of Biomedical Engineerin (ICBME2010)*, 978-981.

Zhao, C. J., Sun, Y. X., Zhu, H. Q., & Liu, X. X. (2015). Axial suspension fuzzy pid control for axial artificial heart pump. *Applied Mechanics and Materials, 703*, 323–326.

Zhao, Q., & Zhan, L. (2005). ECG Feature Extraction and Classification Using Wavelet Transform and Support Vector Machines. *2005 International Conference on Neural Networks and Brain.*

Zhengzhong, G., Fanxue, K., & Xu, Z. (2011). Accurate and Rapid QRS Detection for Intelligent ECG Monitor. *2011 Third International Conference on Measuring Technology and Mechatronics Automation*, 1, 298-301. 10.1109/ICMTMA.2011.76

Chapter 10
Hybrid Multimodality Medical Image Fusion Using Various Fusion Techniques With Quantitative and Qualitative Analysis

Rajalingam B.
Annamalai University, India

Priya R.
Annamalai University, India

Bhavani R.
Annamalai University, India

ABSTRACT

In this chapter, different types of image fusion techniques have been studied and evaluated in the medical applications. The ultimate goal of this proposed method is to obtain the fused image without any loss of similar information and preserve all special features present in the input medical images. This method is used to improve the fused image quality for better diagnosis of critical disease analysis. The fused hybrid multimodal medical image should convey better visual description than the individual input images. This chapter proposes the method for multimodal medical image fusion using the hybrid fusion algorithm. The computed tomography, magnetic resonance imaging, positron emission tomography, and single photon emission computed tomography are the input images used for this experimental work. In this chapter, experimental results discovered that the proposed techniques provide better visualization of fused image and gives the superior results compared to various existing traditional algorithms.

DOI: 10.4018/978-1-5225-7796-6.ch010

INTRODUCTION

Image Fusion

Image fusion is a process to combine similar information present in input images using advanced fusion algorithm. The main purpose is to enhance the information present in the image by integrating the similar and dissimilar data. This leads to more accurate data and increased utility. It is also stated that fused data provides improved classification, robust operational performance, reduced ambiguity, increased confidence and improved reliability. Image fusion is generally applied to digital imagery for the following applications that are valuable in human life.

- Geographical change detection
- Deforestation monitoring
- Glacier monitoring
- Hazards monitoring
- Military target detection
- Border security surveillance
- Early detection of medical symptoms like a cancer
- Urban mapping
- Replace defective data
- Object identification and classification

Multimodal Image Fusion

Multimodal image fusion produces a better visible image by combining two or more images from heterogeneous sources. The fused images can decrease the ambiguity related to a single image. The resultant fused images are used in military and security applications, such as weapon detection, target detection, object tracking, night vision, etc. The multi-sensor data in many fields, such as medical imaging, remote sensing, machine vision, sensor fusion has emerged as a novel and robust research area. It is possible to have several images of the same scene providing different information although the scene is the same. This is because each image has been captured with a different sensor. If we are able to merge the heterogeneous information that is collected from different image sensors, we can obtain a new and improved image which is called a multimodal fusion image. Naturally the image fusion combines most similar information present in input images and achieved a new fused image. Hence, the fused image has better quality than any of the input images. Target detection, urban mapping, medical imaging and remote sensing are some applications multimodal image fusion technique.

Importance and Significance of the Multimodal Medical Image Fusion

Multimodal medical image fusion technique is one of the recent research topics in the medical imaging field. This technique performed to reduce the redundancy in clinical applicability and to increase the relevant information present in the images. The multimodal medical images can be particular organ focused by the different types of modalities which include CT, MRI, PET and SPECT images. In this research work the Neurocysticercosis (NCC) affected multimodality medical images of same patient are used. The NCC is a parasite infection caused by the tapeworm Taenia solium in its larvae stage which affects the central nervous system of the human body. It results in the formation of multiple lesions in the brain at different locations during its various stages. During diagnosis of such symptomatic patients, these lesions can be better visualized using a feature-based fusion of the input multimodality medical images. The hybrid multimodal medical image fusion presented here is a technique of combining CT/MRI/PET and SPECT data.

Findings

The performance of the proposed hybrid multimodality medical image fusion algorithm is evaluated over pairs of CT, MRI, PET and SPECT medical images obtained from patients. Both traditional and hybrid multimodal medical image fusion algorithms are evaluated using several quality metrics including Fusion factor, Fusion symmetry Image quality index, Edge quality measure, Mean structural similarity index measure, Cross entropy and Correlation coefficient.

Applications and Improvements of Multimodal Medical Image Fusion

Through the simulation result, as compared with the traditional fusion techniques, it is concluded that the proposed hybrid fusion techniques gives better results. This work can be used to diagnose any type of abnormalities in all types of medical images (CT/MRI/PET and SPECT).

Challenges and Approaches

There are many different methods in the multimodal medical image fusion. The Brovey Transform (BT), Intensity Hue Saturation (IHS) and Principal Component Analysis (PCA) provide the basis for most commonly used image fusion techniques. The IHS method is the oldest method used in image fusion. BT is based on the chromacity transform. PCA based image fusion methods are similar to IHS methods, without any limitation in the number of fused bands. Some of these techniques improve the spatial resolution while distorting the original chromaticity of the input images, which is a major drawback. Recently, great interests have arisen on new transform techniques that utilize the multiresolution analysis, such as wavelet transform (WT). The multi-resolution decomposition schemes decompose input images into different scales or levels of frequencies. Wavelet based image fusion techniques are implemented by replacing the detail components from one input image with the detail components from another input image. However, the wavelet based fusion techniques are not optimal in capturing two-dimensional singularities from the input images. In the contourlet transform, a Laplacian pyramid (LP) is employed in the first stage, while directional filter banks (DFB) are used in the angular decomposition stage. However, the contourlet transform does not provide shift-invariance and structural information; hence, it may not be the optimum choice for image processing applications such as image fusion. Recently, some approaches have been attempted to introduce image transforms based on the DFB with the capability of both radial and angular decomposition. The octave-band directional filter banks are a new family of directional filter banks that offer an octave-band radial decomposition as well. Another approach is the critically sampled contourlet transform, which is realized using a one-stage non-separable filter bank. Using similar frequency decomposition to that of the contourlet transform, it provides a non-redundant version of the contourlet transform. The second major drawback of the contourlet transform is the occurrence of artifacts that are caused by setting some transform coefficients to zero for nonlinear approximation during the fusion process. These unwanted artifacts occur in the areas with useful information; hence, there is a possibility of losing important characteristics or information after the fusion process is completed. In this research work, a new medical image fusion method is proposed using hybrid wavelet-based non subsampled shearlet transform.

Outline of This Chapter

This research work focuses on the study of multimodal medical image fusion and proposed a novel fusion method using hybrid wavelet-based nonsubsampled shearlet transform. The proposed techniques overcome the major drawbacks in existing techniques and improve the fusion performance. The different types of traditional and hybrid multimodal medical image fusion techniques on the ten set of multimodality medical images are used for the experimental work. Experimental study is conducted to evaluate the performance of the proposed method in each multimodal medical image fusion category using suitable quality metrics.

The chapter organized as follows: Sec. 2 describes the literature survey. Sec. 3 discusses the proposed work on traditional and hybrid multimodal medical image fusion algorithms. Sec. 4 explains the performance evaluation metrics. Sec. 5 describes experimental results and performance comparative analysis. Finally, Sec. 6 concludes the paper.

LITERATURE SURVEY ON MULTIMODAL MEDICAL IMAGE FUSION

Aisha Moin, et.al. (2016) developed a weighted-PCA based multimodal medical image fusion in contourlet domain. B. Rajalingam, B. Rajalingam, Dr. R. Priya (2018) proposed an efficient hybrid multimodal medical image fusion approach based on combining the transform technique with pulse coupled neural network. B. Rajalingam, Dr. R. Priya (2017) proposed a multimodal medical image fusion approach based on curvelet transform with neural network to fuse the input medical images. B. Rajalingam, Dr. R. Priya (2017) proposed an efficient multimodal medical image fusion approach based on both traditional and hybrid fusion techniques are evaluated using several performance metrics. B. Rajalingam, Dr. R. Priya (2018) proposed a neural network and fuzzy logic based hybrid multimodal medical image fusion technique is to improve the quality of fused image. B. Rajalingam, Dr. R. Priya (2018) proposed an efficient multimodal medical image fusion approach based on deep learning convolutional neural networks (CNN) for the fusion process. B. Rajalingam, Dr. R. Priya (2018) proposed the guided image filtering with pulse coupled neural network for the efficient multimodal medical image fusion process. B. Rajalingam, Dr. R. Priya (2018) reviewed the improvement of multimodality medical image fusion based on combined transform techniques. B. Rajalingam, Dr. R. Priya (2018) proposed and examines some of the hybrid multimodality medical image fusion methods and discusses the most essential advantages and disadvantages of these methods to develop hybrid multimodal medical image fusion algorithms. C. T. Kavitha and C. Chellamuthu (2015) proposed the fast discrete curvelet transform to a multiresolution image which is obtained by applying integer wavelet transform to the input multimodal medical images for better clinical disease analysis. C. T. Kavitha, C. Chellamuthu proposed the medical image fusion based on the hybrid intelligence system. C. Karthikeyan, B. Ramadoss (2016) proposed the fusion of multimodal medical images using dual tree complex wavelet transform and self-organizing feature map for better disease diagnosis. Gaurav Bhatnagar, et al. (2015) proposed a novel framework for spatially registered multimodal medical image fusion based on the non-subsampled contourlet transform (NSCT). Heba M. El-Hoseny, et al. (2017) proposed the hybrid technique that enhances the fused image quality using both traditional and hybrid fusion algorithms. Jiao Du, et al. (2016) reviewed the overview of medical image fusion has been widely used in clinical for physicians to comprehend the lesion by the fusion of different modalities medical images. Jyoti Agarwal and Sarabjeet Singh Bedi (2016) introduced the hybrid technique using curvelet and wavelet transform for the medical diagnosis by fusing the CT and MRI image. K.N. Narasimha Murthy and J. Kusuma (2017) proposed the Shearlet Transform to fuse two different multimodal medical images MRI and PET by using the singular value decomposition to improve the information content of the multimodal medical images. Nasrin Amini, et al. (2014) proposed the adding structural information from MRI to functional information of PET images. The multimodal medical images decomposed with nonsubsampled contourlet transform and then two medical images were fused with applying fusion rules. Padma Ganasala, Vinod Kumar (2015) proposed a novel image fusion method utilizing feature-motivated adaptive PCNN in NSST domain for fusion of anatomical images. Periyavattam Shanmugam Gomathi, Bhuvanesh Kalaavathi (2016) proposes the non-subsampled contourlet transform image fusion algorithm for the fusion of multimodal medical images. Rajalingam, R.Priya (2018) introduced the combination of non sub-sampled shearlet transform with non sub-sampled contourelet transform hybrid multimodal medical image fusion techniques for the better fusion process and accurate clinical analysis. Richa Srivastava, et al. (2016) proposed a multimodal medical fusion technique based on curvelet transform. Satishkumar S. Chavan, et al. (2017) proposed the nonsubsampled rotated complex wavelet transform for combining CT and MRI images of the same patient. Shuaiqi Liu, et al. (2015) proposed the combined the advantages of time-frequency separation of complex shearlet (CST) with the feature of guided filtering, a new image fusion algorithm based on CST domain and guided filtering. Xiaojun Xua, et al. (2016) proposed the multimodality medical image fusion algorithm based on discrete fractional wavelet transform. Xingbin Liu, et al. (2017) proposed the structure tensor and nonsubsampled shearlet transform to extract geometric features of multimodal medical images. Yuqian Lia, et al. (2017) proposed an advanced data fusion scheme for brain tumor diagnosis using both MRSI and MRI data to improve the tumor differentiation accuracy of MRSI alone.

PROPOSED WORK

Traditional Multimodal Medical Image Fusion

This research article implements different traditional and hybrid image fusion algorithms for different types of multimodality medical images. Different types of traditional fusion algorithms: (a) Discrete fractional wavelet transform (DFRWT) (b) Curvelet transform (CVT) (c) Guided image filtering (d) Non-subsampled contourlet transform (NSCT) (e) Non-subsampled shearlet transform (NSST)

Discrete Fractional Wavelet Transforms

The DWT can provide better spatial and spectral localization of image information; it has no shift invariant property because of the down-sampling operation. Thus, the fused image of the DWT method cannot efficiently preserve the salient features of the input images and produce pseudo-Gibbs effect. A

Figure 1. Overall structure for wavelet based medical image fusion

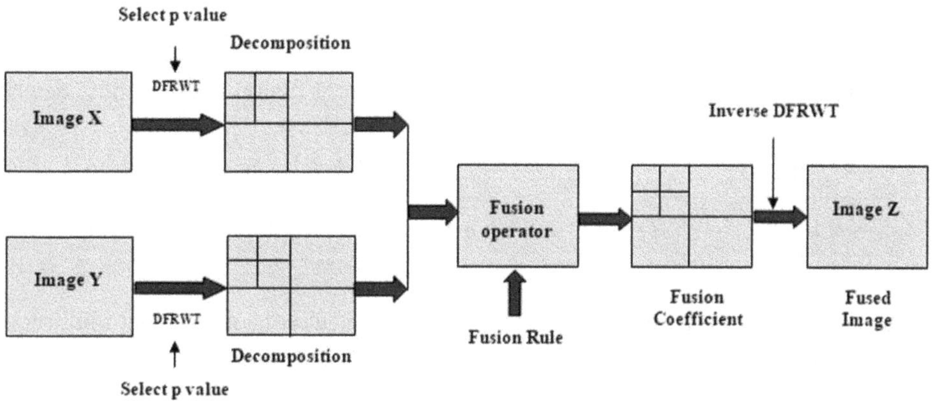

step is added to the DFRWT multimodal medical image fusion method. The input multimodality medical images are first decomposed into low-frequency subbands and a sequence of high-frequency subbands in different scales and orientations and in different p orders. Then, at each position in the transformed sub-bands, the coefficients of both the low-and high-frequency bands are performed with a certain fusion rule. Finally, the fused image is obtained by applying inverse DFRWT transform on the fused sub-bands. From analysis of the previous steps, the decomposition coefficients are a variety of different p orders; the fusion effects are different. This characteristic adds additional flexibility for the DFRWT fusion method and enhances the selection space for the fusion results (X.J. Xu.et al.). In the wavelet medical image fusion method, because of different decomposition coefficients feature in the low-and high-frequency bands, the LF- and HF-subbands are fused using the different combinations of fusion rules. However, in low p order, the decomposition a coefficient of the DFRWT in each subband has the same histogram distribution and shows the same non-sparse characteristics; hence, the authors use identical fusion rule in the LF- and HF-subbands. The Figure 1 shows the overall structure of the discrete fractional wavelet transform based multimodal medical image fusion algorithm.

Procedural Steps for Medical Image Fusion Using DFRWT Algorithm

Step 1: Take the two input multimodal medical images.
Step 2: Resize both images into 256 X 256 dimensions.
Step 3: Take l layer DFRWT of both input multimodal medical images in the same p order and obtain 3l + 1 pieces of the subbands coefficients.
Step 4: Suppose that the region has the size of K × L (which is generally 3 × 3, 5 × 5, and 7 × 7; here, take 3 × 3), and take p(a,b) as the center. The local variance $var_n^m\left(a,b\right)$ is defined as follows:

$$var_n^\tau\left(a,b\right)=\frac{1}{K\,x\,L}\sum_{i=1}^{K}\sum_{j=1}^{L}\left[abs\left(f_n^\tau\left(a+i,b+j\right)-\mu\right)\right]^2 \qquad (1)$$

where $f_n^\tau\left(a,b\right)$ is the subband coefficient at position (i,j) at the nth scale and τ[th] direction. μ is the average of the coefficients in the current local area, K and L are the number of rows and columns of the local area, respectively. Each direction τ (τ = x, v, d, h) local variance of the related pixel is record as $var_{n.X}^{\tau}\left(a,b\right)$, $var_{n.Y}^{\tau}\left(a,b\right)$.

Step 5: According to the regional variance, the weight of current fusion coefficient is determined as

$$\omega_{n.X}^{\tau} = \frac{var_{n.X}^{\tau}\left(A,B\right)}{var_{n.X}^{\tau}\left(A,B\right) + var_{n.Y}^{\tau}\left(A,B\right)},\ \omega_{n.Y}^{\tau} = \frac{var_{n.Y}^{\tau}\left(A,B\right)}{var_{n.X}^{\tau}\left(A,B\right) + var_{n.Y}^{\tau}\left(A,B\right)} \tag{2}$$

where $\omega_{n.X}^{\tau}$ and $\omega_{n.Y}^{\tau}$ are the weights between the DFRWT coefficients of the input multimodal medical images at the nth scale and τth direction, respectively. Supposing that $R_{n.X}^{\tau}$ are the fusion coefficients, researcher use the following formula to compose the pixel.

$$R_{n.X}^{\tau} = f_{n.X}^{\tau}\left(a,b\right) X \omega_{n.X}^{\tau} + f_{n.X}^{\tau}\left(a,b\right) X \omega_{n.X}^{\tau} \tag{3}$$

From the equation (2) and (3), $R_{n.X}^{\tau}$ as the fusion coefficients are dynamically and adaptively fused with the significant features of the input multimodality medical images. This rule can automatically allocate the right weight for each pixel and prominent target combination information according to the characteristics of multimodal medical image.

Step 6: Perform inverse DFRWT on the fused low and high frequency subband coefficients, which are reconstructed into a fused multimodal medical image.

Curvelet Transform

In the current research topic ridgelet transform is one of the new powerful transform techniques. Ridgelet transform is anisotropic in nature and can efficiently capture the global straight line singularities. However, in real medical images, global straight line is not so common. To handle this situation, the whole multimodal medical image is partitioned into small sub multimodality medical images. This partitioning is done in a manner so that the curves and edge lines appear just as a straight line. Ridgelet transform is then applied on each sub medical image. This block-based ridgelet transform is the basic concept of first generation curvelet transform (Candes et al., 2005). The theoretical idea of first generation curvelet is easy to understand, but, its implementation in discrete domain is difficult. Also, it is not quite popular because of its dependency on ridgelet transform whose geometry is very unclear. Discrete version of curvelet transform, which is based on frequency partition. This version of curvelet transform is efficient for representing curves and edges. Unlike wavelet transform, curvelet transform is localised in scale, position and orientation. Due to these properties, curvelet transform can give efficient results for medical image fusion. The traditional wavelet is popular in image processing, but, its isotropic nature makes it inefficient in capturing line singularities. Wavelet representation needs more coefficients than curvelet representation for representing the same curve. Hence, discrete curvelet transform is faster in capturing edges than wavelet and other transforms. The discrete version of curvelet transform can be implemented in two ways. The first one is wrapping-based curvelet transform and the second one is unequally-spaced

Figure 2. Overall structure for Curvelet based medical image fusion

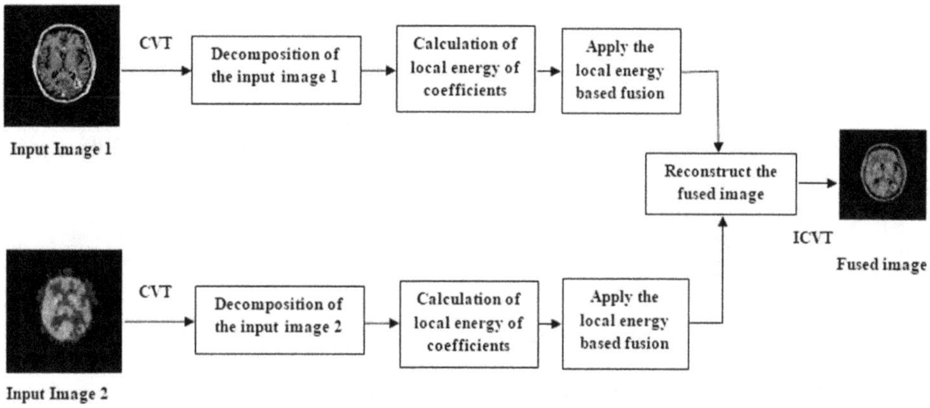

fast Fourier transform (USFFT)-based curvelet transform (Candes et al., 2005). These two implementations use different spatial grids for translation of curvelet at different scales and directions. Figure 2 shows the overall process structure of the curvelet transform based medical image fusion algorithm.

The basic structure of curvelet transform is divided into four steps.

Subband Decomposition

A multimodal medical image MI is divided into several decomposition levels with the help of low-pass filter P_0 and several band-pass filter banks, Δ_s, $S \geq 0$. Medical image MI is decomposed using à trous algorithm

$$MI \rightarrow \left(P_0 MI, \Delta_1 MI, \Delta_2 MI, \ldots.\right) \tag{4}$$

Smooth Partitioning

Each subband is partitioned smoothly into 'squares' of proper scales

$$\Delta_s MI \rightarrow \left(S_Q \Delta_s MI\right)_{Q \int Q_s} \tag{5}$$

where S_Q is smooth window localised around dyadic squares

$$Q = \left[\frac{d_1}{2^s}, \frac{(d_1+1)}{2^s}\right] X \left[\frac{d_2}{2^s}, \frac{\left(d_2+1\right)}{2^s}\right] \tag{6}$$

Renormalisation

The resulting dyadic squares are renormalized into unit scale of $[0, 1]^2$

$$r_Q = (T_Q)^{-1}\left(S_Q \Delta_S MI\right), Q \int Q_s \tag{7}$$

Ridgelet Analysis

The normalized dyadic square is analyzed by ridgelet system. It has basis elements p_λ that make an orthonormal basis for L^2 (R^2)

$$\beta_\mu = \left(r_Q, p_\lambda\right) \tag{8}$$

Procedural Steps for Image Fusion Using Curvelet Transform Algorithm

Step 1: Take the two input multimodal medical images.
Step 2: Resize both images into 256 x 256 dimensions.
Step 3: Decompose the each input multimodal medical image using curvelet transform.
Step 4: Compute the local energy of coefficients.
Step 5: Apply the local energy based medical image fusion rule.
Step 6: Finally, apply the inverse curvelet transform to reconstruct the multimodal medical image.
Step 7: Perform the image reconstruction and get the final fused multimodal medical image.

Guided Image Filtering

In the current research of edge preserving guided image filtering is one of the hotspot in image processing. The guided filtering is the latest weighted least squares filtering and other edge preserving smoothing filtering can do image filtering without blurring strong edges and hence they avoid introducing artificial texture in the process of filtering. The guided filtering is a linear edge preserving filtering algorithm and its computation time does not depend on the size of filtering kernel. Therefore it can be well applied in the field of image processing. Compared to other edge preserving filtering algorithms, the guided filtering is very fast (its time complexity is O (n), and it is easily applied to image fusion. Hence guide filtering is selected to enhance the spatial continuity in our multimodal medical image fusion algorithm. Figure 3 describes the overall structure for guided image filtering based medical image fusion algorithm.

Figure 3. Overall structure for guided image filtering based medical image fusion

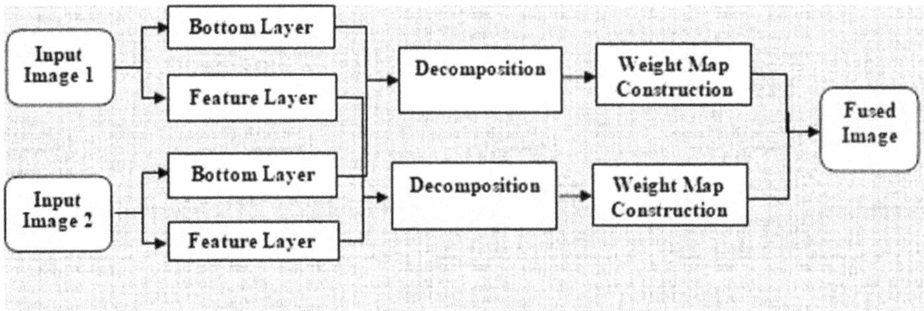

Process of Guided Image Filtering

The process of using the guided filtering involves a guidance image G, an input image X which needs filtering and an output image Y. Image G and Y can be identical. The key assumption of the guided filtering is a local linear model between the guidance G and the filtering output r.

$$r_i = m_k G_i + n_k, \forall i \in \omega_k \tag{9}$$

where i is pixel index, $m_k n_k$ are some linear coefficients, and ω_k is a local square window of radius (2r + 1) centered at the pixel k in the guidance image G . Then the image filtering problem of edge preserving is converted into the optimal problem of minimizing the difference between r and X and satisfying the linear condition in (10) at the same time. That is:

$$T(m_k n_{k)} = \sum_{i\in\omega_k} \left(\left(m_k G_i + n_k - X_i \right)^2 + \varepsilon m_k^2 \right) \tag{10}$$

Here ε denotes a regularization parameter (fuzzy parameter). The solution to formula (11) can be given by linear regression.

$$m_k = \frac{\frac{1}{|\omega|} \sum_{i\in\omega_k} G_i X_i - r_k \overline{X_k}}{\sigma_k^2 + \varepsilon} \tag{11}$$

$$n_k = \overline{X_k} - n_k \mu_k \tag{12}$$

Here, μ_k and σ_k^2 denote the mean and variance of G in local window ω_k , |ω| is the number of pixels in ωk, and $\overline{X_k}$ is the mean of X in ω_k . In order to keep the value of r_i invariant when it is computed in different windows, after working out m_k and n_k for all patches ω_k in the image, researcher use average filter to average all the possible values in local window.

$$r_i = \frac{1}{|\omega|} \sum_{k:i\in\omega_k} \left(m_k G_i + n_k \right) = \overline{m_i} G_i + \overline{n_i} \tag{13}$$

where $\overline{m_i}$ and $\overline{n_i}$ denote the mean of m_k and n_k in local window ω_k , namely

$$\overline{m_i} = \frac{1}{|\omega|} \sum_{k\in\omega_i} m_k, \overline{n_i} = \frac{1}{|\omega|} \sum_{k\in\omega_i} n_k \tag{14}$$

For simplicity, $T_{s,\mu}(X,G)$ denote guided image filtering. Here, s denotes the size of filter kernel, X denotes the input image and G denotes the guidance image.

Procedural Steps for Image Fusion Using Guided Image Filtering

Step 1: Take the two input multimodal medical images.
Step 2: Resize both images into 256 x 256 dimensions.
Step 3: Decompose the input multimodal medical images using average filtering.
Step 4: Separate the input multimodality medical images into bottom layer and feature layer based on multi scale representation.
Step 5: Apply the Gaussian laplacian filters to construct the weight map and saliency map.
Step 6: Perform the image reconstruction and get the final fused multimodal medical image.

Non-Subsampled Contourlet Transform Techniques

The contourlet transform is a multiscale and multidirectional transform, which is capable of capturing the geometrical features of 2D multimodal medical images. It provides flexible number of directions in each scale and satisfies the anisotropic scaling law by just doubling the number of directions in every next higher scale. It utilizes a double filter bank structure. Double filter bank structure has two parts: (i) Multiscale decomposition (ii) Directional decomposition. Multiscale decomposition and directional decomposition are performed by Laplacian pyramid (LP) and directional filter banks (DFBs) respectively. Point discontinuities, present in a multimodality medical image, are captured by multiscale decomposition and local directional decomposition associates these points into continuous edge or contour. Thus, an image is represented by small image segments called contours. Therefore, this transform is called as contourlet transform. The NSCT is based on the theory of Contourlet Transform (CT) which achieves better results in image processing in geometric transformations. The contourlet transform is a shift variant because it contains both down-samplers and up-samplers in the Laplacian Pyramid (LP) and Directional Filter Bank (DFB) stages. NSCT is a shift invariant, multi-scale and multi-directional transform which has a very vibrant implementation. It is obtained by using the Non-subsampled Pyramid Filter Bank (NSP or NSPFB) and the Non-subsampled Directional Filter Bank (NSDFB).

Non-Subsampled Pyramid Filter Bank

The multiscale property is ensured by the non-subsampled pyramid filter bank using two-channel non-subsampled filter bank. At each decomposition level, one low-frequency image and one high-frequency image can be produced. In the subsequent NSP decomposition level, the low-frequency components are decomposed iteratively to capture the singularities in the multimodality medical image. As a result, NSP can result in L + 1 sub-image, which consists of one low frequency medical image and L high frequency medical images where L denotes the number of decomposition levels. The sub-images have the same size as the input multimodality medical image.

Non-Subsampled Directional Filter Bank

The Non-subsampled Directional Filter Bank is a two-channel NSDFB which are constructed by combining the directional fan filter banks. The NSDFB ensures the NSCT with the multi-direction property and provides more directional detail information. The NSDFB is achieved by eliminating downsamplers and upsamplers in each two-channel filter bank in DFB tree structure and upsampling filters accordingly. NSDFB allows the direction decomposition with k levels in each high-frequency subbands from NSPFB and then produces 2 k directional subbands with the same size as the input medical images. Thus, the NSDFB provides the NSCT with multidirectional performance and gives more precise directional detail information to get more accurate results. Therefore, NSCT provides better frequency selectivity and an important property of the shift-invariance on account of non-subsampled operation. The size of sub-images decomposed by NSCT is same and image fusion based on NSCT can mitigate the effects of misregistration in the fused medical images. Therefore, NSCT is more suitable for multimodal medical image fusion. Figure 4 shows the decomposition process of the NSCT.

Procedural Steps for Image Fusion Using NSCT Algorithm

Step 1: Take the two input multimodal medical images.
Step 2: Resize both images into 256 x 256 dimensions.
Step 3: NSCT is applied on the both input images to obtain lowpass subband coefficients and highpass directional subband coefficients at each scale and each direction. NSPFB and NSDFB are used to complete multiscale decomposition and multi-direction decomposition.
Step 4: The transformed coefficients are performed with fusion rules to select NSCT coefficients of the fused image.

Figure 4. NSCT Framework for Decomposition Process

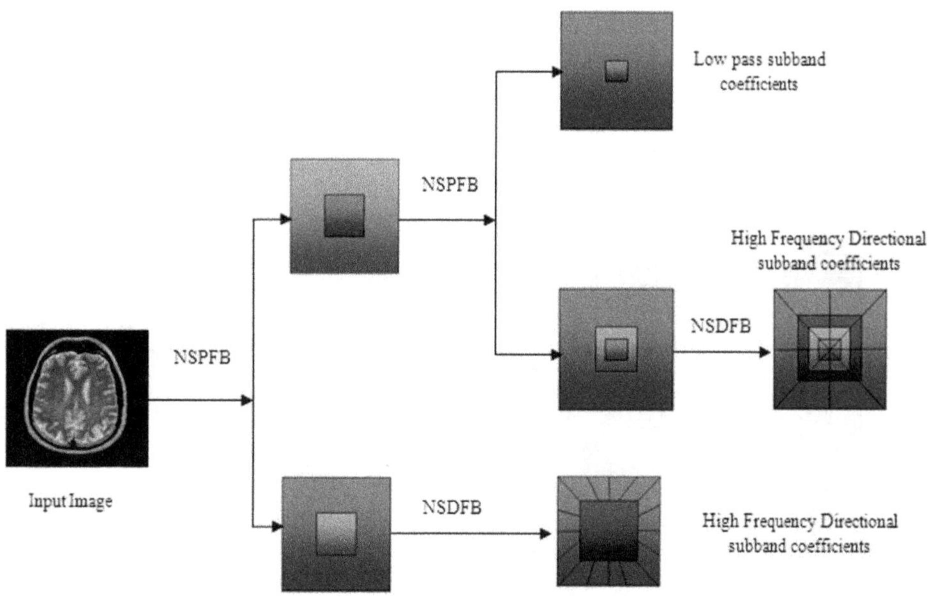

Figure 5. Overall structure for NSCT based medical image fusion

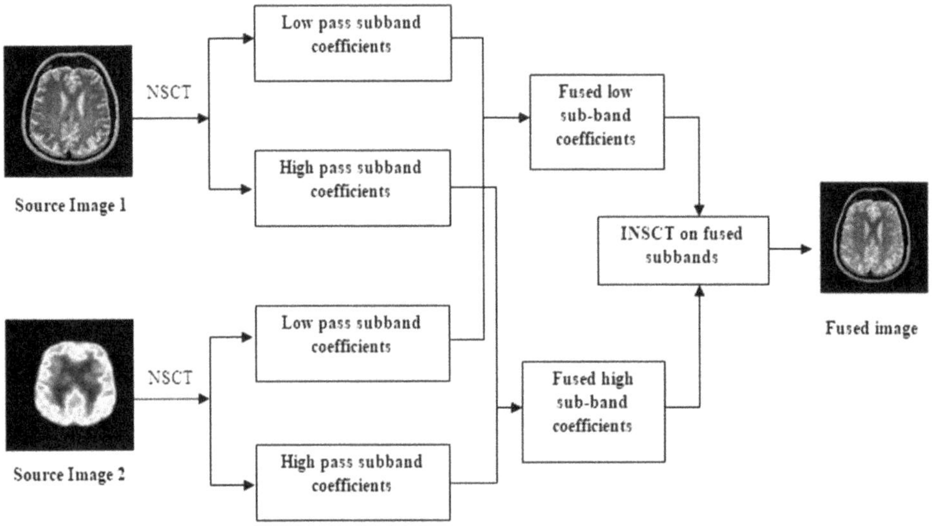

Step 5: The fused image is constructed by performing an inverse NSCT to the selected coefficients obtained from previous step. Figure 5 show the implementation process of the NSCT based multimodal medical image fusion algorithm.

Non-Subsampled Shearlet Transform

The ST is used to encode the features which are varying in direction in many problems. Its primary steps are localization in directions and decomposition is done in multiple scales. There are two types of ST: continuous and discrete which are defined as follows with the fixed resolution level j. Figure 6 show the frequency tilling by the shearlet transform.

Figure 6. Frequency tilling by the shearlet (a) frequency plane (b) frequency size

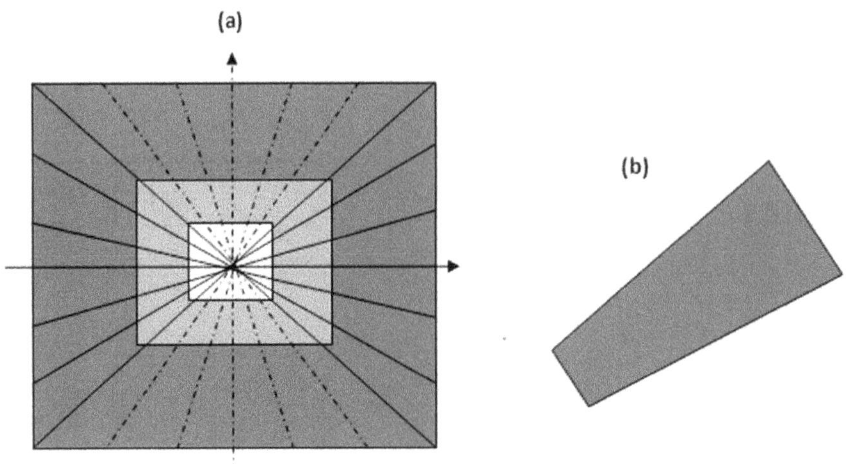

Continuous Shearlet Transform

It is defined as the affine systems which are grouped with the complex dilation which are of the form:

$$Sh_{AB}\left(\Psi\right) = \left\{\Psi_{x,y,z}\left(P\right) = \left|\det A\right|^{x/2}\,\Psi\left(Q^{y}A^{x}P - z\right); x, y \in Z, z \in Z^{2}\right\} \tag{15}$$

where a represents scale, b is orientation, c is cone for 2 dimensions, A and B are 2 × 2 invertible matrices. For the function fn ∈ $M^{2}\left(N^{2}\right)$, is as follows:

$$\sum_{x,y,z}\left|fn,\Psi_{x,y,z}\right|^{2} = fn^{2} \tag{16}$$

For the function fn ∈ $M^{2}\left(N^{2}\right)$, tight frame is formed by the $Sh_{AB}\left(\Psi\right)$. The matrix Pa is related with scale transform and the matrix Qb related with the orientation like shear and rotation. The continuous ST is of the form:

$$\Psi_{x,y,z}\left(P\right) = x^{-3/4}\,\Psi\left(Y_{y}^{-1}X_{x}^{-1}\left(P - z\right)\right) \tag{17}$$

where,

$$X_{x} = \begin{pmatrix} x & 0 \\ 0 & \sqrt{x} \end{pmatrix}, Y_{y} = \begin{pmatrix} y & 0 \\ 0 & \sqrt{y} \end{pmatrix}, \ \Psi \in M^{2}\left(N^{2}\right)$$

where ψ1 is a continuous WT, in, $\Psi_{x,y,z}$,$x, y \in N$ and z ∈ N^2, for any function fn ∈ $M^{2}\left(N^{2}\right)$, for different scales of wavelets. Usually, the values of x = 4 and y = 1.

Discrete Shearlet Transform

There are two steps in discrete shearlet transform: they are directional localization and dividing in different scales. Let for any scale j, the function fn ∈ L Z_{M}^{2}. Initially for ecomposing an image the Laplacian pyramid is applied. Let consider the image as f_{a}^{j}, when Laplacian pyramid is applied on image then it is decomposed into low frequency f_{l}^{j} and high frequency f_{i}^{j}. If another division is needed then the Laplacian pyramid is applied on low frequency f_{l}^{j}. Then for reconstructing these frequencies into images the inverse fast Fourier Transform is applied.

The NSST is a newly established multi-scale geometric analysis tool, which is superior at capturing multidimensional geometry and is optimally well-organized in medical images representation. In the implementation procedure of NSST, non-subsampled laplacian pyramid is adopted to realize multi-scale factorization. Shearing filters are used to complete multi-orientation factorization. As a result, the NSST

Figure 7. Overall structure for NSST for medical image fusion

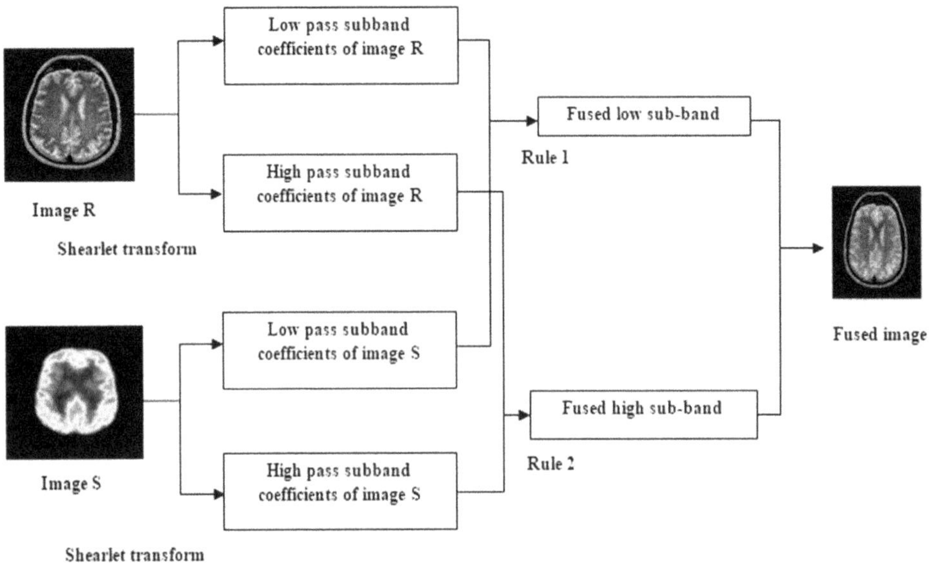

has not only shift invariance property but also a more flexible directional selectivity than other geometric analysis tools. The original multimodal medical image can be decomposed into a low-frequency sub-image and several high-frequency sub-images. Figure 7 shows the overall structure of the NSST based medical image fusion process algorithm.

Procedural Steps for Image Fusion Using NSST Algorithm

Step 1: Take the two input multimodal medical images.
Step 2: Resize both images into 256 x 256 dimensions.
Step 3: Decompose the each input multimodal medical image using shearlet transform.
Step 4: Compute the low and high frequency of Shearlet transform.
Step 5: Fuse the selected low and high frequency of the subband coefficients.
Step 6: Finally apply the Inverse non subsampled shearlet transform (INSST) to reconstruct the multi-modal medical image.
Step 7: Perform the image reconstruction and get the final fused multimodal medical image

Hybrid Multimodal Medical Image Fusion Techniques

Traditional multimodal medical image fusion techniques lack the ability to get high quality images. So, there is a bad need to use hybrid fusion techniques to achieve this objective. The basic idea of the hybrid technique is to combine the discrete fractional wavelet transform with shearlet transforms to improve the performance and increase fused image quality. Another possibility is applying two stage transformations on input images before fusion process. These transformations provide better characterization of input images, better handling of curved shapes and higher quality for fused details. The overall advantages of the hybrid techniques are improving the visual quality of the images and decreasing image artifacts and

Figure 8. Overall structure of the proposed hybrid multimodal medical image fusion

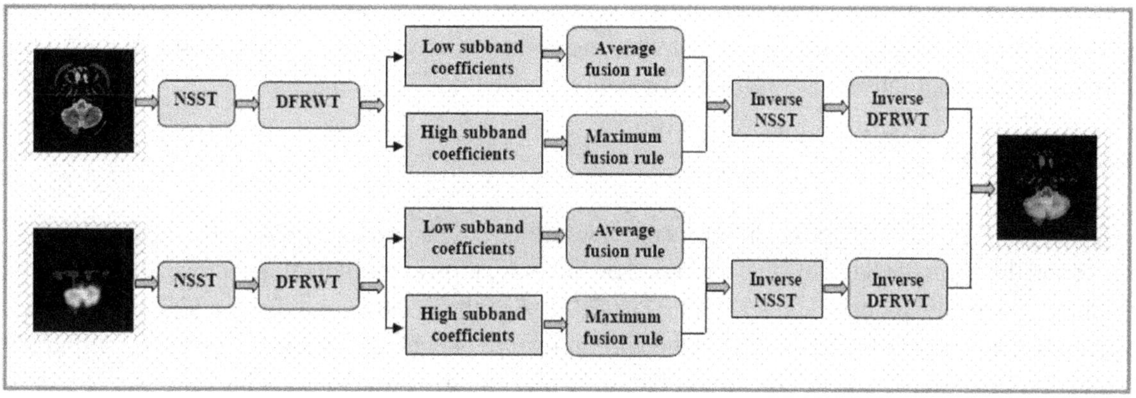

noise. Figure 8 shows the overall structure of the proposed hybrid multimodal medical image fusion techniques.

Proposed Hybrid Multimodal Medical Image Fusion Algorithm (NSST-DFRWT)

In this proposed work NSST and DFRWT techniques are applied on the both input multimodal medical images.

Input: CT, MRI, PET and SPECT are the two inputs of multimodal medical images which need to be processed.

Output: Multimodality medical image which is getting fused.

Step 1: Take the two input multimodal medical images.
Step 2: Resize both images into 256 x 256 dimensions.
Step 3: Compute the low and high frequency of Shearlet transform coefficients.
Step 4: Fuse the selected low and high frequency of the subband coefficients.
Step 5: Apply the discrete fractional wavelet transform maximum and minimum fusion rule in the low-pass and highpass subbands coefficients
Step 6: Decompose the each input multimodal medical image using shearlet transform.
Step 7: Finally take the Inverse shearlet transform (IST) to reconstruct the multimodal medical image.
Step 8: Then, apply the inverse DFRWT to reconstruct the fused image.
Step 9: Perform the image reconstruction and get the final fused multimodal medical image

PERFORMANCE EVALUATION METRICS

The proposed hybrid fusion algorithms are evaluated based on qualitative and quantitative performance parameter analysis. The visual quality of the fused multimodal medical image is estimated based on qualitative analysis and whereas image fusion parameters are estimated as quantitative analysis. Based on the similar and dissimilar features the fused image is compared with input images. The statistical parameters like mean, standard deviation and entropy help analyse the quality of the fused multimodal medical image. The fusion parameters fusion symmetry, image quality index, edge quality measure, mean structural similarity index, cross entropy and correlation coefficient are used for evaluating the qualitative and quantitative analysis of the fused multimodal medical image.

Fusion Factor

Fusion factor (FusFact) is a type of similarity measure which indicates the comparison of the fused medical images and the input medical images. It is based on the estimation of mutual information between original multimodality medical images (CT/MRI/PET/SPECT) and the fused output multimodal medical image as given by Equation (19). Here, $MI_{X,B}$ is the similar feature between X and Y image, $p(.)$ is probability distribution function. The better quality of the fused medical image indicates a higher value of FusFact

$$\text{FusFact} = \text{MI}_{\text{input1,Fu}} + \text{MI}_{\text{input2,Fu}} \tag{18}$$

$$MI_{X,Y} = \sum_{k,l} P_{X,Y}\left(k,l\right) \log \frac{P_X\left(k,l\right)}{P_X\left(k\right) P_Y\left(l\right)} \tag{19}$$

Fusion Symmetry

The fusion symmetry (FuSymt) which indicates the proximity of fused medical image with respect to input medical images. It is also estimated using similar feature between input images and fused image. It is computed using Equation (20). The fused multimodal medical image is visually better if the value of FuSymt is smaller.

$$FuSymt = abs\left[\frac{MI_{input1.Fu}}{MI_{input1.Fu} + MI_{input2.Fu}} - 0.5\right] \tag{20}$$

Image Quality Index

The universal similarity index called as image quality index (IQI) which is computed using Equation (21). It gives similarity measure between two multimodality medical images X and Y. Here, σ stands for standard deviation and μ stands for mean. Average value of IQI for the fused medical image with CT/MRI/PET/SPECT is taken as an index. The value of IQI should be close to 'one' to declare that the fused medical image is of better quality (Wang and Bovik.et al).

$$IQI\left(X,Y\right) = \frac{2\sigma_{X,Y}.2\mu_X\mu_Y}{\left(\sigma_X^2 + \sigma_Y^2\right)\left(\mu_X^2 + \mu_Y^2\right)} \tag{21}$$

Edge Quality Measure

The edges of input medical images are preserved in the fused medical image which is represented as edge quality measure $EQM_{x,y}^{fus}$. Mathematically, it is computed using Equation (22). Here, fus is fused medical image obtained from images x and y. $EQM_{x,fus}$ and $EQM_{y,fus}$ are indices of preservation of edge in the fused multimodal medical image imparted by input medical images. The 'zero' value of $EQM_{x,y}^{fus}$, indicates loss of edge and value 'one' indicates preservation of edge in the fused medical image (C.S. Xydeas.et al).

$$EQM_{x,y}^{fus} = \frac{\sum_{a=0}^{K-1}\sum_{b=0}^{L-1} EQ_{x,fus}\left(a,b\right) w_x\left(a,b\right) + EQ_{y,fus}\left(a,b\right) w_y\left(a,b\right)}{\sum_{m=0}^{K-1}\sum_{n=0}^{L-1} w_x\left(m,n\right) + w_y\left(m,n\right)} \tag{22}$$

Mean Structural Similarity Index Measure

The anatomical closeness of fused multimodal medical image can be estimated using the parameter 'mean structural similarity index measure (mSSIM)'. It is calculated using Equations (23) and (24), where σ is standard deviation and μ is mean. The I_1 and I_2 are the iterative parameter constants. The fused multimodal medical image is structurally similar in comparison with input multimodal medical images (CT/MRI/PET/SPECT) if mSSIM approaches to value 'one' (Wang et al, 2004; Biswas et al, 2015).

$$SSIM\left(k,l\right) = \frac{\left(2\mu_k\mu_l + I_1\right)\left(2\sigma_{k,l} + I_2\right)}{\left(\mu_k^2 + \mu_l^2 + I_1\right)\left(\sigma_k^2 + \sigma_l^2 + I_2\right)} \tag{23}$$

$$mSSIM\left(k,l\right) = \frac{1}{N}\sum_{o=1}^{N} SSIM(k_o, l_o) \tag{24}$$

Cross Entropy

The cross entropy (CE) estimates the relative quality of the fused image with respect to the input images which is given by Equation (25). Here, X and Y are the two input medical images, p(.) is probability distribution function, and N is highest gray value in an image. The fused multimodal medical image is of better quality if CE has lower value (G. Qu, et al).

$$CE\left(X,Y\right) = \sum_{k=0}^{L-1} P_A\left(k\right)\log_2\frac{P_X\left(k\right)}{P_Y\left(k\right)} \tag{25}$$

Correlation Coefficient

The correlation coefficient (CCR) represents the closeness of fused multimodal medical image with input modalities. It is computed using Equation (26). Here, F_i is input medical image and I_{fus} is fused output medical image. The fused image and input images will be similar if CCR is close to value 'one.

$$CCR(k,l) = \frac{2\sum_{k=0}^{M-1}\sum_{l=0}^{N-1} F_i(k,l).I_{fus}(k,l)}{\sum_{k=0}^{M-1}\sum_{l=0}^{N-1}\left|F_i(k,l)\right|^2 + \sum_{k=0}^{M-1}\sum_{l=0}^{N-1}\left|I_{fus}(k,l)\right|^2} \tag{26}$$

RESULTS AND DISCUSSIONS

The implemented results based on two stages. The traditional fusion algorithms applied to ten set of multimodal medical images and the qualitative and quantitative performance metrics are discussed. The experiment is executed in MATLAB R2015b on windows 7 laptop with Intel Core I5 Processor, 4.0 GB

Figure 9. Experimental results of the set 1 to 5

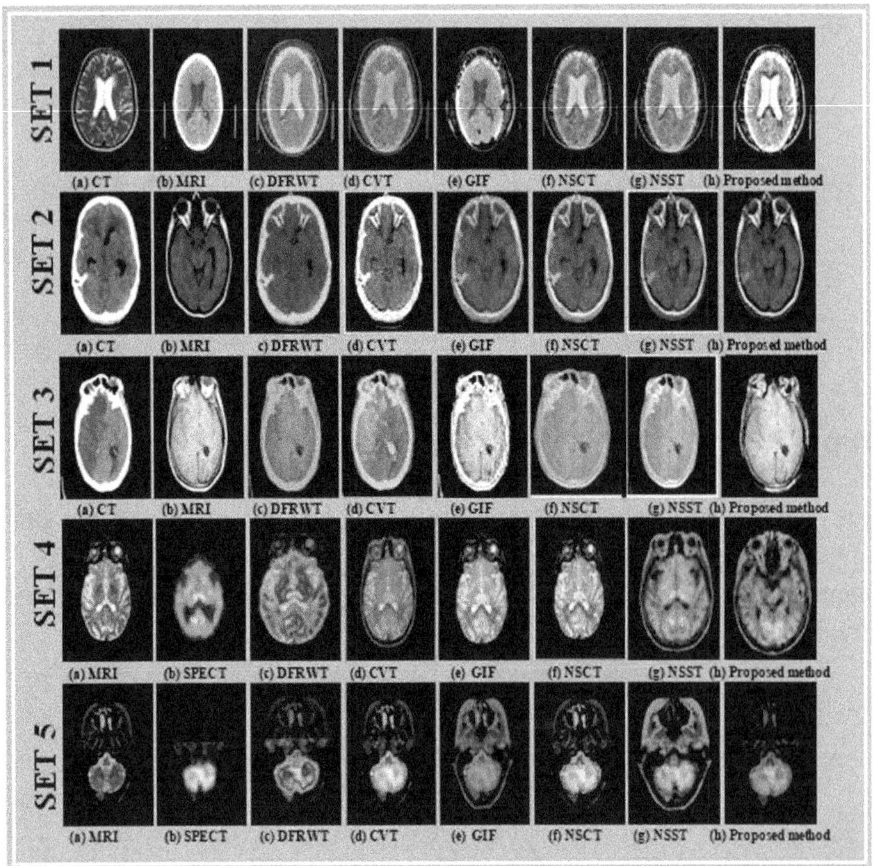

Figure 10. Comparative analysis for experimented medical images performance metrics for set 1

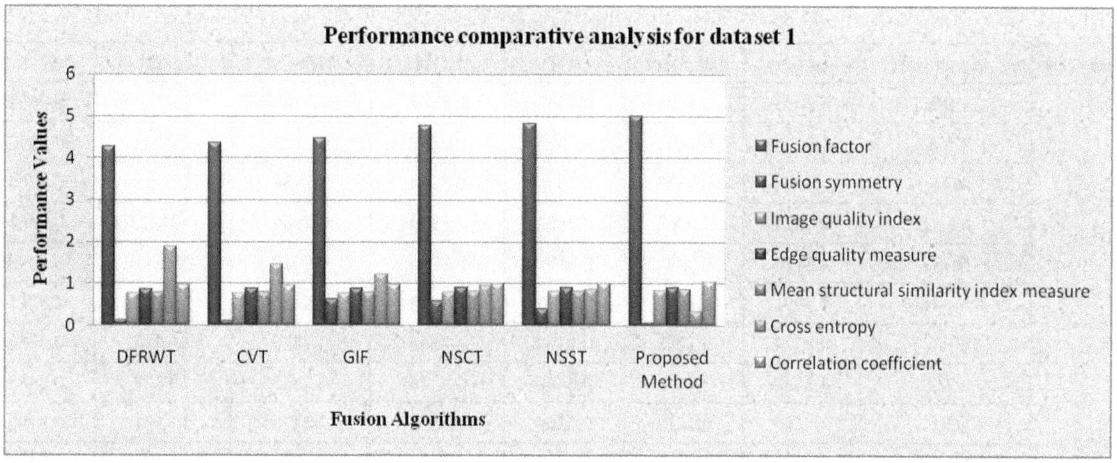

Figure 11. Comparative analysis for experimented medical images performance metrics for set 2

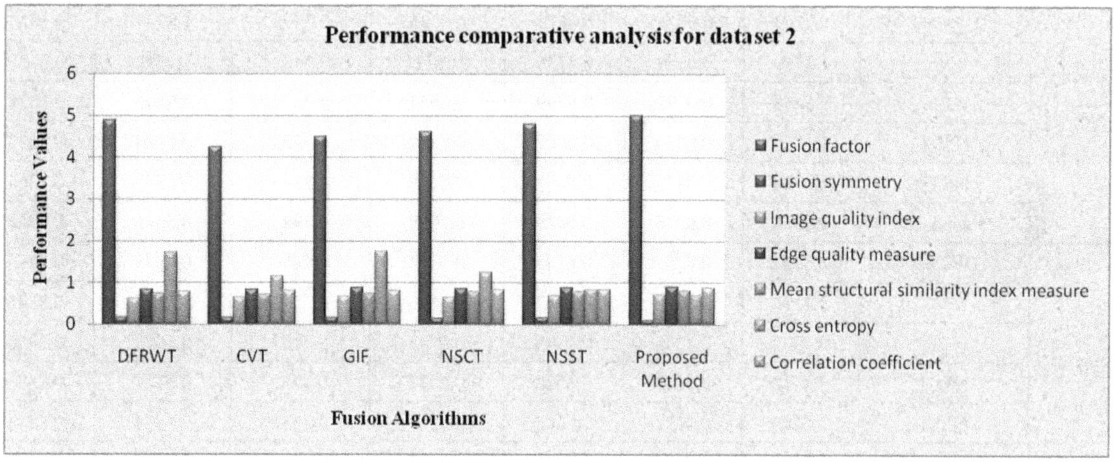

Figure 12. Comparative analysis for experimented medical images performance metrics for set 3

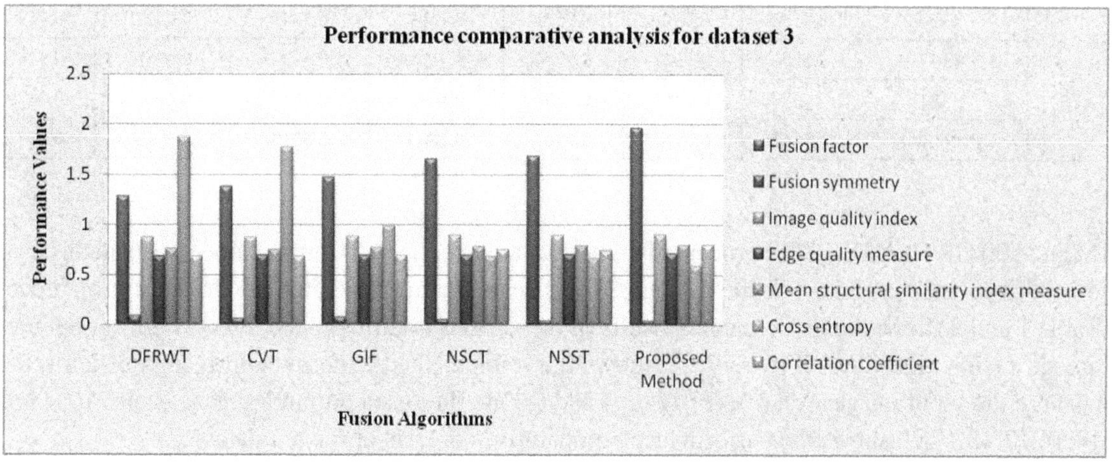

Table 1. Performance metrics values obtained from different multimodal medical image fusion algorithms for Set 1 to 5

Study Set	Algorithm	Fus Fact	Fus Symt	IQI	EQM	MSSIM	CE	CCR
SET 1	DFRWT	4.2687	0.1198	0.7543	0.8587	0.7783	1.8743	0.9587
	CVT	4.3476	0.1043	0.7598	0.8872	0.7823	1.4398	0.9398
	GIF	4.4578	0.6332	0.7676	0.8754	0.7954	1.2194	0.9765
	NSCT	4.7623	0.5762	0.7823	0.8899	0.7985	0.94323	0.9861
	NSST	4.8119	0.3982	0.8199	0.8966	0.8010	0.8541	0.9998
	Proposed	**4.9991**	**0.0652**	**0.8427**	**0.9038**	**0.8476**	**0.3287**	**1.0361**
SET 2	DFRWT	4.8723	0.1788	0.6354	0.8365	0.7376	1.7246	0.7958
	CVT	4.2387	0.1632	0.6489	0.8376	0.7245	1.1537	0.7988
	GIF	4.4845	0.1612	0.6598	0.8658	0.7476	1.7501	0.8102
	NSCT	4.6129	0.1532	0.6543	0.8598	0.7774	1.2498	0.8265
	NSST	4.7982	0.1587	0.6872	0.8712	0.7856	0.8367	0.8299
	Proposed	**4.9898**	**0.1076**	**0.7104**	**0.8975**	**0.7999**	**0.6954**	**0.8654**
SET 3	DFRWT	1.2764	0.0875	0.8674	0.6799	0.7598	1.8734	0.6834
	CVT	1.3769	0.0649	0.8735	0.68721	0.7487	1.7698	0.6756
	GIF	1.4698	0.0772	0.8799	0.6934	0.7694	0.9843	0.6876
	NSCT	1.6522	0.0533	0.8867	0.6879	0.7753	0.6784	0.7433
	NSST	1.6788	0.0423	0.8891	0.6999	0.7856	0.6573	0.7365
	Proposed	**1.9589**	**0.0376**	**0.9029**	**0.7098**	**0.7984**	**0.5846**	**0.7968**
SET 4	DFRWT	3.3237	0.8287	0.6145	0.6734	0.7466	0.4875	0.8793
	CVT	3.2389	0.3267	0.6287	0.6856	0.7591	0.4637	0.8845
	GIF	3.4322	0.7845	0.6345	0.6792	0.7667	0.6389	0.8736
	NSCT	3.4412	0.5643	0.6523	0.6577	0.7756	0.5721	0.8893
	NSST	3.5726	0.4572	0.6645	0.6967	0.7643	0.5524	0.8974
	Proposed	**3.9975**	**0.0474**	**0.6834**	**0.7047**	**0.7988**	**0.4289**	**0.9029**
SET 5	DFRWT	2.6733	0.1326	0.9377	0.7145	0.7697	0.6743	0.9145
	CVT	2.4356	0.2467	0.9478	0.7564	0.7734	0.6532	0.9287
	GIF	2.4188	0.2674	0.9671	0.7599	0.7845	0.6421	0.9176
	NSCT	2.5658	0.1342	0.9874	0.7691	0.7936	0.6389	0.9387
	NSST	2.6674	0.2854	0.9754	0.7693	0.7903	0.6308	0.9478
	Proposed	**2.9863**	**0.0916**	**0.9967**	**0.7863**	**0.8019**	**0.5979**	**0.9874**

RAM and 500 GB Hard Disk. The processed input images are collected from radiopedia.org and Harvard Medical School medical image online database. The size of the image is 256 × 256 for execution process.

Table 1 and 2 shows the experimental results of the various traditional and hybrid multimodal medical image fusion algorithms. Figure 9, 15 shows the implemented experimental results of ten set: (a) and (b) are the input images (c), (d), (e), (f), (g) and (h) are the fused output images. Figure 10, 11, 12, 13,14,16,17,18,19,20 shows the performance comparative analysis of the ten dataset.

Table 2. Performance metrics values obtained from different multimodal medical image fusion algorithms for Set 6 to 10

Study Set	Algorithm	Fus Fact	Fus Symt	IQI	EQM	MSSIM	CE	CCR
SET 6	DFRWT	4.5768	0.3546	0.7299	0.7793	0.7236	1.2637	0.9467
	CVT	4.7891	0.3659	0.7411	0.7844	0.7389	013784	0.9566
	GIF	4.7791	0.3288	0.7536	0.7963	0.7424	1.3598	0.9521
	NSCT	4.8716	0.3841	0.7365	0.8194	0.7504	1.2951	0.9128
	NSST	4.3452	0.3475	0.7537	0.8338	0.7639	1.5821	0.9236
	Proposed	**5.1915**	**0.2923**	**0.7986**	**0.8845**	**0.76.48**	**0.8734**	**0.9975**
SET 7	DFRWT	4.1541	0.0263	0.7623	0.7218	0.7538	0.5110	0.9123
	CVT	4.2651	0.0242	0.7589	0.7484	0.7682	0.4814	0.9327
	GIF	4.4122	0.0182	0.7426	0.7699	0.7859	0.4626	0.9267
	NSCT	4.5311	0.0096	0.7589	0.7329	0.7855	0.4783	0.9582
	NSST	4.6123	0.0173	0.7714	0.7826	0.7901	0.4692	0.9472
	Proposed	**5.1421**	**0.0031**	**0.7992**	**0.7987**	**0.8112**	**0.4374**	**0.9956**
SET 8	DFRWT	3.2011	0.2361	0.9872	0.4672	0.7512	0.9901	0.8243
	CVT	3.3915	0.2278	0.9813	0.4529	0.7488	0.9511	0.8346
	GIF	3.4121	0.2741	0.9743	0.4421	0.7911	0.9428	0.8517
	NSCT	3.7419	0.2631	0.9856	0.4589	0.7819	0.9218	0.7939
	NSST	3.6623	0.2923	0.9622	0.5611	0.7331	0.9852	0.8123
	Proposed	**4.1213**	**0.1391**	**0.9982**	**0.6982**	**0.8264**	**0.9015**	**0.8917**
SET 9	DFRWT	4.3766	0.0314	0.7319	0.6982	0.7192	2.2199	0.7144
	CVT	4.2196	0.0321	0.7421	0.7269	0.7166	2.2752	0.7373
	GIF	4.4178	0.0699	0.8152	0.7901	0.7238	1.5025	0.7685
	NSCT	4.48864	0.07236	0.9275	0.8891	0.7394	1.9091	0.7639
	NSST	4.5818	0.0522	0.9769	0.9019	0.7359	1.7381	0.7917
	Proposed	**5.4821**	**0.0224**	**1.1045**	**0.9483**	**0.8105**	**0.8879**	**0.9128**
SET 10	DFRWT	2.7161	0.0637	0.8331	0.6268	0.7867	1.1179	0.8714
	CVT	2.7519	0.0782	0.8492	0.7616	0.7729	1.0752	0.8637
	GIF	2.7416	0.0559	0.9512	0.7896	0.7482	0.9225	0.8765
	NSCT	2.7819	0.0612	0.9928	0.8138	0.7899	0.9619	0.8763
	NSST	2.7998	0.0552	0.9826	0.8199	0.7755	0.9731	0.8891
	Proposed	**2.8515**	**0.0102**	**1.0184**	**0.8848**	**0.8995**	**0.9011**	**0.9422**

Figure 13. Comparative analysis for experimented medical images performance metrics for set 4

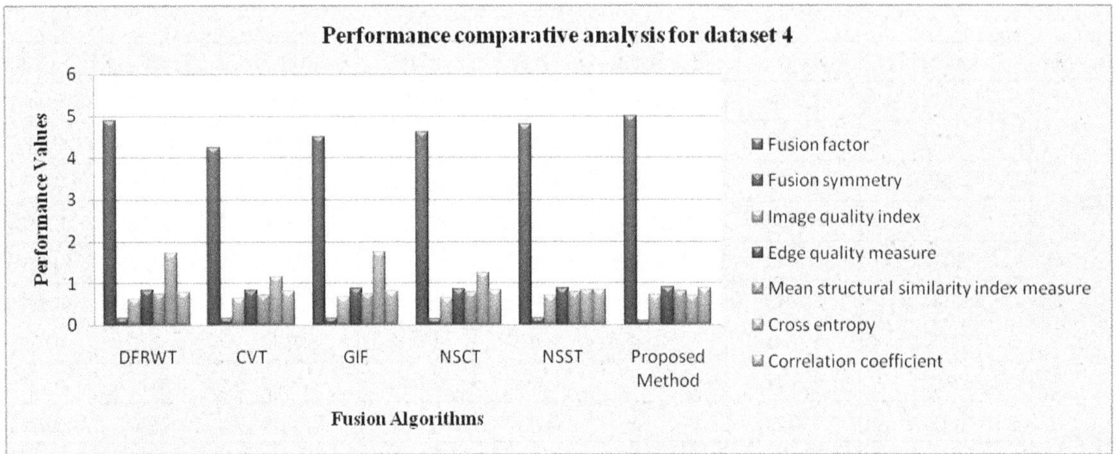

Figure 14. Comparative analysis for experimented medical images performance metrics for set 5

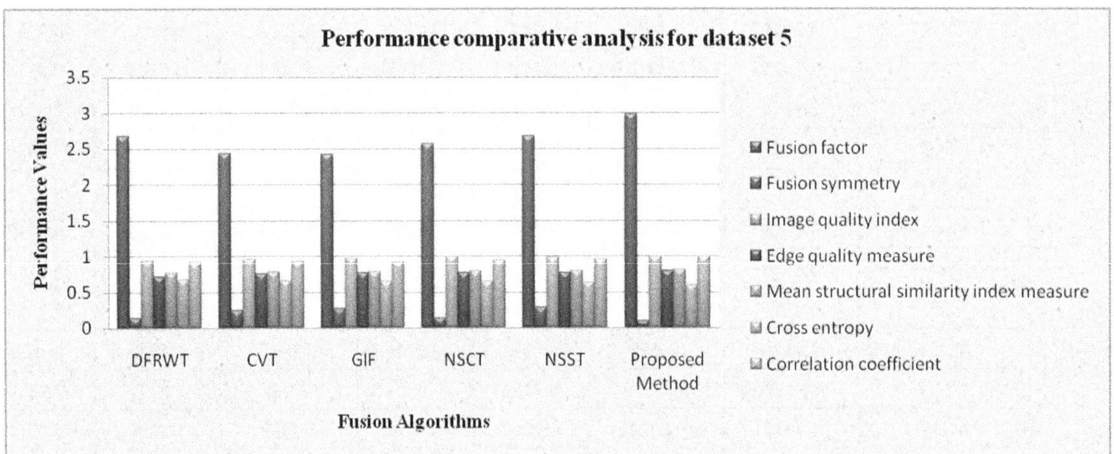

CONCLUSION

In this chapter, various types of image fusion algorithm have been discussed and evaluated to fulfill the requirements medical imaging. The main objective of this proposed method is to obtain the fused image without any loss of similar information and preserve all special features present in the input medical images to improve the fused image quality for better diagnosis of critical diseases. The fused hybrid multimodal medical image should convey better visual description than the individual input images. This method is the process of fusing medical images obtained from two different multimodal medical images for better diagnosis. This research work proposes a method for multimodality medical image fusion using the hybrid fusion algorithms. The implemented proposed technique discovered results provide the better visualization of fused output images gives the higher qualitative and quantitative performance metrics of the hybrid fusion algorithms compared with various existing traditional fusion algorithms.

Figure 15. Experimental results of the set 6 to 10

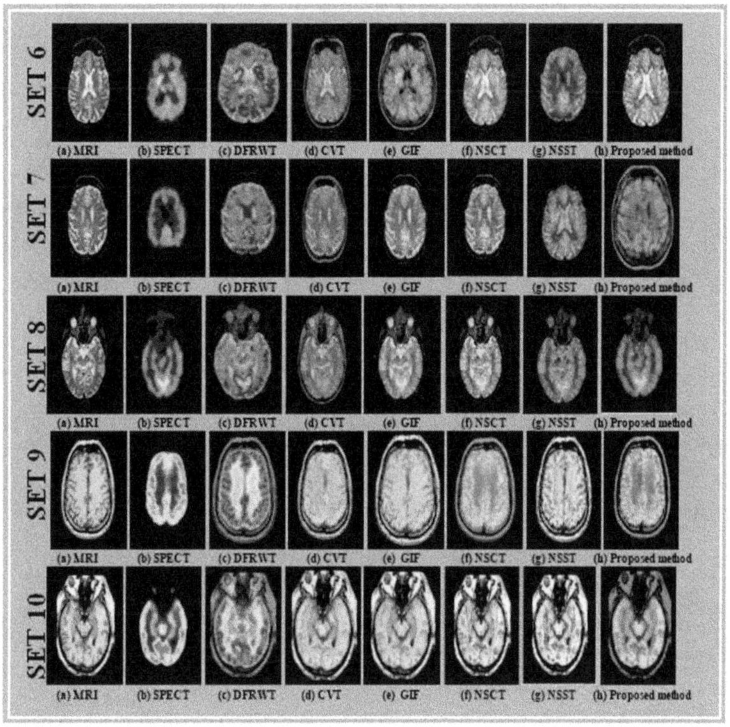

Figure 16. Comparative analysis for experimented medical images performance metrics for set 6

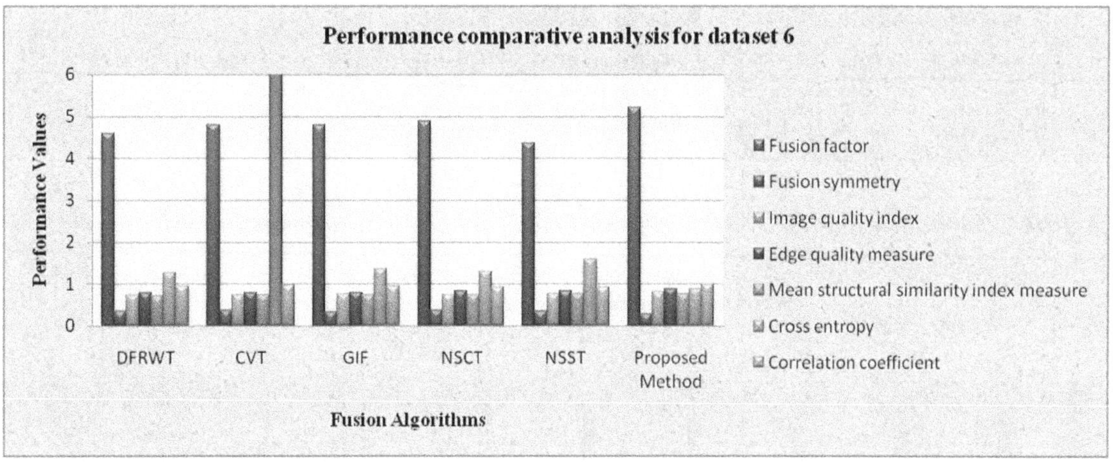

Figure 17. Comparative analysis for experimented medical images performance metrics for set 7

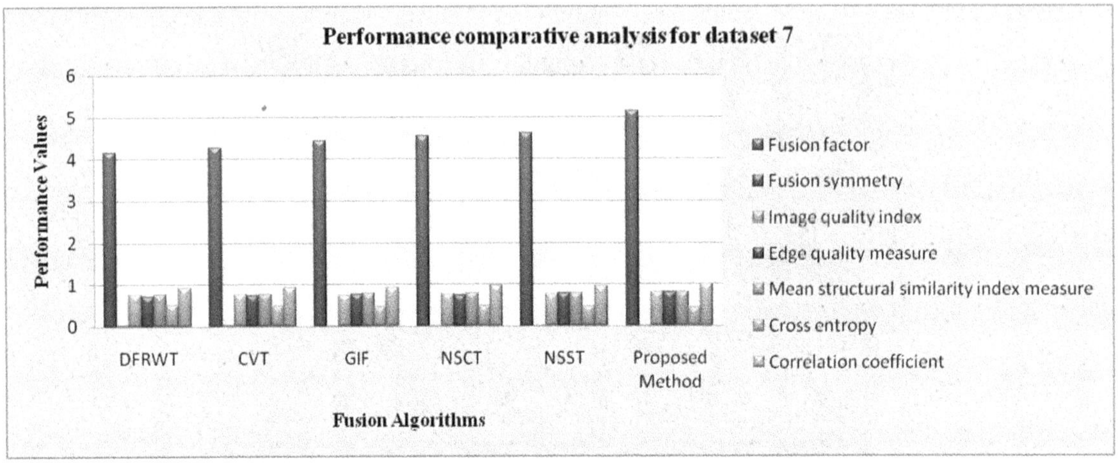

Figure 18. Comparative analysis for experimented medical images performance metrics for set 8

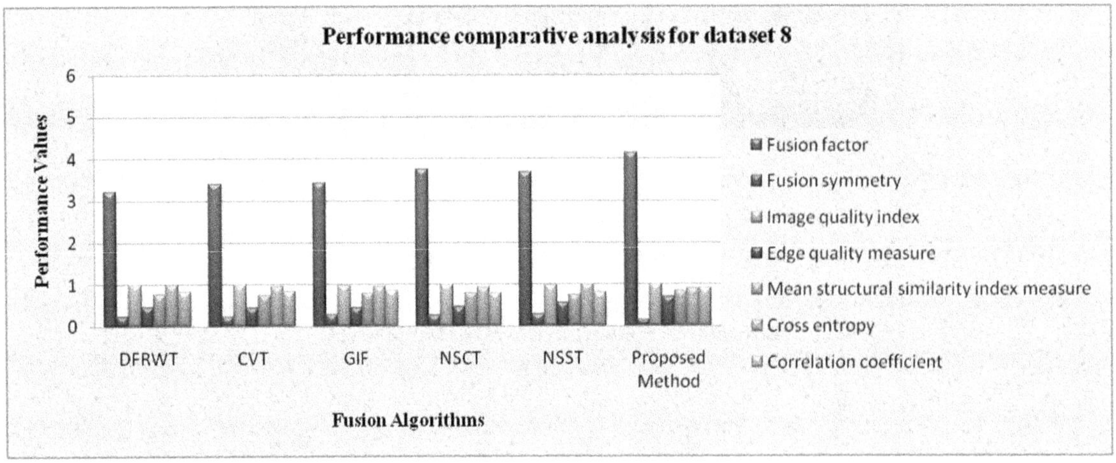

Figure 19. Comparative analysis for experimented medical images performance metrics for set 9

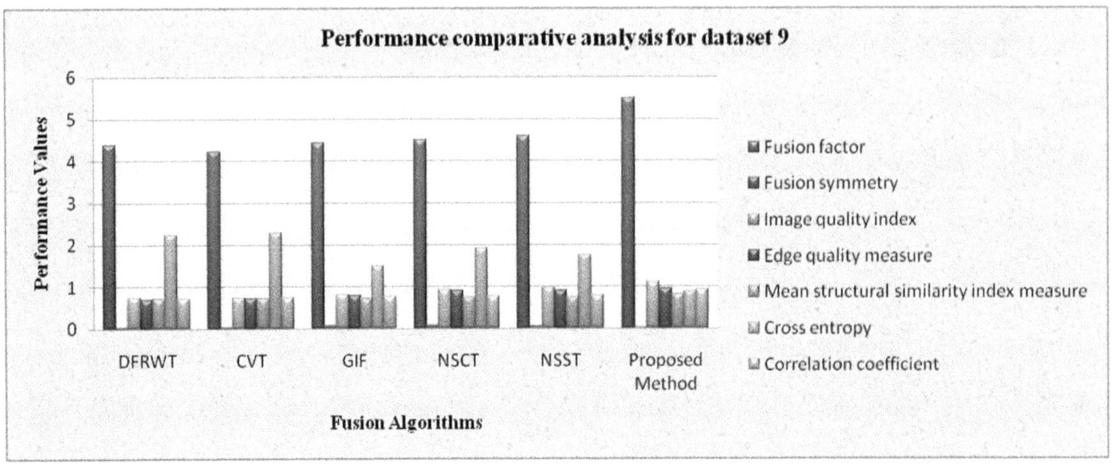

Figure 20. Comparative analysis for experimented medical images performance metrics for set 10

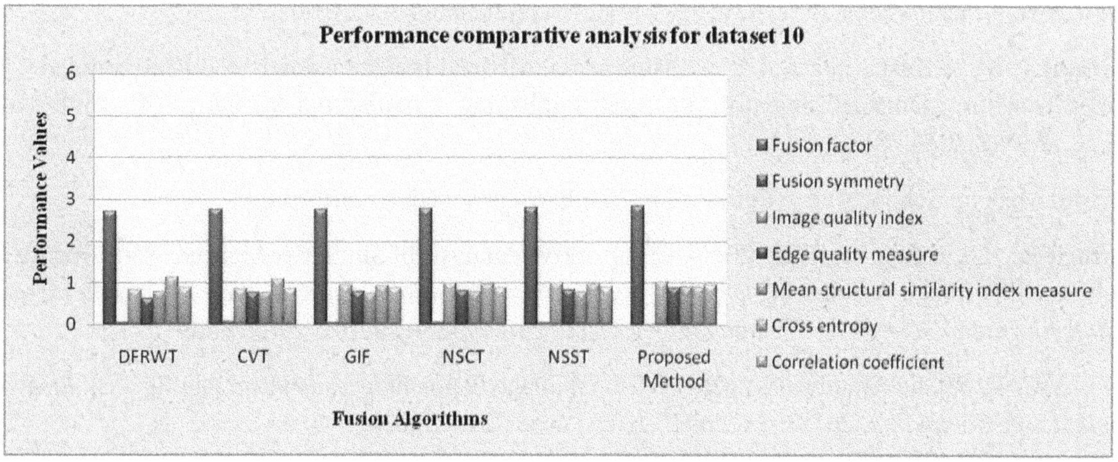

REFERENCES

Agarwal & Bedi. (2016). *Implementation of hybrid image fusion technique for feature enhancement in medical diagnosis.* Springer.

Biswas, R., Sarawadekar, K., Varna, S., & Banerjee, S. (2015). An FPGA-based architecture of DSC-SRI Units specially for motion blind ultrasound systems. *Journal of Real-Time Image Processing, 10*(3), 573–595. doi:10.100711554-012-0289-y

Candes, E., Demanet, L., Donoho, D., & Ying, L. (2006). Fast discrete curvelet transform. *Multiscale Modeling & Simulation, 5*(3), 861–899. doi:10.1137/05064182X

Candes, E. J., & Donoho, D. L. (2005). Continuous curvelet transform: I. Resolution of the wavefront set. *Appl. Comput. Harmon., 19*(2), 162–197. doi:10.1016/j.acha.2005.02.003

Candes, E. J., & Donoho, D. L. (2005). Continuous curvelet transform: II. Discretization and frame. *Applied and Computational Harmonic Analysis, 19*(2), 198–222. doi:10.1016/j.acha.2005.02.004

Chen, D. (2014). Image fusion method based on edge feature detection in electricalcapacitance tomography. *Int. J. Signal Process. Image Process. Pattern Recognit, 7*(1), 67–76.

Chen, G., & Gao, Y. (2013). Multisource images adaptive fusion based on double density dual-tree complex wavelet transform. *J. Conv. Inf. Technol, 8*(1), 548–557.

Du, J., Li, W., Lu, K., & Xiao, B. (2016). An Overview of Multi-Modal Medical Image Fusion, *Elsevier. Neurocomputing, 215*, 3–20. doi:10.1016/j.neucom.2015.07.160

El-Hoseny, El-Sayed, El Rabaie, Elrahman, & El-Samie. (2017). Medical Image Fusion Techniques Based on Combined Discrete Transform Domains. In *34th National Radio Science Conference.* IEEE.

Ganasala, P., & Kumar, V. (2015). Feature-Motivated Simplified Adaptive PCNN-Based Medical Image Fusion Algorithm in NSST Domain. *Journal of Digital Imaging.* PMID:26032980

Gaurav Bhatnagar, Q. M. (2015). A new contrast based multimodal medical image fusion framework, *Elsevier. Neurocomputing*, *157*, 143–152. doi:10.1016/j.neucom.2015.01.025

Gomathi, P. S., & Kalaavathi, B. (2016). Multimodal Medical Image Fusion in Non-Subsampled Contourlet Transform Domain" Scientific Research Publishing. *Circuits and Systems*, *7*(8), 1598–1610. doi:10.4236/cs.2016.78139

Harvard Medical School. (n.d.). Retrieved from http://www.med.harvard.edu

Karthikeyan, C., & Ramadoss, B. (2016). Comparative Analysis of Similarity Measure Performance for Multimodality Image Fusion using DTCWT and SOFM with Various Medical Image Fusion Techniques. *Indian Journal of Science and Technology*, *9*(22). doi:10.17485/ijst/2016/v9i22/95298

Kavitha, C. T., & Chellamuthu, C. (2014). Medical image fusion based on hybrid intelligence, *Elsevier. Applied Soft Computing*, *20*, 83–94. doi:10.1016/j.asoc.2013.10.034

Kavitha, C. T., & Chellamuthu, C. (2015). Fusion of SPECT and MRI images using integer wavelet transform in combination with curvelet transform. *Imaging Science Journal*, *63*(1), 17–23. doi:10.1179/1743131X14Y.0000000092

Lia, Y., Liu, X., Wei, F., Sima, D. M., Van Cauter, S., Himmelreich, U., ... Van Huffel, S. (2017). An advanced MRI and MRSI data fusion scheme for enhancing unsupervised brain tumor differentiation. *Elsevier. Computers in Biology and Medicine*, *8*, 121–129. doi:10.1016/j.compbiomed.2016.12.017

Liu, Shi, Zhu, & Zhao. (2015). *Image fusion based on complex-shearlet domain with guided filtering,* Springer.

Liu, X., Mei, W., & Du, H. (2017). Structure tensor and nonsubsampled sheasrlet transform based algorithm for CT and MRI image fusion, *Elsevier. Neurocomputing*, *235*, 131–139. doi:10.1016/j.neucom.2017.01.006

Moin, A., Bhateja, V., & Srivastava, A. (2016). Weighted-PCA Based Multimodal Medical Image Fusion in Contourlet Domain. *Proceedings of the International Congress on Information and Communication Technology, Advances in Intelligent Systems and Computing*, 439.

Narasimha Murthy, K. N., & Kusuma, J. (2017). Fusion of Medical Image Using STSVD. *Proceedings of the 5th International Conference on Frontiers in Intelligent Computing: Theory and Applications*, *516*, 69-79.

Nasrin Amini, E. (2015). MRI-PET image fusion based on NSCT transform using local energy and local variance fusion rules. *Journal of Medical Engineering & Technology*, *38*(4), 211–219. doi:10.3109/03091902.2014.904014 PMID:24758393

Qu, G., Zhang, D., & Yan, P. (2002). Information measure for performance of image fusion. *Electronics Letters*, *38*(7), 313–315. doi:10.1049/el:20020212

Radiopaedia. (n.d.). Retrieved from https://radiopaedia.org

Rajalingam, B., & Priya, R. (2017a). A Novel approach for Multimodal Medical Image Fusion using Hybrid Fusion Algorithms for Disease Analysis. *International Journal of Pure and Applied Mathematics*, *117*(15), 599–619.

Rajalingam, B., & Priya, R. (2017b). Multimodality Medical Image Fusion Based on Hybrid Fusion Techniques. *International Journal of Engineering and Manufacturing Science*, *7*(1).

Rajalingam, B., & Priya, R. (2018a). Hybrid Multimodality Medical Image Fusion based on Guided Image Filter with Pulse Coupled Neural Network. *International Journal of Scientific Research in Science. Engineering and Technology*, *5*(3), 86–100.

Rajalingam, B., & Priya, R. (2018b). Hybrid Multimodality Medical Image Fusion Technique for Feature Enhancement in Medical Diagnosis. *International Journal of Engineering Science Invention*, *2*, 52–60.

Rajalingam, B., & Priya, R. (2018c). Combining Multi-Modality Medical Image Fusion Based on Hybrid Intelligence for Disease Identification. *International Journal of Advanced Research Trends in Engineering and Technology*, *5*(12), 862–887.

Rajalingam, B., & Priya, R. (2018d). Enhancement of Hybrid Multimodal Medical Image Fusion Techniques for Clinical Disease Analysis. *International Journal of Computer Vision and Image Processing*, *8*(3), 17–40. doi:10.4018/IJCVIP.2018070102

Rajalingam, B., & Priya, R. (2018e). Multimodal Medical Image Fusion based on Deep Learning Neural Network for Clinical Treatment Analysis. *International Journal of Chemtech Research*, *11*(6), 160–176.

Rajalingam, B., & Priya, R. (2018f). Multimodal Medical Image Fusion Using Various Hybrid Fusion Techniques For clinical Treatment Analysis. *Smart Construction Research*, *2*(2), 1–20.

Rajalingam, B., & Priya, R. (2018g). Review of Multimodality Medical Image Fusion Using Combined Transform Techniques for Clinical Application. *International Journal of Scientific Research in Computer Science Applications and Management Studies*, *7*(3).

Srivastava, R., Prakash, O., & Khare, A. (2016). Local energy-based multimodal medical image fusion in curvelet domain. *IET Computer Vision*, 1–16.

Wang, Z., & Bovik, A. C. (2002). A universal image quality index. *IEEE Signal Processing Letters*, *9*(3), 81–84. doi:10.1109/97.995823

Wang, Z., Bovik, A. C., Sheikh, H. R., & Simoncelli, E. P. (2004). Image quality assessment: From error visibility to structural similarity. *IEEE Transactions on Image Processing*, *13*(4), 600–612. doi:10.1109/TIP.2003.819861 PMID:15376593

Xin, Z., & Chen, W. (2014). Medical image fusion based on weighted Contourlet transformation coefficients. *J. Image Graphics*, *19*(1), 133–140.

Xu, X., Wang, Y., & Chen, S. (2016). Medical image fusion using discrete fractional wavelet transform, *Elsevier. Biomedical Signal Processing and Control*, *27*, 103–111. doi:10.1016/j.bspc.2016.02.008

Xu, X. J., Wang, Y. R., & Chen, S. (2014). Novel image fusion method based on down sampling fractional wavelet transform. *Yiqi Yibiao Xuebao*, *35*(9), 2061–2069.

Xydeas, C. S., & Petrovic, V. (2000). Objective image fusion performance measure. *Electronics Letters*, *36*(4), 308–309. doi:10.1049/el:20000267

Chapter 11
Comparative Study of Various Machine Learning Algorithms for Prediction of Insomnia

Ravinder Ahuja
Jaypee Institute of Information Technology Noida, India

Vishal Vivek
Jaypee Institute of Information Technology Noida, India

Manika Chandna
Jaypee Institute of Information Technology Noida, India

Shivani Virmani
Jaypee Institute of Information Technology Noida, India

Alisha Banga
Satyug Darshan Institute of Engineering and Technology Faridabad, India

ABSTRACT

An early diagnosis of insomnia can prevent further medical aids such as anger issues, heart diseases, anxiety, depression, and hypertension. Fifteen machine learning algorithms have been applied and 14 leading factors have been taken into consideration for predicting insomnia. Seven performance parameters (accuracy, kappa, the true positive rate, false positive rate, precision, f-measure, and AUC) are used and for implementation. The authors have used python language. The support vector machine is giving higher performance out of all algorithms giving accuracy 91.6%, f-measure is 92.13, and kappa is 0.83. Further, SVM is applied on another dataset of 100 patients and giving accuracy 92%. In addition, an analysis of the variable importance of CART, C5.0, decision tree, random forest, adaptive boost, and XG boost is calculated. The analysis shows that insomnia primarily depends on the factors, which are the vision problem, mobility problem, and sleep disorder. This chapter mainly finds the usages and effectiveness of machine learning algorithms in Insomnia diseases prediction.

DOI: 10.4018/978-1-5225-7796-6.ch011

INTRODUCTION

Insomnia is a subjective complaint of sleep disorder in which the patient has a difficulty to fall asleep or remain sleeping as long as desired. Insomniac usually have low energy, less concentrating power, less appetite, and mood swings, leading to low performance throughout the day at work (Mulaffer, Shahin, Glos, Penzel & Ahmed, 2017). Insomnia is mainly categorized into the following types on the basis of duration of disturbed sleep timings (Chouvarda et al., 2013): (i) Acute Insomnia: It prevails for a short duration of time (Maximum for a month). The main cause for its existence could be bizarre life events such as a stressful environment at work, jet lags due to traveling or existence of a certain problem at home. This does not require severe medical treatment and can be cured by general meditation (National Sleep Foundation, n.d; Saddichha, 2010) (ii) Chronic Insomnia: A person is said to be facing chronic insomnia if he/she suffers from a disturbed sleep more than 3 days a week and continuously for 3 or more months. The main causes are depression, anxiety, chronic stress, and pain or discomfort at night. Often it requires behavioral therapies; sleep restriction therapies, relaxation exercises and reconditioning for its cure (Zhang, Mo & Zhang, 2017) and, (iii) Comorbid Insomnia: It is also known as secondary insomnia. It is said to prevail when a person faces insomnia due to medical or psychiatric conditions or intake of drugs. Treatment of comorbid insomnia is done by separately treating insomnia and the co-morbid mental illness. Treatment and medication are suggested by the psychiatrist (Hu, 2017; Neikrug, 2010; Skaer, 2018).

According to Global health and an aging report presented by WHO in 2016, it was reported that the population of people with age group 65 or more was 524 million in 2010 which counts nearly 8.5% and is expected to increase up to 1.6 billion till 2050 that is 17% of the total population ("Global health ag-ing", n.d). In America, it is projected that the population with age group 65 or above will nearly double over 3 decades that is 48 million to 88 million by 2050. The global population of elderly people (age 80 or above) is expected to be three times higher during 2015 and 2050 as estimated by the national institute of aging (United Nations, 2010). In India, the increase in decrepit patients rose from about 7% in 2000 to 9% in 2015.

Comparing the data of the previous 35 years, we find that each year the percentage of elderly people is increasing linearly around the globe, in India too we see a similar trend in the increase of the population of elderly patients. According to a survey of 1.1 million Individuals, people who sleep between 6.5 to 7.5 hours a day have been found to have the least mortality rate; whereas those who sleep under 6 hours or above 8 hours are found to have higher mortality rates (Kinsella, 2009; "Global health aging" n.d). Although till date it is not clear why sleeping more than 7.5 hours is associated with higher mortality (Banno & Kryger, 2006). According to research by the National Center for Biotechnology information, 50% of decrepit patients generally complain about deprived sleep, not just due to increased aging; but also due to factors like increased medication, stressful life, etc. These above-mentioned mortality factors can be responsible for insomnia, either is it acute, chronic or comorbid insomnia. Studies show that around 1 out of 3 people face either of the symptoms of insomnia. Owing to the seriousness of the situation, The American Academy of Sleep Medicine has declared Insomnia Awareness Day on March 12, 2018 (American Academy of Sleep Medicine, n.d).

The National Sleep Foundation, in 2005, carried a survey on American population and reported that 76% of the decrepit population thinks that they have a sleep problem. Surveys also reveal that nearly 70% of population experience at least one symptom of insomnia ("Sleep findings data" n.d)(Waking up too early, inconsistent sleep, Difficulty falling asleep, Tension, Headache, Unhealthy stomach and many more). In the 1991 National Sleep Foundation conducted a multicenter epidemiologic polling on a sample size of 1000 patients in which people of age group 18 years or older were taken and further divided into 6 age groups (15-19, 18-24, 25-34, 35-44, 45-54, 55-64, and ≥65). The result of which it was observed that approximately 9% of the patients reported chronic insomnia, and out of which 20% in the group ≥ 65 years reported chronic insomnia, the highest among all age groups (Morin, 2011).

According to the World Health Organization (WHO), being healthy does not merely mean the absence of a disease, but it means complete soundness of the physical and mental state of our body. Change in mental health and thought the process of a person with age is very common. With increasing age, generally, a person gets more mature, responsible and less carefree. The reasons can be many, it can be family issues, job-related issues, income issues or living spouse and it also depends on how much value does the person gives to address these issues (I. J. I. P. 2016). For example: if a person is working, he/she will be busy with work and have a big social circle thus will not focus much on small family-related issues; whereas if the person sits at home all day long with less interaction with people around, he/she will go through a continuous thought process over and over again for a small issue. All these thought processes cause deprived sleep leading to insomnia and hence leading to anxiety and depression and several heart-related issues. Although there is no as such exact treatment for insomnia, the only cure could be behavioral changes to maintain the quality of sleep and few drugs such as Zaleplon and Ramelteon (Li, 2011; Yang, 2011) would also help which can make a person stay asleep for a few hours and could help.

That is why detection of insomnia at a very first stage is necessary. In developing countries like India sleep disorder or insomnia is very highly prevalent due to the above-mentioned reasons. It contributes to approximately 12% of the global population and thus its urge of time to deal with issues like insomnia with the help of prediction tools using Machine Learning (ML) in order to avoid other serious health-related problems like anxiety, depression, hypertension, and heart-related problems. Considering the rapid increase in the world population of an insomniac and thus leading to increased patients with anxiety and depression World Sleep Society (WSS) announced world sleep day in March each year (sleep data, Chouvarda et al., 2012; de León, 2008). The major contribution of this study is, firstly we find out effectiveness and application of machine learning technique (15 classification algorithms) in Insomnia disease prediction. Secondly, by using the variable importance of each classifier, we can easily identify which factors out of 14 are playing an important role in Insomnia diseases. The main objective of this chapter to explore the machine learning algorithms in the prediction of Insomnia disease.

RELATED WORK

Despite the rapid increase in the number of an insomniac in decrepit population, a number of reports/papers discussed the prediction of insomnia with the help of socio-demographic factors and previous medical history. In the paper (Chaparro-Vargas, 2016) insomnia has been detected using the hypnogram generation of sleep onset patterns. Although we know the only sleep pattern is not enough to detect insomnia. Few researchers have also focused on detecting insomnia only by considering sleep to wake transition (Dissanyaka, 2016; Chouvarda, 2007). In some of the previous studies, Hjorth parameters extracted from the electroencephalogram (EEG) has been taken into account (Subhani, 2017), but we cannot justify our result based on one pattern only. Some studies have focused on distinguishing insomniac and healthy patients based on eye movements which are of two types: Non-Rapid Eye Movement (NREM) and Rapid Eye Movement (REM). Depending on these two eye movement states different measures are recorded in physiological signals: Electroencephalogram (EEG), Electrooculogram (EOG), Electrocardiogram (ECG) (Hamida, 2015) and based on these signals insomniac has been distinguished from healthy patients. But only eye movements are not responsible for insomnia. A lot of studies has been done only to predict insomnia with the mapping of EEG signals (Attaran, 2018). One of the researches include predicting insomnia but only SVM classifier had been used, also it lacks in attributes compared to our work (Dissanyaka, 2016). Respiratory signals have been used to classify different stages of sleep. Some studies have detected mental stress at multiple levels using the machine learning framework with the help of EEG signals (Thapliyal et al., 2017; Jáuregui, 2017). After having a glance to several types of research and papers we observed that almost all studies focus on predicting insomnia either by using only one or two features, or few algorithms have only been applied, whereas we have considered all fourteen major factors as well socio-demographic factors and the past medical history of patients. In the paper (Shahin, 2017), they have predicted anxiety and depression relating to deprived sleep. But we must consider the root causes of insomnia in order to build a relevant predictive model and hence we have considered almost all causes in the form of attributes and predicted insomnia by applying 15 classification algorithms. In the paper (Rashid & Abdullah, 2018), authors have proposed a hybrid model of Artificial Bee Colony, artificial neural network, and a genetic algorithm for classifying and diagnosing Diabetic Mellitus. They have considered two datasets i.e primary and secondary dataset. The primary data set consists of 31 features of 501 patients and the second dataset is Pima dataset. Three experiments were performed considering single artificial neural network, an artificial neural network trained with Artificial Bee Colony method, and artificial neural network with mutation-based Artificial Bee Colony. In a paper (Rashid, Abdullah & Abdullah, 2016), authors have explored the relationship between chronic diseases and blood sugar rate. The complete process is divided into two modules. In the first module, the artificial neural network is applied to predict the fasting sugar rate and in second module decision tree is used to describe the impact of fasting sugar rate and symptoms on the patient's health. In a paper (Rashid, Abdullah & Abdullah, 2016), the authors proposed an approach for doctors and physicians to provide good health treatment. They have applied four algorithms i.e artificial neural networks, C 4.5, regression tree and self-organizing map and found that artificial neural network is best out of all these.

MATERIALS AND METHODS

Data Collection

Data is collected from 500 OPD patients for their various medical problems with their consent at R.G. Kar Medical College and Hospital, Kolkata (A. Sau and I. Bhakta, 2017). The authors have applied a ten-fold cross-validation method, which is best suited for small datasets to increase the dataset and cross verify the result.

Also, we have selected attributed in dataset after consulting with the psychiatrists from different recognized hospitals on the basis of their knowledge of insomnia. Our dataset includes (i) Personal attributes(age, sex) (ii) Socio-Demographic Attributes (Literacy, Residence, Marital Status, Recent bereavement) (iii) Economic Conditions (Employment Status, Socio-Economic Status, PI) (iv) Past Medical History (The previous history of Anxiety and Depression) (v) Any kind of Addiction (vi) Current Medical Condition (Pain at multiple sites, Diabetes, HTN, Hearing Aid, Visual Impairment, Mobility impairment). These features represent different probable causative dimensions of insomnia among decrepit patients.

Table 1. Insomnia severity index scale

ISI Score Intervals	Severity of Insomnia
0—7	Not Insomniac
8—14	Partially Insomniac
15—21	Moderately Insomniac (Need clinical treatment)
22—28	Severely Insomniac (Need clinical treatment)

Attribute Selection

The attributes of our dataset have been selected in such way that it matches the seven questionnaires of insomnia severity index (ISI) so that the final result can be verified by matching the gold standards set by insomnia severity index scale. Insomnia severity index is a scale used to figure out the extent of insomnia disease in patients. Taking these attributes in our dataset will help to predict the outcome closer to the gold standards set by insomnia severity index, and finally, the result can be a match using an ISI scale for the reliability of the result. Overall, the authors have considered 14 leading factors in our dataset keeping in mind the symptoms of disease and questionnaires of ISI. Also, the authors have selected attributed in dataset after consulting with the psychiatrists from different recognized hospitals on the basis of their knowledge of insomnia.

Insomnia Severity Index

Insomnia severity index is a widely used scale used to measure the extent of insomnia disease in a patient. ISI contains seven different questionnaires (Begum, Chakraborty & Sarkar, 2015), on the basis of the answer of the question, a score (Zero to four) is assigned and finally, the score is summed up, and

Table 2. Methodology in tabular form

Involved Steps	Explanation
Collection of Data	The data of 500 patients are collected
Attributes	The following features are used: Age, Sex, Living spouse, Family types, Literacy, Occupation, Substance abuse, Personal income, Diabetic Mellitus (DM), Hypertension (HTN), Hearing problem, Vision problem, Mobility problem, and Sleep problem.
Algorithms Applied	Classification Algorithms: K Nearest Neighbors(KNN), Support Vector Machine(SVM), Logistic Regression, Random Forest (RF), Naïve Bayes(Bernoulli), Bayesian Network, C 5.0, CART, AdaBoost, XGBoosting, Decision Tree, Multi-Layer Perceptron, Random Tree, Gradient Boosting, Gaussian Naïve Bayes
Result Validation	Confusion matrix corresponding to each algorithm was created after the ten-fold cross-validation method was applied, and finally, the respective accuracies were calculated.
Result Justification	A test data if 100 new patients Were given as test data to SVM classifier and results matched with ISI scale.
Variable importance is applied to Adaptive Boosting, XG Boosting, Decision Tree, Random Forest, C 5.0, and CART algorithms to find out important factors contributing to Insomnia	

Figure 1. Flowchart depicting methodology in a nutshell

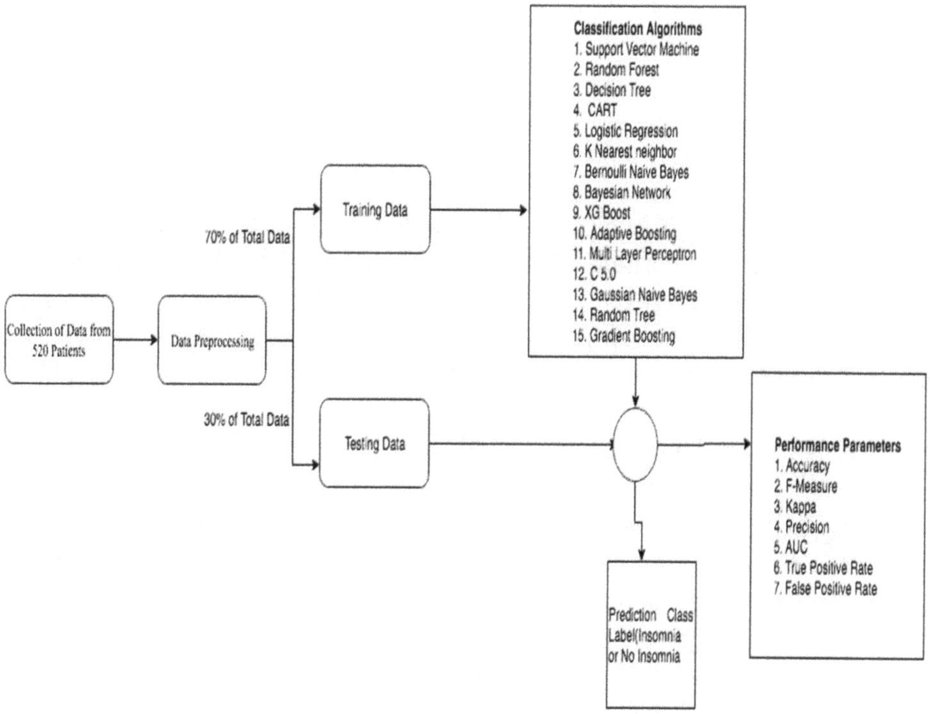

the final score ranges from zero to twenty-eight as shown in Table 1. If the score is zero to seven then it is No insomnia. If the score is eight to fourteen then it is sub-threshold insomnia. If the score is fifteen to twenty-one then it is clinical insomnia (moderate severity). If the score is twenty-two to twenty-eight then it is clinical insomnia (Severe) (Pandey, 2017). A research was organized in India in Jamia Millia Islamia, New Delhi, in which sample data were students of their university, which clearly suggests that ISI has excellent consistency and reliability. Hence, ISI can prove to be an outstanding tool for the prediction of insomnia.

The detailed methodology as shown in Table 2 has several steps (i) Data collection (ii) Attribute selection (iii) Apply classification algorithms and (iv) Result validation (v) Cross verification of the SVM model is done on data set of 100 new patients.

CLASSIFICATION MODELS

Classification is one of the promising domains used to solve trending problems in today's era. In classification usually, we assign a class label among the existing class values which are mapped to unseen instances comprising the set of variables. A learning algorithm is applied on a training set which consists of past instances and an equivalent variable set. In classification models, the authors already know the class level of each instance which is mentioned in the training set. After the model is trained, the prediction accuracy of the corresponding classifier is evaluated on an unknown testing set. In our case, the binary class classification algorithm is most suitable. In a binary class classification problem usually,

Table 3. Confusion matrix of KNN

KNN	Predicted Insomnia (Yes)	Predicted Insomnia (No)
Actual Insomnia (Yes)	248	21
Actual Insomnia (No)	111	160

the focus is on binary result i.e. either a person has insomnia (unhealthy) or no insomnia (healthy). We have applied the following 15 algorithms: **1.** K Nearest Neighbors (KNN) **2.** Support vector machine (SVM) **3.** Bernoulli Naïve Bayes (BNB) **4.** Logistic Regression (LR) 5. Decision tree (DT) **6.** Random Forest (RF) **7.** Multi-layer perceptron (MLP) **8.** Bayesian Network (BN) **9.** Adaptive Boost (AB) **10.** XG Boost (XGB) **11.** C5.0 **12.** CART **13.** Random Tree **14.** Gaussian Naïve Bayes **15.** Gradient Boosting

Algorithm 1: K Nearest Neighbors (KNN)

This algorithm is applied to N training vectors; it identifies the k nearest neighbors of test data by computing the Euclidean distance of test data from the training vectors. Then the authors predict the class value of test data by finding the maximum class represented in the k nearest neighbors. We have taken k=5. We find the 5 nearest neighbors of the test data. Among the 5 neighbors, if 3 of them belong to category 1 and 2 of them belong to category 2, then the test data belongs maximum numbers in both and hence goes to the category 1 (Nugrahaeni, 2016)

The Steps for KNN algorithm would be:-

1. Classify (A, B, c) // A: training data, B: the data label of A, c: testing sample
2. for i=1 to m
3. do

   Calculate Euclidean distance d (Ai, c)

4. end
5. Calculate set I containing all indices for k smallest distances d (Ai, c).
6. Return the majority label for (Bi where ε I)

After applying this algorithm the authors obtained the following confusion matrix.

Algorithm 2: Support Vector Machine (SVM)

It is used in classification as well as regression problems (commonly used in classification). The main agenda is to plot the data in an n dimension plane wherein n is the number of features taken into consideration. Once this is done, the authors find the hyperplane with maximum margin by performing classification and ignoring the outliers (Liu, 2017)

The Steps for SVM would be:-

1. Initialize reduced data set by randomly choosing data from the training data.

Table 4. Confusion matrix of SVM

SVM	Predicted Insomnia (Yes)	Predicted Insomnia (No)
Actual Insomnia (Yes)	246	20
Actual Insomnia (No)	22	249

2. Calculate the reduced kernel matrix
3. For each data point which is not in the reduced dataset, calculate their kernel vectors.
4. Calculate distance from these kernel vectors to the current reduced kernel matrix.
5. The authors form the reduced set by adding those points which have exceeded the threshold.
6. Repeat the above steps until the reduced set remains the same.

Algorithm 3: Bernoulli Naïve Bayes (BNB)

It is a simple probabilistic classifier which is based on Bayes theorem (conditional probability) with strong independent assumptions made amongst the features. Gaussian NB is used when the features have continuous values, whereas Bernoulli NB is used when the features are independent (Bhargava, K., et. Al, 2017)

$$P\left(\frac{A}{B}\right) = \frac{P\left(\frac{B}{A}\right) * P(A)}{P(B)} \text{P(B)} \neq 0 \quad (1)$$

Steps for BNB would be:-

1. A frequency table is made for all the features corresponding to the training data.
2. Calculate the probabilities and conditional probabilities of each element of the frequency table.

where, Conditional probability = No. of distinct feature values * No. of target values

Algorithm 4: Logistic Regression (LR)

It is the appropriate regression analysis to conduct when there are more independent variables. The output is always measured in a dichotomous variable. The logistic function is used similarly to sigmoid function (Ying et al., 2015)

Table 5. Confusion matrix of Bernoulli Naïve Bayes

Bernoulli Naïve Bayes	Predicted Insomnia (Yes)	Predicted Insomnia (No)
Actual Insomnia (Yes)	172	41
Actual Insomnia (No)	37	290

Table 6. Confusion matrix of logistic regression

Logistic Regression	Predicted Insomnia (Yes)	Predicted Insomnia (No)
Actual Insomnia (Yes)	215	49
Actual Insomnia (No)	101	175

Steps for LR would be:-
Recursively:
{Calculate Gradient Average

1. Multiply by Average Learning Rate (α)
2. Subtract from Weights}

After applying this algorithm the authors obtained the following confusion matrix.

Algorithm 5: Decision Tree (DT)

It is used for decision analysis. Decision trees where target values can take continuous values are known as the regression trees. Considering in the tree, input values are represented in a path from the root to the leaves, each leaf represents the target variable (Zhang, Y., et. al., 2018)

The Steps for DT would be:-

1. Form a tree with its nodes as features.
2. Select 1 feature to predict the output from the input, where the root node is that which contains the highest information gain.
3. Repeat the above steps to form subtrees based on features which are not used in the above nodes.

Algorithm 6: Random Forest (RF)

It is a further approach to Decision Tree. In this classifier algorithm, rather than considering a single tree, the authors consider numerous decision trees, thus forming a forest, the denser the forest, i.e. the higher the number of trees, the higher will be the accuracy rate (El Majd, Y. A., El Ghazi, H., & Nahhal, T., 2017)

Steps for RF are as follows:

1. From a total of n features, randomly m features are selected. $m<<n$

Table 7. Confusion matrix of decision tree

Decision Tree	Predicted Insomnia (Yes)	Predicted Insomnia (No)
Actual Insomnia (Yes)	235	22
Actual Insomnia (No)	40	243

Table 8. Confusion matrix of random forest

Random Forest	Predicted Insomnia (Yes)	Predicted Insomnia (No)
Actual Insomnia (Yes)	226	29
Actual Insomnia (No)	36	249

2. A node d, which belongs to the set of m nodes, is calculated using the best split point.
3. Further, d is split into daughter nodes using the best split method.
4. Repeat steps 1-3 until a tree is formed with a root node and having the target as the leaf node.
5. Steps 1-4 represent the creation of a tree. Repeat them the number of times to create a forest.

Algorithm 7: Multi-Layer Perceptron (MLP)

One hidden layer and three network layers used (Zhou, Q., 2017)
The Steps for MLP would be:-

1. Randomly initialize the weights of labels.
2. For each training example compute error
3. 3. Compute error

Error = Predicted value – Actual value

4. Compute change in weight for all the weights from the hidden layer to the output layer.
5. Compute change in weight for all the weights from the input layer to the hidden layer.
6. Update the weights of the network.
7. Return network

Algorithm 8: Bayesian Network (BN)

It is a concept based on parameter learning. In this case, the authors are not very clear about the conditional probabilities but know the network very well. Formally, it is similar to the Directed Acyclic Graph (DAC). Human beings are not very comfortable with reasoning problems thus such a machine is designed. If Y= $\{A_{1,}A_{2,}A_{3\ldots}A_n\}$ as the universe of variables in the Bayesian network and P (A_i) is a parent of A_i then probability function (joint) is given by P (X) as shown below (Fonseca-Delgado & Gomez-Gil, 2013; Dixit & Sahu, 2017)

Table 9. Confusion matrix of multi-layer perceptron

MLP	Predicted Insomnia (Yes)	Predicted Insomnia (No)
Actual Insomnia (Yes)	220	26
Actual Insomnia (No)	64	230

Table 10. Confusion matrix of bayesian network

Bayesian Network	Predicted Insomnia (Yes)	Predicted Insomnia (No)
Actual Insomnia (Yes)	196	64
Actual Insomnia (No)	44	236

Table 11. Confusion matrix of adaptive boosting

AdaBoost	Predicted Insomnia (Yes)	Predicted Insomnia (No)
Actual Insomnia (Yes)	290	63
Actual Insomnia (No)	30	157

Table 12. Confusion matrix of XGBoost

XGBoost	Predicted Insomnia (Yes)	Predicted Insomnia (No)
Actual Insomnia (Yes)	236	26
Actual Insomnia (No)	29	249

Algorithm 9: Adaptive Boosting (AdaBoost)

It is the first Boosting algorithm discovered. It is an ensemble classifier which is similar to Random Forest. It is most preferably used for binary classification. Its output converges to the logarithmic likelihood ratio. The idea is to use weak classifiers in succession repeatedly for more accurate predictions.

Algorithm 10: XGBoost

A self-contained derivation of Gradient Boosting. It is a software library and focuses on computational speed and model performance. Algorithm implementation includes Sparse Aware, Block Structure, and Continued Training. Trees are constructed individually in an organized manner which leads to decreased training time and high performance.

Algorithm 11: C 5.0

It is a tree classifier algorithm, an extended version of a decision tree algorithm. It solves the problem of overfitting and error pruning. Using this algorithm relevant attributes can be identified. It acknowledges noise and missing data which helps improve performance.

Table 13. Confusion matrix of C 5.0

C 5.0	Predicted Insomnia (Yes)	Predicted Insomnia (No)
Actual Insomnia (Yes)	223	22
Actual Insomnia (No)	32	262

Table 14. Confusion matrix of the CART

CART	Predicted Insomnia (Yes)	Predicted Insomnia (No)
Actual Insomnia (Yes)	236	27
Actual Insomnia (No)	32	245

Algorithm 12: CART (Classification and Regression Trees)

A binary decision tree is constructed. Recursive binary splitting (greedy method) is used for the construction of the trees. Prediction for the new input after training is done by traversing the tree from root to leaf node where the predicted output is stored.

Algorithm 13: Random Tree (RT)

It is a classification algorithm where there are random trees i.e. a collection of tree predictors. The classifier classifies each feature with each tree and gives a result according to the maximum number of votes. The plus point in this algorithm is that accuracy estimation is not required to be done externally; it is done through the training process internally (Susanti, S. P., & Azizah, F. N., 2017)

Steps for RT would be:-

1. From a total of n features, randomly m features are selected. m<<n
2. A node d, which belongs to the set of m nodes, is calculated using the best split point.
3. Further, d is split into daughter nodes using the best split method.
4. Repeat steps 1-3 until a tree is formed with a root node and having the target as the leaf node.

Algorithm 14: Gaussian Naïve Bayes (GNB)

It is a special Naïve Bayes classification algorithm, particularly used when features have continuous values and follow a normal distribution (Bhargava, K., & Katarya, R., 2017)

Steps for GNB would be:

1. A frequency table is made for all the features corresponding to each patient.
2. For each patient, the probability is calculated corresponding to each feature.
3. The conditional probability for all the patients is calculated using the given formula:

Table 15. Confusion matrix of Random Tree

Random Tree	Predicted Insomnia (Yes)	Predicted Insomnia (No)
Actual Insomnia (Yes)	224	39
Actual Insomnia (No)	37	240

Table 16. Confusion matrix of Gaussian Naïve Bayes

Gaussian Naïve Bayes	Predicted Insomnia (Yes)	Predicted Insomnia (No)
Actual Insomnia (Yes)	219	27
Actual Insomnia (No)	38	256

Table 17. Confusion matrix of gradient boosting

Gradient Boosting	Predicted Insomnia (Yes)	Predicted Insomnia (No)
Actual Insomnia (Yes)	250	46
Actual Insomnia (No)	44	200

Algorithm 15: Gradient Boosting

The idea is to use weak classifiers in succession repeatedly for more accurate predictions. It involves 3 steps: 1. Loss Function: It uses a logarithmic loss function. 2. Weak Learner: Decision Trees are constructed using the best split points in a greedy manner. 3. Additive Model: Trees are added one by one and the previous trees are not changed.

10-Fold Cross-Validation of Classifiers

Ten-fold Cross-validation: In ten-fold cross-validation method our original data set of 500 patients is partitioned into ten equal-sized sub-segments (50 patients in each segment). Out of all 10 sub-segments, one partition as testing data and remaining nine as training data. This cross-validation technique is repeated 10 times, where each sub partition is taken as testing data at least once. These ten results obtained from the above repetitions are averaged or otherwise combined to produce a single estimation. The advantage of using this validation method is that every single data is used for training as well as testing the model which increases and each entry in the dataset is used for validation of the result at least once (Tong, Kan & Yang, 2018). After ten-fold cross-validation the authors calculated the performance metrics (accuracy, Kappa Coefficients, Sensitivity (TPR), Specificity, the False Positive rate (FPR), Recall, Precision) to measure the performance of each classifier for comparing different classification algorithms.

PERFORMANCE PARAMETERS

1. Accuracy corresponds to a fraction of the result that is predicted correctly by our model. It is a ratio of the number of correct predictions to total prediction.

$$\text{Accuracy} = \frac{\text{number of correct prediction}}{\text{total prediction}} \tag{2}$$

$$\text{Accuracy} = \frac{TP + TN}{TP + TN + FP + FN} \tag{3}$$

2. Cohen's Kappa coefficient gives a quantitative measure of agreement in any situation in which two or more observers are evaluating the same thing (Tong, W., 2018). It is the ratio of the difference of total accuracy and random accuracy divided by 1 - random accuracy.

$$\text{kappa}=\frac{\text{total accuracy-random accuracy}}{\text{1-random accuracy}} \tag{4}$$

$$\text{Random Accuracy}=\frac{\left(TN + FP\right) * \left(TN + FN\right) + \left(FN + TP\right) * \left(FP + TP\right)}{\left(TP + TN + FP + FN\right)^2} \tag{5}$$

3. Sensitivity is defined as a number of predicted true which are actually true. It is also known as the True positive rate (TPR). It estimates how many positives have been actually predicted as positive. It is also known as Recall.

$$\text{Sensitivity} = \frac{\text{predicted YES}\left(\text{TP}\right)}{\text{actual YES}\left(\text{P}\right)} \tag{6}$$

4. False positive rate means the expectancy of false positive ratio. It estimates how many negatives have been actually predicted as negative.

$$\text{FP rate} = \frac{\text{predicted NO}\left(\text{FP}\right)}{\text{actual NO}\left(\text{TN} + \text{FP}\right)} \tag{7}$$

5. Precision is a fraction of actually positive which have been predicted positive.

$$\text{Precision} = \frac{TP}{TP + FP} \tag{8}$$

6. Specificity is the ratio of predicted true negatives to actual negatives (TN+FP). It is a measure of how many negatives have been predicted correctly from actual negatives.

$$\text{Specificity} = \frac{TN}{TN + FP} \tag{9}$$

7. F-measure is the harmonic mean of precision and Recall (sensitivity). It is provided as a measurement tool for the test's accuracy.

$$\mathrm{F-measure} = \frac{2^{*}\mathrm{precision}^{*}\mathrm{recall}}{\mathrm{precision} + \mathrm{recall}} \tag{10}$$

8. AUC (Area Under Cover): It relates the hit rate to the false alarm rate. It gives the probability that a randomly chosen positive instance gets the higher rank than a randomly chosen negative instance.

TP-True Positive TN-True Negative FP-False Positive FN-False Negative

RESULTS

As per research conducted by us for 500 decrepit patients among which 277(55.4%) were males and 223(44.3%) were females. The mean age of our data set is 66.5%. Among 540 decrepit patients, 45.6% of patients were suffering from at least one or the other symptom of insomnia. Personal information (PI) as a feature was not considered, the reason being people in India believe in certain cultural and social norms and thus are not comfortable to share such information. All these 14 attributes were applied on 15 classifiers. For each algorithm, a confusion matrix was created after applying ten-fold cross-validation. With the help of confusion matrix further true Positive (TP), False Positive (FP), the true positive rate (TPR), false positive rate (FPR), accuracy, precision, sensitivity, specificity (Recall), Cohen's kappa coefficient, F measure (F1 Score), and Area under the Curve (AUC) were calculated for each algorithm for comparison purpose as shown in table 19. The authors found that the support vector machine (SVM) is the best possible classifier with the highest Accuracy of 91.6% because the dataset is small and SVM works better in smaller dataset. Also, for SVM the TP rate is 91.3%, the FP rate is 8.06%, Precision is 93.05%, F-Measure is 91.72% and AUC is 92.85%. At last, the authors took a new data set of 100 decrepit patients and passed as testing data to the SVM classifier. A new confusion matrix was created and hence its performance matrix was also created, the final result was compared with the ISI scale for which accuracy came out to be 92%.

Variable importance represents the statistical significance of each feature in the data with respect to its effect on the calculated output. It is calculated by a sum of the decrease in error when split by a feature, the relative importance is the variable importance divided by the highest variable importance (0…1).

Table 18. Test data matched with ISI standard

SVM	Insomnia Severity Index(ISI)		Total
	Predicted Insomnia (Yes)	**Predicted Insomnia (No)**	
Actual Insomnia (Yes)	44	6	50
Actual Insomnia (No)	3	47	50
Total	47	53	100

Table 19. Performance of different measures

	Classification Algorithms	Percentage of Different Matrix						
		Accuracy	TPR	FPR	F-Measure	Precision	AUC	Kappa
1	Logistic Regression	72.22	81.43	36.59	74.13	68.03	85.71	0.45
2	KNN	75.55	92.19	40.95	78.97	69.08	75.71	0.52
3	SVM	91.6	92.48	8.11	92.13	91.79	92.85	0.83
4	Random Forest	87.9	88.6	12.63	87.4	86.25	75.71	0.75
5	Bernoulli Naïve Bayes	85.55	80.75	11.31	71.61	82.29	85.71	0.71
6	Decision Tree	88.5	91.4	14.13	88.32	85.45	65.71	0.59
7	MLP	83.33	89.43	21.76	79.3	77.46	83.34	0.77
8	Bayesian Network	80	75.38	15.71	75.3	81.67	72.43	0.71
9	Adaptive Boost	82.76	82.15	16.04	86.17	90.62	91.32	0.76
10	XG Boost	89.89	90.07	10.43	89.55	89.05	87.63	0.72
11	C 5.0	90.06	91.02	10.88	89.19	87.45	85.43	0.56
12	Gaussian Naïve Bayes	87.9	89.02	12.92	87.07	85.21	75.71	0.76
13	Gradient Boosting	83.33	84.46	18.03	83.33	83.33	82.86	0.68
14	Random Tree	85.9	85.17	13.35	85.49	85.82	88.09	0.71
15	CART	89	89.73	11.55	88.88	88.05	87.91	0.69

Figure 2. Performance measures of different classification algorithms

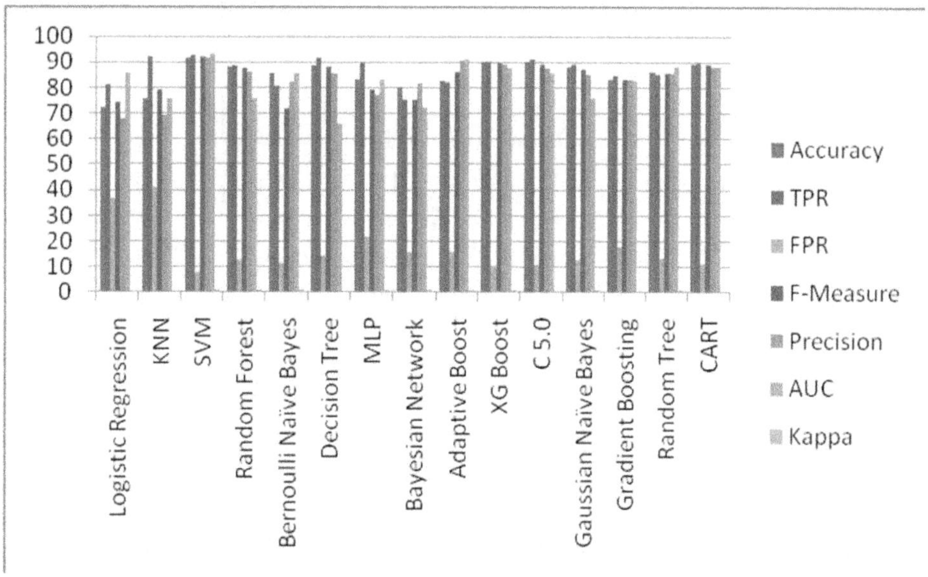

The Variable importance of Ad boost algorithm is given in Figure 3; the most important three factors are factor 8, 13, and 5. In XG boosting, the authors find out that the most important three factors are factor 12, factor 8, and factor 2 as shown in Figure 4. According to the decision tree algorithm, the three most important factors are 14, 12, and 9 as shown in Figure 5. As shown in Figure 6, according to

Figure 3. The importance of factors with adaptive boosting

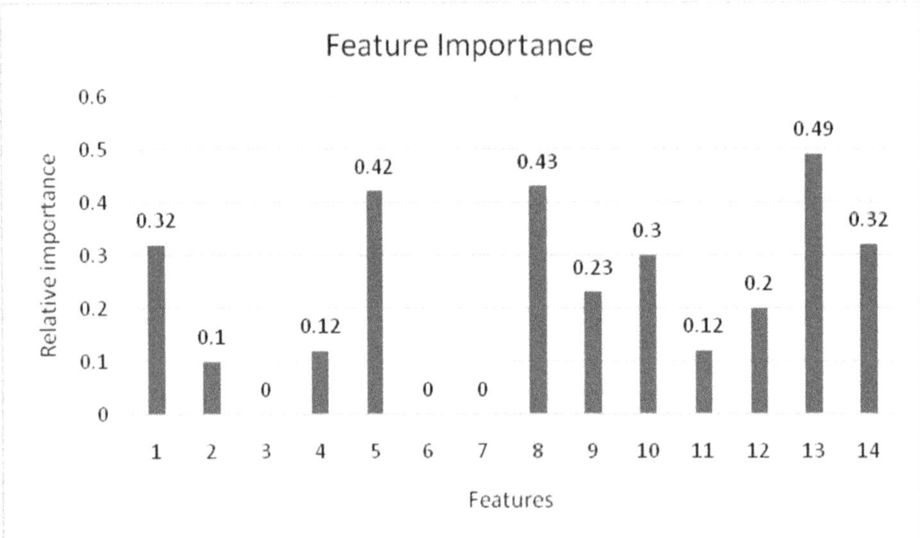

Figure 4. Importance of the factors with XG boosting

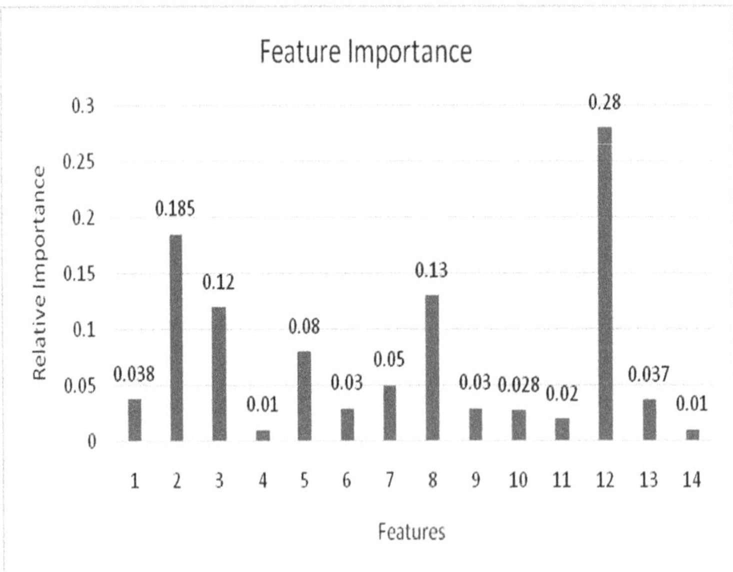

the Random forest, the most important three factors are 14, 13, and 12. As shown in Figure 7, according to C 5.0 algorithm, the most important factors are 11, 14, and 12. According to CART, the three most important factors are 13, 12, and 14. Hence when the authors analyze the variable importance of all these algorithms, the authors find out that factor 14 i.e sleep disorder, factor 13 i.e mobility problems, and factor 12 i.e vision problems are the major factors contributing to Insomnia diseases that are common in all graphs of variable importance.

Figure 5. Importance of the factors with decision tree

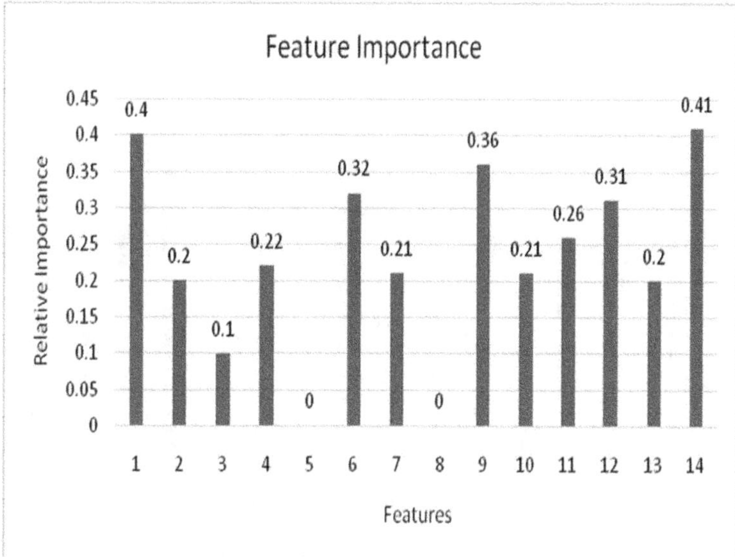

Figure 6. Importance of the factors in random forest

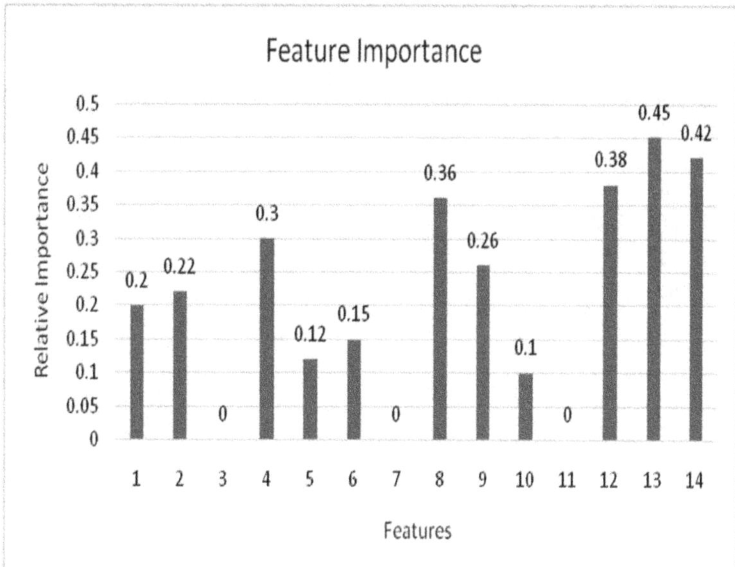

DISCUSSION

Machine Learning is considered to be one of the most promising tools for predicting a disease based on a given dataset. In this chapter, the authors have identified a new problem of predicting insomnia using existing machine learning algorithms. For the first time insomnia prediction is done using 14 leading factors and fifteen classification algorithms. After applying 15 classification algorithms we found the

Figure 7. Importance of the factors in C 5.0

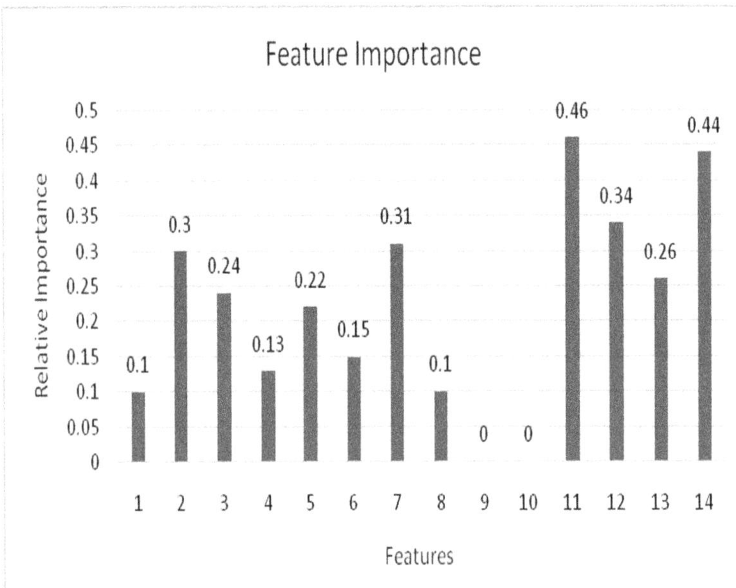

Figure 8. Importance of the factors in the CART

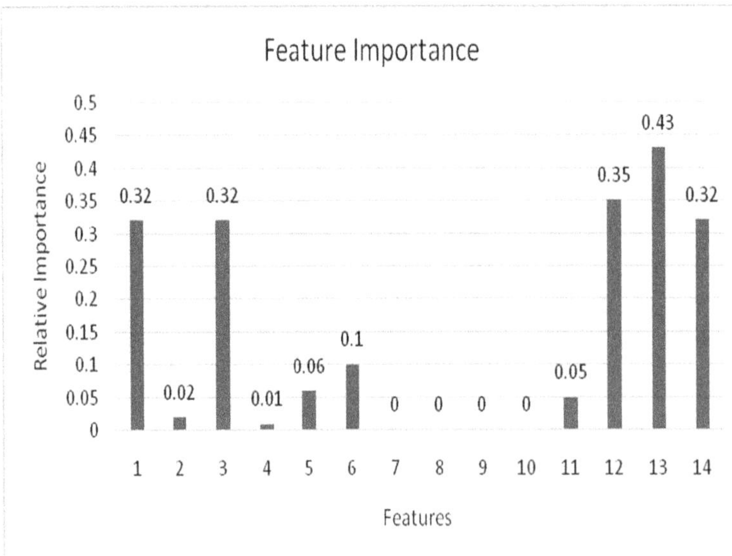

highest accuracy of 91.6% using SVM. The result was a cross verified in two layers; (i) Using the ten-fold cross-validation method, (ii) SVM model was tested on a new dataset of 100 decrepit patients. Evaluated results of these 100 patients matched with the Gold Standards set by Insomnia Severity Index (ISI) with the accuracy of 92%. However, previous and ongoing researches have been in the realm of psychological signals associated with EEG and EOG signals. The comparison of our research with previous studies is as follows: Insomnia has been characterized using hypnogram to Graph spectral theory (Chaparro-Vargas, R, 2016) which differentiates between healthy and insomniac using only one classifier, i.e. logistic regression model. The above study comprises of overnight polysomnogram of 16 healthy and 16 insomniac samples. Wherein our research consists of 15 classifiers, also rather than focusing on a single overnight hypnogram collection, the authors have considered data set in which past medical history and 14 leading factors of insomnia have been considered for better results. Another study classifies insomnia based on the wake to sleep transition, according to this study they generated psychological signals based on rapid eye movements (REM) and non-rapid eye movements (NREM) (Dissanyaka et al., 2016). But the authors can't build a relevant predictive model based on only sleep to wake transition; therefore, the authors have considered hypertension, Diabetic Mellitus (DM) along with sleep which helps to build a better predictive model than existing. One more study involves Hjorth parameter extracted from EEG signals for identification of insomnia (Hamida, Ahmed & Penzel, 2015). We conclude from above researches that results of previous studies are dependent on a single overnight data of psychological signals (EEG and EOG), but insomnia is not an overnight issue, but it is a prolonged disease. So in order to detect insomnia properly, at least the authors should consider data of past six months along with the previous history. Also, insomnia is accompanied by behavioral changes in a person. So, there is a need to include the behavior of a person in our dataset. Insomnia also depends on the socio-demographic factors like living spouse, family type (nuclear or joint family), etc. Therefore sociodemographic factors have been included in the dataset. No researches have applied the standards of medical science (Scales for measuring insomnia) in their research. The authors have understood the importance of gold standards and therefore included the seven questionnaires of ISI scale in the prediction of insomnia. So after including all the above factors and fifteen classification algorithms the authors ended up with 91.6% accuracy using the SVM classifier. The result was also cross-validated using a ten-fold cross-validation method, and a new test data of 100 decrepit patients. None of the studies has matched their result with any standard scale, but we have matched our result with gold standards set by ISI scale.

CONCLUSION

Our Research provides the usages of machine learning algorithms in the prediction of Insomnia disease. The prediction of disease is applied to the dataset of 500 patients. Our dataset includes 14 essential features. Among all the classification algorithms SVM was found to have the maximum accuracy of 91.6%, precision of 93.05%, with the sensitivity of 91.3%, specificity of 91.2%, Kappa with 0.83. These results were also cross verified using the ten-fold cross-validation method. Finally, SVM was tested on a new data set of 100 decrepit patients and its accuracy was 92% with a 9.5% FP rate. Thus, the authors can say that SVM algorithm can be best suited to predict insomnia diseases. The variable importance of six algorithms is calculated and the authors find out that the most contributing factors to Insomnia are the sleep disorder, vision problems, and mobility problems.

The Contribution of this study to literature can be summarized as follows: firstly, the effectiveness of machine learning algorithms has been shown in real-world data to predict Insomnia. Secondly, variable importance analyses show that three major factors contributing to Insomnia are a sleep disorder, mobility problems, and vision problems. By focusing on these three parameters Insomnia diseases can be avoided.

REFERENCES

American Academy of Sleep Medicine. (n.d.). Dates of insomnia day. *American Academy of Sleep Medicine.* Retrieved on July 13, 2018 available at https://aasm.org/

Attaran, N., Puranik, A., Brooks, J., & Mohsenin, T. (2018). Embedded Low-Power Processor for Personalized Stress Detection. *IEEE Transactions on Circuits and Wystems. II, Express Briefs*, 1. doi:10.1109/TCSII.2018.2799821

Banno, K., & Kryger, M. H. (2006). Comorbid insomnia. *Sleep Medicine Clinics*, *1*(3), 367–374. doi:10.1016/j.jsmc.2006.06.003

Begum, S., Chakraborty, D., & Sarkar, R. (2015, December). Data classification using feature selection and kNN machine learning approach. In *Computational Intelligence and Communication Networks (CICN), 2015 International Conference on* (pp. 811-814). IEEE.

Bhargava, K., & Katarya, R. (2017, October). An improved lexicon using logistic regression for sentiment analysis. In *Computing and Communication Technologies for Smart Nation (IC3TSN), 2017 International Conference on* (pp. 332-337). IEEE.

Chaparro-Vargas, R., Ahmed, B., Wessel, N., Penzel, T., & Cvetkovic, D. (2016). Insomnia Characterization: From Hypnogram to Graph Spectral Theory. *IEEE Transactions on Biomedical Engineering*, *63*(10), 2211–2219. doi:10.1109/TBME.2016.2515261 PMID:26742123

Chaparro-Vargas, R., Ahmed, B., Wessel, N., Penzel, T., & Cvetkovic, D. (2016). Insomnia Characterization: From Hypnogram to Graph Spectral Theory. *IEEE Transactions on Biomedical Engineering*, *63*(10), 2211–2219. doi:10.1109/TBME.2016.2515261 PMID:26742123

Chouvarda, I., Grassi, A., Mendez, M. O., Bianchi, A. M., Parrino, L., Milioli, G., . . . Cerutti, S. (2013, July). Insomnia types and sleep microstructure dynamics. In *Engineering in Medicine and Biology Society (EMBC), 2013 35th Annual International Conference of the IEEE* (pp. 6167-6170). IEEE. 10.1109/EMBC.2013.6610961

Chouvarda, I., Mendez, M. O., Rosso, V., Bianchi, A. M., Parrino, L., Grassi, A., & Maglaveras, N. (2012). Cyclic alternating patterns in normal sleep and insomnia: Structure and content differences. *IEEE Transactions on Neural Systems and Rehabilitation Engineering*, *20*(5), 642–652. doi:10.1109/TNSRE.2012.2208984 PMID:22855235

Chouvarda, I., Papadelis, C., Domis, N., Staner, L., & Maglaveras, N. (2007, August). Insomnia treatment assessment based on physiological data analysis. In *Engineering in Medicine and Biology Society, 2007. EMBS 2007. 29th Annual International Conference of the IEEE* (pp. 6694-6696). IEEE.

de León, F. S., Nicklin, P., Rhodesf, C., & Kwankam, S. Y. (2008). *Promoting appropriate eHealth technologies in the developing world: The Sharing eHealth Intellectual Property for Development (SHIPD) initiative*. World Health Organization.

Dissanyaka, C., Cvetkovic, D., Abdullah, H., Ahmed, B., & Penzel, T. (2016, December). Classification of healthy and insomnia subjects based on wake-to-sleep transition. In *Biomedical Engineering and Sciences (IECBES), 2016 IEEE EMBS Conference on* (pp. 480-483). IEEE.

Dixit, D., & Sahu, P. R. (2017, September). Outage Probability of Cooperative Relay Networks in eta-µ, kappa-µ, and Mixed Fading Channels. In *Vehicular Technology Conference (VTC-Fall), 2017 IEEE 86th* (pp. 1-5). IEEE. 10.1109/VTCFall.2017.8288003

El Majd, Y. A., El Ghazi, H., & Nahhal, T. (2017, November). PaRRT: Parallel rapidly-exploring random tree (RRT) based on MapReduce. In *Electrical and Information Technologies (ICEIT), 2017 International Conference on* (pp. 1-5). IEEE.

Fonseca-Delgado, R., & Gomez-Gil, P. (2013, September). An assessment of ten-fold and Monte Carlo cross validations for time series forecasting. In *Electrical Engineering, Computing Science and Automatic Control (CCE), 2013 10th International Conference on* (pp. 215-220). IEEE.

Global health aging report of the elderly population. (n.d.). Available at http://www.who.int/ageing/publications/global_health.pdf

Global health aging report of the total population. (n.d.). Available at http://www.who.int/ageing/publications/global_health.pdf

Hamida, S. T. B., Ahmed, B., & Penzel, T. (2015, December). A novel insomnia identification method based on Hjorth parameters. In *Signal Processing and Information Technology (ISSPIT), 2015 IEEE International Symposium on* (pp. 548-552). IEEE.

Hu, F., Qiao, Y., Xie, G., Zhu, Y., Jia, Y., & Huang, P. (2017, October). Symptom Distribution Regulation of Core Symptoms in Insomnia Based on Informap-SA Algorithm. In *Distributed Computing and Applications to Business, Engineering and Science (DCABES), 2017 16th International Symposium on* (pp. 229-232). IEEE.

Jáuregui, D. A. G., Castanier, C., Chang, B., Val, M., Cottin, F., Le Scanff, C., & Martin, J. C. (2017, October). Toward automatic detection of acute stress: Relevant nonverbal behaviors and impact of personality traits. In *Affective Computing and Intelligent Interaction (ACII), 2017 Seventh International Conference on* (pp. 354-361). IEEE.

Kinsella, K., & He, W. (2009). *An aging world: 2008: International population reports.* US Government Printing Office.

Li, Y., Xu, B., Chen, S., Liu, P., Ou, A., Xu, Y., . . . Zeng, L. (2011, November). A randomized, controlled study of efficacy and safety on mild to moderate insomnia intervened by Chinese medicine in the integrated program. In *Bioinformatics and Biomedicine Workshops (BIBMW), 2011 IEEE International Conference on* (pp. 732-739). IEEE.

Liu, P., Yu, H., Xu, T., & Lan, C. (2017, December). Research on archives text classification based on Naive Bayes. In *Technology, Networking, Electronic and Automation Control Conference (ITNEC), 2017 IEEE 2nd Information* (pp. 187-190). IEEE.

Morin, C. M., Belleville, G., Bélanger, L., & Ivers, H. (2011). The Insomnia Severity Index: Psychometric indicators to detect insomnia cases and evaluate treatment response. *Sleep*, *34*(5), 601–608. doi:10.1093leep/34.5.601 PMID:21532953

Mulaffer, L., Shahin, M., Glos, M., Penzel, T., & Ahmed, B. (2017, July). Comparing two insomnia detection models of clinical diagnostic techniques. In *Engineering in Medicine and Biology Society (EMBC), 2017 39th Annual International Conference of the IEEE* (pp. 3749-3752). IEEE.

National Sleep Foundation. (n.d.). *Types of Insomnia*. National Sleep Foundation. Available at https://sleepfoundation.org/insomnia/content/what-are-different-types-insomnia

Neikrug, A. B., & Ancoli-Israel, S. (2010). Sleep disorders in the older adult–a mini-review. *Gerontology*, *56*(2), 181–189. doi:10.1159/000236900 PMID:19738366

Nugrahaeni, R. A., & Mutijarsa, K. (2016, August). Comparative analysis of machine learning KNN, SVM, and random forests algorithm for facial expression classification. In *Technology of Information and Communication (semantic), International Seminar on Application for* (pp. 163-168). IEEE.

Pandey, P. S. (2017, July). Machine learning and iot for prediction and detection of stress. In *Computational Science and Its Applications (ICCSA), 2017 17th International Conference on* (pp. 1-5). IEEE.

Rashid, T. A., Abdulla, S. M., & Abdulla, R. M. (2016). Decision support system for diabetes mellitus through machine learning techniques. *Database, 7*.

Rashid, T. A., & Abdullah, S. M. (2018). A Hybrid of Artificial Bee Colony, Genetic Algorithm, and Neural Network for Diabetic Mellitus Diagnosing. *ARO-The Scientific Journal of Koya University*, *6*(1), 55–64. doi:10.14500/aro.10368

Rashid, T. A., Abdullah, S. M., & Abdullah, R. M. (2016). An intelligent approach for diabetes classification, prediction, and description. In *Innovations in Bio-Inspired Computing and Applications* (pp. 323–335). Cham: Springer. doi:10.1007/978-3-319-28031-8_28

Saddichaa, S. (2010). Information about acute insomnia. *Annals of Indian Academy of Neurology*, *13*(2). Available at https://www.ncbi.nlm.nih.gov/pmc/articles/PMC2924526/

Sau, A., & Bhakta, I. (2017) Predicting anxiety and depression in elderly patients using machine learning technology. Healthcare Technology Letters, 4(6), 238-243.

Shahin, M., Ahmed, B., Hamida, S. T. B., Mulaffer, F. L., Glos, M., & Penzel, T. (2017). Deep Learning and Insomnia: Assisting Clinicians With Their Diagnosis. *IEEE Journal of Biomedical and Health Informatics*, *21*(6), 1546–1553. doi:10.1109/JBHI.2017.2650199 PMID:28092583

Skaer, T. L. (n.d.). *Treatment of Insomnia with Comorbid Mental Illness*. Retrieved from http://cdn.intechopen.com/pdfs/32274.pdf

Subhani, A. R., Mumtaz, W., Saad, M. N. B. M., Kamel, N., & Malik, A. S. (2017). Machine learning framework for the detection of mental stress at multiple levels. *IEEE Access: Practical Innovations, Open Solutions*, *5*, 13545–13556. doi:10.1109/ACCESS.2017.2723622

Susanti, S. P., & Azizah, F. N. (2017, November). Imputation of missing value using the dynamic Bayesian network for multivariate time series data. In *Data and Software Engineering (ICoDSE), 2017 International Conference on* (pp. 1-5). IEEE.

Thapliyal, H., Khalus, V., & Labrado, C. (2017). Stress detection and management: A survey of wearable smart health devices. *IEEE Consumer Electronics Magazine*, *6*(4), 64–69. doi:10.1109/MCE.2017.2715578

Tong, W., Kan, C., & Yang, H. (2018, March). Sensitivity analysis of wearable textiles for ECG sensing. In *Biomedical & Health Informatics (BHI), 2018 IEEE EMBS International Conference on* (pp. 157-160). IEEE.

United Nations. (2010). World population data available at United Nations. *World Population Prospects: The 2010.* Retrieved on July 13, 2018 available at http://esa.un.org/unpd/wpp

Yang, X. B., Yan, S. X., Zhou, Z. Y., Li, G. Z., Li, Y., & Guo, X. F. (2011, November). Balance-bagging-PRFS algorithm for feature optimization on insomnia data intervened by traditional Chinese Medicine. In *Bioinformatics and Biomedicine Workshops (BIBMW), 2011 IEEE International Conference on* (pp. 854-857). IEEE.

Ying, K., Ameri, A., Trivedi, A., Ravindra, D., Patel, D., & Mozumdar, M. (2015, November). Decision tree-based machine learning algorithm for in-node vehicle classification. In *Green Energy and Systems Conference (IGESC)* (pp. 71-76). IEEE. 10.1109/IGESC.2015.7359454

Zhang, J. A., Mo, G., & Zhang, K. (2017, October). The design and clinical application of sleep disorder treatment system. In *Image and Signal Processing, Biomedical Engineering and Informatics (CISP-BMEI), 2017 10th International Congress on* (pp. 1-5). IEEE.

Zhang, Y., Cao, G., Li, X., & Wang, B. (2018). Cascaded Random Forest for Hyperspectral Image Classification. *IEEE Journal of Selected Topics in Applied Earth Observations and Remote Sensing*, *11*(4), 1082–1094. doi:10.1109/JSTARS.2018.2809781

Zhou, Q., Zhao, M., & Bian, G. (2017, December). An HFC-based Bayesian Network Structure Learning Algorithm. In *2017 International Conference on Industrial Informatics-Computing Technology, Intelligent Technology, Industrial Information Integration (ICIICII)* (pp. 104-107). IEEE.

Section 3
Others

Chapter 12
Smart Technologies to Build Healthcare Models for Vision Impairment

Shikha Singhal
Jaypee Institute of Information Technology, India

Shubham Jain
Jaypee Institute of Information Technology, India

Megha Rathi
Jaypee Institute of Information Technology, India

Adwitiya Sinha
Jaypee Institute of Information Technology, India

ABSTRACT

Technology has broadened the perspective healthcare delivery. Computer vision is such an enhanced spectrum of scientific revolution that imparts automated intelligence to assist patients with full or partial vision difficulties. This discipline engages machine acumen with learning and mining techniques to substitute impairment with clarity in vision. This helps people suffering from visionary ailments to see the world and experience its elegance through machine intelligence. The chapter surveys the recent and smartly configured technologies for building models and related applications, which could be useful for managing health problems in case of visually challenged ones. Several intelligent systems are analyzed and highlighted that can be utilized for providing sub-optimal cure to the concerned patients who mostly confront problems in plight of accessing relevant information, thereby receiving severely limited healthcare facilities. The chapter also illustrates several methods and mechanisms that can be applied to tailor treatment strategies as per the criticality and need towards customized clinical care for vision impairment.

DOI: 10.4018/978-1-5225-7796-6.ch012

INTRODUCTION

Any adaptive service or device, which increases achievement, participation or independence for a person suffering from a disability, is known as an Assistive Technology. AT can help anyone who has impaired vision (with and without additional disabilities) to improve their connection with the world and boost their confidence. It is necessary to give it a thought regarding which tools, technologies and devices will prove suitable to meet a person's unique and individual needs.

Healthcare Sector

Healthcare sector provide services like medical aid, creation and installation of medical equipments, medicines, life insurance, health policies, and aid to day to day operations of hospital management. India's one of biggest sector is healthcare in terms of income generation and job opportunities. Services provided by healthcare organization includes: hospital management, healthcare equipments, clinical tests, outsourcing, telemedicine, health tourism, e-health, and health insurance. Quality of Indian health services are upgrading day by day due to the usage of advanced medical informatics, tools, e-services. Healthcare wraps the advanced mechanism for disease diagnosis, treatment options, disease prevention, visual and other kind of impairments (Briggs & Gray, 1999). Also, healthcare sector generates massive amount of medical data including electronic health records, medical tests findings, and management reports (McLaughlin & Fitzgerald, 2001). Medical data is further utilized for detailed analysis for effective decision making. Data mining is the most widely used technique for extracting valuable information from medical data. Data mining is basically used for assisting doctors in diagnosis, treatment options, drug suggestion. Machine learning is another field which is widely used to provide effective healthcare services. Machine learning possess great potential for health science for using medical data and analyze it to find out inefficiencies and adopt best practices that enhance overall quality, care and reduce cost. Computer Vision also made substantial progress in health science. It plays vital role for creating applications for impaired patients.

Vision Impairment

Vision Impairment (VI) is the consequence of a functional loss of vision rather than the eye disorder itself. It is not necessary therefore, to define VI in terms of the catalogue of permanent conditions or chronic diseases that result in a loss of vision (Wickramasinghe, 2010; Espique, 2010). However, the impact may be described through 3 terms:

- **Low Vision:** A person can see, but not well, and full vision cannot be enabled by surgery
- **Legally Blind:** Someone lacking visual perception due to physiological or neurological factors so that they can't see well or have minimal vision e.g. they can't see at 6 meters what others can see at 60 m
- **Totally Blind:** Someone who cannot see at all (less than 20/200 vision in their better eye), and who must therefore depend on their other senses

Assistive Technologies in Healthcare

Imagine talking to an app instead of seeing your doctor when in pain or ache. Post listening to your description (symptoms), the app retrieves the most modern research it might require to examine about how to diagnose and treat your disease/problem. Lastly, a computer server examining your medical records and family history, comparing it with the finest and most current study to advise a healing procedure to your doctor that is precisely personalized to your requirements. AI in healthcare and medicine for visually impaired people can organize patient paths and curing plans better providing doctors with literally all the data they require to make a worthy choice. This consummates for the requirement for Assistive Technology (AI).

Implementations of AT

One implementation for visually disabled people uses a sighted Artificial intelligence application in their mobile phones that functions with Pivot-head glasses while they discover the world surrounding them. The glasses are attached with a camera that handovers visual data into auditory signals (Chang, 2015). With this help, a visually disabled person can read the expressions of persons surrounding him/her, read what is there in any eatery's menu using the same sighted AI application. One firm is using Cognitive services, which is an assemblage of APIs, which allows the server to hear, speak, see, interpret and understand our needs by means of natural methods of communication. Whenever visually disabled people will be more inspired to participate in a joint debate or commotion, being able to read their co workers' facial expressions and respond during the conversation, using such smart Artificial Intelligence applications will positively allow them to overcome all communication problems making them feel alike in the chat (Masud, et al., 217). According to initial work on ATs conducted by the Lincoln Centre for Autonomous Systems, their team strategies to use depth and color sensor technology in new tablets and smart-phones, like the new Tango Project by Google, to permit localization and 3D mapping, navigation with objects recognition. The same team will develop the finest UI to communicate that to consumers, whether it be vibration, sound or the verbal words.

The research team is aiming to develop an arrangement, which will identify optical signs in a setting. This information (huge in size) will be sensed through the camera device and will be used to recognize the room type as the consumer travels around the area. An important feature of the arrangement will be its ability to familiarize with distinct users' experiences, adjusting the supervision it offers as the mechanism acquires from its setting and from the human communication. With the user becoming further habituated to the technology, the earlier and relaxed, it will be to recognize the location using machine learning.

Much visual assistance is presently available from wearable devices to guide dogs to cameras. Distinctive difficulties with the former are acceptability and usability (Kwon et al., 2010). Should people be able to use technology implanted in their devices like smart-phones, it will not necessitate them to wear additional equipment that could make them feel uncomfortable. There are many prevailing smartphone applications, which for example speak to describe places or recognize an object, but the sensors implanted in those devices are still not entirely utilized. The aim is to create an arrangement with 'human-in-the-loop' that delivers worthy customization significant to visually disabled users and most significantly, that comprehends how people perceive and identify specific features of their surroundings. Most machine learning systems are extremely data ravening, necessitating millions of observations to reach satisfactory performance ranks. In addition to that, prejudices in data gathering can considerably disturb both generalizability and performance. Lactate may be a decent forecaster of the risk of death, but only a minor sample of patients gets their lactate levels tested. Progressive telecare service providers recognize that they are well positioned to extend their level of provision to include people with disabilities and to include relevant smart assistive devices in their inventories. They understand sensory issues and the technology applications that they can offer to meet their needs.

LITERATURE SURVEY AND BACKGROUND STUDY

The following section encompasses through several significant aspects required for developing smart health care models. This includes viability to extended human vision impairment with computer vision and brain computing technology.

Computer Vision

Computer vision, as the name suggests, is the vision of the computer, that is, how the computer visualizes our environment and surroundings. This technology is very much helpful and assistive to visually impaired people as it enables them to walk, navigate and know about their environment and surroundings (Espique, 2010). A recent work on this is done by Google and they named it Project Tango. It has embedded sensors in it for measurement of color and depth, in new phones and devices, which enables object mapping, object localization, object navigation and object recognition, all in the 3-D space. Therefore, these devices can fully guide and navigate the visually impaired people through their path by sending vibrations, sounds and spoken words. Many other visual aids are available such as guide dogs, cameras and wearable sensors. But the problem with these devices is usability and acceptability. If people are able to use technology embedded in their smart phones, then there is no requirement to wear extra equipment which could make them feel self-conscious (Coughlan & Miele, 2017). The most important feature of the computer vision VI system is "human-in-the-loop" which provides good localization relevant to the VI person and which understands how people observe and recognize particular features of their environment.

Brain Computing

Brain computing is making a brain-computer interface so that computer can send signals to the brain and can communicate with the brain. There are some high-tech devices available for visually impaired people, which work on brain computing and help them to sense what is in front of them. Brainport is a brain computing device which is developed by Wicab, a Wisconsin company. The person using this device wears sunglasses which have a video camera in it, and a small mouthpiece, which consists of 400 electrodes, is planted in the person's mouth. The device translates information from video camera into a pattern of tiny electrical shocks on the mouthpiece. The person reads these electrical shocks with his tongue. However, learning to interpret these sensations require extensive training, but has many advantages for a visually impaired person because he will be able to identify objects in front of him, he will be able to walk, even up and down the stairs without the need of cane, he will be able to read short words such as bus stop signs. It opens up a world of large number of possibilities for the visually impaired person, which would otherwise be impossible to do. Some devices being developed by other companies include the vOICe, which converts visual information into a soundscape, and the AuxDeco, which delivers a pattern of electrical shocks to the skin of the forehead.

Data Mining and Machine Learning

Data mining is retrieving useful information from data by using different data mining and machine learning techniques such as pre-processing, clustering, classification, etc. There are a number of sources of healthcare data. We can get healthcare data from hospitals, colleges and institutions, social networks, other medical services, and even from IOT devices. This is a large amount of mixed type of data and thus we need to have proper data mining and machine learning tools to extract useful information from it. Thus data mining and machine learning techniques are very important to be applied to the data, so that we can successfully deal with the unstructured and mixed type of data and can extract good amount of useful information from this large data, thus providing information which can be very helpful to the healthcare industry (Sivan & Darsan, 2016; Lodh et al., 2016).

Big Data

Data of health patients generated is increasing day-by-day. This data includes electronic health records, treatment follow-ups, medical records, data on syndrome, medicines, exercises, prescriptions, diet, laboratory reports, machine related data from MRI, ultrasound, digital microscopy, CT scans, X-rays, ECG, etc. Moreover, wearable health devices which are IOT devices are also generating continuous data. All this data possesses the characteristics of the 5 V's of big data. It is of different types generating from different sources (variety), growing dramatically (volume), generating at a large speed (velocity), having different quality, pertinence and meaning (veracity), can be analyzed to give valuable outcomes and unknown insights (value). Thus, big data analytics in healthcare can be applied to analyze this data and predict the outcomes (Wickramasinghe, 2010).

Big data technologies have evolved very much in the modern world. Tools and analytics of big data are very useful in processing and analyzing this large amount of healthcare data and this will provide us with many benefits:

- Medical related judgements can be made for accurate health predictions.
- A generalised and accurate treatment procedure can be made for the patients having a particular disease by analysing all the medical data of all the patients who already suffered from the same disease or are suffering from the same disease. In this way, an exact and specific treatment plan can be made for the patients for a particular disease.
- Number of readmissions of patients can be reduced. Readmissions of patients are caused by misunderstanding, mismanagement and lack of access to all the pertinent data and socioeconomic health of the patient. Large number of readmissions lead to the doctors spending lesser time on new patients and thus leading to loss of revenue to the hospital. Using predictive analytics, number of readmissions can be reduced to a large extent and thus freeing physician's times (Kwon et al., 2010).
- Data from different machines can be analysed using computer models to get graphical results which can help track trends and diagnoses and thus provide with better treatment to the patients.
- Healthcare analytics can be used to detect commonalities between the patients and thus making diagnosis and treatment easier and more accurate.

- By doing analytics on patient's data, we can detect diseases at earlier stages, detect healthcare abuse and fraud faster, reduce costs, detect individuals that need proactive care or need change in their lifestyle to avoid health condition degradation.
- Collecting different data from different sources can help improve research, knowledge and awareness about new diseases, symptoms, therapies and treatments.
- Healthcare providers can recognise high risk population and can propose preventive acts, thus, enhancing the patient experience.
- Due to the increasing patient load, the time available for each patient is reduced largely as compared to the past years. Healthcare analytics are very useful in such a scenario to provide with effective solutions in lesser time.
- Big data analytics in healthcare will provide us with large distributed storage to store the large amount of patient's data, thus reducing data loss and providing the identification of the key factors in providing care to the patients, thus reducing additional hospital visits, and additional costs for both the patients and the healthcare organisations (Sun & Reddy, 2013).

Research Contribution in Advanced Healthcare Delivery

Low or no vision people find it very difficult to complete daily routine tasks. Their life is affected in almost all aspects from shopping in a crowded area to crossing the roads, reading books or newspaper, or cooking food. There is need of some advanced gadgets or sensors which makes their life easy. Recent Technological tools needed to complete and engaged in daily routine tasks. Few fields are emerging which can aid in development of recent tools for no visually impaired people. Computer Vision, Big Data, Brain Computing, Machine Learning, Data Mining are name few. Glasses for face recognition, Braille keyboard embed in smart watches, health android apps; body wearable sensors are some technological advancement in latest technologies for visually impaired patients.

Assistive Technology: Principles, Practice and Application

Assistive technology device is a hardware system or an equipment which helps in assisting a disabled person in all aspects of life, which in turn, increases the achievement, participation, independence and autonomy for a person with disabilities. This means that AT device can be as simple as a pencil with a special grip for students with writing disabilities and can be as complex as a device which helps in communicating ideas of a disabled person by taking input from him (Coughlan & Miele, 2017). AT is a special need for people with learning disabilities, hearing impairments, visual impairments or other physical limitations. AT has been used in many classrooms around the world to help students with disabilities to learn, write and explore the things in their daily lives (Cernazanu-Glavan et al., 2014; Kwon et al., 2010; Zhang et al., 2014), AT helps teachers to instruct students with disabilities more successfully. AT not only helps teachers to achieve specific needs of learning but also helps to provide a sense of personal achievement and success in the students with learning disabilities. Some of the AT devices with their applications are explained below:

- Hearing aids for persons with hearing disabilities.
- Wheelchairs, scooters, walkers, cranes, crutches for people with mobility disabilities.

- Automatic page turners, book holders and adapted pencil grips to help disabled students in the classroom to participate in educational activities.
- Kitchen utensils with large cushioned grips to help people with weakness or arthritis in their hands.
- Automatic door openers, ramps, grab bars and wider doorways in buildings and workplaces.
- Speech recognition software, audio books, variable speed tape recorders, word processing programs, alternate keyboards, graphic organisers and outlining for students with learning disabilities (Lodh et al., 2016; De Souza Veriscimo & Bernardes, 2015).

Assistive Technology for Developing Advanced Healthcare Systems

In the modern era, large numbers of assistive devices is already made and are currently being made for providing assistance for specific types of illnesses or diseases and also for aged people. These technologies are very advanced because they require robotics, special computers, advanced sensors and other types of advanced tech stuff to build them (Ahmed et al., 2017; Geman & Chiuchisan, 2015). Some of them are explained in the following section.

AT For Persons With Multiple Sclerosis

Multiple Sclerosis (MS) is an autoimmune disease in which the myelin sheath encasing neurons in the central nervous system are destroyed by auto-reactive T-cells. The exposed neurons are not able to move the information encoded in the form of electrical signals as efficiently, thus, slowing the motor function and reducing cognitive abilities.

AT devices can make the life with MS much easier. They can help with tasks like walking, dressing and bathing and make use less energy. Some of those devices are listed below:

1. Leg braces and walkers for those having weakness in their leg muscles. Canes can be useful if having one leg weaker than the other, or, when having mild problems with balance.
2. Tub bench and hand-held shower head for bathing.
3. Bedside commode and grab bars near the toilet.
4. Velcro, buttons, zippers and hooks on clothing.
5. Utility cart with wheels, electric can opener and pot stabilizer for cooking purposes.
6. Electric beds or mattresses for sleeping.
7. Special grips for pens and pencils and wrist supports for writing.

AT For People With Dementia

The term dementia refers to a set of symptoms which includes loss of memory, confusion, mood changes and difficulties with communication and reasoning. It is a progressive disease, i.e., it develops gradually over time. Early diagnosis and treatment is necessary to slow down the progression of the disease. There is currently no cure for dementia.

AT can improve the lives of people living with dementia providing it is introduced early into their lives. AT gives them the opportunity to engage in daily activities and participate in their life and home community. Virtual reality, for instance, has been proven to soothe individuals by placing them in a calm environment. An interactive and engaging ipad-based activity helps them to stay connected to the outside world. Moreover, they can receive emails and photos from their loved ones which help them to stay in touch. It is seen that musical environment keeps them motivated and helps them to stay relaxed. They can also use interactive games which help them to stay focused and mentally stimulated.

AT For Aged People

Recent advancements in AT provide great help to elderly people at home or in institutions. AT devices improve older people's safety, security and capability to cope at home (Espique, 2010). Some of the AT devices for elderly people are listed below:

1. Community alarms which enables a person to remain safe and independent in his own home.
2. Video-monitoring for keeping an eye on the aged people so that they can be given any assistance when needed.
3. Health monitors for constantly monitoring the pulse, skin temperature and movement of the aged people.
4. Fall detectors for reducing fall related injuries and giving immediate care to the aged people in case of any fall.
5. Hip protectors for reducing the risk of hip fracture in case a person falls onto their hip.
6. Smoke alarms and fire alarms for detecting an early presence of fire. These are for people who are smokers and people who do cooking at home.
7. Dawn/dusk lights to prevent falls at night. These are beneficial for people who require to go to toilet at night.
8. Door alerts for those who wander at night. They can generate an alarm, or video-call a relative who lives some distance away.
9. Electronic calendars/speaking clocks for those who repeatedly ask the date or time.

Mobile Based Smart Technologies

There are various mobile based assistive technologies which are published by many researchers (Cernazanu-Glavan et al., 2014; Nalavade et al., 2014). Some of them are explained below:

DeeDee System

This system is designed to assist a type-1 diabetic person through his daily life. This system is deployed on the phone which is required to be carried by the person throughout the day. The main application of the system is that it does the prediction of glycaemia. Current systems which do prediction of glycaemia, require that patient is to be monitored continuously in an environment which is controlled by the doctors and physicians (Cernazanu-Glavan et al., 2014). The benefit of keeping the patient in such environment is that a complete set of data can be collected on patient's life for a particular time interval. Using this data, predictions can be made for blood glucose concentration levels for a specific time. So the patient has to remain in the hospital, takes food at fixed intervals of time and is kept separated from everyday life. If patients are removed from the hospital and placed in everyday life, then a large decrease in data collection will occur and the data will become completely unreliable. So to solve these problems, DeeDee system is designed to help a diabetic to collect blood glucose concentration values, CHO values and other parameters. This system maintains several profiles of the patients which are triggered according to the patient's circumstance at a particular time. Each profile is uniquely characterised by its context data: instances of time when the profile can be triggered, schedule of the user, geographic context, level of physical activity and the emotional factors. The BGC prediction module and the knowledge extraction module of the system make use of these profiles and predicts the possible advent of hyperglycaemia periods in the near future. This is achieved by doing the analysis of BGC variation for the future interval of time and the user profile which can be triggered at that time. Thus the user is provided with a credible information.

Resource-Aware Mobile-Based Health Monitoring

Monitoring of heart diseases requires performing the measurements of electrocardiogram signals at different intervals of time and in different circumstances (Chang, 2015). This can only be possible using mobile devices so as to cope with the mobility of the patients. However, these mobile devices are energy-aware, their computational resources (speed, memory and CPU) are limited, and can lose connectivity with network which makes it very hard to monitor the patient continuously. So some researchers have proposed a solution for this problem by giving a new approach. First the data is collected from the patient using WSBN (wireless body sensor networks), then this data is transmitted to a mobile device using protocols like Wifi, GPRS, 3G, 4G, Bluetooth. The whole task of monitoring is divided into several subtasks and these subtasks are either executed on the mobile device or on a backend server. SDSM (smart decision support module) is deployed on the mobile device which has a resource meter that measures the device's availability of resources (memory, CPU, battery). According to these values, it decides where to process each subtask: on the device itself or on a backend server. This can also be a combined decision which means some subtasks are to be executed on device and rest are executed on the backend server. All the mathematical computations for making these decisions are done on the mobile device. Finally, all the results are shown on the mobile device.

Ubiquitous Health System

IT field technologies are being merged with the technologies of other fields. Even the medical field technology is merged with the IT field technology which results in a system called Ubiquitous health system (U-health system). This system uses sensors to determine the condition of the patient and the patient's family members and the medical staff has to directly analyze the data to get results. This has many disadvantages as the family members and the medical staff are not able to manage rightly because of the occurrence of malfunction and accidental situation on the sensor equipment. Thus, some researchers enhances the U-health system to increase reliability and to correctly diagnose patient's condition and judge any abnormal sign or emergency situation by applying the disease-identification algorithm to the U-health system. The patient has to wear several sensors based on USN (Ubiquitous Sensor Network) and the data extracted from these sensors is used by the DCAP (Disease Combination Appearance Probability) algorithm to predict the incidence of emergency situation (Ahmed et al., 2017). Also, this system makes it possible for the family members and medical institution to cope promptly by sending a text message if any emergency situation occurs and enhances speed by offering mobile service so that the patient's information can be searched through smart phone using wireless network.

Assistive Technology for Vision Impairment

Vision Impairment is the consequence of a functional loss of vision rather than the eye disorder itself. It is not necessary therefore, to define visual impairment in terms of the catalogue of permanent conditions or chronic diseases that result in a loss of vision. However, the impact may be described through 3 terms:

- **Low Vision:** A person can see, but not well, and full vision cannot be enabled by surgery
- **Legally Blind**: Someone lacking visual perception due to physiological or neurological factors so that they can't see well or have minimal vision e.g. they can't see at 6 meters what others can see at 60 m
- **Totally Blind:** Someone who cannot see at all (less than 20/200 vision in their better eye), and who must therefore depend on their other senses

There are various technological tools and devices developed specifically to assist people with any kind of visual impairment (Zhang et al., 2014; Espique, 2010). Many of them are listed below:

Non-Optical Low Vision Devices

- Acetate or colour filters increases contrast and darken the print when placed on printed page.
- Bold line paper provides darker lines.
- Typoscopes for students who find it difficult to focus on a word or a line of text. They block the surrounding text so that students can focus on what they are reading.
- Stand boards provide automatic magnification of text when the student is close enough to the board. They are also useful for students who need to look closely in order to read, because they bring material closer to the eyes so as to reduce neck pain and postural fatigue.
- Felt tip pens provide darker lines and increased contrast.
- Large print keyboards for students who have cognitive delays or are physically not able to use touch typing skills.
- Low vision watches for students with low vision who are learning time management skills.
- Task lighting for students who have problems when seeing in bright lights and glares, providing light directed on the print, thus increasing clarity and assisting the students on seeing in dimmed lights during board presentations.

Optical Devices for Near Viewing

- Hand-held magnifiers provide illumination by directing light directly on the source. They require to be held by hand at a certain distance from the source.
- Stand mounted and dome magnifiers are placed directly on the page and provide a fixed distance between the lens and the source. They are useful for those who have difficulty holding hand-held magnifiers.
- Illuminated magnifiers are for students who require supplementary lighting or those who want to avoid reflections from ceiling lights. They put the focus on the source creating more light and higher contrast. They are available in hand-held and stand magnifiers and require batteries to operate.

- Pocket magnifiers can be used to read labels in the kitchen, price tags in the market and menu items in the restaurant. They are lightweight and easy to use but they offer a narrow field of view and a short working distance.

Optical Devices for Distance Viewing

- Monocular are useful for spotting information such as on the board, restaurant menus, street signs, scoreboards but their visual field is restricted.
- Binoculars provide a larger visual field and are useful when students have vision in both the eyes and can fuse an image. They are generally used for short-term viewing and make it easier to find the targets but they are heavier and larger as compared to monocular.

Video Magnifiers

- Stand video magnifiers project the image of the material onto a television screen at the student's eye level. Hence, students are able to view more information at a time.
- Video magnifiers with distance capabilities allow to toggle between near and distance, thus allowing students to view the screen at a distance without holding monocular or binoculars.
- Portable video magnifiers are for students who have more movement during the school day. They are portable and lightweight, thus allowing students to carry them as they transition to different environments.
- Optical Character Recognition (OCR) software scans a text or image, then it converts it into the recognisable characters or words and then produce a synthetic speech that read the text or image. Thus, students are able to scan a text or image and then listen to the synthetic speech that reads the text or image.

Braille Technology

- Refreshable Braille display translates, what is appearing on the computer screen, to Braille, one line at a time. It connects to computer using a cable. It does translation to Braille by electronically lowering and raising different combination of pins.
- Braille printer/embosser is a printer attached to a computer to produce Braille copy of a text. Students can use it to print Braille copy of their personal notes and written work.
- Braille translation software for converting text into Braille. Converted text can then be printed using Braille embosser.
- Electronic Braille note takers can be used by a student for taking notes in the class using either a Braille keyboard or a standard keyboard. These notes can then be transferred to computer for storage or can be printed in Braille format.

AT's to Support Orientation and Mobility

- Cane allows to have safe and independent travel through all the environments for the blind or visually impaired persons.

- Talking compass is a hand-held device and it provides visual, tactile or auditory cues related to direction.
- Electronic Travel Aids (ETA)and GPS devices: Both of these two types of devices provide guidance, directions or feedback related to movement but the difference is that ETA uses radar and sonar technology to detect obstacles and thus providing feedback while GPS uses the global positioning technology to give directions according to the position and location coordinates (Khan et al., 2015).

Auditory Access Devices

- Recording devices can be used by the students to record any classroom lecture for studying and note-taking purposes. These recordings can then be played using any CD player, MP3 player, tape recorders, etc.
- Auditory books are the recordings of the texts being read. These are useful for people with visual impairment because they can listen to the reading of text instead of reading themselves.
- Screen reading software is a software which reads the information on the computer screen (Khan et al., 2015). Using this software student can access the internet, word processing programs and other printed material without having to see the computer screen.
- Talking calculators which speak out each entry and calculated result.
- Talking watches for visually impaired students who are learning time management skills.

ASSISTIVE TECHNOLOGY: METHODS AND MODELS

No vision can have unfortunate effect on health and its commonness is expanding day by day. Visual impaired patients can have restricted access to health information and medical facilities. For treatment of such kind of patients skilled staff is required as they are aware of special needs of no vision sufferer, which is generally not available in most of the hospitals. Extending the role of technology, we can create devices or mobile apps which support blind people and provide quality medical services at their door step. Loss of vision is a distressing condition. For reducing stress effective healthcare services are mandate which help visually impaired people to independently enjoy their life. Now days mobile apps are for every basic need. Innovative ideas are merged with mobile technologies for creating applications for visually impaired patients. One can online monitor his pulse rate, blood pressure; insulin level, heart beat etc. also find solution to various health problems online. With the usage of assistive technologies visually impaired patients can now online detect disease, they just need to input some attribute values and result outcome is in front of them. Convert is required which convert you voice to text and take further action accordingly.

Overview of Smart Healthcare Systems

The term "visual impairment" refers to low vision or incapability to sense the external environment through vision. The visual impairment can be partial loss in vision or complete blindness. The visual impairment is not a disease but might be caused due to congenital reasons or due to severe accident. Visually impaired people face lots of problems in their daily routine. The main concern for visually impaired people is "Mobility". Mobility refers two basic needs such as accessibility and self-dependent. They would be able to access all facilities which are used by normal people. They would be able to move self dependently. The best way to help visually disabled people is to provide them these basic needs. Now a days, new technologies have developed, to use new life concept where visually impaired people are not blind but they have different abilities (Nalavade et al., 2014). With the help of upgrading technology, an assistive systems or devices can be designed in such a manner to make independent life possible for visually impaired people. Assistive systems are smart healthcare systems for feeble people which build physical perception of external environment by using sensors. These systems provide the users refined or optimized information of external environment to make them safe and secure by any harm. These systems can be implemented by using several technologies such as ultra sonic waves, laser waves, infrared waves, cameras, sensors. The main task of assistive healthcare devices is to provide efficient and safe perception of surroundings for mobility with autonomy. These systems provide navigation, localization, orientation, tracking indoor and outdoor obstacles facilities with the help of bluetooth, sensors, and some other new technologies (Emiliani & Stephanidis, 2005). The use of assistive device has increased for urban mobility (navigation, localization, orientation). Some tools which are available in market and used for navigation such as white cane, tactile floor. These tools only provide some part of information for mobility. The sensors which are used to design assistive device must be able to detect range, dimensions, height of the objects for safe mobility. Assistive devices must be wearable or flexible. Portable devices are usually compact, lightweight, they can easily carried by the user and require constant hand interaction. For example: tactile display, electronic canes, mobile phones, laptop computers, etc. Figure 1 presents the overview of smart technologies for Disease Detection.

To design number of wearable assistive devices as per user requirement is a task. Assistive devices provide solution for activities like travelling from one location to another location without the help of other human, reading. Assistive devices create a new communication channel through touch and hearing for blind people. Devices are placed on the body parts such as feet, tongue, wrist, fingers, hands, chest, ear, etc (Jothi et al., 2017). The potential of these devices is based on some important factors:

Figure 1. Intelligent techniques for disease diagnosis for personalized medicine system

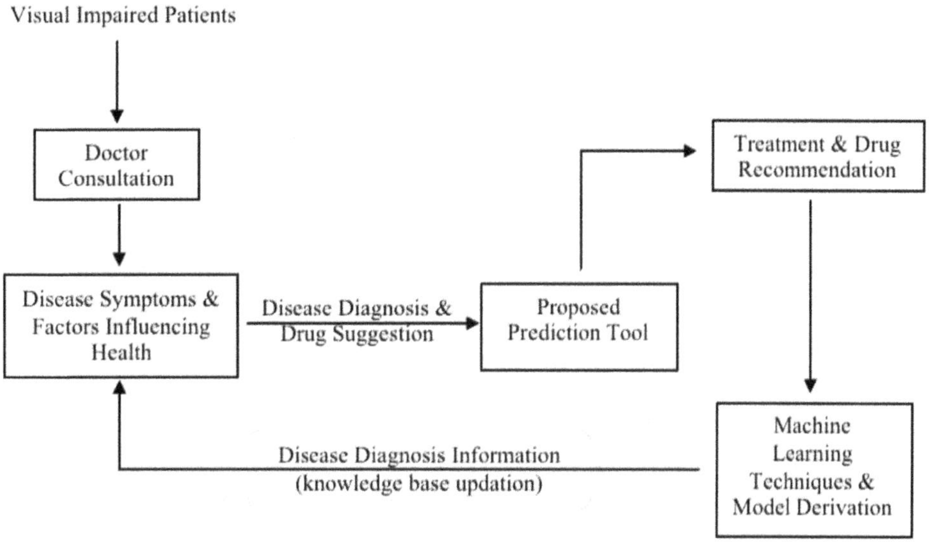

- **Performance:** It depends on the functioning of assistive devices on time.
- **Wireless Connectivity:** The wearable devices must be wirelessly connected with server to store and exchange the necessary information.
- **Reliable:** Wearable devices must be satisfied their specifications and functions for both software and hardware.
- **Simple:** Assistive devices must be user friendly. GUI should be simple and easy to use. Interface of the device can make use of it easier to the user.
- **Wearable:** Assistive devices must be comfortable and flexible in use. Users want to wear assistive devices rather than carry it.
- **Economically Accessible:** Devices must be economically accessible for users so that everybody can afford it. These devices help the users to enhance their quality of life. In order to make it accessible by all users, it should economically available at reasonable rate.

METHODOLOGIES

Healthcare sector facilitates storage of cumbersome and massive amount of information like clinical examination, treatment record, electronic patient reports, medicine etc. about individual patients. This section highlights predominant technologies, including intelligent mining, learning and processing of huge medical data.

Machine Learning and Big Data

The huge volume of collected data is impossible to analyze by human beings. Due to unmanageable amount of data, the quality of decision making is getting affected. This difficulty has been resolved by the use of machine learning techniques in healthcare sector. Machine learning provides a way to analyze the patterns from collected data which permits the healthcare professionals to offer personalized care at real time. Machine learning helps healthcare industries to decrease the risk and improve the standard of care to generate good amount of revenue. Machine learning is fast- growing trend in healthcare sector (Bhardwaj, et al., 2017). Assistive devices and sensors use the sensed data to access the patient's health information at real time and this technology also allow medical professionals to analyze the data for improving the diagnose and treatment of patient. There are so many ways to use machine learning technology in healthcare sector. Machine learning can apply to classify or filter the sensed data present in a particular environment. The goal of machine learning is to analyze the unstructured or structure data.

Machine learning with big data comes into existence. It plays a vital role in healthcare sector. Machine learning with big data provides the optimal or précised information because devices has huge amount of data to learn and make decision precisely. Machine learning with big data collects enormous volume of domain specific data which contains useful information about patient's health and then analyze the précised information to provide personalized care. Machine learning is a domain of artificial intelligence. Some popular machine learning methods are supervised learning, unsupervised learning, semi- supervised learning, reinforcement learning. These techniques learn automatically through experience and also improve the performance of learning data with each experience. These methods build a model based on input data which make a precise prediction for new data in real time (Nambiar et al., 2013). Machine

Table 1. Training data example

TRAINING DATA SET					
Age	**Pulse Rate**	**Heart Rate**	**Blood Pressure**	**Insulin Level**	**Class**
45	110	77	156/70	Yes	Yes
56	80	64	110/78	No	No
34	120	78	160/75	Yes	Yes
45	100	80	150/70	No	Yes

learning techniques identify patterns from enormous volume of data sets that allows medical experts to predict and make decision process for diagnosis and treatment planning.

Data Mining

The importance of data miming in healthcare sector is increasing significantly day by day. Data mining techniques are necessary to analyze health data. Analyzing the huge amount of health data is essential for providing personalized care at real time. Data mining is a strong analysis tool which is useful to extract knowledge from large data sets and find the patterns or attributes of data which is related to each other. In healthcare sector, data mining is sometimes called "Text Mining of Health Data" which is capable of analyzing doctor's prescription (Crasto et al., 2003). The use of data mining in healthcare sector is ubiquitous and it is useful to detect valuable and hidden information from medical data. Data mining is the core process of knowledge discovery of medical data. Data mining techniques have divided into two categories: predictive model and descriptive model. Predictive model is based on supervised learning. This model generates predictive rules to classify or extract the patterns of useful medical data based on specific target data. Descriptive model attempts to extract the similarity of records and find the patterns and relation between the data. Assistive devices collected data from real time environment. This collected information has its own specific characteristics can be refined by the help of data mining techniques to assist the user from current environment. To achieve useful and reliable information for blind people from data mining process, it requires the collected data of good quality. Generally, assistive devices collect health related data from different sources. This gathered information contains missing information, erroneous data, miscoding, and incorrectness. Data mining is necessary to refine it and provide related features to predict the next movement of blind person (Cios, 2000). Classification is the most commonly used data mining approach for prediction. It is the process of prediction future outcome based on past historical data. Table 1 and 2 presents few instances of test and training dataset example. Train data is used to train the classification algorithm and test data is used to validate the real time performance of designed classification algorithm. Person age, pulse rate, heart rate, insulin level, blood pressure are few core attributes to detect heart related disease. Classifier start training based on these attributes and validated on test data.

Performance of classification technique is judged using the term known as Accuracy. Accuracy is defined as the measure to identify class labels correctly or percentage of rightly identifies tuples. Error is defined as the percentage of incorrectly identified tuples. Table 3 presents the confusion matrix which depicts how predictions on instances are tabulated (Cabena et al., 1997).

Table 2. Test data example

TEST DATA SET					
Age	**Pulse rate**	**Heart Beat**	**Blood Pressure**	**Diabetes**	**Heart problem?**
55	89	70	110/78	No	No
66	110	78	160/78	No	Yes
45	115	78	155/70	Yes	Yes
56	80	67	100/78	Yes	No

Table 3. Matrix to measure classifier performance

	Predicted Label	
	Positive	**Negative**
Positive	a True Positive (TP)	b False Negative (FN)
Negative	c False Positive (FP)	d True Negative (TN)

Deep Learning

Deep learning is a branch of machine learning with algorithms which is inspired by functions of human brain called ANN. It is a multilayer neural network which learns complex patterns from enormous volume of data. Deep learning is an approach of artificial intelligence which learns relationships of data from the large data sets. Deep learning approach is domain expertise approach which transforms raw data into suitable representation of data for decision making process of medical experts. Deep learning has an ability to extract features from raw data automatically (Ker et al., 2018). That is why deep learning is also known as Hierarchical Feature Learning. Deep learning allows a model that is composed of multi-processing layers called artificial neural network to learn representation of data with multiple levels of abstraction. Deep learning is basically multilayer perceptron networks. A deep neural network processes the inputs in layer-wise manner with some hidden layers to learn the deep structure and representation of data from large data sets. The use of deep learning in healthcare devices is increasing at an alarming rate. Deep learning algorithms need one-time training. Once a model gets train, it can work itself and improve the performance of system continuously. Wearable device which works on the principle of deep learning learns the representation of medical data through multilayer and it functions like a human brain. Assistive device for blind person needs deep representation of current environment data to predict the next movement in real time so deep learning approach is very helpful in these devices (Ravı et al, 2017).

Advanced Mobile Technology

Mobile technology is the technology used for cellular communication and use of mobile computing. Mobile technology includes wireless communication, WiFi, Bluetooth, 3G, 4G, location tracking, GPS, GPRS, Messaging service (MMS, SMS). Mobile technology allows the devices to communicate and access data and information remotely [AbdulRasool & Sabra, 2011). The technology has a feature of mobility which allows the user to communicate anytime, anywhere. It is battery operated technology that can be used anywhere without electric. It allows wireless communication, accessing and sharing of information through internet. The devices based on mobile technology are portable, access and store the data at very high speed. In modern era, mHealth app is fast growing trend. Health related apps access the information in real time and provide medical experts advice also. Wearable devices or assistive devices are using mobile technology for mobility and for wireless communication at anytime and anywhere. Mobile technology in assistive devices is used to giving treatment, making diagnosis, monitoring of health time to time, self-management, promoting health tips. Wearable devices with some algorithms and mobile technology are able to gather accurate information about health to provide personalized care in real time. Mobile technology combines with some important technology such as remote monitoring technology, advanced monitoring devices, and personalized care management (Billi et al., 2010).

Natural Language Processing for Medical Data

In the last few decades medical data is growing exponentially, which is generated from saved and is considered as massive source of medical information (Ding et al., 2001). Techniques have been developed by researchers to extract relevant information from medical literature like prescription, reports etc (Leonard et al., 2002). Text mining is used to retrieve vital information from medical literature. For the discovery of new health information smart Electronic Health Records are utilized for finding out the novel health vision for future and hence upgrading the decision and quality of healthcare framework for blind people. All medical data like patient health record, blood test reports, pathology reports are saved in digital format, so for extracting valuable information text mining is required.

Present day challenges in smart healthcare system involve collection of genuine medical history, which eventually becomes much more significant as compared to analysis and interpretation of the collected medical data. Such health-related data can be effectively sampled using multi-sensor embedded electronic devices deployed pervasively around the patient, thereby creating smart health monitoring environment. The sensors may also accommodate health data in different languages, which may require in-built natural language interpreters. The entire health heuristics generated produce huge repositories of medical data of numerous patients suffering from different types of ailments and exhibiting same or distinct symptoms. Such colossal amount of data needs to be managed, thus forming the urge to build knowledge management system that may incorporate intelligent mining over the diversified knowledge base.

Vision Impairment Healthcare Management

Healthcare Management System needs real-time, authentic, dependable, and accurate diagnostic results provided by monitoring devices for vision impairment, which could be further applied to monitor patients remotely, whether he is in hospital, clinic, or at home. Visually impaired patients face several challenges every day, especially in activities like commuting, reading, texting, etc. In order to provide better health care services, it is necessarily important to develop and implement new technologies at affordable prices for people and to ensure maximum comfort, and independency of patients [Sujith & Safeeda, 2014). Health care monitoring devices permits patients to stay at home rather than in expensive hospitals. These devices provide a systematic and cost-effective way to assist health of vision impaired people at home while monitoring real time health related information.

Home Assistant for Health-Related Problems

Ubiquitous health care is available for every vision impaired patients which is independent of time and location. There is need of remote health care monitoring assistant at home for moving one location to another location independently and diagnoses of all health related problems at home. Home assistant is necessary in many ways such as:

- To provide remotely health related information
- To provide personalized and independent services
- To be flexible and reliable in any environment
- To make decision automatically
- To response any disease or health situation in real time
- To diagnose results of health information timely
- To provide security in information exchanging between devices and servers
- To collect data related to health regularly

Wearable sensors devices are best to use as automated home assistant. These devices are physically and technologically very flexible, reliable, and enable to monitor natural environment (Velázquez, 2010). They have potential to collect and store a huge amount of information that can lead the better understandings of wellness and diseases, which in resulting the better treatment and health outcomes. Today's generation is completely dependent on smart phones and devices. These resources are become easier to access anywhere and anytime. With these smart electronic devices, life quality of vision impaired people has also improved. There are many apps which can help to make a difference to everyday life of

Table 4. Priority domain for smart healthcare model for visually impaired

Priority Areas	Functionality
Daily Routine Activity and fitness applications	Healthcare app is able to assist blind people in daily routine activities and also helps in following daily exercise routine that leads to healthy lifestyle for blind patients.
Diet Recommendation	Diet is very important in context of health. Right diet leads to good health status. App is also able to recommend diet based on patient profile.
Health status: Mentally and physically	Smart technologies can be used to find out mental and abnormal condition so that one can take preventive action. Intelligent mining techniques can be used to detect any mental abnormality in blind patients.
Privacy, Security	Biometric systems must be added to improve privacy of crucial data. Proper alarms must be there in order to enhance security of blind patient.
Educational Programs	Braille input, text to speech, and speech to text converter is required for providing online education to blind patients so that he can address his issue/ problem to his mentor.
Diagnosis & Treatment module for severe and priority diseases: Heart, diabetes, cancer.	App can diagnose disease just after inputting certain attributes. User can select or enter data and disease outcome is in front of them.
Medical Precautionary services	Proper notification for all medical precautionary services
Automatic dialing and messaging in case of urgency	In case of emergency option of automatic dialing to some fixed numbers must be addressed by smart healthcare app.
Maternity and child health	In case mother is blind app can assist her in baby monitoring task along with reminder of all vaccines and medical precautions to be taken

low vision people and also make them more independent. Some apps like Be My Eyes, AppleVis Aipoly Vision, Light Detector, Magnifying Glass with Light, DAISY Talk and many more. Table shown below presents the priority domains that must be addressed while designing healthcare app for blind patients.

Online Monitoring of Severe Health Issues

In the area of healthcare services, online monitoring or use of mobile technologies has great impact on world (Kakria et al., 2015) . Health experts are taking the benefits of mobile technologies to improve the health care. Online monitoring-based health systems provides health experts who are able to access central database and patient's health information timely. Online monitoring devices are used to monitor the conditions of patients with chronic diseases. Two types of online monitoring devices are: mobile devices and agent-based system without agent. Online monitoring has various advantages which resolve all health issues, which includes following [Hii & Chung, 2011):

- To facilitate self Care anywhere, anytime
- To promote new lifestyle
- To improve the quality of life
- To prevent unnecessary hospitalization
- To provide mobility to do daily routines works
- To permits free consultation at home
- To get the knowledge of medicine and treatment anywhere
- To track patient's disease symptoms and response to therapy on time

Furthermore, the online monitoring is affordable for patients with severe various health issues in real time environment. Figure 2 presents the overall smart healthcare architecture for vision impaired patients.

Figure 2. Overall architecture of smart healthcare delivery for vision impaired patients

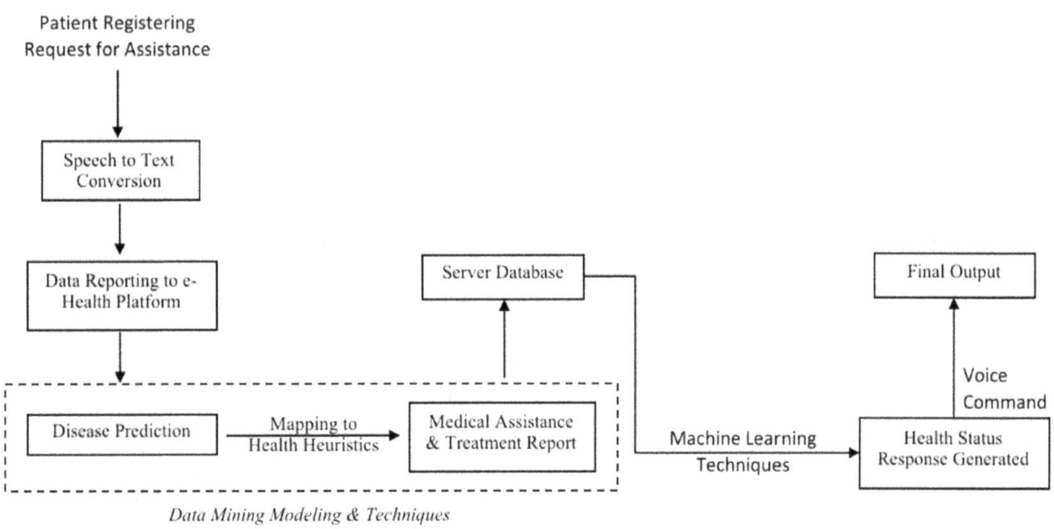

Diagnosis, Consultation, and Follow-Up

Artificial intelligence (AI) has rapid progress in health care management. AI aims to perform human cognitive functions and has applications in various health care devices for diagnosis. AI has an ability to handle any type of data (structured or unstructured data). AI has some popular techniques for handling structured data such as machine learning, deep learning, neural network and natural processing language for unstructured data. These applications have ability to early detection of diseases, diagnosis, consultation, treatment, follow-up, outcome prediction. AI is leading to transformational change in the world of medicine. It can help health experts to make faster and more accurate diagnose. The main concern of AI applications is to predict the risk of disease in time and to prevent it. AI can also help health experts how variations in genes or hormones can lead to disease. It can analyze medical data to treat diseases and provide personalized medicine on the basis of diagnosis results. At the early stage, accurate diagnosis of any diseases plays a most important role in patient's health and care. The performance of AI applications depends on training data. In order to provide most precise result, AI must have to use good quality of training data (Boegl et al., 2004). After accurate diagnosis, health experts can easily treat the patient and provide consultation on time.

Treatment Strategy

Identifying the novel treatment and accurate medicine is challenging task. Treatment strategies depend on collected data set of current environment and diagnosis results. In order to provide most precise treatment for any chronic diseases, an assistive device must be able to perceive data in real time. Several AI applications help to understand the perceiving information of current environment to provide better treatment of any diseases (Snae & Brueckner, 2008). Health experts use this generalized information to provide treatment and medicine in real time at anywhere. Treatment strategies are time-oriented. Some health experts using "trial and error" strategy provide effective drugs to patients based on collective and diagnosis information of patient's health during that time. Health experts often do not possess prior patient's history; hence they provide drugs only on the basis of current situation. This method is not sufficient for long term purpose as it becomes expensive and laborious to conduct tests repetitively. Another strategy used by health experts is "identifying effective drug". In this approach, health experts have prior patient's history. They provide medicine or any type of drugs to patient which is highly related in future treatment also. They find the specific drug combinations to treat the detected diseases.

Personalized Medicine System

Machine Learning is rapidly evolving in drug discovery that applies pattern recognition algorithms to discover the relationship between the drugs molecules and biological activities which is highly useful to treat (Dilsizian & Siegel, 2014). Health experts could suggest drugs according to patient profile. Drug discovery is very important to suggest the drugs to treat the patients. Some patients have side effects of some biological and chemical activities so before suggesting the drug to patients there is a need of patient profile. Machine Learning Approaches apply on history of patient to get the precise result in order to discover precise medicine for patient. Even some AI programs are developed that can accurately find the composition between chemical and biological behaviour of drug. Health experts use analysis reports of drugs to suggest them to patients based on their profile. Some experts use Un-supervised learning to identify the patterns in data without prediction (Khemmarat & Gao, 2015).

Recommendation System for Diet, Exercise, and Daily Health Routine

Recommender models for diet, exercise and healthy routine is essential in today's era. Developing personalized recommendation system is the requirement of quality healthcare services. These systems provide functional modules to track daily nutritional and healthy consumption as well as suggesting diets according to user profile (Li, et al., 2010). In today's world with no time constraint people usually do not care about their health. Therefore, there is desperate need of advanced model which can recommend healthy diet, exercise and personal health routines. Owing to bad eating habits people suffers from various diseases. Food like fast food, high cholesterol food, alcohol may increase the chance of having heart related diseases and if someone is so sensitive he/she may be diagnosed with severe heart related disease. Design and implementation of personalized recommender system using Machine Learning or AI help us to improve our health status. Healthy and right selection of exercise is also crucial in building right health status. High medical cost and health risks switches people from health treatment to disease prevention.

Voice Assistant

Voice assistant is an innovative and unfamiliar system for low vision people which acts as voice assistant for them. Visually impaired people can access most important features of phone and computer using voice assistant. This system helps to convert speech into text and makes low vision people life easier. This system has all features such as messaging, inbox, sent item, dialer, notes, reminder, wireless connection, battery level checking. Visually impaired people can perform all function by speech or voice. This system helps to user to tell their current position and read all the inbox messaging along with sender's name and date and time. This system helps to take medicine on time by using reminder service. Mobile technology is most abundant technology using across the world. Generally, people used to use mobile technology (Chaudhry et al, 2008). This system innovates novel way to access mobile technology for people with poor vision.

Healthcare Services for Visual Impaired Patients

Healthcare sector offers various services but the issue arise when blind people comes into picture. To access medical information and services is the major concern for visual impaired patients. It is desirable for medical care professional to understand that visual impaired patients will encounter problem in every services offered by healthcare organizations (Quigley, et al., 2018). While designing healthcare model for blind people main emphasis must be on enhancing the means of informing visual impaired patients regarding various medical services. All medical information and data must be open access and is easily available to blind patients (Pittman, 2010).

Listed are some important points that must be addressed or considered while designing healthcare model for blind patients. Healthcare organizations such as clinics, pathology labs, hospitals etc. generate massive amount of data regarding hospital in-stay, regular patients visit, health checkups and preventive medical programmes (Steinwachs & Hughes, 2008). Awareness has been paid by medical professionals to make this information easily accessible to visual impaired patients (Naidu, 2009). Such attention

Figure 3. Healthcare services for vision impaired patients

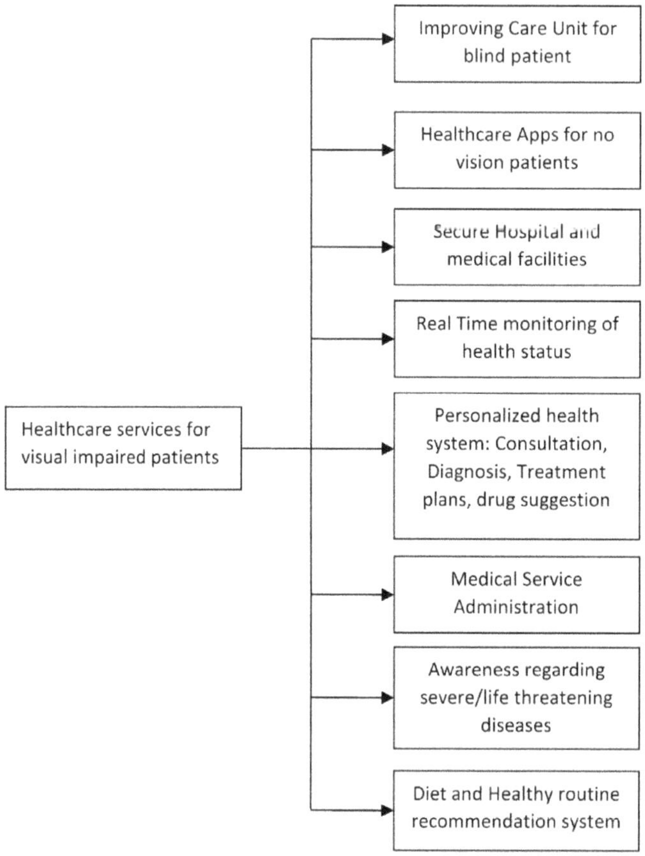

leads to great access to all medical related information and could help in enhancing the health status of low or blind vision people.

Figure 3 presents the core medical services required for visual impaired patients:

- Specialized treatment and diagnosis procedures are required for meeting the expectation of blind people. Still most of the hospitals and pathology labs do not have active strategy and arrangement for dealing with person with vision disability (Mosadeghrad, 2014). Healthcare sector created some strategies and protocols for blind people but rarely was it utilized by the hospitals. Owing to the blind sufferers face frightening situation especially when dealing with severe health issues (Lee et al., 2006).
- Reading material like not to do list during pregnancy, infants care literature, or diagnosed with severe disease like cancer, AIDS etc. is easily accessible to normal patients but what about patients with no vision. Models are required which can read the selected information from a given resource so that one may take preventive measures (Kasper et al., 1992).
- No vision patients face major challenges in getting safe medical care which is cost and time effective and is of high quality. Four major concern of blind people are: Respect, communication medium, receiving prescription or other laboratory reports in inaccessible format (i.e. not in Braille

text), and last interaction with hospital staff and doctors. Higher quality mobile based or e-tools are required which incorporate all these basic needs of blind patients. Awareness about issues associated with blind patients is vital for designing good healthcare model for visual impaired patients (O'day et al., 2004). Advanced computational techniques must be utilized for information access, medical facilities, disease diagnosis, communication medium and administrative strategies; text to speech and speech to text enabled systems are required to meet individual needs.

Performance Evaluation Methods

The evaluation of any model, apps, assisting devices is very significant task to understand the quality of methods, models, techniques, training data, learning algorithms, refining parameters for the given set of data. Evaluation methods are benchmark to examine the efficiency and performance of any assisting devices. Evaluating the performance of machine learning techniques and learning algorithms is an elementary feature of AI. Some evaluation methods are: Cross validation, hold out method, random sub sampling, bootstrap, confusion matrix. Some evaluation criteria enhance the performance of assisting devices are highlighted as following:

- **Scalability**: It is the ability of a model which can effectively work on given large dataset. Assisting devices perceive huge amount of data from current environment in real time so the devices must be able to perform effectively on it.
- **Simplicity**: Assisting devices must be as simple as they can easily be operated by visually impaired people. Simplicity of any system is dependable on its size, GUI, dependency on other system, coupling, and cohesion. To make it easier to use, assisting devices should be simple to operate.
- **Reliability**: The electronic assisting devices must also be reliable to work in any situation. These devices must be authentic and genuine.
- **Usability**: As the model is intended for visually impaired people it must be easy to use. These mobile based technologies are easy to use and must possess text to speech and speech to text converter for the ease of blind patients so that one can call or send messages in case of emergency.

CONCLUSION

Researchers are gaining attention for developing smart healthcare apps for visually impaired patients. Recent technological advances in wearable devices, mobile technologies, sensors, data structure and algorithm and embedded technology clutch assurance to develop latest vision technology that can address the basic health need of visually impaired patients. Main conclusion of this study is to address smart technologies for creating healthcare model for blind patients. One can create and use smart healthcare models for no vision patients. Main idea is to connect them with their smart phones with voice assistant for navigating into the system. Main emphasis is on the designing of prototype for mobile apps that can be easily operated by blind patients and assist them in solving their health-related issues like they can consult doctor online, suggestion of drugs, automatic calling to some predefined numbers in case of urgency, disease diagnosis etc. Development of smart health apps would help in smoothing the way for healthy lifestyle for visually impaired patients and assist them in case of severe health issues or emergency.

REFERENCES

AbdulRasool, D., & Sabra, S. (2011, June). Mobile-embedded smart guide for the blind. In *International Conference on Digital Information and Communication Technology and Its Applications* (pp. 571-578). Springer.

Ahmed, T., Hoyle, R., Shaffer, P., Connelly, K., Crandall, D., & Kapadia, A. (2017). Understanding the Physical Safety, Security, and Privacy Concerns of People with Visual Impairments. *IEEE Internet Computing*, *21*(3), 56–63. doi:10.1109/MIC.2017.77

Bhardwaj, R., Nambiar, A. R., & Dutta, D. (2017, July). A Study of Machine Learning in Healthcare. In *Computer Software and Applications Conference (COMPSAC), 2017 IEEE 41st Annual* (Vol. 2, pp. 236-241). IEEE.

Billi, M., Burzagli, L., Catarci, T., Santucci, G., Bertini, E., Gabbanini, F., & Palchetti, E. (2010). A unified methodology for the evaluation of accessibility and usability of mobile applications. *Universal Access in the Information Society*, *9*(4), 337–356. doi:10.100710209-009-0180-1

Boegl, K., Adlassnig, K. P., Hayashi, Y., Rothenfluh, T. E., & Leitich, H. (2004). Knowledge acquisition in the fuzzy knowledge representation framework of a medical consultation system. *Artificial Intelligence in Medicine*, *30*(1), 1–26. doi:10.1016/S0933-3657(02)00073-8 PMID:14684262

Briggs, A., & Gray, A. (1999). Methods in health service research: Handling uncertainty in economic evaluations of healthcare interventions. *BMJ (Clinical Research Ed.)*, *319*(7210), 635–638. doi:10.1136/bmj.319.7210.635 PMID:10473486

Cabena, P., Hadjinian, P., Stadler, R., Verhees, J., & Zanasi, A. (1997). Discovering data mining: from concept to implementation. Prentice Hall PTR.

Cernazanu-Glavan, C., Todinca, D., & Precup, R. E. (2014, May). DeeDee-A mobile intelligent system able to assist a type 1 diabetic through the daily life. In *Applied Computational Intelligence and Informatics (SACI), 2014 IEEE 9th International Symposium on* (pp. 343-347). IEEE.

Chang, H. (2015). Book Review: Data-Driven Healthcare & Analytics in a Big Data World. *Healthcare Informatics Research*, *21*(1), 61. doi:10.4258/hir.2015.21.1.61

Chaudhry, M., Kamran, M., & Afzal, S. (2008). Speaking monuments—design and implementation of an RFID based blind friendly environment. In *Electrical Engineering, 2008. ICEE 2008. Second International Conference on* (pp. 1-6). IEEE.

Cios, K. J. (2000). From the guest editor medical data mining and knowledge discovery. *IEEE Engineering in Medicine and Biology Magazine*, *19*(4), 15–16. doi:10.1109/MEMB.2000.853477 PMID:10916728

Coughlan, J. M., & Miele, J. (2017). AR4VI: AR as an Accessibility Tool for People with Visual Impairments. In *Mixed and Augmented Reality (ISMAR-Adjunct), 2017 IEEE International Symposium on* (pp. 288-292). IEEE.

Crasto, C. J., Marenco, L. N., Migliore, M., Mao, B., Nadkarni, P. M., Miller, P., & Shepherd, G. M. (2003). Text mining neuroscience journal articles to populate neuroscience databases. *Neuroinformatics*, *1*(3), 215–237. doi:10.1385/NI:1:3:215 PMID:15046245

De Souza Veriscimo, E., & Bernardes, J. L. (2015). A New 3D Interaction Technique Accessible to the Visually Impaired. In *2015 XVII Symposium on Virtual and Augmented Reality (SVR)* (pp. 208-211). IEEE. 10.1109/SVR.2015.37

Dilsizian, S. E., & Siegel, E. L. (2014). Artificial intelligence in medicine and cardiac imaging: Harnessing big data and advanced computing to provide personalized medical diagnosis and treatment. *Current Cardiology Reports*, *16*(1), 441. doi:10.100711886-013-0441-8 PMID:24338557

Ding, J., Berleant, D., Nettleton, D., & Wurtele, E. (2001). Mining MEDLINE: Abstracts, sentences, or phrases? *InBiocomputing*, *2002*, 326–337. PMID:11928487

Emiliani, P. L., & Stephanidis, C. (2005). Universal access to ambient intelligence environments: Opportunities and challenges for people with disabilities. *IBM Systems Journal*, *44*(3), 605–619. doi:10.1147j.443.0605

Espique, F. P. (2010). Notice of Retraction Provisions of computer technology in the learning development of students with visual impairment. In *Computer Engineering and Technology (ICCET), 2010 2nd International Conference on* (Vol. 7, pp. V7-547). IEEE.

Geman, O., & Chiuchisan, I. (2015). A health care self-monitoring system for patients with visual impairment using a network of sensors. In E-Health and Bioengineering Conference (EHB), 2015 (pp. 1-4). IEEE.

Hii, P. C., & Chung, W. Y. (2011). A comprehensive ubiquitous healthcare solution on an Android™ mobile device. *Sensors (Basel)*, *11*(7), 6799–6815. doi:10.3390110706799 PMID:22163986

Jothi, R., Kayalvizhi, M., & Sagadevan, K. (2017). Smart walking stick for visually challenged people. *Asian J. Appl. Sci. Technol*, *1*, 274–276.

Kakria, P., Tripathi, N. K., & Kitipawang, P. (2015). A real-time health monitoring system for remote cardiac patients using smartphone and wearable sensors. *International Journal of Telemedicine and Applications*, *2015*, 8. doi:10.1155/2015/373474 PMID:26788055

Kasper, J. F., Mulley, J. A. Jr, & Wennberg, J. E. (1992). Developing shared decision-making programs to improve the quality of health care. *QRB. Quality Review Bulletin*, *18*(6), 183–190. doi:10.1016/S0097-5990(16)30531-0 PMID:1379705

Ker, J., Wang, L., Rao, J., & Lim, T. (2018). Deep learning applications in medical image analysis. *IEEE Access: Practical Innovations, Open Solutions*, *6*, 9375–9389. doi:10.1109/ACCESS.2017.2788044

Khan, M. N. H., Arovi, M. A. H., Mahmud, H., Hasan, M. K., & Rubaiyeat, H. A. (2015). Speech based text correction tool for the visually impaired. In *Computer and Information Technology (ICCIT), 2015 18th International Conference on* (pp. 150-155). IEEE.

Khemmarat, S., & Gao, L. (2015). Supporting drug prescription via predictive and personalized query system. In *Pervasive Computing Technologies for Healthcare (PervasiveHealth), 2015 9th International Conference on* (pp. 9-16). IEEE.

Kwon, O. Y., Shin, S. H., Shin, S. J., & Kim, W. S. (2010). Design of U-health system with the use of smart phone and sensor network. In *Ubiquitous Information Technologies and Applications (CUTE), 2010 Proceedings of the 5th International Conference on* (pp. 1-6). IEEE.

Lee, P. M., Khong, P., & Ghista, D. N. (2006). Impact of deficient healthcare service quality. *The TQM Magazine*, *18*(6), 563–571. doi:10.1108/09544780610707075

Leonard, J. E., Colombe, J. B., & Levy, J. L. (2002). Finding relevant references to genes and proteins in Medline using a Bayesian approach. *Bioinformatics (Oxford, England)*, *18*(11), 1515–1522. doi:10.1093/bioinformatics/18.11.1515 PMID:12424124

Li, X., Liu, X., Zhang, Z., Xia, Y., & Qian, S. (2010). Design of Health Eating System Based on Web Data Mining. In *Information Engineering (ICIE), 2010 WASE International Conference on* (Vol. 1, pp. 346-349). IEEE.

Lodh, T., Subramaniam, A., & Paswan, A. K. (2016). Ultrasound based assistive mobility devices for the visually-impaired. In *Power India International Conference (PIICON), 2016 IEEE 7th* (pp. 1-6). IEEE.

Masud, M., Adel Serhani, M., & Navaz, A. (2017). Resource-Aware Mobile-Based Health Monitoring. *IEEE Journal of Biomedical and Health Informatics*, *21*(2), 349–360. doi:10.1109/JBHI.2016.2525006 PMID:26863682

McLaughlin, C., & Fitzgerald, C. (2001). Converging genetics and information technologies and the emerging healthcare system. *International Journal of Healthcare Technology and Management*, *3*(5/6), 498. doi:10.1504/IJHTM.2001.001125

Mosadeghrad, A. M. (2014). Factors influencing healthcare service quality. *International Journal of Health Policy and Management*, *3*(2), 77–89. doi:10.15171/ijhpm.2014.65 PMID:25114946

Naidu, A. (2009). Factors affecting patient satisfaction and healthcare quality. *International Journal of Health Care Quality Assurance*, *22*(4), 366–381. doi:10.1108/09526860910964834 PMID:19725209

Nalavade, K. C., Bharmal, F., Deore, T., & Patil, A. (2014). Use of ultrasonic sensors, GPS and GSM technology to implement alert and tracking system for blind man. *Proceedings of the International Conference of Advance Research and Innovation (ICARI)*, 272-274.

Nambiar, R., Bhardwaj, R., Sethi, A., & Vargheese, R. (2013). A look at challenges and opportunities of big data analytics in healthcare. In *Big Data, 2013 IEEE International Conference on* (pp. 17-22). IEEE.

O'day, B. L., Killeen, M., & Iezzoni, L. I. (2004). Improving health care experiences of persons who are blind or have low vision: Suggestions from focus groups. *American Journal of Medical Quality*, *19*(5), 193–200. doi:10.1177/106286060401900503 PMID:15532911

Ocampo, M. G., Leal, E. H., Cadavid, J. M., Gómez, D. E., & Méndez, N. D. (2016). Application of a technical tool to support the inclusion process of people with visual impairment in an educational web platform. In *Learning Objects and Technology (LACLO), Latin American Conference on* (pp. 1-5). IEEE.

Pittman, P. (2010). Health Services Research in 2020: data and methods needs for the future. *Health Services Research, 45*(5), 1431-1441.

Quigley, D. D., Elliott, M. N., Setodji, C. M., & Hays, R. D. (2018). Quantifying Magnitude of Group-Level Differences in Patient Experiences with Health Care. *Health Services Research*, *53*, 3027–3051. doi:10.1111/1475-6773.12828 PMID:29435975

Ravı, D., Wong, C., Deligianni, F., Berthelot, M., Andreu-Perez, J., Lo, B., & Yang, G. Z. (2017). Deep learning for health informatics. *IEEE Journal of Biomedical and Health Informatics*, *21*(1), 4–21. doi:10.1109/JBHI.2016.2636665 PMID:28055930

Sivan, S., & Darsan, G. (2016). Computer Vision based Assistive Technology for Blind and Visually Impaired People. In *Proceedings of the 7th International Conference on Computing Communication and Networking Technologies* (p. 41). ACM. 10.1145/2967878.2967923

Snae, C., & Brueckner, M. (2008). Personal health assistance service expert system (PHASES). *International Journal of Biological and Medical Sciences*, *1*(2), 109–112.

Steinwachs, D. M., & Hughes, R. G. (2008). *Health services research: Scope and significance*. Academic Press.

Sujith, B., & Safeeda, V. (2014). Computer Vision-Based Aid for the Visually Impaired Persons-A Survey and Proposing New Framework. *International Journal of Innovative Research in Computer and Communication Engineering*.

Sun, J., & Reddy, C. K. (2013, August). Big data analytics for healthcare. In *Proceedings of the 19th ACM SIGKDD international conference on Knowledge discovery and data mining* (pp. 1525-1525). ACM. 10.1145/2487575.2506178

Velázquez, R. (2010). Wearable assistive devices for the blind. In *Wearable and autonomous biomedical devices and systems for smart environment* (pp. 331–349). Berlin: Springer. doi:10.1007/978-3-642-15687-8_17

Wickramasinghe, N. (2010). The Role for Knowledge Management in Modern Healthcare Delivery. *International Journal of Healthcare Delivery Reform Initiatives*, *2*(2), 1–9. doi:10.4018/jhdri.2010040101

Zhang, S., McClean, S. I., Nugent, C. D., Donnelly, M. P., Galway, L., Scotney, B. W., & Cleland, I. (2014). A predictive model for assistive technology adoption for people with dementia. *IEEE Journal of Biomedical and Health Informatics*, *18*(1), 375–383. doi:10.1109/JBHI.2013.2267549 PMID:24403437

Chapter 13
Despeckling Algorithms for Optical Coherence Tomography Images: A Review

Anoop B. N.
National Institute of Technology Karnataka, India

G. N. Girish
National Institute of Technology Karnataka, India

Sudeep P. V.
National Institute of Technology Calicut, India

Jeny Rajan
National Institute of Technology Karnataka, India

ABSTRACT

Optical coherence tomography (OCT) is a non-invasive imaging technique widely used in ophthalmology. The presence of speckle affects the quality of OCT images. Despeckling is necessary to improve its visual quality, and it is an integral part of software packages used for the computerized analysis of OCT. Even though a few methods for despeckling OCT are available in the literature, a cross-comparison of their performance is not known to be available. In this chapter, the techniques available in the literature for despeckling the OCT images have been identified. The results of the despeckling algorithms are compared both qualitatively and quantitatively by concerning the noise suppression capability and feature preservation. Among the available techniques, iterative adaptive unbiased (IAUB) filter is found to be superior as far as its performance regarding despeckling on retinal OCT images.

DOI: 10.4018/978-1-5225-7796-6.ch013

INTRODUCTION

Second, to the brain, the eyes are the most complex organ in human body (Gregory, 2015). The eye consists of complex mechanisms and pathways and with the help of several structures like the cornea, retina, iris, pupils, optic nerves and the ciliary muscles. All these parts work together to help the eye function properly and make our vision perfect.

The retina is a thin layered tissue (Gupta et al., 2016). It is situated near to the optic nerve. Retina collects the light focused by the lens and converts the luminance into nerve impulse. Nerve impulses are transmitted through the optic nerve to the visual cortex to establish the vision. The retina contains a layer of photoreceptor cells on its surface. These cells are light-sensitive cells, capable of detecting physical quantities such as color and luminous intensity. The retina processes the information gathered by the photoreceptor cells and sends this information to the visual cortex of the brain through the optic nerve. Due to the retina's critical role in vision, its degradation may cause permanent blindness.

The normal retina comprises retinal pigment epithelium and neuroretina. The neuroretina includes inner and outer segments of photoreceptors (rods and cones), outer nuclear layer, nerve fiber layer, inner nuclear layer, outer plexiform layer, external limiting membrane, ganglion cell layer, inner plexiform layer, and internal limiting membrane. Commonly found retinal pathologies include degenerations (notably age-related macular degeneration), neoplasms, toxicities, inflammatory diseases, congenital abnormalities, retinal detachment, retinal vascular diseases, dystrophies, retinal involvement of systemic diseases and trauma. The thickness of the retina measured from OCT is helpful to characterize many diseases. The retinal layer thickness can be used as a potential biomarker to understand the progression of the diseases and the underlying pathologies (Gupta et al., 2016).

OCT is a non-invasive imaging technology (Drexler et al., 2001), widely used in ophthalmology (Aum et al., 2015; Chiu et al., 2010; Fabritius et al., 2009) for the diagnosis of chronic diseases like macular degeneration (Guillonneau et al., 2017), glaucoma (Khaing & Aimmanee, 2017), cataract (Zhang et al., 2017) and retinal detachment (Wu et al., 2017). As per the report of World Health Organization (WHO) (Blindness and visual impairment, 2018, retrieved from http://www.who.int/news-room/fact-sheets/detail/blindness-and-visual-impairment) 84% of the visual impairments results from the diseases mentioned earlier (Delcourt et al., 2010; Isar; Yorston, 2003; Shah, 2009). Mainly, OCT is helpful to quantify the

Figure 1. (a) Zeiss Cirrus HD OCT machine, (b) The crossectional visualization of the human eye using OCT

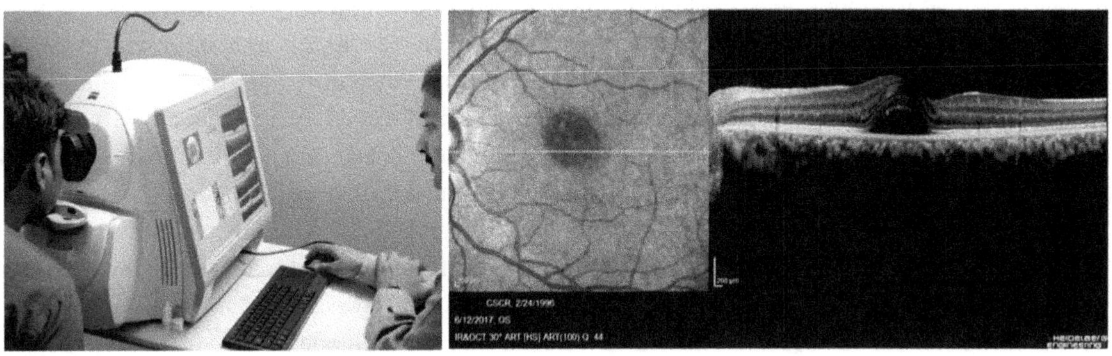

(a) (b)

thickness of retinal layers (Mayer et al., 2008; Chiu et al., 2010) and for the diagnosis of Cystoid Macular Edema (CME) (Girish et al., 2017; Girish et al., 2018a; Girish et al., 2018b; Samagaio et al., 2018) and age-related macular degeneration(Muftuoglu et al., 2018). It is extensively employed in neonates and pediatric cases to characterize the development of the retina (Lee et al., 2013). Another interesting fact about OCT is that it uses coherent light to catch micrometre or sub-micrometre resolution (Carrasco et al., 2006; Povazay et al., 2002). The capturing of retinal layers using Zeiss Cirrus HD OCT machine is shown in Figure 1 (a). The crossectional visualization of the human eye using OCT is given in Figure 1(b).

In principle, OCT works similar to ultrasound (US) imaging systems, based on interferometric techniques. However, in practice, OCT make use of light beams in position of sound profiles in US system (Kennedy et al., 2010). As in US imaging, speckle noise hampers the quality of OCT and limits its clinical utility. Speckle arises because of the coherence of optical waves (Schmitt, 1999; Bashkansky & Reintjes, 2000) and destroys the edges of the retinal layers and the cystic boundaries. Hence, despeckling of OCT images is a significant preprocessing stage for the proper diagnosis of the retinal disorders and its quantification. The objective of the chapter is to study the methods available in the literature to remove the speckle present in the OCT.

The remaining part of the chapter is arranged as follows. Section 2 discusses the speckle models and despeckling schemes available in the literature. Section 3 compares the performance of the despeckling schemes available in the literature. Finally, Section 4 ends up with a course summary.

BACKGROUND

The literature addressing the removal of speckle in OCT can be classified into two categories, models governing the speckle and algorithms for its elimination.

Speckle Models

Prior knowledge about the statistical behaviour of noise present in the OCT is necessary before designing despeckling techniques. According to Schmitt (1999) when a more quantity of polarized quasi-monochromatic waves with random phase fuse, well developed speckle patterns are formed. Schmitt (1999) also stated that the speckle follows a decaying exponential distribution. Bashkansky and Reintjes (2000) calculated the statistics of speckle directly from the statistical field on the detector and suggested that speckle follows a Gaussian distribution. Pircher et al. (2003) used the field back-scattered from the illuminated sample to model the speckle instead of the statistical field on the detector and employed Rayleigh distribution to express the statistical behaviour of the speckle. Karamata et al. (2005) also agreed with the Rayleigh distribution of speckle. After few years, Vegas et al. (2010) showed that Gamma distribution is suitable for the speckles present in the ultrasound images. In accordance with the Vegas et al. (2010), Sudeep et al. (2016) proposed a denoising method based on Gamma distribution for the speckle reduction in OCT. It was demonstrated that the Gamma distribution could adapt to the standard distributions like exponential, normal, Chi-square, and Rayleigh. Figure 3 depicts the distribution of homogeneous regions of real OCT images (Figure 2) obtained from different scanners. Comparison with the actual Gamma distribution with parameters computed out of a few selected similar fields indicates that the distribution can be approximated with a Gamma PDF based model.

Figure 2. OCT scans of different vendors from OPTIMA dataset, (a) Spectralis, (b) Nidek, (c) Topcon, (d) Cirrus

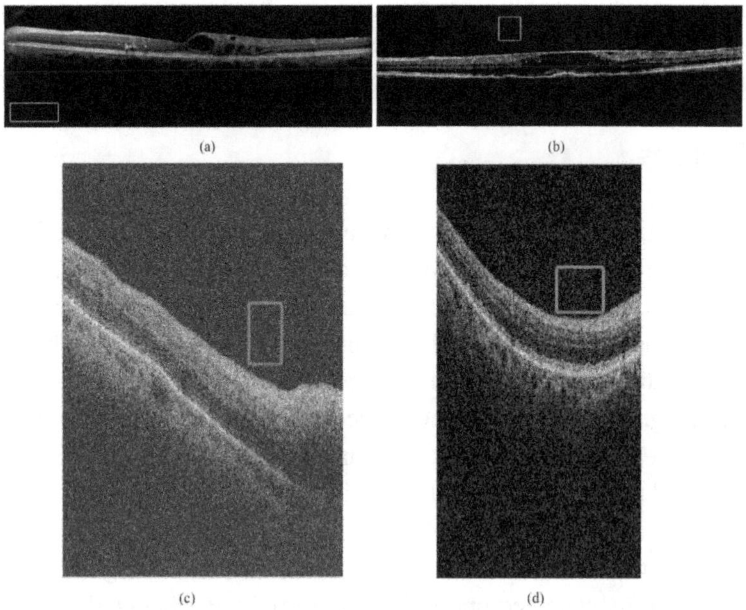

Figure 3. The distribution of homogeneous regions(in red box) of real OCT images, (a) Spectralis, (b) Nidek, (c) Topcon, (d) Cirrus

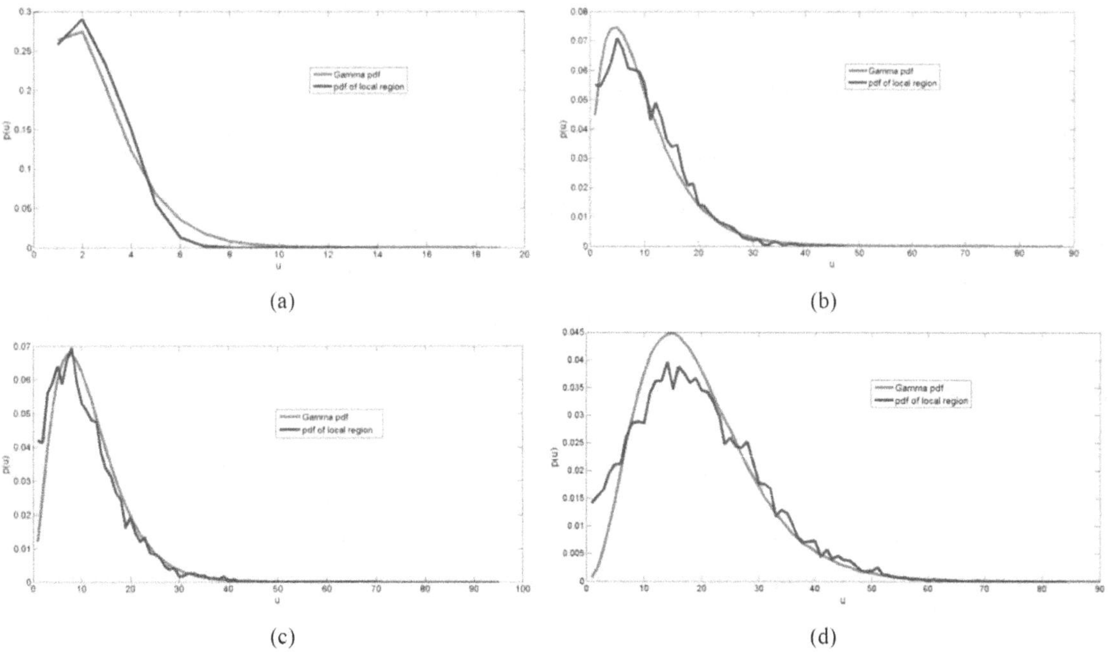

Despeckling Schemes

The despeckling schemes can be broadly classified into two, hardware modification termed as complex domain methods and analytical manipulations. The analytical methods are usually done at the post-processing stage, termed as magnitude domain methods (Kafieh et al., 2015).

Hardware Modifications

In this approach, noise is mitigated through hardware modifications before the image formation. The modifications meant for reducing the noise can be either in the optical setup or in the imaged subject itself.

Modification in the optical setup refers to alterations made on the incident angle of the laser beam. One of the approaches in this category was by Bashkansky & Reintjes (2000). They detected the optical signal in the exact backscattered direction and averaged it over different angles of incidence. Angular compounding by path length encoding was the choice of Iftimia et al. (2003). Ramrath et al. (2008) averaged the images obtained from different incident angles to alleviate the effect of speckle. Desjardins et al. (2006) also expressed the confidence that alteration in the recording angle of the reflected light is helpful for reducing the speckle.

Other design modifications available in the literature include sequential angular compounding proposed by Hughes et al. (2010) and frequency compounding put forth by Pircher et al. (2003). The averaging of multiple projections (Sander et al. (2005)) or their co-registration (Jrgensen et al. (2007); Ferguson et al. (2004)) are among the most popular techniques. A polarization sensitive OCT system proposed by Gotzinger et al. (2005) is another sophisticated technique for eliminating speckle.

Post-Processing Filters

Traditional methods for despeckling includes mean filter (Ishikawa et al., 2005; Mayer et al., 2008; Hee et al., 1995; Huang et al., 1991), median filter (George et al., 2000; Koozekanani et al., 2001; Rogowska & Brezinski, 2002; Baroni et al., 2007; Herzog et al., 2004; Shahidi et al., 2005; Boyer et al., 2006; Srinivasan et al., 2008), Lee filter (Lee et al., 2013), enhanced Lee filter (Ozcan et al., 2007), Wiener filter (Ozcan et al., 2007), and geodesic denoising (Varnousfaderani et al., 2016). In the mean filter, each pixel in the image is substituted by the average of its neighbourhood pixels. In the median filter, the median of the neighbourhood pixels is taken into account instead of mean. Unlike mean and median filters, Lee filter (Lee et al., 2013) is a local statistic filter which uses the mean and variance of pixels within a neighbourhood window of arbitrary radius. In one of the extensions of Lee filter termed as enhanced Lee filter, the filter is applied separately on pre-segmented heterogeneous regions.

Similar to Lee filter, the restored intensity in a Wiener filter is computed from mean and variance of gray levels in the neighbourhood window and from the global estimate of the noise. There is another practice of computing the restored intensity by averaging the similar pixels or patches from the entire image, rather than from a neighbourhood of restricted dimension. This practice is usually called as Nonlocal Means (NLM) denoising. Recently, Varnousfaderani et al. (2016) have used Geodesic denoising for despeckling OCT images. In this scheme, the patch distributions were computed initially via cluster sampling. It was assumed that the two patches are similar and the geodesic distance between them is minimum when the patch distributions are identical. The Geodesic weighted average of random samples from the patches identical to the patch corresponding to the noisy pixel was considered as the restored intensity. Aum et al. (2015), Liu et al. (2016) and Cuartas-Vélez et al. (2018) also used the potential of NLM filter for despeckling OCT. Double Gaussian anisotropic kernels were used as an alternative for the conventional homogeneous kernel in NLM. Chen et al. (2015, 2018) suggested that a horizontally stretched rectangular search window is optimal for NLM when used on OCT. Methods based on bilateral filter for denoising OCT is also proposed in the literature. In the bilateral filter, a neighbourhood pixel is believed to be similar to the contextual pixel if it is near to the contextual pixel both radiometrically and spatially. Anantrasirichai et al. (2014) employed a cascade of wavelet shrinkage and bilateral filter for despeckling application. Sudeep et al. (2016) tried out the iterative version of the bilateral filter for speckle removal in multiframe OCT data. Anisotropic diffusion filter (AD) (Fernandez et al., 2004; Gregori & Knighton, 2004; Garvin et al., 2008; Puvanathasan & Bizheva, 2009; Zhang et al., 2017; Bernardes et al., 2010; Salinas & Fernandez, 2007; Cheng et al., 2014) is another nonlinear spatial filter. In AD filter the average of a fraction of local gradients is added to the contextual pixel such that the contextual pixel comes closer to its neighbourhood pixels in greyscale space.

Apart from bilateral, AD, and NLM filters, Total variational (TV) minimization is one of the most popular edge preserving filtering technique. Duan et al. (2015) proposed split Bregman algorithm based variational model for image decomposition model for OCT despeckling. In this procedure, the noisy image is decomposed into noise-free data, edge map, and noise. Duan et al. (2016) proposed a second order total generalized variation decomposition for despeckling OCT. Ren et al. (2016) also made use of the method of variational image decomposition in which OCT is decomposed into cartoon part, texture and speckle. I-Divergence regularization (Marks et al., 2005), is another extension of TV despeckling approach. Inline with these efforts, Schirrmacher et al. (2017), tried to solve median filter regularization problem under Huber data fidelity constraints with the help of augmented Lagrangian optimization.

Apart from linear and nonlinear spatial filters and frequency domain filters, wavelet domain techniques (Adler et al., 2004; Zlokolica et al., 2007; Gupta et al., 2008; Pizurica et al., 2008; Quellec et al., 2010; Isar; Mayer et al., 2012; Stankiewicz et al., 2017; Chitchian et al., 2009; Rabbani et al., 2013) are also suggested for despeckling OCT. In wavelet despeckling, the fundamental procedure is wavelet thresholding in which the wavelet coefficients in the selected sub-bands with magnitude greater than an arbitrary threshold are attenuated. Wavelet thresholding is otherwise called wavelet shrinkage. As mentioned, all the wavelet denoising techniques are based on wavelet shrinkage. They differ only in the selection of mother wavelet and the method for determining the threshold. The most popular choices of mother wavelet while despeckling OCT is haar wavelet (Mayer et al., 2012; Stankiewicz et al., 2017), dual tree wavelet transform (DTCWT) (Forouzanfar & Moghaddam, 2007; Kajic et al., 2012; Kajic et al. 2010), Contourlet Transform (Dong et al., 2013), Curvelet Transform (Jian et al., 2009, 2010), and wave atom transform (Du et al., 2014). The Adaptive method for defining the threshold available in literature includes bishrink (Isar) and Circular symmetric Laplacian Mixture Model (Kafeh et al., 2013).

Another practice of despeckling OCT is based on the principal component analysis (PCA) (Luan & Wu, 2013; Bian et al., 2015; Baghaie et al., 2015). This method decomposes the image into a low-rank matrix of a denoised image and a sparse matrix of speckle. Liu et al. (2016) adopted a two-stage patch based despeckling technique which makes use of singular value decomposition followed by optimization using the noisy prior. It's well known that SVD is based on PCA. Inline with this, the dictionary-based denoising proposed by Kafeh et al. (2015) was based on K-SVD, a decomposition model based on generalized *k*-means. K-SVD makes use of the directional sensitivity of DT-CWT. Fuller et al. (2007) demonstrated that Support Vector Machine is useful in soft computing based despeckling. Bayesian denoising available for OCT denoising is a similar approach (Wong et al., 2010; Rajabi & Zirak, 2016). The speckle reduction algorithm based on an ensemble framework of Multi-Layer Perceptron (MLP) proposed by Adabi et al. (2016, 2018), make use of local statistics of the neighbourhood pixels and features of the wavelet sub-bands of the block obtained via decomposition. The denoising scheme put forth by Fang et al. (2012), (2013) is also multiscale sparsity-based method. Meiniel et al. (2017) proposed a Total variation Sparsity-based image reconstruction based on compressed sensing for enhancing the quality of OCT images. The despeckling scheme introduced by Lv et.al. (2018), Muramatsu et al. (2015), is based on dictionary learning which uses non-separable oversampled lapped transform and iterative hard thresholding. Amini & Rabbani (2017) employed a despeckling scheme based on the spatially constrained Gaussian mixture model. The graph-based despeckling proposed by Bogunovic et al. (2014), is based on random sample consensus which makes use of a transform. Other despeckling schemes available for OCT are rotating kernel based transform (Rogowska & Brezinski, 2002), directional filtering approach (Bagci et al., 2008), and Adaptive vector-valued kernel (Mishra et al., 2009).

COMPARATIVE STUDY

Experimental Setup

From the above discussed despeckling algorithms, six recently proposed methods are chosen to study and compare the efficiency of despeckling OCT images. These methods are implemented on MATLAB 2017b platform, which is been installed on a workstation with a 64bit windows 10 operating system, Intel Xeon processor E5-2650 (Intel, Mountain View, CA), solid state hard drive and 64 GB of RAM.

Dataset

The performance of the despeckling algorithms were analysed by performing experiments using three different datasets. The test images used for the first experiment are the standard noise-free phantom of size 512x512, simulated via the modified Shepp-Logan algorithm (Shepp & Logan (1974)). Qualitative and quantitative analysis of the selected methods were performed on this image. The second is the Duke dataset (Fang et al. (2013)). This dataset contains 18 patients' information. They are acquired from Bioptigen, Inc. (Durham, NC, USA) by 840-nm wavelength SDOCT imaging systems with an axial resolution of ~4.5μm per pixel in tissue. Each patient's information is associated with synthetically generated ground truth images by averaging multiple near-noise free frames. The third is the OPTIMA challenge dataset (OPTIMA cyst segmentation challenge (2015)). It Contains OCT images from four different vendors, namely Spectralis Heidelberg, Topcon, Zeiss Cirrus and Nidek. The images of the different OCT vendors is shown in Figure 2.

Methodology

This section describes the flow of the experiments conducted on the three different datasets (Figure 4.). The first is despeckling experimentation process with phantom images of size 512x512. The noise-free phantom image is generated using the modified Shepp-Logan algorithm. These noise-free phantom image pixel intensities are further normalised into the pixel intensities of range 0-255. Then these pixel intensities are mixed with multiplicative noise which follows the Gamma pdf.

Figure 4. Block diagram showing the various steps involved in the despeckling experimentation process

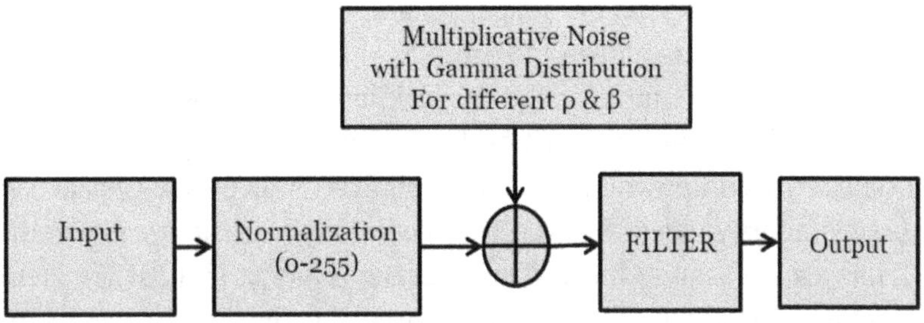

The Gamma distribution (Sudeep et al. 2016) with respect to the shape (ρ) and scale (β) are described as,

$$f\left(x;\rho,\beta\right)=\frac{x^{\rho-1}e^{\frac{-x}{\beta}}}{\beta^{\rho}\Gamma\left(\rho\right)}\,for\,x>0,and\,\rho,\beta>0 \tag{1}$$

where $\Gamma(\rho)$ is the Gamma function (Dubey,1970) defined as,

$$\Gamma\left(\rho\right)=\int_{0}^{\infty}x^{\rho-1}e^{-x}dx \tag{2}$$

Figure 5. (a) Noise-free phantom, (b) phantom images after adding speckle noise with (ρ=3 β=2), (c) phantom images after adding speckle noise with (ρ=4 β=3), (d) phantom images after adding speckle noise with (ρ=4 β=4), (e) phantom images after adding speckle noise with (ρ=6 β=6), (f) phantom images after adding speckle noise with (ρ=8 β=7)

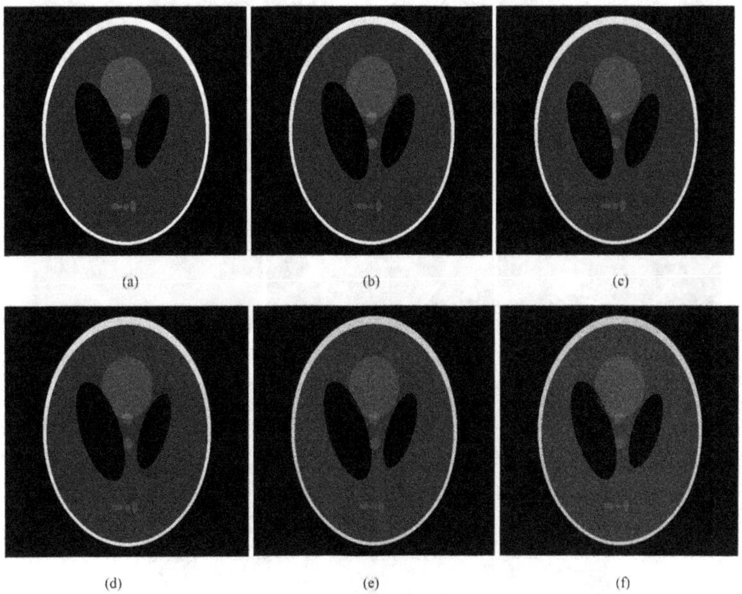

Following the noise generation procedure proposed by Sudeep et al. (2016), five different images of noisy-phantom are generated by varying the shape (ρ) and scale (β) parameters of Gamma pdf and the images with different noise levels are shown in Figure 5.

These noisy phantom images are input to the despeckling algorithms selected for comparison. The outputs of the despeckling filters are analysed both qualitatively and quantitatively. The quantitative analysis is made possible by well-known image quality analysis indices like as peak signal to noise ratio (PSNR) and structured similarity index (SSIM). The second experiment is with synthetic OCT images. The synthetic OCT images are acquired from Duke dataset (Fang et al. (2013)). Here the only change in the experimental setup is the usage of a different dataset. The third experiment is with real OCT images. The performance evaluation of the despeckling algorithms on the real 3D OCT data generated by different vendors is made possible with the help of OPTIMA dataset.

Qualitative Analysis

In this section, the performance of the state-of-the art techniques for despeckling OCT, available in the literature, is compared objectively and qualitatively. The techniques whose despeckling performance is compared are TGV, wavelet-based denoising, curvature anisotropic diffusion, KSVD with DTCWT,

Figure 6. (a) Noise-free phantom, (b) phantom images after adding speckle noise with (ρ=4 β=4), (c) despeckled image with TGV, (d) despeckled image with Wavelet thresholding, (e) despeckled image with Curvature anisotropic diffusion, (f) despeckled image with KSVD with DTCWT (g), despeckled image with OBNLM, (h) despeckled image with IAUB.

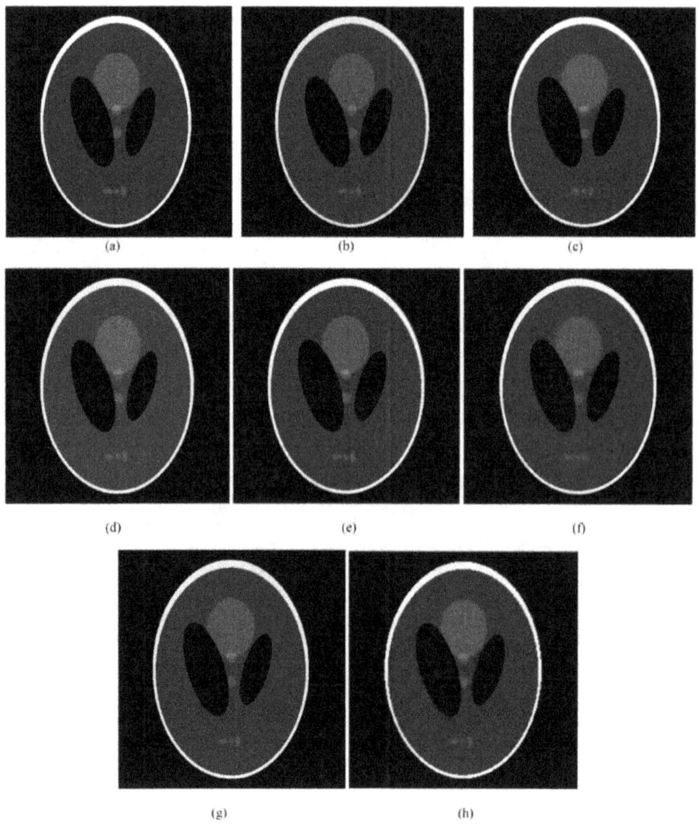

OBNLM and IAUB. The performance of these despeckling schemes is compared on two kinds of test images. The test images of the first kind are produced by mixing speckle noise with standard noise-free phantom, simulated via modified Shepp-logan algorithm (Shepp & Logan (1974)). To produce test images of different noise levels, the shape parameter ($\rho = 4$) and scale parameter ($\beta = 4$) in the noise model (Sudeep et al. (2016)) for simulating speckle noise are varied. The second kind of test images is real-time OCT images (Fang et al. (2013)) with a known noise-free ground truth. Images of the noise-free phantom, phantom images after introducing speckle noise ($\rho = 4$, $\beta = 4$) and despeckled images from the above mentioned despeckling schemes are shown in Figure 6.

The zoomed portions of images of the noise-free phantom, phantom images after introducing speckle noise ($\rho = 4$, $\beta = 4$) and the despeckled images from the above mentioned despeckling schemes are shown in Figure 7.

It can be observed that speckle is not fully suppressed and noise is left in the images denoised with Wavelet thresholding (Figure 6(d) and Figure 7(d)), Curvature anisotropic diffusion (Figure 6(e) and

Figure 7. Zoomed portions of (a) noise-free phantom, (b) phantom images after adding speckle noise with (β=4 ρ=4), (c) despeckled image with TGV, (d) despeckled image with Wavelet thresholding, (e) despeckled image with Curvature anisotropic diffusion, (f) despeckled image with KSVD with DTCWT, (g) despeckled image with OBNLM, (h) despeckled image with IAUB.

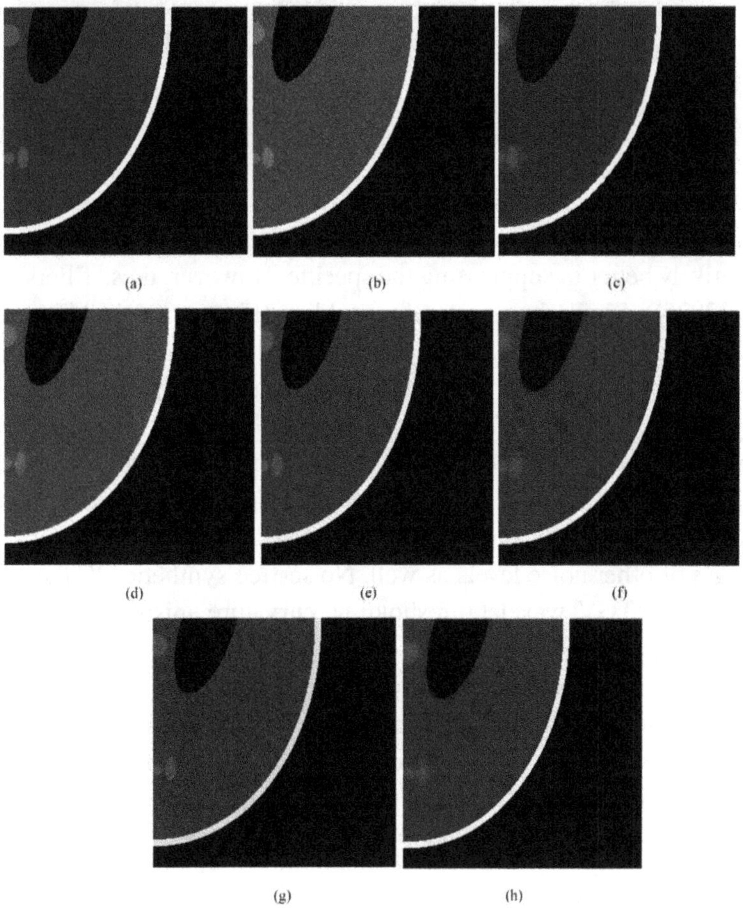

Figure 8. (a) Noise-free synthetic OCT image, (b) noisy OCT, (c) despeckled image with OBNLM, (d) despeckled image with Wavelet thresholding, (e) despeckled image with TGV, (f) despeckled image with Curvature anisotropic diffusion, (g) despeckled image with KSVD with DTCWT, (h) despeckled image with IAUB.

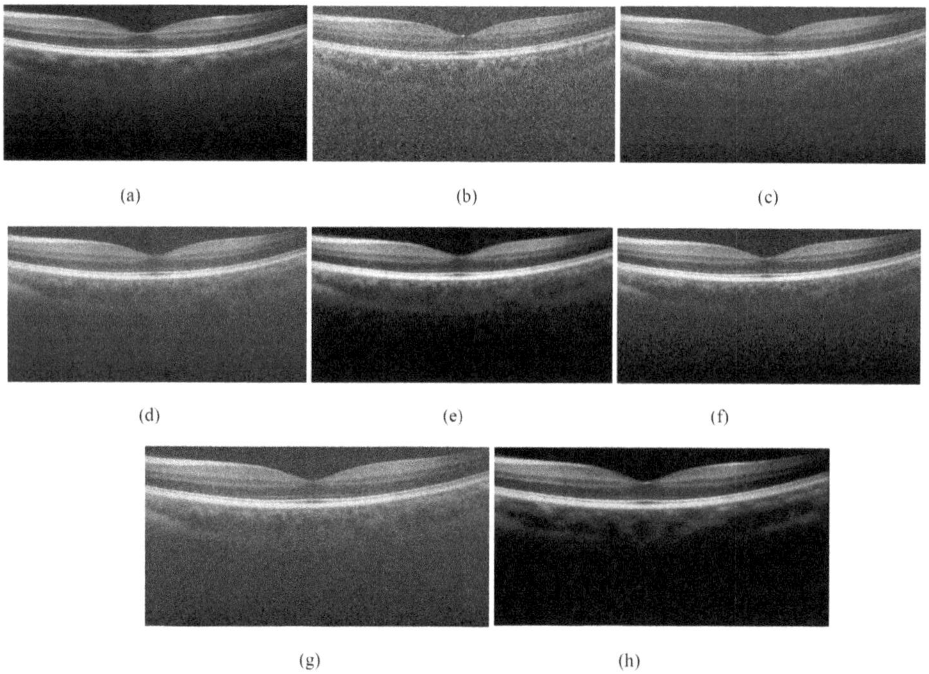

Figure 7(e)), and OBNLM (Figure 6(g) and Figure 7(g)). The despeckling performance of TGV (Figure 6(c) and Figure 7(c)), KSVD (Figure 6(f) and Figure 7(f)) and IAUB (Figure 6(h) and Figure 7(h)) seems to be comparatively better in suppressing the speckle. However, these filters suffer from Cartoon artifacts (Elad et al. (2005)). Similarly, wavelet thresholding (Figure 6(d) and Figure 7(d)) suffers from staircase artifact (Bach et al. (1997)). It can be noticed in the despeckled images with TGV (Figure 6(c) and Figure 7(c)), Wavelet thresholding (Figure 6(d) and Figure 7(d)), KSVD (Figure 6(f) and Figure 7(f)) and IAUB (Figure 6(h) and Figure 7(h)) that edges get blurred during despeckling. While considering the artifacts and noise suppression capability of the despeckling schemes together, IAUB (Figure 6(h) and Figure 7(h)) seems to be comparatively better. In the image despeckled with IUAB (Figure 6(h) and Figure 7(h)), speckle is fully suppressed, and artifact is marginal. The observations are found to be valid with images of other noise levels as well. Noise-free synthetic OCT image, noisy OCT and the despeckling outcome of TGV, wavelet thresholding, curvature anisotropic filter, KSVD, OBNLM, and IAUB are shown in Figure 8.

The experiments on real-time OCT images show that denoising results of the IAUB (Figure 8(h)) are superior to other despeckling techniques. IAUB can selectively suppress the speckles in homogeneous areas of the image without affecting the strength of true edges. In the image despeckled with curvature anisotropic diffusion filter (Figure 8(e)), true edges seem to be blurred. The remaining filters fail to suppress speckle completely. On both Phantom images and real-time OCT images IAUB is observed to

Figure 9. (a) OCT image from Cirrus vendor (OPTIMA, 2015), (b) despeckled image with OBNLM, (c) despeckled image with Wavelet thresholding, (d) despeckled image with TGV, (e) despeckled image with Curvature anisotropic diffusion, (f) despeckled image with KSVD with DTCWT, (g) despeckled image with IAUB.

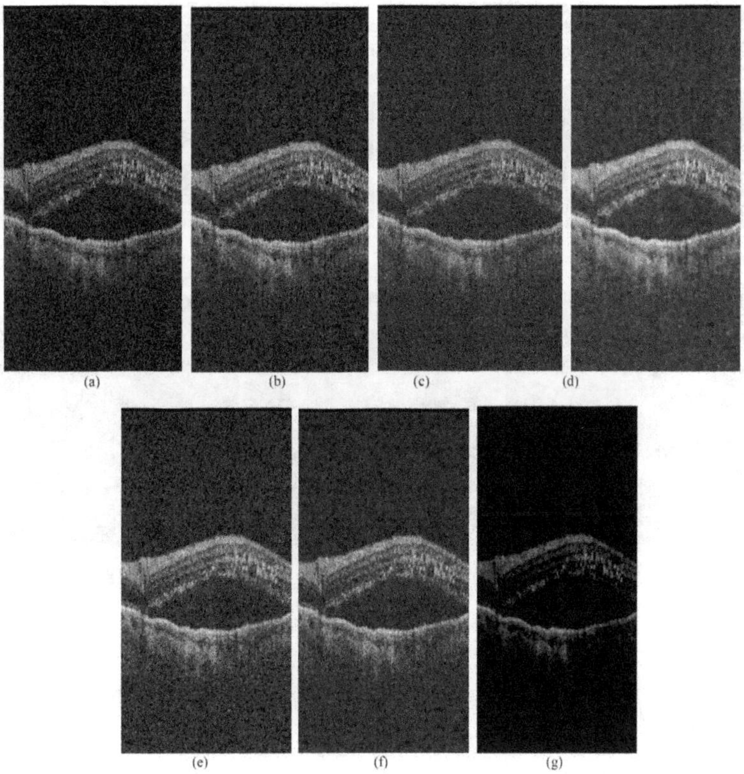

be superior to its alternatives. These observations were found to be valid on 18 real-time OCT images. Figure 9-12 are the inputs and corresponding outputs of despeckling algorithms on the all four vendors of OPTIMA dataset.

Table 1. PSNR values of noise-free synthetic Phantom with respect to synthetic Phantom images mixed with Gamma noise with different values of ρ & β and the images restored with different despeckling filters

Noise Levels	ρ=3 β=2	ρ=4 β=3	ρ=4 β=4	ρ=6 β=6	ρ=8 β=7
Ground truth	31.66	26.36	25.16	20.42	18.52
TGV	33.26	33.06	32.79	31.92	30.72
Wavelet thresholding	31.45	26.11	23.67	16.76	12.96
Curvature anisotropic diffusion	32.58	26.62	24.11	17.07	13.22
KSVD with DTCWT	32.33	26.47	24.01	16.98	13.07
OBNLM	35.79	31.39	29.94	25.08	22.62
IAUB	53.68	48.29	44.78	40.66	38.23

Figure 10. (a) OCT image from Spectralis vendor (OPTIMA, 2015), (b) despeckled image with OBNLM, (c) despeckled image with Wavelet thresholding, (d) despeckled image with TGV, (e) despeckled image with Curvature anisotropic diffusion, (f) despeckled image with KSVD with DTCWT, (g) despeckled image with IAUB.

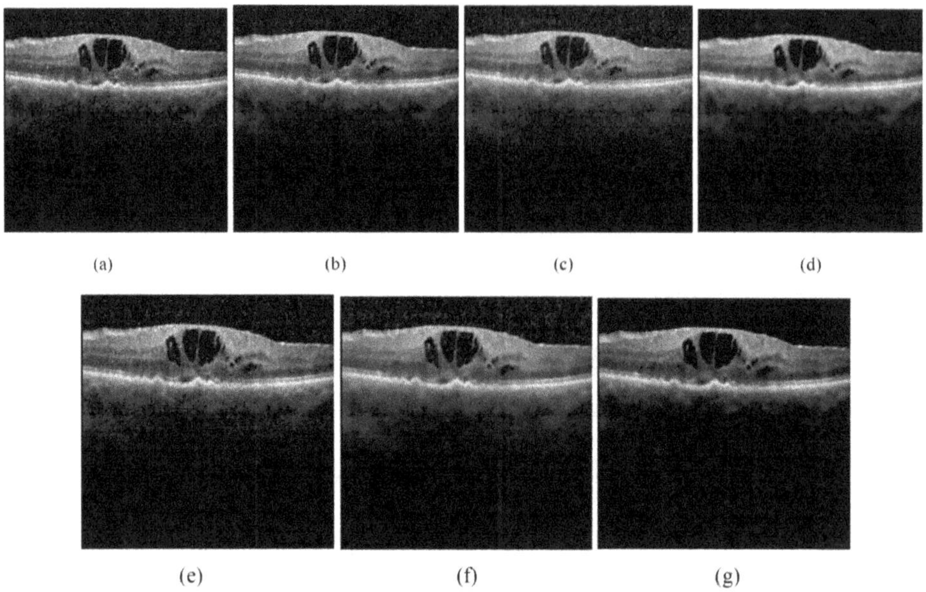

Figure 11. (a) OCT image from Nidek vendor (OPTIMA, 2015), (b) despeckled image with OBNLM, (c) despeckled image with Wavelet thresholding, (d) despeckled image with TGV, (e) despeckled image with Curvature anisotropic diffusion, (f) despeckled image with KSVD with DTCWT, (g) despeckled image with IAUB.

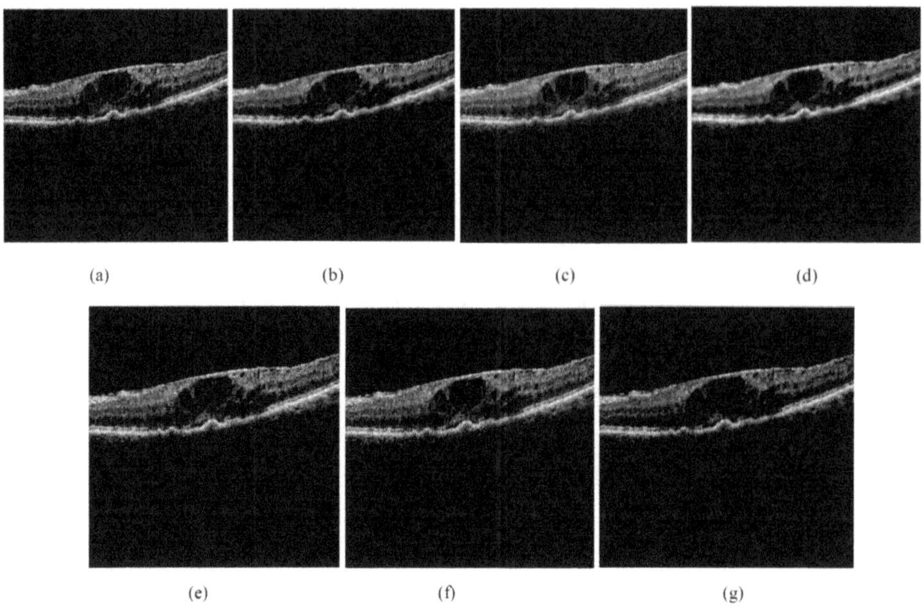

Figure 12. (a) OCT image from Topcon vendor (OPTIMA, 2015), (b) despeckled image with OBNLM, (c) despeckled image with Wavelet thresholding, (d) despeckled image with TGV, (e) despeckled image with Curvature anisotropic diffusion, (f) despeckled image with KSVD with DTCWT, (g) despeckled image with IAUB.

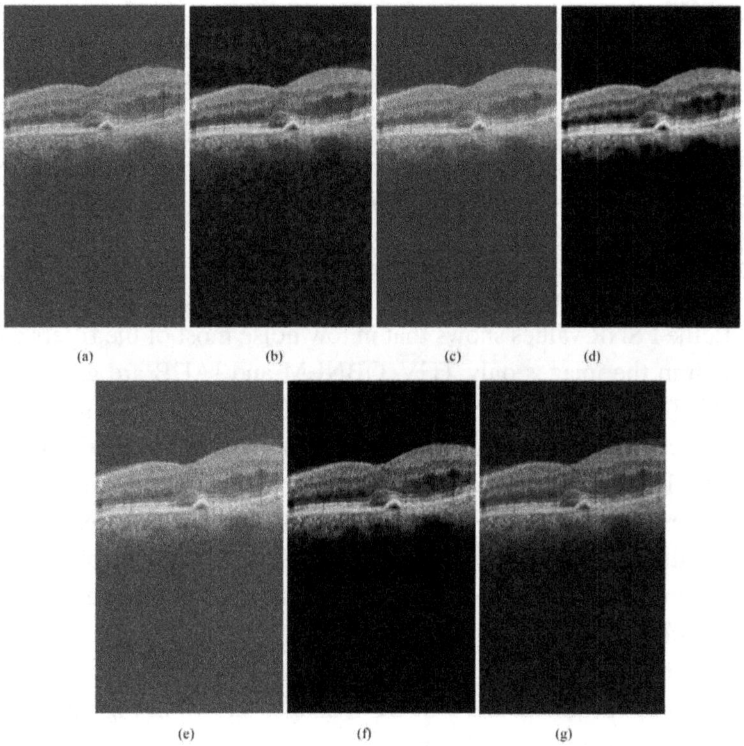

Quantitative Analysis

PSNR values of noise-free synthetic OCT with respect to synthetic OCT images mixed with Gamma noise with different values of ρ and β and the images restored with different despeckling filters are furnished in Table 1.

The PSNR between the ground truth and the despeckled images is greater than the PSNR between ground truth and the noisy images regardless of the type of despeckling scheme and noise level. This is a clear indication that despeckling is helpful for improving SNR. The PSNR value between the ground truth and the despeckled image for IAUB is consistently greater than the PSNR between ground truth and images despeckled with other despeckling schemes at different noise levels. This justifies that, regarding noise suppression capability, IAUB is superior to other despeckling schemes available in the literature. MSSIM values between noise free synthetic OCT and the images restored with different despeckling filters are furnished in Table 2.

The MSSIM value between the ground truth and the despeckled image for IAUB is consistently greater than the MSSIM between ground truth and images despeckled with other despeckling schemes at different noise levels. This justifies that, in terms of the feature preservation also, IAUB is superior to other despeckling schemes available in the literature. SSIM is a full reference image similarity metric

Table 2. MSSIM values between noise- free synthetic OCT and the images restored with different despeckling filters

Noise levels	ρ=3 β=2	ρ=4 β=3	ρ=4 β=4	ρ=6 β=6	ρ=8 β=7
TGV	0.98	0.96	0.89	0.77	0.66
Wavelet thresholding	0.56	0.49	0.47	0.37	0.29
Curvature anisotropic diffusion	0.58	0.50	0.47	0.39	0.32
KSVD with DTCWT	0.57	0.51	0.49	0.43	0.33
OBNLM	0.58	0.57	0.54	0.50	0.48
IAUB	0.99	0.98	0.96	0.91	0.88

with its ideal value 1. A value of 1 represents that the contextual image is exactly alike to the reference image. From Table 1., the PSNR values shows that in low noise most of the filters are performing well. But if the noise is high in the images only TGV, OBNLM and IAUB are giving better performance. From Table 2., the MSSIM values of TGV, OBNLM, and IAUB is higher. In this, the values obtained for the IAUB filter is much better compared to other filters used here. The high value of SSIM exhibited by IAUB justifies that it has appreciable feature preservation capability on real-time OCT also, as observed in Phantom images. The experiments on both simulated images and real-time OCT confirm that IAUB is superior to its alternatives in terms of feature preservation and the ability to suppress speckle. The observations made in the quantitative evaluations are in correspondence to the observations made in the qualitative evaluation.

As a further stratagem for evaluation, the expert scoring from a retinal surgeon on the quality of the despeckled outputs in the synthetic and real OCT images shown in Figure. 8, 9, 10, 11 and 12 are given in Table.3. Remember that, the ophthalmologists have ranked the outputs on a scale of 1–5, for which1and 5 are used to indicate the low and best results, respectively. From Table 3., it is clear that through visual inspection KSVD with DTCWT, OBNLM and IAUB is giving better results. In this, the performance of the IAUB is constant over all the datasets. It can also be observed via visual evaluation that the contrast of the output image is much better for IAUB technique compared to other despeckling schemes. The qualitative results, quantitative results, and the expert evaluation pointing the goodness of IAUB for despeckling.

Table 3. Expert evaluation

	Data sets				
Method	**Cirrus**	**Nidek**	**Spectralis**	**Topcon**	**Duke**
Curvature anisotropic diffusion	4	3	2	2	4
KSVD with DTCWT	3	4	2	4	3
OBNLM	3	3	2	3	3
TGV	1	2	1	2	1
Wavelet thresholding	2	2	1	2	3
IAUB	3	3	3	3	3

CONCLUSION

The techniques for despeckling OCT, available in the literature, have been identified and compared both qualitatively and objectively regarding their noise suppression capability and feature preservation. The possible approaches for modelling the behaviour of speckle were also reviewed. The approaches for despeckling include hardware modification, traditional linear filters (mean, median, Gaussian etc.), nonlinear spatial filters (anisotropic, bilateral, NLM and TV) and advanced techniques based on PCA (SVD and KSVD), soft-computing (MLP, SVM) and probabilistic methods (MLE). For despeckling post-processing techniques are more suitable than hardware modifications. Out of the post-processing techniques, IAUB was found to be better than its alternatives. The influence of the selection of operational parameters involved in the despeckling algorithms is a context which needs further study. Perhaps, the optimization of operational parameters can be helpful for improving the performance of the available despeckling schemes.

Despeckling is always a trade-off between noise suppression and loss of information. It is, therefore, desirable to keep as much important information as possible. The methods proposed for despeckling OCT relay on arbitrary parameters. The arbitrary parameters include the size of kernel, search area, decay control parameter, the gradient of diffusion, Photometric distance, radiometric distance, number of iteration, thresholding, etc.. The adaptive technique to find out the optimal parameters is available in the literature. But these approaches are time-consuming and failed to produce the same performance on different vendor data. A convolutional autoencoder based despeckling scheme may overcome these drawbacks because they will learn the features automatically, rather than engineered by the human.

ACKNOWLEDGMENT

The research was supported by the Science and Engineering Research Board (Department of Science and Technology, India) through project funding EMR/2016/002677.

We are thankful to Dr. Abhishek Kothari, Consultant Ophthalmologist and Vitreoretinal Surgeon, Pink City Eye and Retina Center, Jaipur, India for giving his evaluation of different techniques on real and synthetic OCT images used in this research.

REFERENCES

Adabi, S., Conforto, S., Clayton, A., Podoleanu, A. G., Hojjat, A., & Avanaki, M. R. (2016). An intelligent speckle reduction algorithm for optical coherence tomography images. In *4th International Conference on Photonics, Optics and Laser Technology (PHOTOPTICS), 2016* (pp. 1–6). IEEE.

Adabi, S., Rashedi, E., Clayton, A., Mohebbi-Kalkhoran, H., Chen, X. W., Conforto, S., & Nasiriavanaki, M. (2018). Learnable despeckling framework for optical coherence tomography images. *Journal of Biomedical Optics*, *23*(1), 016013. doi:10.1117/1.JBO.23.1.016013 PMID:29368458

Adler, D. C., Ko, T. H., & Fujimoto, J. G. (2004). Speckle reduction in optical coherence tomography images by use of a spatially adaptive wavelet filter. *Optics Letters*, *29*(24), 2878–2880. doi:10.1364/OL.29.002878 PMID:15645810

Amini, Z., & Rabbani, H. (2017). Optical coherence tomography image denoising using Gaussianization transform. *Journal of Biomedical Optics*, *22*(8), 086011. PMID:28853244

Anantrasirichai, N., Nicholson, L., Morgan, J. E., Erchova, I., Mortlock, K., North, R. V., ... Achim, A. (2014). Adaptive-weighted bilateral filtering and other pre-processing techniques for optical coherence tomography. *Computerized Medical Imaging and Graphics*, *38*(6), 526–539. doi:10.1016/j.compmedimag.2014.06.012 PMID:25034317

Aum, J., Kim, J. H., & Jeong, J. (2015). Effective speckle noise suppression in optical coherence tomography images using nonlocal means denoising filter with double Gaussian anisotropic kernels. *Applied Optics*, *54*(13), D43–D50. doi:10.1364/AO.54.000D43

Bach, M., Meigen, T., & Strasburger, H. (1997). Raster-scan cathode-ray tubes for vision research-limits of resolution in space, time and intensity, and some solutions. *Spatial Vision*, *10*(4), 403–414. doi:10.1163/156856897X00311 PMID:9176948

Bagci, A. M., Shahidi, M., Ansari, R., Blair, M., Blair, N. P., & Zelkha, R. (2008). Thickness profiles of retinal layers by optical coherence tomography image segmentation. *American Journal of Ophthalmology*, *146*(5), 679–687. doi:10.1016/j.ajo.2008.06.010 PMID:18707672

Baghaie, A., D'souza, R. M., & Yu, Z. (2015, April). Sparse and low rank decomposition based batch image alignment for speckle reduction of retinal OCT images. In *12th International Symposium on Biomedical Imaging (ISBI), 2015 IEEE* (pp. 226-230). IEEE.

Baroni, M., Fortunato, P., & La Torre, A. (2007). Towards quantitative analysis of retinal features in optical coherence tomography. *Medical Engineering & Physics*, *29*(4), 432–441. doi:10.1016/j.medengphy.2006.06.003 PMID:16860587

Bashkansky, M., & Reintjes, J. (2000). Statistics and reduction of speckle in optical coherence tomography. *Optics Letters*, *25*(8), 545–547. doi:10.1364/OL.25.000545 PMID:18064106

Bernardes, R., Maduro, C., Serranho, P., Araújo, A., Barbeiro, S., & Cunha-Vaz, J. (2010). Improved adaptive complex diffusion despeckling filter. *Optics Express*, *18*(23), 24048–24059. doi:10.1364/OE.18.024048 PMID:21164752

Bian, L., Suo, J., Chen, F., & Dai, Q. (2015). Multiframe denoising of high-speed optical coherence tomography data using interframe and intraframe priors. *Journal of Biomedical Optics*, *20*(3), 036006. doi:10.1117/1.JBO.20.3.036006 PMID:25751163

Bogunović, H., Sonka, M., Kwon, Y. H., Kemp, P., Abràmoff, M. D., & Wu, X. (2014). Multi-surface and multi-field co-segmentation of 3-D retinal optical coherence tomography. *IEEE Transactions on Medical Imaging*, *33*(12), 2242–2253. doi:10.1109/TMI.2014.2336246 PMID:25020067

Boyer, K. L., Herzog, A., & Roberts, C. (2006). Automatic recovery of the optic nervehead geometry in optical coherence tomography. *IEEE Transactions on Medical Imaging*, *25*(5), 553–570. doi:10.1109/TMI.2006.871417 PMID:16689260

Carrasco, S., Nasr, M. B., Sergienko, A. V., Saleh, B. E., Teich, M. C., Torres, J. P., & Torner, L. (2006). Broadband light generation by noncollinear parametric downconversion. *Optics Letters*, *31*(2), 253–255. doi:10.1364/OL.31.000253 PMID:16441047

Chen, H., Fu, S., Wang, H., Lv, H., & Zhang, C. (2018). Speckle attenuation by adaptive singular value shrinking with generalized likelihood matching in optical coherence tomography. *Journal of Biomedical Optics*, *23*(3), 036014. doi:10.1117/1.JBO.23.3.036014 PMID:29595018

Chen, Q., de Sisternes, L., Leng, T., & Rubin, D. L. (2015). Application of improved homogeneity similarity-based denoising in optical coherence tomography retinal images. *Journal of Digital Imaging*, *28*(3), 346–361. doi:10.100710278-014-9742-8 PMID:25404105

Cheng, J., Duan, L., Wong, D. W. K., Akiba, M., & Liu, J. (2014, August). Speckle reduction in optical coherence tomography by matrix completion using bilateral random projection. In *36th Annual International Conference of the Engineering in Medicine and Biology Society (EMBC), 2014* (pp. 186-189). IEEE.

Chitchian, S., Fiddy, M. A., & Fried, N. M. (2009). Denoising during optical coherence tomography of the prostate nerves via wavelet shrinkage using dual-tree complex wavelet transform. *Journal of Biomedical Optics*, *14*(1), 014031. doi:10.1117/1.3081543 PMID:19256719

Chiu, S. J., Li, X. T., Nicholas, P., Toth, C. A., Izatt, J. A., & Farsiu, S. (2010). Automatic segmentation of seven retinal layers in SDOCT images congruent with expert manual segmentation. *Optics Express*, *18*(18), 19413–19428. doi:10.1364/OE.18.019413 PMID:20940837

Cuartas-Vélez, C., Restrepo, R., Bouma, B. E., & Uribe-Patarroyo, N. (2018). Volumetric non-local-means based speckle reduction for optical coherence tomography. *Biomedical Optics Express*, *9*(7), 3354–3372. doi:10.1364/BOE.9.003354 PMID:29984102

Delcourt, C., Korobelnik, J. F., Barberger-Gateau, P., Delyfer, M. N., Rougier, M. B., Le Goff, M., ... Dartigues, J. F. (2010). Nutrition and age-related eye diseases: The Alienor (Antioxydants, Lipides Essentiels, Nutrition et maladies OculaiRes) Study. *The Journal of Nutrition, Health & Aging*, *14*(10), 854–861. doi:10.100712603-010-0131-9 PMID:21125205

Desjardins, A. E., Vakoc, B. J., Tearney, G. J., & Bouma, B. E. (2006). Speckle reduction in OCT using massively-parallel detection and frequency-domain ranging. *Optics Express*, *14*(11), 4736–4745. doi:10.1364/OE.14.004736 PMID:19516630

Dong, F., Guo, Q., Sun, S., Ren, X., Wang, L., Feng, S., & Gao, B. Z. (2013). Directional Weight Based Contourlet Transform Denoising Algorithm for Oct Image. *Intelligent Automation & Soft Computing*, *19*(4), 525–535. doi:10.1080/10798587.2013.869110

Drexler, W., Morgner, U., Ghanta, R. K., Kärtner, F. X., Schuman, J. S., & Fujimoto, J. G. (2001, April). Ultrahigh-resolution ophthalmic optical coherence tomography. *Nature Medicine*, *7*(4), 502–507. doi:10.1038/86589 PMID:11283681

Du, Y., Liu, G., Feng, G., & Chen, Z. (2014). Speckle reduction in optical coherence tomography images based on wave atoms. *Journal of Biomedical Optics*, *19*(5), 056009. doi:10.1117/1.JBO.19.5.056009 PMID:24825507

Duan, J., Lu, W., Tench, C., Gottlob, I., Proudlock, F., Samani, N. N., & Bai, L. (2016). Denoising optical coherence tomography using second order total generalized variation decomposition. *Biomedical Signal Processing and Control*, *24*, 120–127. doi:10.1016/j.bspc.2015.09.012

Duan, J., Tench, C., Gottlob, I., Proudlock, F., & Bai, L. (2015). New variational image decomposition model for simultaneously denoising and segmenting optical coherence tomography images. *Physics in Medicine and Biology*, *60*(22), 8901–8922. doi:10.1088/0031-9155/60/22/8901 PMID:26553577

Dubey, S. D. (1970). Compound gamma, beta and F distributions. *Metrika*, *16*(1), 27–31. doi:10.1007/BF02613934

Elad, M., Starck, J. L., Querre, P., & Donoho, D. L. (2005). Simultaneous cartoon and texture image inpainting using morphological component analysis (MCA). *Applied and Computational Harmonic Analysis*, *19*(3), 340–358. doi:10.1016/j.acha.2005.03.005

Fabritius, T., Makita, S., Miura, M., Myllylä, R., & Yasuno, Y. (2009). Automated segmentation of the macula by optical coherence tomography. *Optics Express*, *17*(18), 15659–15669. doi:10.1364/OE.17.015659 PMID:19724565

Fang, L., Li, S., McNabb, R. P., Nie, Q., Kuo, A. N., Toth, C. A., ... Farsiu, S. (2013). Fast acquisition and reconstruction of optical coherence tomography images via sparse representation. *IEEE Transactions on Medical Imaging*, *32*(11), 2034–2049. doi:10.1109/TMI.2013.2271904 PMID:23846467

Fang, L., Li, S., Nie, Q., Izatt, J. A., Toth, C. A., & Farsiu, S. (2012). Sparsity based denoising of spectral domain optical coherence tomography images. *Biomedical Optics Express*, *3*(5), 927–942. doi:10.1364/BOE.3.000927 PMID:22567586

Ferguson, R. D., Hammer, D. X., Paunescu, L. A., Beaton, S., & Schuman, J. S. (2004). Tracking optical coherence tomography. *Optics Letters*, *29*(18), 2139–2141. doi:10.1364/OL.29.002139 PMID:15460882

Fernández, D. C., Villate, N., Puliafito, C. A., & Rosenfeld, P. J. (2004). Comparing total macular volume changes measured by optical coherence tomography with retinal lesion volume estimated by active contours. *Investigative Ophthalmology & Visual Science*, *45*(13), 3072–3072.

Forouzanfar, M., & Moghaddam, H. A. (2007, April). A directional multiscale approach for speckle reduction in optical coherence tomography images. In *International Conference on Electrical Engineering, 2007. ICEE'07.* (pp. 1-6). IEEE.

Fujimoto, J., & Drexler, W. (2008). Introduction to optical coherence tomography. In *Optical coherence tomography* (pp. 1–45). Berlin: Springer. doi:10.1007/978-3-540-77550-8_1

Fuller, A., Zawadzki, R., Choi, S., Wiley, D., Werner, J., & Hamann, B. (2007). Segmentation of three-dimensional retinal image data. *IEEE Transactions on Visualization and Computer Graphics*, *13*(6), 1719–1726. doi:10.1109/TVCG.2007.70590 PMID:17968130

Gargesha, M., Jenkins, M. W., Rollins, A. M., & Wilson, D. L. (2008). Denoising and 4D visualization of OCT images. *Optics Express*, *16*(16), 12313–12333. doi:10.1364/OE.16.012313 PMID:18679509

Garvin, M. K., Abràmoff, M. D., Kardon, R., Russell, S. R., Wu, X., & Sonka, M. (2008). Intraretinal layer segmentation of macular optical coherence tomography images using optimal 3-D graph search. *IEEE Transactions on Medical Imaging*, *27*(10), 1495–1505. doi:10.1109/TMI.2008.923966 PMID:18815101

George, A., Dilienseger, J. L., Weber, M., & Pechereau, A. (2000, March). Optical coherence tomography image processing. In Investigative Ophthalmology & Visual Science (Vol. 41, No. 4, pp. S173-S173). Assoc Research Vision Ophthalmology Inc.

Girish, G. N., Anima, V. A., Kothari, A. R., Sudeep, P. V., Roychowdhury, S., & Rajan, J. (2018a). A benchmark study of automated intra-retinal cyst segmentation algorithms using optical coherence tomography B-scans. *Computer Methods and Programs in Biomedicine*, *153*, 105–114. doi:10.1016/j.cmpb.2017.10.010 PMID:29157443

Girish, G. N., Kothari, A. R., & Rajan, J. (2017). Marker controlled watershed transform for intra-retinal cysts segmentation from optical coherence tomography b-scans. Pattern Recognition Letters. ISSN 0167-8655, https://doi.org/10.1016/j.patrec.2017.12.019

Girish, G. N., Thakur, B., Chowdhury, S. R., Kothari, A. R., & Rajan, J. (2018 b). Segmentation of Intra-Retinal Cysts from Optical Coherence Tomography Images using a Fully Convolutional Neural Network Model. *IEEE Journal of Biomedical and Health Informatics*, 1. doi:10.1109/JBHI.2018.2810379 PMID:29994161

Götzinger, E., Pircher, M., & Hitzenberger, C. K. (2005). High speed spectral domain polarization sensitive optical coherence tomography of the human retina. *Optics Express*, *13*(25), 10217–10229. doi:10.1364/OPEX.13.010217 PMID:19503236

Gregori, G., & Knighton, R. W. (2004). A robust algorithm for retinal thickness measurements using optical coherence tomography (Stratus OCT). *Investigative Ophthalmology & Visual Science*, *45*(13), 3007–3007.

Gregory, R. L. (2015). *Eye and brain: The psychology of seeing*. Princeton University Press.

Guillonneau, X., Eandi, C. M., Paques, M., Sahel, J. A., Sapieha, P., & Sennlaub, F. (2017). On phagocytes and macular degeneration. *Progress in Retinal and Eye Research*, *61*, 98–128. doi:10.1016/j.preteyeres.2017.06.002 PMID:28602950

Gupta, M. P. (2016). *Retinal anatomy and pathology. In Retinal Pharmacotherapeutics* (Vol. 55, pp. 7–17). Karger Publishers. doi:10.1159/000431128

Gupta, V., Chan, C. C., Poh, C. L., Chow, T. H., Meng, T. C., & Koon, N. B. (2008, May). Computerized automation of wavelet based denoising method to reduce speckle noise in OCT images. In *International Conference on Information Technology and Applications in Biomedicine, 2008* (pp. 120-123). IEEE.

Hee, M. R., Izatt, J. A., Swanson, E. A., Huang, D., Schuman, J. S., Lin, C. P., ... Fujimoto, J. G. (1995). Optical coherence tomography of the human retina. *Archives of Ophthalmology*, *113*(3), 325–332. doi:10.1001/archopht.1995.01100030081025 PMID:7887846

Herzog, A., Boyer, K. L., & Roberts, C. (2004). Robust extraction of the optic nerve head in optical coherence tomography. In *Computer Vision and Mathematical Methods in Medical and Biomedical Image Analysis* (pp. 395–407). Berlin: Springer. doi:10.1007/978-3-540-27816-0_34

Huang, D., Swanson, E. A., Lin, C. P., Schuman, J. S., Stinson, W. G., Chang, W., ... & Puliafito, C. A. (1991). Optical coherence tomography. *Science, 254*(5035), 1178-1181.

Hughes, M., Spring, M., & Podoleanu, A. (2010). Speckle noise reduction in optical coherence tomography of paint layers. *Applied Optics*, *49*(1), 99–107. doi:10.1364/AO.49.000099 PMID:20062495

Iftimia, N., Bouma, B. E., & Tearney, G. J. (2003). Speckle reduction in optical coherence tomography by. *Journal of Biomedical Optics*, *8*(2), 260–264. doi:10.1117/1.1559060 PMID:12683852

Isar, C. S. C. A. (n.d.). Optical Coherence Tomography Speckle Reduction in the Wavelets Domain. *Editorial Board*, 3.

Ishikawa, H., Stein, D. M., Wollstein, G., Beaton, S., Fujimoto, J. G., & Schuman, J. S. (2005). Macular segmentation with optical coherence tomography. *Investigative Ophthalmology & Visual Science*, *46*(6), 2012–2017. doi:10.1167/iovs.04-0335 PMID:15914617

Jian, Z., Yu, L., Rao, B., Tromberg, B. J., & Chen, Z. (2010). Three-dimensional speckle suppression in optical coherence tomography based on the curvelet transform. *Optics Express*, *18*(2), 1024–1032. doi:10.1364/OE.18.001024 PMID:20173923

Jian, Z., Yu, Z., Yu, L., Rao, B., Chen, Z., & Tromberg, B. J. (2009). Speckle attenuation in optical coherence tomography by curvelet shrinkage. *Optics Letters*, *34*(10), 1516–1518. doi:10.1364/OL.34.001516 PMID:19448806

Jørgensen, T. M., Thomadsen, J., Christensen, U., Soliman, W., & Sander, B. A. (2007). Enhancing the signal-to-noise ratio in ophthalmic optical coherence tomography by image registration—method and clinical examples. *Journal of Biomedical Optics*, *12*(4), 041208. doi:10.1117/1.2772879 PMID:17867797

Kafieh, R., Rabbani, H., Abramoff, M. D., & Sonka, M. (2013). Curvature correction of retinal OCTs using graph-based geometry detection. *Physics in Medicine and Biology*, *58*(9), 2925–2938. doi:10.1088/0031-9155/58/9/2925 PMID:23574790

Kafieh, R., Rabbani, H., & Selesnick, I. (2015). Three dimensional data-driven multi scale atomic representation of optical coherence tomography. *IEEE Transactions on Medical Imaging*, *34*(5), 1042–1062. doi:10.1109/TMI.2014.2374354 PMID:25934998

Kajić, V., Esmaeelpour, M., Považay, B., Marshall, D., Rosin, P. L., & Drexler, W. (2012). Automated choroidal segmentation of 1060 nm OCT in healthy and pathologic eyes using a statistical model. *Biomedical Optics Express*, *3*(1), 86–103. doi:10.1364/BOE.3.000086 PMID:22254171

Kajić, V., Považay, B., Hermann, B., Hofer, B., Marshall, D., Rosin, P. L., & Drexler, W. (2010). Robust segmentation of intraretinal layers in the normal human fovea using a novel statistical model based on texture and shape analysis. *Optics Express*, *18*(14), 14730–14744. doi:10.1364/OE.18.014730 PMID:20639959

Karamata, B., Hassler, K., Laubscher, M., & Lasser, T. (2005). Speckle statistics in optical coherence tomography. *JOSA A*, *22*(4), 593–596. doi:10.1364/JOSAA.22.000593 PMID:15839265

Kennedy, B. F., Hillman, T. R., Curatolo, A., & Sampson, D. D. (2010). Speckle reduction in optical coherence tomography by strain compounding. *Optics Letters, 35*(14), 2445–2447. doi:10.1364/OL.35.002445 PMID:20634858

Khaing, T. T., & Aimmanee, P. (2017, May). Optic disk segmentation in retinal images using active contour model based on extended feature projection. In *2017 8th International Conference of Information and Communication Technology for Embedded Systems (IC-ICTES)* (pp. 1-6). IEEE.

Koozekanani, D., Boyer, K., & Roberts, C. (2001). Retinal thickness measurements from optical coherence tomography using a Markov boundary model. *IEEE Transactions on Medical Imaging, 20*(9), 900–916. doi:10.1109/42.952728 PMID:11585207

Lee, H., Sheth, V., Bibi, M., Maconachie, G., Patel, A., McLean, R. J., ... Gottlob, I. (2013). Potential of handheld optical coherence tomography to determine cause of infantile nystagmus in children by using foveal morphology. *Ophthalmology, 120*(12), 2714–2724. doi:10.1016/j.ophtha.2013.07.018 PMID:24161406

Liu, X., Yang, Z., & Wang, J. (2016, October). A novel noise reduction method for optical coherence tomography images. In *Image and Signal Processing, BioMedical Engineering and Informatics (CISP-BMEI), International Congress on* (pp. 167-171). IEEE.

Luan, F., & Wu, Y. (2013). Application of RPCA in optical coherence tomography for speckle noise reduction. *Laser Physics Letters, 10*(3), 035603. doi:10.1088/1612-2011/10/3/035603

Lv, H., Fu, S., Zhang, C., & Zhai, L. (2018). Speckle noise reduction for optical coherence tomography based on adaptive 2D dictionary. *Laser Physics Letters, 15*(5), 055401. doi:10.1088/1612-202X/aaaeb0

Marks, D. L., Ralston, T. S., & Boppart, S. A. (2005). Speckle reduction by I-divergence regularization in optical coherence tomography. *JOSA A, 22*(11), 2366–2371. doi:10.1364/JOSAA.22.002366 PMID:16304722

Mayer, M. A., Borsdorf, A., Wagner, M., Hornegger, J., Mardin, C. Y., & Tornow, R. P. (2012). Wavelet denoising of multiframe optical coherence tomography data. *Biomedical Optics Express, 3*(3), 572–589. doi:10.1364/BOE.3.000572 PMID:22435103

Mayer, M. A., Tornow, R. P., Bock, R., Hornegger, J., & Kruse, F. E. (2008). Automatic nerve fiber layer segmentation and geometry correction on spectral domain OCT images using fuzzy C-means clustering. *Investigative Ophthalmology & Visual Science, 49*(13), 1880–1880.

Meiniel, W., Gan, Y., Olivo-Marin, J. C., & Angelini, E. (2017, August). A sparsity-based simplification method for segmentation of spectral-domain optical coherence tomography images. In *Wavelets and Sparsity XVII* (Vol. 10394, p. 1039406). International Society for Optics and Photonics. doi:10.1117/12.2274126

Mishra, A., Wong, A., Bizheva, K., & Clausi, D. A. (2009). Intra-retinal layer segmentation in optical coherence tomography images. *Optics Express, 17*(26), 23719–23728. doi:10.1364/OE.17.023719 PMID:20052083

Muftuoglu, I. K., Ramkumar, H. L., Bartsch, D. U., Meshi, A., Gaber, R., & Freeman, W. R. (2018). Quantitative analysis of the inner retinal layer thicknesses in age-related macular degeneration using corrected optical coherence tomography segmentation. *Retina (Philadelphia, Pa.)*, *38*(8), 1478–1484. doi:10.1097/IAE.0000000000001759 PMID:28650925

Muramatsu, S., Choi, S., & Kawamura, T. (2015, December). 3-D OCT data denoising with nonseparable oversampled lapped transform. In *Signal and Information Processing Association Annual Summit and Conference (APSIPA), 2015 Asia-Pacific* (pp. 901-906). IEEE.

Ozcan, A., Bilenca, A., Desjardins, A. E., Bouma, B. E., & Tearney, G. J. (2007). Speckle reduction in optical coherence tomography images using digital filtering. *JOSA A*, *24*(7), 1901–1910. doi:10.1364/JOSAA.24.001901 PMID:17728812

Pircher, M., Götzinger, E., Leitgeb, R. A., Fercher, A. F., & Hitzenberger, C. K. (2003). Speckle reduction in optical coherence tomography by frequency compounding. *Journal of Biomedical Optics*, *8*(3), 565–570. doi:10.1117/1.1578087 PMID:12880365

Pizurica, A., Jovanov, L., Huysmans, B., Zlokolica, V., De Keyser, P., Dhaenens, F., & Philips, W. (2008). Multiresolution denoising for optical coherence tomography: A review and evaluation. *Current Medical Imaging Reviews*, *4*(4), 270–284. doi:10.2174/157340508786404044

Povazay, B., Bizheva, K., Unterhuber, A., Hermann, B., Sattmann, H., Fercher, A. F., ... Russell, P. S. J. (2002). Submicrometer axial resolution optical coherence tomography. *Optics Letters*, *27*(20), 1800–1802. doi:10.1364/OL.27.001800 PMID:18033368

Puvanathasan, P., & Bizheva, K. (2009). Interval type-II fuzzy anisotropic diffusion algorithm for speckle noise reduction in optical coherence tomography images. *Optics Express*, *17*(2), 733–746. doi:10.1364/OE.17.000733 PMID:19158887

Quellec, G., Lee, K., Dolejsi, M., Garvin, M. K., Abramoff, M. D., & Sonka, M. (2010). Three-dimensional analysis of retinal layer texture: Identification of fluid-filled regions in SD-OCT of the macula. *IEEE Transactions on Medical Imaging*, *29*(6), 1321–1330. doi:10.1109/TMI.2010.2047023 PMID:20363675

Rabbani, H., Sonka, M., & Abramoff, M. D. (2013). Optical coherence tomography noise reduction using anisotropic local bivariate Gaussian mixture prior in 3D complex wavelet domain. *Journal of Biomedical Imaging*, *2013*, 22. PMID:24222760

Rajabi, H., & Zirak, A. (2016). Speckle noise reduction and motion artifact correction based on modified statistical parameters estimation in OCT images. *Biomedical Physics & Engineering Express*, *2*(3), 035012. doi:10.1088/2057-1976/2/3/035012

Ramrath, L., Moreno, G., Mueller, H., Bonin, T., Huettmann, G., & Schweikard, A. (2008, September). Towards multi-directional OCT for speckle noise reduction. In *International Conference on Medical Image Computing and Computer-Assisted Intervention* (pp. 815-823). Springer. 10.1007/978-3-540-85988-8_97

Ren, H., Qin, L., & Zhu, X. (2016). Speckle reduction and cartoon-texture decomposition of ophthalmic optical coherence tomography images by variational image decomposition. *Optik-International Journal for Light and Electron Optics*, *127*(19), 7809–7821. doi:10.1016/j.ijleo.2016.05.088

Rogowska, J., & Brezinski, M. E. (2002). Image processing techniques for noise removal, enhancement and segmentation of cartilage OCT images. *Physics in Medicine and Biology*, *47*(4), 641–655. doi:10.1088/0031-9155/47/4/307 PMID:11900196

Salinas, H. M., & Fernández, D. C. (2007). Comparison of PDE-based nonlinear diffusion approaches for image enhancement and denoising in optical coherence tomography. *IEEE Transactions on Medical Imaging*, *26*(6), 761–771. doi:10.1109/TMI.2006.887375 PMID:17679327

Samagaio, G., Estévez, A., de Moura, J., Novo, J., Fernandez, M. I., & Ortega, M. (2018). Automatic Macular Edema Identification and Characterization Using OCT Images. *Computer Methods and Programs in Biomedicine*, *163*, 47–63. doi:10.1016/j.cmpb.2018.05.033 PMID:30119857

Sander, B., Larsen, M., Thrane, L., Hougaard, J. L., & Jørgensen, T. M. (2005). Enhanced optical coherence tomography imaging by multiple scan averaging. *The British Journal of Ophthalmology*, *89*(2), 207–212. doi:10.1136/bjo.2004.045989 PMID:15665354

Schirrmacher, F., Köhler, T., Husvogt, L., Fujimoto, J. G., Hornegger, J., & Maier, A. K. (2017, September). Quasi: Quantile sparse image prior for spatio-temporal denoising of retinal oct data. In *International Conference on Medical Image Computing and Computer-Assisted Intervention* (pp. 83-91). Springer. 10.1007/978-3-319-66185-8_10

Schmitt, J. M. (1999). Optical coherence tomography (OCT): A review. *IEEE Journal of Selected Topics in Quantum Electronics*, *5*(4), 1205–1215. doi:10.1109/2944.796348

Schmitt, J. M., & Knüttel, A. (1997). Model of optical coherence tomography of heterogeneous tissue. *JOSA A*, *14*(6), 1231–1242. doi:10.1364/JOSAA.14.001231

Schmitt, J. M., Xiang, S. H., & Yung, K. M. (1999). Speckle in optical coherence tomography. *Journal of Biomedical Optics*, *4*(1), 95–106. doi:10.1117/1.429925 PMID:23015175

Shah, S. (2009). Blindness and visual impairment due to retinal diseases. *Community Eye Health*, *22*(69), 8. PMID:19506713

Shahidi, M., Wang, Z., & Zelkha, R. (2005). Quantitative thickness measurement of retinal layers imaged by optical coherence tomography. *American Journal of Ophthalmology*, *139*(6), 1056–1061. doi:10.1016/j.ajo.2005.01.012 PMID:15953436

Shepp, L. A., & Logan, B. F. (1974). The Fourier reconstruction of a head section. *IEEE Transactions on Nuclear Science*, *21*(3), 21–43. doi:10.1109/TNS.1974.6499235

Srinivasan, V. J., Monson, B. K., Wojtkowski, M., Bilonick, R. A., Gorczynska, I., Chen, R., ... Fujimoto, J. G. (2008). Characterization of outer retinal morphology with high-speed, ultrahigh-resolution optical coherence tomography. *Investigative Ophthalmology & Visual Science*, *49*(4), 1571–1579. doi:10.1167/iovs.07-0838 PMID:18385077

Stankiewicz, A., Marciniak, T., Dąbrowski, A., Stopa, M., Rakowicz, P., & Marciniak, E. (2017). Denoising methods for improving automatic segmentation in OCT images of human eye. *Bulletin of the Polish Academy of Sciences. Technical Sciences*, *65*(1), 71–78. doi:10.1515/bpasts-2017-0009

Sudeep, P. V., Niwas, S. I., Palanisamy, P., Rajan, J., Xiaojun, Y., Wang, X., ... Liu, L. (2016). Enhancement and bias removal of optical coherence tomography images: An iterative approach with adaptive bilateral filtering. *Computers in Biology and Medicine*, *71*, 97–107. doi:10.1016/j.compbiomed.2016.02.003 PMID:26907572

Varnousfaderani, E. S., Vogl, W. D., Wu, J., Gerendas, B. S., Simader, C., Langs, G., . . . Schmidt-Erfurth, U. (2016, March). Geodesic denoising for optical coherence tomography images. In Medical Imaging 2016: Image Processing (Vol. 9784, p. 97840K). International Society for Optics and Photonics.

Vegas-Sánchez-Ferrero, G., Martín-Martínez, D., Aja-Fernández, S., & Palencia, C. (2010, April). On the influence of interpolation on probabilistic models for ultrasonic images. In *Biomedical Imaging: From Nano to Macro, 2010 IEEE International Symposium on* (pp. 292-295). IEEE.

Wong, A., Mishra, A., Bizheva, K., & Clausi, D. A. (2010). General Bayesian estimation for speckle noise reduction in optical coherence tomography retinal imagery. *Optics Express*, *18*(8), 8338–8352. doi:10.1364/OE.18.008338 PMID:20588679

Wu, M., Chen, Q., He, X., Li, P., Fan, W., Yuan, S., & Park, H. (2018). Automatic Subretinal fluid segmentation of retinal SD-OCT images with neurosensory retinal detachment guided by enface fundus imaging. *IEEE Transactions on Biomedical Engineering*, *65*(1), 87–95. doi:10.1109/TBME.2017.2695461 PMID:28436839

Yorston, D. (2003). Retinal diseases and vision 2020. *Community Eye Health*, *16*(46), 19–20. PMID:17491850

Zhang, L., Li, J., Han, H., Liu, B., Yang, J., & Wang, Q. (2017, May). Automatic cataract detection and grading using Deep Convolutional Neural Network. In *Networking, Sensing and Control (ICNSC), 2017 IEEE 14th International Conference on* (pp. 60-65). IEEE.

Zlokolica, V., Jovanov, L., Pižurica, A., De Keyser, P., Dhaenens, F., & Philips, W. (2007, October). Wavelet-based denoising for 3D OCT images. In *Applications of Digital Image Processing XXX* (Vol. 6696, p. 66960P). International Society for Optics and Photonics. doi:10.1117/12.734286

Chapter 14
Advances in Ultrasound Despeckling:
An Overview

Sudeep P. V.
National Institute of Technology Calicut, India

Palanisamy P.
National Institute of Technology Tiruchirappalli, India

Jeny Rajan
National Institute of Technology Karnataka, India

ABSTRACT

The B-mode ultrasound images are corrupted due to the presence of speckle noise. Hence, the speckle removal in the ultrasound images is essential for proper clinical examination and quantitative assessments. The speckle pattern varies with several imaging parameters as well as the anatomical structure in the image. It is hard to avoid speckle by performing averaging and low noise system designs. An excessive speckle reduction diminishes the visibility of small anatomical structures and thereby makes the image understanding complicated. This chapter is intended to encapsulate various techniques for reducing speckle in medical ultrasound images and improving the image quality for visual inspection and/or computer-assisted diagnosis of ultrasound images. In addition, the chapter surveys the papers published between 2015 and 2018 to highlight the latest trends in the despeckling of ultrasound images. The chapter also presents the performance comparison of a few popular algorithms to despeckle medical ultrasound images.

INTRODUCTION

Ultrasound is a modern medical diagnostic instrument for imaging organs, muscles, and tissues or for obtaining measures that are good biomarkers in the clinical diagnosis and therapeutic procedures (Araki et al., 2016; Acharya et al., 2014; Loizou et al., 2005). It is preferred due to its merits such as economi-

DOI: 10.4018/978-1-5225-7796-6.ch014

cal, real-time nature, safe and easy to use in practice. Ultrasound is useful in invasive and non-invasive medical applications (Suri, 2008; Saba et al., 2014; Del Cura et al., 2012; Christodoulou et al., 2002).

A conventional ultrasound system produces images using the principle of echo imaging. The use of echo localization for medical purposes has been initiated in the mid-1950s. In principle, the ultrasound system transmits acoustic (pressure) waves with frequencies that lie in the range from 1 to 20 MHz into the patient's body (Tole & Ostensen, 2005). When the acoustic wave hits the tissue barriers (scatters) exist in a specified size of medium (resolution cell), backscattering of the wave (echo) occurs. An ultrasonic probe detects the echoes and integrates to develop 1D acoustic line (A-line) signal. An envelope detector produces a low-frequency envelope signal from the high-frequency A-line signal. Then, the logarithmic compression and nonlinear processing of the envelope signal is performed. The procedure repeats for all the A lines usually arranged in a sequential order and interpolates to create a Cartesian image of the ultrasound B-scan (Sudeep et al., 2016).

Even though recent advances in technology have improved the functionality of ultrasound, it still possesses severe limitations in the following aspects: (i) Ultrasound scans of the brain, lungs and the abdominal region are limited due to the obstruction of sound waves by bone or air, (ii) it is difficult to produce clinically relevant images on patients with obesity, and (iii) its effectiveness heavily depends upon the expertise of the technician or physician conducting the examination (Patel, 2010).

In fact, the speckle generated by the intervention of back-scattered waves leads to quality degradation of ultrasound images. The granular pattern of speckle masks small anatomical structures in the image. Therefore, it complicates interpretations from the image. In (Goodman, 1975), speckle is modeled as the summation of many complex phasors, called a *complex random walk*. Among them, the phasors that possess destructive relationships interfere to form the speckle. Therefore, the relative phase between the back-scattered waves determines its degree of seriousness.

Based on the scatter number density (SND) per resolution cell, we can classify the speckle into 4 groups, which are (i) fully developed (ii) fully resolved (iii) partially developed and (iv) partially resolved (Seabra J. C. R., 2011). When SND is high, the envelope becomes Rayleigh distributed due to the contamination of *fully developed speckle* and it happens in blood regions. For the Gaussian distributed complex echo envelope with standard deviation σ and the absolute envelope amplitude u, the Rayleigh probability density function (PDF) is expressed as (Sudeep et al., 2016):

$$f\left(u,\sigma\right)=\frac{u}{\sigma^{2}}e^{-\frac{u^{2}}{2\sigma^{2}}} \tag{1}$$

If the random walk possesses an extra deterministic component, *fully resolved* speckle arises and the Rician distribution fits well with the envelope. Usually, it happens in regions of tremendous echolucent response like myocardium. The Rician distribution PDF is (Sudeep et al., 2016):

$$f\left(u\mid v,\sigma\right)=\frac{u}{\sigma^{2}}e^{-\frac{(u^{2}+v^{2})}{2\sigma^{2}}}I_{0}\left(\frac{uv}{\sigma^{2}}\right) \tag{2}$$

where $I_0\left(\cdot\right)$ is the modified Bessel function of the first kind with order zero and v is the noise-free envelope magnitude value.

In practice, the most common forms of speckle are fully developed and fully resolved. Nonetheless, the nonlinear post-processing step such as the upsampling operation to form Cartesian image changes the data intensities and the observed distributions in the ultrasound images differ from Rayleigh or Rician distribution (Vegas-Sanchez-Ferrero et al., 2010). Consequently, many statistical models such as Nakagami, generalized Nakagami, Rician inverse Gaussian (RiIG), Gamma or Weibull have been investigated in literature to model ultrasound images (Tao et al., 2006). Latest articles indicate that Gamma distribution accurately fits ultrasound images (Vegas-Sanchez-Ferrero et al., 2010a).

In this section, we begin by briefly recalling the principle of ultrasound imaging and then discussed the speckle formation process in the ultrasound system. The major objective of this chapter is to provide a general explanation of various terms and techniques on the image quality of ultrasound images. Also, we compare a few popular despeckling methods using the ultrasound datasets.

BACKGROUND

The image quality improvement in ultrasound is broadly classified as preprocessing and post-processing techniques (see Figure 1). Preprocessing methods include the fine-tuning of the data with the physical properties of the associated signals during image acquisitions. Post-processing quality improvement of ultrasound images refers to the techniques in which adjustments to enhance the image quality is applied after storage of the digitized data. Therefore, there is no major requirement of hardware modification in post-processing strategies.

Ultrasound Image Quality Improvement via Preprocessing Techniques

The different preprocessing techniques of ultrasound images are given below:

- **Beamforming Techniques:** It is a signal processing technique to control the timing and the shape of the US beams and thereby, to diminish side-lobes and speed of sound errors, and to improve penetration without the cost of resolution (Ortiz et al., 2012). A few modern beamforming techniques are discussed below:

Figure 1. Classification of ultrasound image quality improvement techniques

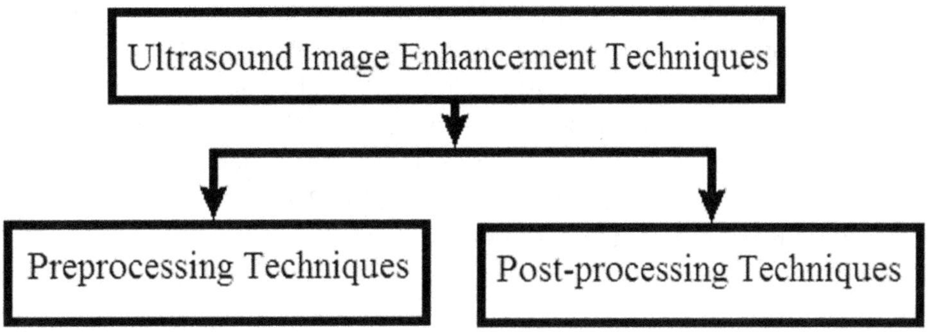

Figure 2. Taxonomy of preprocessing techniques

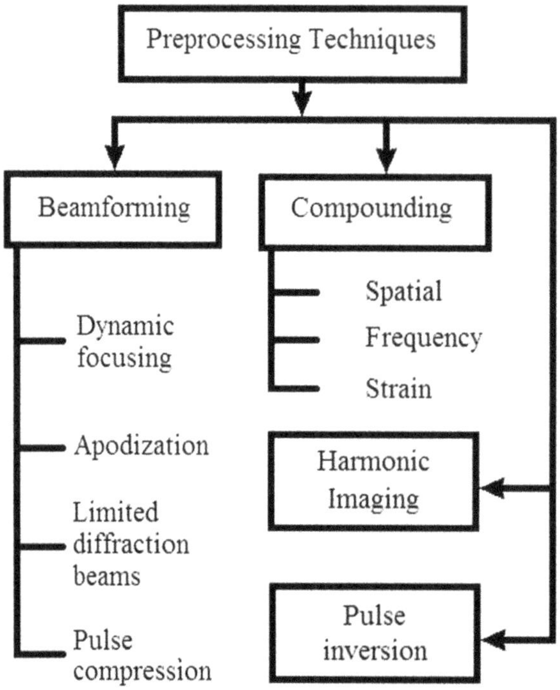

- **Dynamic Focusing:** The purpose of dynamic focusing is to expand the depth of field without affecting the low side lobes by using the automated adjustment of the focal length of the receiving beam. In addition, the transmission by means of many pulse sequences with different focal lengths can provide an extra improvement in the depth of field (Del Cura et al., 2012).
- **Apodization:** The technique of improving resolution and achieving sidelobe reduction by using aperture-weighting functions in ultrasound scanners (Guenther et al., 2007).
- **Limited Diffraction Beams:** These beams improve the depth of field. At the same time, the beams produce very high sidelobes and hence, reductions in image contrast (Lu et al., 1994).
- **Pulse Compression:** In ultrasound imaging systems having pulse compression approaches, pulse with longer duration and lower amplitude is used in transmission and compress the returning energy into a short duration during the reception. It improves the SNR of output ultrasound images (Ortiz et al., 2012).

- **Compounding (Averaging):** It fuses multiple images to produce a better quality image.
  - **Spatial Compounding:** It combines images acquired from multiple angles by rotating transducer in the ultrasound imaging system (Jespersen et al., 1998). Different operators such as mean, median, maximum, geometric mean, mean excluding maximum and root mean square have been discussed in the literature for combining the images. Usually, images at different angles are registered (aligned) before compounded. The motion of the transducer can be either in the horizontal or in the elevational direction.

  - **Frequency Compounding:** Frequency compounding achieves quality improvement by combining images at different frequencies. Images at different frequencies are acquired by using numerous sources at separate frequencies or by using sub-bands produced by splitting the entire RF spectrum of the echoes (Trahey et al., 1986).
  - **Strain Compounding:** Li and Chen (Li et al., 2002) proposed another method of compounding called strain compounding. Herein the external forces are used to introduce tissue motion and the images in different strain states are obtained. After the in-plane motion correction, all the images are combined for speckle suppression without the cost of in-plane spatial resolution.
- **Harmonic Imaging:** The principle behind harmonic imaging is that the harmonics of the transmitted fundamental frequency in the ultrasound back-scattered signal can be used to form the image with better spatial and contrast resolution. Nowadays, it finds application in the field of breast, abdominal and cardiac imaging (Ortiz et al., 2012).
- **Pulse Inversion:** It is the method developed for contrast imaging and offers an improved resolution. This method analyzes the variations in the echo generated by the transmission ultrasound wave and an echo due to its inverted replica.

Ultrasound Image Quality Improvement via Post-Processing Techniques

Figure 3 shows the classification of different post-processing approaches and in which, most of the methods are associated with the class speckle reduction filtering. The purpose of speckle reduction filtering is the suppression of speckle noise introduced in the image acquisition process without disturbing different spatial features in the ultrasound image. Otherwise, the speckle in the ultrasound image affects the visual inspection as well as image processing techniques like segmentation, registration or tissue classification (Soorajkumar et al., 2016).

We have already discussed that many speckle reduction methods modeled the nature of the noise as multiplicative. In (Zong et a., 1998), it has found that the noise is composed of a multiplicative part and additive part, instead of multiplicative noise alone. In fact, the multiplicative component is the predominant one over the additive part (Zhang et al., 2015). Nevertheless, the multiplicative model does not consider the nonlinear processing such as logarithmic compression commonly applied to ultrasound data. So, different assumptions on the empirical distributions of ultrasound data have seen in the literature (Tao et al., 2006).

Different post-processing techniques can be classified based on different criteria or parameters associated with it. For e.g.

- **Based on Noise Model/Distribution:** As discussed earlier, different methods in literature have been adopted different empirical distributions to model the nature of the noise such as Nakagami, Fisher Tippett, Gamma or Weibull (Tao et al., 2006).
- **Based on the Internal Organ to be Photographed:** In practice, speckle is an unavoidable phenomenon during ultrasound imaging of an internal organ. However, different speckle reduction methods are proposed in the literature in application to different organs in the body, like pelvic, kidneys, spleen, stomach, liver, gallbladder, pancreas, intestines, inferior vena cava, carotid arteries and others such as breast and fetus (Perperidis, 2016; Loizou &Pattichis, 2015).

- **Based on the Processing Domain:** The image pixels are modified in the image plane itself in spatial domain filters. Nonetheless, the transform domain filters work on the coefficients obtained by transforming an image into a transform domain and finally, the results procured back into the spatial domain.

Referred to Figure 3, the filters for speckle suppression in ultrasound images can be divided into four categories (i) spatial domain filters (ii) Transform domain filters (iii) statistical filters and (iv) hybrid filters.

In the literature, many despeckling approaches use linear filtering based on local statistics. In linear filtering, the linear combination of neighboring pixel values substitutes the target pixel in the input image. A linear convolutional filter performs a convolutional mask operation by computing a weighted sum of the pixel intensities in a patch around the target pixel position. Contrasts to linear filters, nonlinear filters perform a nonlinear operation to find the filtered output. Also, the nonlocal filtering takes the advantage of redundancy in the image to suppress the speckle noise.

Earlier attempts to despeckle ultrasound images with filters, such as mean and median, resulted in a loss of relevant diagnostic information due to the blurring in the edges of anatomic structures. In (Loizou &Pattichis, 2015), the authors compared twenty despeckling filters that include the linear and nonlinear spatial despeckling filters and a wavelet-based transform domain filter. In (Loizou &Pattichis, 2015), the first order linear despeckling filters such as mean and variance local statistics filter and Wiener despeckle filter and nonlinear filters such as median filter, hybrid median filter, geometric filter, homomorphic filter, and diffusion despeckling filters have been used. In addition, the authors have made a Matlab toolbox available online for these speckle reduction techniques and the details are given in (Loizou et al., 2014). The homomorphic filter first applies the logarithmic transform on images with multiplicative noise and uses additive white Gaussian model for noise removal. In (Biradar et al., 2015), Biradar *et al.* compared 48 denoising filters quantitatively.

Figure 3. Classification of post-processing techniques

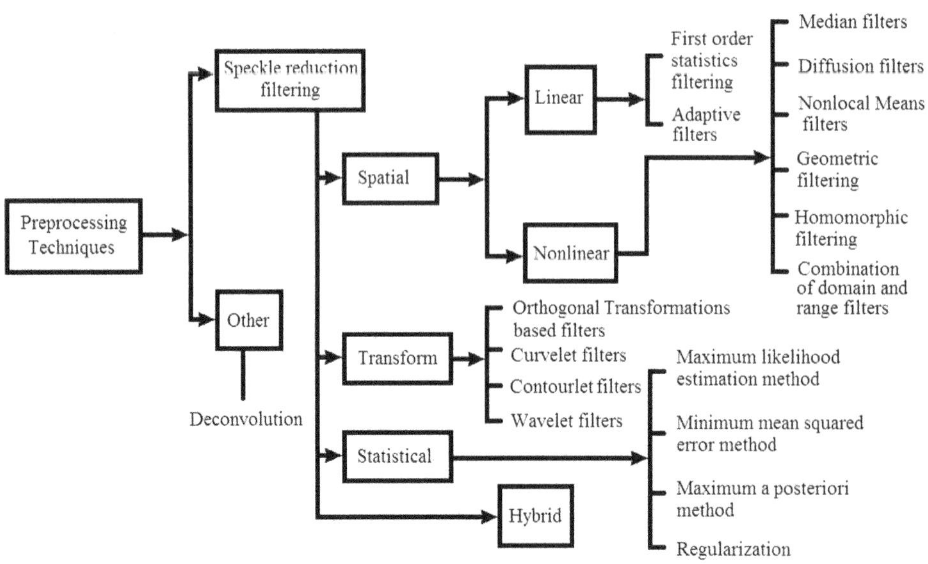

Generally, spatial adaptive filters that rely on local statistics derived from the processed image by modifying some filter parameters like weighting, size, and shape of the filter applied to the image accordingly. The early spatial adaptive filters like Lee's filter (Lee, 1980), Frost's filter (Frost et al., 1982), and Kuan's filter (Kuan et al., 1985) are popular only to suppress the speckle noise without preserving edges very well. These filters use the multiplicative model for the speckle noise. Lopes *et al.* (Lopes et al., 1990) modified the filters in (Lee, 1980; Frost et al., 1982) by arranging the pixels in separate groups in which specific operation is defined.

Another class of speckle reduction filtering is the diffusion despeckle filters. Perona and Malik (Perona & Malik, 1990) first developed the concept of anisotropic diffusion, where the diffusion formulates the smoothening process and the process ceases at object boundaries according to the local gradient strengths in different directions. Thus, the filter is able to achieve a remarkable improvement in the image quality by suppressing noise in uniform regions, maintaining object boundaries and edge sharpening. Diffusion filters like SRAD filter (Yu & Acton, 2002) and its advanced forms in (Aja-Fernández & Alberola-López, 2006) achieve speckle suppression by solving a partial differential equation (PDE) (Perona & Malik, 1990). The diffusion filter in (Vegas-Sanchez-Ferrero et al., 2010) sustains the statistics of tissues and gives better solution compared to the aforementioned filters.

Recently, an effective patch based spatial filtering approach called nonlocal means (NLM) filter and its variants that adapted to an ultrasound noise model are proposed in the literature (Coupé et al., 2008; Coupé et al., 2009). The probabilistic patch based filter (Deledalle et al., 2009) and optimized Bayesian NLM (OBNLM) filter (Coupé et al., 2009) are also employed for speckle reduction.

It is an established fact that the bilateral filter uses both the geometric and photometric spreads to smooth the noise while preserving edges. In (Balocco et al., 2010), the authors present a fully automatic bilateral filter for despeckling ultrasound images. The non-iterative, despeckling trilateral filter (Yu et al., 2011) combines the spatial closeness, intensity similarity and the coefficient of variation component. The trilateral filter makes use of the geometric, photometric and the local structural similarities to smooth the images.

In the past, different filters using transforms such as wavelet, dual-tree complex wavelet (Rabbani et al., 2008; Khare et al., 2010), contourlet (Hiremath et al., 2010; Parthiban & Subramanian, 2006) and curvelet (Devarapu et al., 2010) have been proposed for speckle reduction in ultrasound images. The wavelets based multi-scale techniques are popular transform domain filters and can be categorized into three groups as wavelet thresholding approaches (Donoho & Johnstone, 1994; Coifman & Donoho, 1995), Bayesian approaches and approaches that use coefficients correlation (Pizurica et al, 2006). In (Achim et al., 2001; Gupta et al., 2005; Bhuiyan et al., 2007), the noise reduction in images with non-Gaussian statistics has tested by using Bayesian estimation with the wavelet thresholding successfully. Pizurica *et al.* (Pizurica et al., 2003) introduced *GenLik* filtering which has implemented in the wavelet transform domain by using a generalized likelihood ratio formulation and without prior statistics for speckle and data. Other transform domain filtering of ultrasound images include orthogonal transformations like principal component analysis (PCA) and singular value decomposition (SVD) (Mauldin, 2011).

In addition, different statistical methods such as maximum likelihood (ML) (Shahdoosti & Rahemi, 2018), Maximum-A-Posteriori estimation (MAP) (Achim et al., 2001a), minimum mean squared error (MMSE) (Forouzanfar et al., 2007; Forouzanfar et al., 2010) and Regularization methods such as total variation (TV) (Bioucas-Dias & Figueiredo, 2009) are applied for speckle suppression in ultrasound images. The Rayleigh ML (R-ML) filter in (Aysal & Barner, 2007) that implemented with the Rayleigh density model perform the ML estimation to solve the estimation problem. In Rayleigh Log Euclidean

TV method, a TV regularization was performed on the logarithmically compressed image and Newton's method has been used to solve the convex optimization problem (Seabra et al., 2008).

The class of hybrid methods includes many despeckling filters that combine the advantages of different filters to provide better performance. For example, the filtering output improves when the transform domain filter combines with a linear or nonlinear filter as in (Gupta et al, 2015; Zhang et al, 2015a; Fu et al., 2015; Abrahim et al., 2012). The hybrid filter in (Ogier et al, 2006) uses a PDE-based method in the wavelet-transformed domain. Also, different hybrid filters can be implemented by combining wavelets and statistical methods (Gupta et al., 2004; Achim et al., 2001).

Deconvolution is another post-processing method, which makes use of the point spread function (PSF) of the image scanner to improve the resolution in ultrasound images. Since PSF represents the system response in the frequency domain, the image is modeled in the spatial domain by convolving the PSF and the tissue reflectivity function or by multiplying corresponding Fourier transforms in the frequency domain. Thus, it can mitigate the effect of the PSF in the image.

Recent Post-Processing Approaches for Enhancing Ultrasound Images

In this section, we investigate the major contributions in the past four years starting from 2015 to 2018 for reducing speckle and for enhancing ultrasound images. The study is intended to list different methods in the literature. It may help a large number of people in the ultrasound imaging research community in understanding the research trends in recent years and pave the way for future research.

In 2015, Homogeneity Map Method (HMM) based speckle reduction technique was introduced. It improves ultrasound image quality through the speckle reduction and edge preservation capabilities of a filter and compared the results with SRAD and OBNLM filters for validation (Gungor & Karagoz, 2015). HMM produce better smoothing of homogeneous regions in the image without edge loss. An anisotropic diffusion filter (Ramos-Llordén et al., 2015) was proposed based on probabilistic models to avoid the over-filtering, which occurs with the progressive loss of original information during the course of diffusion. Also, the filtering process is assisted by a memory mechanism with a delay differential equation (DDE) for the diffusion tensor to maintain significant structural information in the image. The diffusion flux function associated with the DDE follows a tissue-selective Volterra equation. The method in (Uddin et al., 2015) assumed a Rayleigh model for the noisy data and suppress the noise through a cascade forward back propagation neural network based algorithm. It estimates the wavelet features of the ultrasound image using the dual-tree complex wavelet transform. In (Fu et al., 2015), an adaptive despeckling algorithm was proposed using a Bayesian framework that incorporates a quantum-inspired thresholding function derived using DTCWT coefficients.

The framework in (Kishore et al., 2015) reduces speckle in the ultrasound images and then restores the degraded object boundaries during denoising. Also, it employs block-based thresholding of wavelet coefficients for denoising and wavelet coefficient fusion of object in the original and denoised ultrasound images for restoration. The idea of TV regularization was applied for speckle filtering in (Bioucas-Dias & Fugueiredo, 2010; Seabra J. et al., 2008). The method has been extended in (Afonso & Sanches, 2015) with an alternating direction method of multipliers (ADMM). It relies on the Rayleigh distribution of speckle noise.

In 2016, Chen *et al.* proposed an ADMM-based compressive deconvolution approach for ultrasound imaging systems and claimed that it is the first compressive deconvolution method for ultrasound images (Chen et al., 2016). It utilizes a regularizer to impose the sparsity of the target image in the transform domain and the other regularizer imposes generalized Gaussian distributed statistics to model the tissue reflectivity function. In the adaptive fuzzy logic filter approach (Babu & Sudha, 2016), the system adaptively performs proper filtering to different areas of the image classified with fuzzy logic technique on the coefficients of variation obtained from the noisy log transformed image. Sudeep *et al.* proposed an unbiased NLM speckle filter (Sudeep et al., 2016) based on Gamma statistics. In (Yang et al., 2016), the NLM based hybrid filter uses a similarity measure by amalgamating the local and non-local information derived from the image.

In 2017, a hybrid algorithm (Singh et al., 2017) has been proposed with a non-iterative three-stage process. First, a guided filter suppress the speckle using the local statistics. Second, there is a bilateral filter having good speckle reducing capability to deal with multiplicative noise. Finally, the goodness of bilateral and NLM filters has used to reconstruct the diffused edges and thus efficient speckle reduction. Shao *et al.* (Shao et al., 2017) proposed a despeckling filter using fractional partial differential equations. In (Wang et al., 2018), Wang *et al.* employed regularization as a blend of TV and high-order TV and used a generalized Kullback Leibler divergence for the data fidelity term. This approach overcomes staircase artifacts in the TV method by utilizing ADMM. In (Baselice, 2017), the NLM method finds the pixel similarity with the Kolmogorov-Smirnov distance. The latest Eigen based clutter filter (Song et al., 2017) can effectively separate tissue, blood, and noise via singular value cutoff thresholds computed adaptively based on local data statistics.

In 2018, Shahdoosti *et al.* (Shahdoosti & Rahemi, 2018) developed a new NLML filter with the Pearson distance based similarity for obtaining speckle reduction. The method in (Gai et al., 2018) employs monogenic wavelet transform (MWT) and the Bayesian framework. Also, Laplace mixture distribution and Rayleigh distribution are used to modeling the MWT coefficients of the ground truth signal and the noisy signal, respectively. The speckle noise reduction is attained with a new Bayesian minimum mean square error estimator.

The most important limitations of the speckle reduction approaches discussed so far can be encapsulated as follows: (1) Some approaches suffer from over-smoothing or generate images with artificial appearances (2) The performance of a few despeckling algorithms varies with ultrasound images from different organs. Hence, a precise tuning of the implementation parameters is necessary for each input image to get the best results (Mishra et al., 2018). (3) Many methods have high computation burden. (4) The methods with oversimplified assumptions result in suboptimal performances (5) A few approaches are based on inadequate noise models.

MAIN FOCUS OF THE CHAPTER

Till now, we described various techniques for the enhancement of ultrasound images in this literature. Also, this chapter includes the literature review of the filtering approaches in the past four years starting from 2015 to 2018 for reducing speckle and for enhancing ultrasound. Next section is devoted to comparing a few state-of-the-art despeckling techniques using simulated data and real ultrasound data.

PERFORMANCE ANALYSIS OF DESPECKLING FILTERS ON ULTRASOUND DATA

This section examines the results of some popular despeckling filters on simulated and real ultrasound images through objective and subjective analyses.

Noise Model

To achieve an accurate statistical characterization of ultrasound signals and thereby, to improve the despeckling, various distributions have been recommended in the past (Aysal & Barner, 2007). In ultrasound data with fully developed speckle and without compression, the interpolated ultrasound B-scans can be approximated with Gamma distribution (Vegas-Sanchez-Ferrero et al., 2010a). Gamma shows decent fitting for the weighted addition of Rayleigh variables. Thus, in this chapter, the recently proposed Gamma model in (Sudeep et al., 2016) is considered suitable for images having speckle noise.

The generation of Gamma distributed simulated image J is mathematically expressed as (Sudeep et al., 2016):

$$J = I + N_g \tag{3}$$

where I and N_g represent the ground truth and Gamma random noise, respectively.

Methods

The different filters chosen for the comparative study are given below:

- **Bayesian Method (Wong et al., 2010):** The algorithm proposed by Wong *et al.* in [80] uses a conditional posterior sampling approach to select relevant data from the noisy image to find the posterior distribution associated with Bayesian least squares estimation and helps to reduce the loss of structural detail in the despeckled image. The authors assumed the noise is multiplicative and hence, projected the observed noisy image v into the logarithmic space to separate the noiseless data $u_l = \log\{u\}$ and the speckle noise $n_l - \log\{u\}$. In the logarithmic space, the noisy image v_l is given as:

$$v_l = u_l + n_l \tag{4}$$

After computing general Bayesian least squares estimate $\hat{u}_l$, the noiseless data u can be created by back-projecting the Bayesian estimate of u_l using:

$$\hat{u} = \exp\{\hat{u}_l\} \tag{5}$$

- **Wiener Filter (Lim, 1990):** Initially, the filter computes local mean μ_L and standard deviation σ_L from the neighborhood ζ of the target pixel in the noisy image v. The noise standard deviation σ_g is computed by averaging all the local estimated variances. Then, the noise-less image $\hat{u}$ pixel at (n_1, n_2) is estimated as:

$$\hat{u}(n_1, n_2) = \mu_L + \frac{\sigma_L^2 - \sigma_g^2}{\sigma_L^2}\left(v(n_1, n_2) - \mu_L\right) \tag{6}$$

- **Bilateral Filter (Tomasi & Manduchi, 1998):** This nonlinear method is a prevalent spatial filter for removing noise while retaining the edges. The output of the bilateral filter at a pixel location p is:

$$\hat{u}(p) = \frac{1}{C}\sum_{q \in N(p)} K_d(p,q) K_r(p,q) v(p,q) \tag{7}$$

where $N(p)$ denotes the neighborhood around the position p, and q is the position in the neighborhood. The constant C is given by:

$$C = \sum_{q \in N(p)} K_d(p,q) K_r(p,q) \tag{8}$$

where the kernels K_d and K_r form the domain filter and the range filter of the bilateral filter, respectively. The kernels K_d and K_r measure the photometric similarity and the radiometric similarity of a pixel around its neighborhood, respectively.

- **SBF (Tay et al., 2006):** The squeezebox filter is an iterative filtering method and each iteration starts by finding outliers which are the set of locations of local maxima and local minima. In each iteration, it smooths the outliers locally by replacing them with the local mean computed without including the outliers in its computation.
- **SRAD (Yu & Acton, 2002):** Perona and Malik performed anisotropic diffusion technique that uses the concept of time-dependent heat diffusion equation to reduce noise by keeping significant image parts such as edges or lines (Perona & Malik, 1990). The diffusion equation of an image with continuous variables over time $J(i, j, t)$ has the form:

$$J(i, j, t) = div\left(c_v(i, j, t)\nabla J(i, j, t)\right) \tag{9}$$

where $div(\cdot)$ is the divergence operator and ∇ is the gradient operator. In (Yu & Acton, 2002), the authors substituted the coefficient of variation c_v with the instantaneous coefficient of variation $c_{v,inst}$ in Eq. 9 to obtain the SRAD filter. The parameter $c_{v,inst}$ is used to control the smoothing operation.

- **OBNLM (Coupé et al., 2009):** The Bayesian nonlocal-means speckle filter in (Coupé et al., 2009) uses a relevant ultrasound noise model. In the paper, the authors preferred its blockwise implementation to reduce the computational burden.
- γ **NLM (Sudeep et al., 2016):** This NLM filter uses Gamma distribution to fit ultrasound data. Suppose i.i.d. random variables $\boldsymbol{y} = y_1, y_2, \cdots y_t$ from a Gamma distribution with the shape and scale parameters ρ and β, respectively. An ML estimator based on three-parameter Gamma function calculates the parameters ρ and β from the noisy image locally and the estimator is given by:

$$\left\{\hat{\rho}, \hat{\beta}\right\} = \arg\max_{\rho,\beta}\left(\log \mathcal{L}\right) \tag{10}$$

where,

$$\log\mathcal{L} = \left(\rho - 1\right)\sum_{i=1}^{t}\log(y_i - \mu_y + \rho\beta) - \frac{1}{\beta}\sum_{i=1}^{t}(y_i - \mu_y + \rho\beta) - t\left[\log(\text{“}(\rho) + \rho\log\left(\beta\right)\right] \tag{11}$$

and μ_y is the mean of the distribution. Then, an unbiased NLM filter is developed to estimate the noise-free image.

Experimental Setup

In this study, we have performed the comparison of seven despeckling methods in ultrasound images. All of them are implemented on MATLAB R2018a (Version 9.4) installed on a desktop computer with a 64-bit windows 10 operating system, Intel i7 processor and 16 GB of RAM. The default values for different filter parameters are listed below:

1. **Bayesian (Wong et al., 2010):** $\sigma_{spatial}$=1.5; window size = 3×3; number of samples = 70; Sigma factor = 2.
2. **Wiener filter (Lim, 1990):** size of $\zeta = 5 \times 5$.
3. **Bilateral filter (Tomasi & Manduchi, 1998):** Half-width = 5; σ_d=1.7; σ_r=0.1.
4. **SBF (Tay et al., 2006):** Window size = 3×3; 45 iterations; Gaussian noise $\left(\sigma = 0.1\right)$ added at every 5th iteration.
5. **SRAD (Yu & Acton, 2002):** 80 iterations; time step=0.3.
6. **OBNLM (Coupé et al., 2009):** Search area size = 11×11; patch size = 3×3; smoothing parameter = 0.7.
7. γ **NLM Filter (Sudeep et al., 2016):** Search window size = 11×11; similarity window size = 3×3.

Dataset

To perform the comparison of the abovementioned despeckling methods, the experiments are conducted on simulated data and real data. The modified Shepp Logan phantom image with size 256×256 has been used to perform the qualitative analysis using simulated data and the quantitative analysis. In (Zukal et al., 2011), the public ultrasound dataset comprises common carotid artery (CCA) images acquired with Sonix OP ultrasound scanner. There are 84 B-mode ultrasound images of CCA in longitudinal section. During our experiments on real data, we used two images of the public ultrasound dataset as shown in Fig. 6 (a) and Fig. 7 (a) with size 339×446 and 340×538 respectively. In Fig. 8, we have shown the results obtained from the experiment conducted on the real ultrasound image of CCA with size 482×466 available with the despeckling toolbox in (Loizou et al, 2014a).

Experiments on Simulated Images

In this section, qualitative and quantitative assessment of a simulated phantom image has presented. Also, the objective image quality evaluation metrics like PSNR (Fisher, 2012), mean SSIM (Wang, 2004) and Bhattacharrya coefficient (BC) (Bhattacharyya, 1943) are used for the assessment.

Figure 4 shows the despeckled images obtained with different algorithms on a corrupted modified Shepp Logan phantom image with Gamma noise ($\rho \times \beta = 56$) and corresponding residual images are displayed in Figure 5. To create simulated images, we altered the modified Shepp Logan phantom image with Gamma-distributed random noise produced for different ρ and β values and hence, with various values of bias, $\rho \times \beta = 6$ to 54. For quantitative assessment, we computed PSNR, mean SSIM and BC for the outputs obtained with different despeckling methods and the results are encapsulated in Table 1, Table 2 and Table 3. We can observe from Figure 4, Figure 5, Table 1, Table 2 and Table 3 that the γ NLM outperforms other state-of-the-art approaches.

Experiments on Real Ultrasound Images

For comparison, we conducted experiments on three real B-mode ultrasound images by applying different despeckling algorithms. The first two images are obtained from the public dataset in (Zukal et al., 2011) and the one is available with the despeckling toolbox in (Loizou et al., 2014a). The estimated values for parameters ρ and β with the images in Figure 6 (a), Figure 7 (a) and Figure 8 (a) are $\left(\hat{\rho}_{ML}, \hat{\beta}_{ML}\right)$ = (2,2), $\left(\hat{\rho}_{ML}, \hat{\beta}_{ML}\right)$ = (2,2) and $\left(\hat{\rho}_{ML}, \hat{\beta}_{ML}\right)$ = (4,3), respectively. The experiment results are displayed in Figure 6, Figure 7 and Figure 8, respectively.

In Figure 6, Figure 7 and Figure 8, the different layers and the lumen associated with CCA are present. Nonetheless, the over-smoothing of an image can hide the closely spaced layers in the wall of CCA. It can be observed from the results on simulated as well as real data that γ NLM filter is showing a remarkable speckle reduction in ultrasound images and outperforms other approaches in edge preservation. It is obvious that the selection of a proper noise model, the excellent quantification of bias and its elimination are actually contributed to the improved despeckling property of the γ NLM.

Our experiments by varying similarity window size of the γ NLM indicate that smaller similarity window gives a better despeckling performance. In addition, a similar experiment by varying the search

Figure 4. Outputs for different despeckling methods on the phantom image corrupted with Gamma noise (ρ = 8; β = 7) (a) Original phantom image (b) Noisy image (c) Bayesian estimation method(d) Wiener Filter (e) Bilateral Filter (f) SBF (g) SRAD (h) OBNLM and (i) γ NLM.

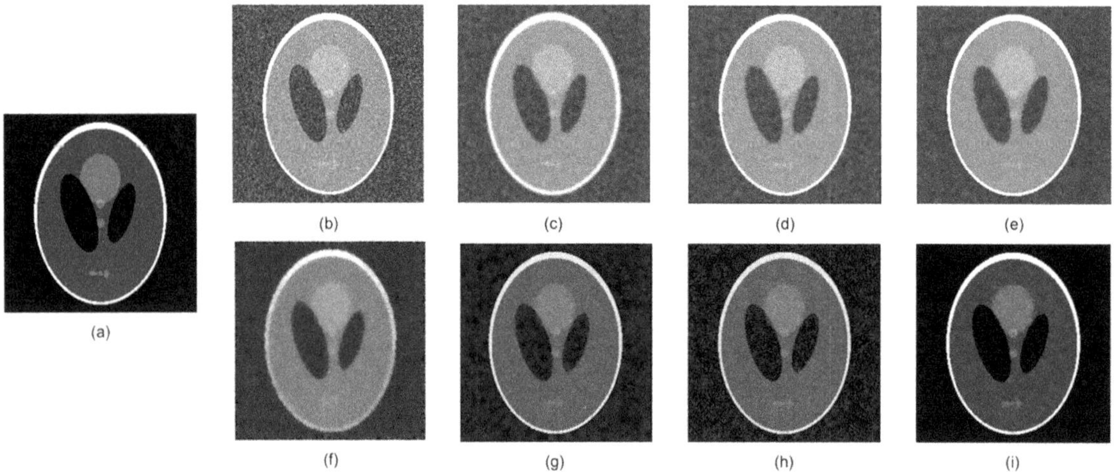

Figure 5. Residual images computed using the original phantom image and different despeckled images in Figure 4. Figure 5 (a) –(g) corresponds to Figure 4 (c) –(i) (scale 0-70).

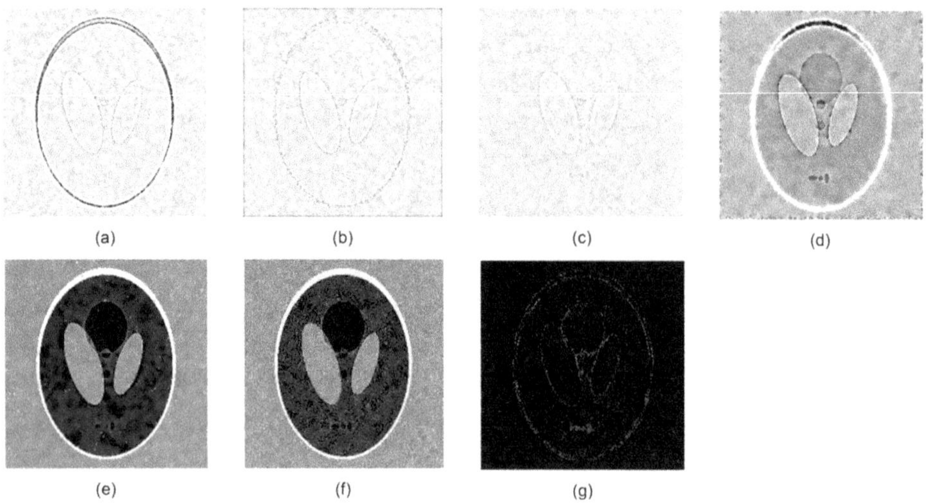

window alone showed that the result is improved when a big search window is used. The disadvantage of the γ NLM is its computational burden, which is almost equal to that of the NLM filter in (Coupé et al., 2009). However, extra computation is involved for the ML estimation of the Gamma parameters and thus, for the quantification of the noise level.

Table 1. Performance comparison of different despeckling techniques based on PSNR

Filter	PSNR(dB)			
	ρ = 3; β = 2	ρ = 4; β = 3	ρ = 6; β = 6	ρ = 8; β = 7
Bayesian	21.6607	20.7055	15.8067	12.6280
Wiener	31.3761	26.1854	16.9627	13.1628
Bilateral	32.3628	26.5226	17.1037	13.2508
SBF	20.3896	19.7618	17.1330	15.5278
SRAD	33.3607	28.4792	21.3094	19.0669
OBNLM	33.1554	28.5730	21.4568	19.1919
γNLM	48.2571	44.8810	37.1887	34.5019

Table 2. Performance comparison of different despeckling techniques based on mean SSIM

Filter	MSSIM			
	ρ = 3; β = 2	ρ = 4; β = 3	ρ = 6; β = 6	ρ = 8; β = 7
Bayesian	0.5020	0.4381	0.3562	0.3046
Wiener	0.5574	0.4899	0.4039	0.3501
Bilateral	0.5729	0.5048	0.4101	0.3336
SBF	0.5274	0.4506	0.3845	0.3578
SRAD	0.5925	0.5235	0.4601	0.4387
OBNLM	0.5954	0.5285	0.4499	0.3806
γNLM	0.9851	0.9735	0.8637	0.7989

Table 3. Performance comparison of different despeckling techniques based on BC

Filter	BC			
	ρ = 3; β = 2	ρ = 4; β = 3	ρ = 6; β = 6	ρ = 8; β = 7
Bayesian	0.5020	0.4381	0.3562	0.3046
Wiener	0.5574	0.4899	0.4039	0.3501
Bilateral	0.5729	0.5048	0.4101	0.3336
SBF	0.5274	0.4506	0.3845	0.3578
SRAD	0.5925	0.5235	0.4601	0.4387
OBNLM	0.5954	0.5285	0.4499	0.3806
γNLM	0.9851	0.9735	0.8637	0.7989

Figure 6. Outputs for different despeckling methods applied to the first real B-mode ultrasound image of CCA (Zukal et al., 2011) (a) Real Image $\left(\hat{\rho}_{ML} = 2,\ \hat{\beta}_{ML} = 2\right)$ *(b) Bayesian estimation method (c) Wiener Filter (d) Bilateral Filter (e) SBF (f) SRAD (g) OBNLM (h)* γ *NLM.*

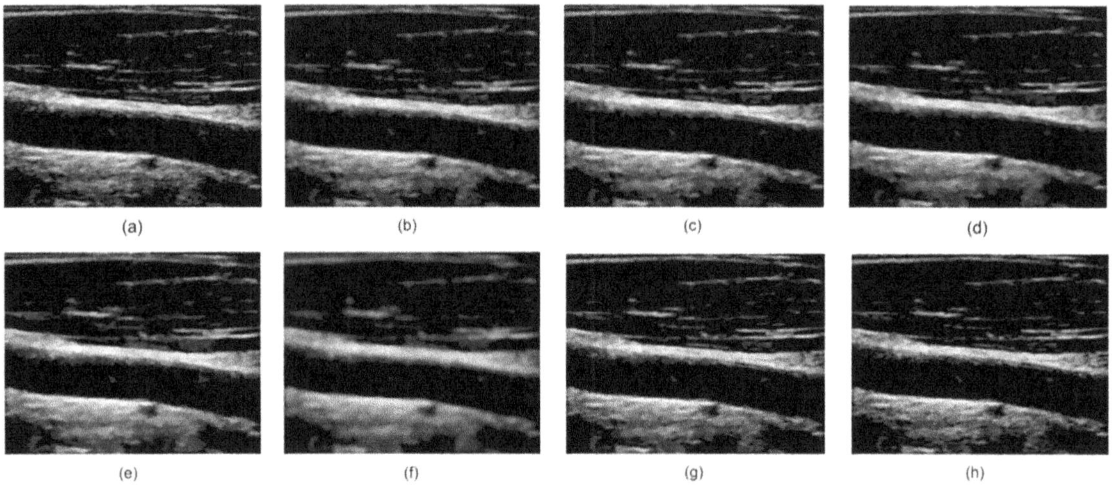

Figure 7. Outputs for different despeckling methods applied to the first real B-mode ultrasound image of CCA (Zukal et al., 2011) (a) Real Image $\left(\hat{\rho}_{ML} = 2,\ \hat{\beta}_{ML} = 2\right)$ *(b) Bayesian estimation method (c) Wiener Filter (d) Bilateral Filter (e) SBF (f) SRAD (g) OBNLM (h)* γ *NLM.*

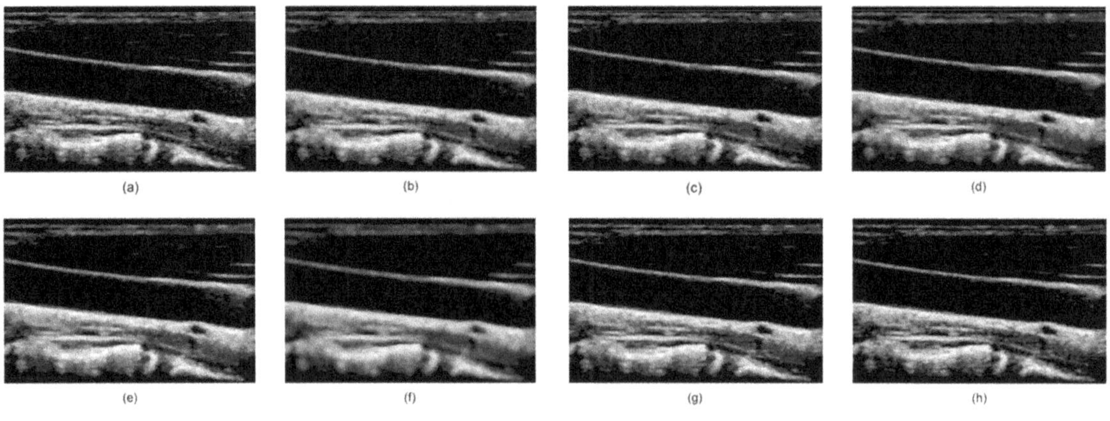

FUTURE RESEARCH DIRECTIONS

In recent years, machine learning algorithms are used for medical image processing and analysis. A machine learning algorithm can learn from data and allows computers to make proper estimations of results without being explicitly programmed. Deep learning is a large class of machine learning methods that learn in supervised or unsupervised modes. It uses artificial neural network layers with better capabilities. A few deep learning approaches have been examined for despeckling ultrasound images.

Figure 8. Outputs for different despeckling methods applied to the third real B-mode ultrasound image of CCA [88] (a) Real Image $\left(\hat{\rho}_{ML} = 4,\ \hat{\beta}_{ML} = 3\right)$ *(b) Bayesian estimation method (c) Wiener Filter (d) Bilateral Filter (e) SBF (f) SRAD (g) OBNLM (h)* γ *NLM.*

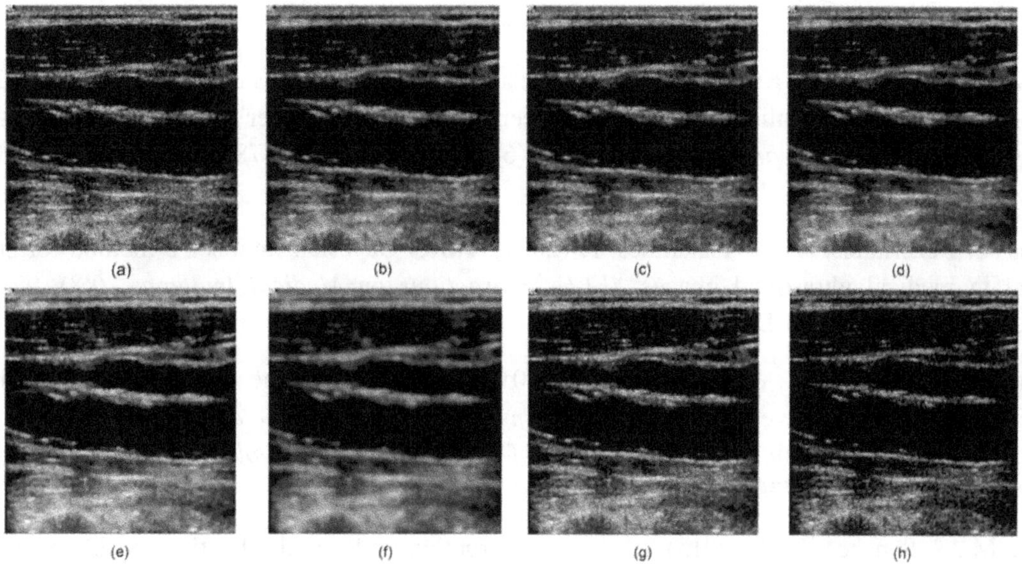

Recently, some deep learning approaches have been examined for despeckling ultrasound images. In 2018, Deepak Mishra et al. proposed a deep unsupervised learning method (Mishra et al., 2018) to reduce speckle and to preserve the relevant anatomical information in the image. The authors first trained a deep residual network to reproduce the inputs. Then, it is combined with the adversarial loss imposed by a discriminator network and trained to suppress speckle in ultrasound images. Also, a structural loss term is used to act as a regularizer and helps in producing the desired outputs. In (Vedula et al., 2017), the authors showed that the proposed multiresolution convolutional neural network is able to reconstruct computed tomography (CT) quality images (apart from despeckling) from ultrasound images. For the purpose, the networks were trained and tested on pairs of CT and the corresponding ultrasound images. However, in practice, the CT- Ultrasound paired data is difficult to obtain. In future, different machine learning techniques can be employed to enhance the image quality in ultrasound.

CONCLUSION

In this chapter, we have discussed many methods for enhancing the medical ultrasound images via speckle reduction. Also, we categorize different ultrasound image enhancement methods such as preprocessing and post-processing techniques. The different classes of each of the techniques are discussed. In addition, the chapter compares some recent filtering techniques for ultrasound image enhancement. We observe that the summary of the ultrasound enhancement techniques discussed so far will help a large number of people in the ultrasound imaging research community to make easier to understand the trends and pave the way for future research.

REFERENCES

Abrahim, B. A., Mustafa, Z. A., Yassine, I. A., Zayed, N., & Kadah, Y. M. (2012). Hybrid total variation and wavelet thresholding speckle reduction for medical ultrasound imaging. *Journal of Medical Imaging and Health Informatics*, *2*(2), 114–124. doi:10.1166/jmihi.2012.1072

Acharya, U. R., Sree, S. V., Kulshreshtha, S., Molinari, F., Koh, J. E. W., Saba, L., & Suri, J. S. (2014). GyneScan: An improved online paradigm for screening of ovarian cancer via tissue characterization. *Technology in Cancer Research & Treatment*, *13*(6), 529–539. doi:10.7785/tcrtexpress.2013.600273 PMID:24325128

Achim, A., Bezerianos, A., & Tsakalides, P. (2001). Novel Bayesian multiscale method for speckle removal in medical ultrasound images. *IEEE Transactions on Medical Imaging*, *20*(8), 772–783. doi:10.1109/42.938245 PMID:11513028

Achim, A., Bezerianos, A., & Tsakalides, P. (2001a). Ultrasound image denoising via maximum a posteriori estimation of wavelet coefficients. In *Engineering in Medicine and Biology Society, 2001. Proceedings of the 23rd Annual International Conference of the IEEE* (*Vol. 3*, pp. 2553-2556). IEEE. 10.1109/IEMBS.2001.1017300

Afonso, M., & Sanches, J. M. (2015). Image reconstruction under multiplicative speckle noise using total variation. *Neurocomputing*, *150*, 200–213. doi:10.1016/j.neucom.2014.08.073

Aja-Fernández, S., & Alberola-López, C. (2006). On the estimation of the coefficient of variation for anisotropic diffusion speckle filtering. *IEEE Transactions on Image Processing*, *15*(9), 2694–2701. doi:10.1109/TIP.2006.877360 PMID:16948314

Araki, T., Ikeda, N., Shukla, D., Londhe, N. D., Shrivastava, V. K., Banchhor, S. K., ... Suri, J. S. (2016). A new method for IVUS-based coronary artery disease risk stratification: A link between coronary & carotid ultrasound plaque burdens. *Computer Methods and Programs in Biomedicine*, *124*, 161–179. doi:10.1016/j.cmpb.2015.10.022 PMID:26707374

Aysal, T. C., & Barner, K. E. (2007). Rayleigh-maximum-likelihood filtering for speckle reduction of ultrasound images. *IEEE Transactions on Medical Imaging*, *26*(5), 712–727. doi:10.1109/TMI.2007.895484 PMID:17518065

Babu, J. J. J., & Sudha, G. F. (2016). Adaptive speckle reduction in ultrasound images using fuzzy logic on Coefficient of Variation. *Biomedical Signal Processing and Control*, *23*, 93–103. doi:10.1016/j.bspc.2015.08.001

Balocco, S., Gatta, C., Pujol, O., Mauri, J., & Radeva, P. (2010). SRBF: Speckle reducing bilateral filtering. *Ultrasound in Medicine & Biology*, *36*(8), 1353–1363. doi:10.1016/j.ultrasmedbio.2010.05.007 PMID:20691924

Baselice, F. (2017). Ultrasound image despeckling based on statistical similarity. *Ultrasound in Medicine & Biology*, *43*(9), 2065–2078. doi:10.1016/j.ultrasmedbio.2017.05.006 PMID:28651920

Bhattacharyya, A. (1943). On a measure of divergence between two statistical populations defined by their probability distributions. *Bulletin of the Calcutta Mathematical Society*, *35*, 99–109.

Bhuiyan, M. I. H., Ahmad, M. O., & Swamy, M. N. S. (2007, May). New spatially adaptive wavelet-based method for the despeckling of medical ultrasound images. In *Circuits and Systems, 2007. ISCAS 2007. IEEE International Symposium on* (pp. 2347-2350). IEEE.

Bioucas-Dias, J. M., & Figueiredo, M. A. (2009, November). Total variation restoration of speckled images using a split-Bregman algorithm. In *Image Processing (ICIP), 2009 16th IEEE International Conference on* (pp. 3717-3720). IEEE.

Bioucas-Dias, J. M., & Figueiredo, M. A. (2010). Multiplicative noise removal using variable splitting and constrained optimization. *IEEE Transactions on Image Processing, 19*(7), 1720–1730. doi:10.1109/TIP.2010.2045029 PMID:20215071

Biradar, N., Dewal, M. L., & Rohit, M. K. (2015). Speckle noise reduction in B-mode echocardiographic images: A comparison. *IETE Technical Review, 32*(6), 435–453. doi:10.1080/02564602.2015.1031714

Chen, Z., Basarab, A., & Kouamé, D. (2016). Compressive deconvolution in medical ultrasound imaging. *IEEE Transactions on Medical Imaging, 35*(3), 728–737. doi:10.1109/TMI.2015.2493241 PMID:26513780

Christodoulou, C. I., Loizou, C., Pattichis, C. S., Pantziaris, M., Kyriakou, E., Pattichis, M. S., . . . Nicolaides, A. (2002). De-speckle filtering in ultrasound imaging of the carotid artery. In *Engineering in Medicine and Biology, 2002. 24th Annual Conference and the Annual Fall Meeting of the Biomedical Engineering Society EMBS/BMES Conference, 2002. Proceedings of the Second Joint* (*Vol. 2*, pp. 1027-1028). IEEE. 10.1109/IEMBS.2002.1106259

Coifman, R. R., & Donoho, D. L. (1995). Translation-invariant de-noising. In *Wavelets and statistics* (pp. 125–150). New York, NY: Springer. doi:10.1007/978-1-4612-2544-7_9

Coupé, P., Hellier, P., Kervrann, C., & Barillot, C. (2008, May). Bayesian non local means-based speckle filtering. In *Biomedical Imaging: From Nano to Macro, 2008. ISBI 2008. 5th IEEE International Symposium on* (pp. 1291-1294). IEEE. 10.1109/ISBI.2008.4541240

Coupé, P., Hellier, P., Kervrann, C., & Barillot, C. (2009). Nonlocal means-based speckle filtering for ultrasound images. *IEEE Transactions on Image Processing, 18*(10), 2221–2229. doi:10.1109/TIP.2009.2024064 PMID:19482578

Del Cura, J. L., Seguí, P., & Nicolau, C. (Eds.). (2012). *Learning Ultrasound Imaging*. Springer Science & Business Media. doi:10.1007/978-3-642-30586-3

Deledalle, C. A., Denis, L., & Tupin, F. (2009). Iterative weighted maximum likelihood denoising with probabilistic patch-based weights. *IEEE Transactions on Image Processing, 18*(12), 2661–2672. doi:10.1109/TIP.2009.2029593 PMID:19666338

Devarapu, K. V., Murala, S., & Kumar, V. (2010, February). Denoising of ultrasound images using curvelet transform. In *Computer and Automation Engineering (ICCAE), 2010 The 2nd International Conference on* (Vol. 3, pp. 447-451). IEEE.

Donoho, D. L., & Johnstone, J. M. (1994). Ideal spatial adaptation by wavelet shrinkage. *Biometrika, 81*(3), 425-455.

Fisher, Y. (2012). *Fractal image compression: theory and application.* Springer Science & Business Media.

Forouzanfar, M., Moghaddam, H. A., & Dehghani, M. (2007, June). Speckle reduction in medical ultrasound images using a new multiscale bivariate Bayesian MMSE-based method. In Signal Processing and Communications Applications, 2007. SIU 2007. IEEE 15th (pp. 1-4). IEEE.

Forouzanfar, M., Moghaddam, H. A., & Gity, M. (2010). A new multiscale Bayesian algorithm for speckle reduction in medical ultrasound images. *Signal, Image and Video Processing*, *4*(3), 359–375. doi:10.100711760-009-0126-3

Frost, V. S., Stiles, J. A., Shanmugan, K. S., & Holtzman, J. C. (1982). A model for radar images and its application to adaptive digital filtering of multiplicative noise. *IEEE Transactions on Pattern Analysis and Machine Intelligence*, *PAMI-4*(2), 157–166. doi:10.1109/TPAMI.1982.4767223 PMID:21869022

Fu, X., Wang, Y., Chen, L., & Tian, J. (2015). An image despeckling approach using quantum-inspired statistics in dual-tree complex wavelet domain. *Biomedical Signal Processing and Control*, *18*, 30–35. doi:10.1016/j.bspc.2014.11.005

Gai, S., Zhang, B., Yang, C., & Yu, L. (2018). Speckle noise reduction in medical ultrasound image using monogenic wavelet and Laplace mixture distribution. *Digital Signal Processing*, *72*, 192–207. doi:10.1016/j.dsp.2017.10.006

Goodman, J. W. (1975). Statistical properties of laser speckle patterns. In *Laser speckle and related phenomena* (pp. 9–75). Berlin: Springer.

Guenther, D. A., & Walker, W. F. (2007). Optimal apodization design for medical ultrasound using constrained least squares part I: Theory. *IEEE Transactions on Ultrasonics, Ferroelectrics, and Frequency Control*, *54*(2). PMID:17328330

Gungor, M. A., & Karagoz, I. (2015). The homogeneity map method for speckle reduction in diagnostic ultrasound images. *Measurement*, *68*, 100–110. doi:10.1016/j.measurement.2015.02.047

Gupta, D., Anand, R. S., & Tyagi, B. (2015). Despeckling of ultrasound medical images using ripplet domain nonlinear filtering. *Signal, Image and Video Processing*, *9*(5), 1093–1111. doi:10.100711760-013-0540-4

Gupta, S., Chauhan, R. C., & Saxena, S. C. (2005). Locally adaptive wavelet domain Bayesian processor for denoising medical ultrasound images using Speckle modelling based on Rayleigh distribution. *IEE Proceedings. Vision Image and Signal Processing*, *152*(1), 129–135. doi:10.1049/ip-vis:20050975

Gupta, S., Chauhan, R. C., & Sexana, S. C. (2004). Wavelet-based statistical approach for speckle reduction in medical ultrasound images. *Medical & Biological Engineering & Computing*, *42*(2), 189–192. doi:10.1007/BF02344630 PMID:15125148

Hiremath, P. S., Akkasaligar, P. T., & Badiger, S. (2010). Speckle reducing contourlet transform for medical ultrasound images. *Int J Compt Inf Engg*, *4*(4), 284–291.

Jespersen, S. K., Wilhjelm, J. E., & Sillesen, H. (1998). Multi-angle compound imaging. *Ultrasonic Imaging*, *20*(2), 81–102. doi:10.1177/016173469802000201 PMID:9691367

Khare, A., Khare, M., Jeong, Y., Kim, H., & Jeon, M. (2010). Despeckling of medical ultrasound images using Daubechies complex wavelet transform. *Signal Processing*, *90*(2), 428–439. doi:10.1016/j.sigpro.2009.07.008

Kishore, P. V. V., Kumar, K. V. V., Prasad, M. V. D., Goutham, E. N. D., Rahul, R., Krishna, C. V., & Sandeep, Y. (2015). Twofold processing for denoising ultrasound medical images. *SpringerPlus*, *4*(1), 775. doi:10.118640064-015-1566-6 PMID:26697285

Krissian, K., Westin, C. F., Kikinis, R., & Vosburgh, K. G. (2007). Oriented speckle reducing anisotropic diffusion. *IEEE Transactions on Image Processing*, *16*(5), 1412–1424. doi:10.1109/TIP.2007.891803 PMID:17491469

Kuan, D. T., Sawchuk, A. A., Strand, T. C., & Chavel, P. (1985). Adaptive noise smoothing filter for images with signal-dependent noise. *IEEE Transactions on Pattern Analysis and Machine Intelligence*, *PAMI-7*(2), 165–177. doi:10.1109/TPAMI.1985.4767641 PMID:21869255

Lee, J. S. (1980). Digital image enhancement and noise filtering by use of local statistics. *IEEE Transactions on Pattern Analysis and Machine Intelligence*, *PAMI-2*(2), 165–168. doi:10.1109/TPAMI.1980.4766994 PMID:21868887

Li, P. C., & Chen, M. J. (2002). Strain compounding: A new approach for speckle reduction. *IEEE Transactions on Ultrasonics, Ferroelectrics, and Frequency Control*, *49*(1), 39–46. doi:10.1109/58.981382 PMID:11833890

Lim, J. S. (1990). *Two-dimensional signal and image processing*. Englewood Cliffs, NJ: Prentice Hall.

Loizou, C. P., & Pattichis, C. S. (2015). Despeckle filtering for ultrasound imaging and video, Volume I: Algorithms and software. *Synthesis Lectures on Algorithms and Software in Engineering*, *7*(1), 1–180. doi:10.2200/S00641ED1V01Y201504ASE014

Loizou, C. P., Pattichis, C. S., Christodoulou, C. I., Istepanian, R. S., Pantziaris, M., & Nicolaides, A. (2005). Comparative evaluation of despeckle filtering in ultrasound imaging of the carotid artery. *IEEE Transactions on Ultrasonics, Ferroelectrics, and Frequency Control*, *52*(10), 1653–1669. doi:10.1109/TUFFC.2005.1561621 PMID:16382618

Loizou, C. P., Pattichis, C. S., Christodoulou, C. I., Istepanian, R. S., Pantziaris, M., & Nicolaides, A. (2014a). *Image despeckle filtering (IDF) toolbox.* Retrieved from http://www.medinfo.cs.ucy.ac.cy/doc/toolboxes/IDF.zip

Loizou, C. P., Theofanous, C., Pantziaris, M., & Kasparis, T. (2014). Despeckle filtering software toolbox for ultrasound imaging of the common carotid artery. *Computer Methods and Programs in Biomedicine*, *114*(1), 109–124. doi:10.1016/j.cmpb.2014.01.018 PMID:24560276

Lopes, A., Touzi, R., & Nezry, E. (1990). Adaptive speckle filters and scene heterogeneity. *IEEE Transactions on Geoscience and Remote Sensing*, *28*(6), 992–1000. doi:10.1109/36.62623

Lu, J. Y., Zou, H., & Greenleaf, J. F. (1994). Biomedical ultrasound beam forming. *Ultrasound in Medicine & Biology*, *20*(5), 403–428. doi:10.1016/0301-5629(94)90097-3 PMID:7941100

Mauldin, F. W., Lin, D., & Hossack, J. A. (2011). The singular value filter: A general filter design strategy for PCA-based signal separation in medical ultrasound imaging. *IEEE Transactions on Medical Imaging*, *30*(11), 1951–1964. doi:10.1109/TMI.2011.2160075 PMID:21693416

Mishra, D., Chaudhury, S., Sarkar, M., & Soin, A. S. (2018). *Unsupervised Despeckling*. arXiv preprint arXiv:1801.03318

Ogier, A., Hellier, P., & Barillot, C. (2006, March). Restoration of 3D medical images with total variation scheme on wavelet domains (TVW). In Medical Imaging 2006: Image Processing (Vol. 6144, p. 61441E). International Society for Optics and Photonics.

Ortiz, S. H. C., Chiu, T., & Fox, M. D. (2012). Ultrasound image enhancement: A review. *Biomedical Signal Processing and Control*, *7*(5), 419–428. doi:10.1016/j.bspc.2012.02.002

Parthiban, L., & Subramanian, R. (2006, December). Speckle noise removal using contourlets. In *Information and Automation, 2006. ICIA 2006. International Conference on* (pp. 250-253). IEEE. 10.1109/ICINFA.2006.374121

Perona, P., & Malik, J. (1990). Scale-space and edge detection using anisotropic diffusion. *IEEE Transactions on Pattern Analysis and Machine Intelligence*, *12*(7), 629–639. doi:10.1109/34.56205

Perperidis, A. (2016). Postprocessing approaches for the improvement of cardiac ultrasound B-mode images: A review. *IEEE Transactions on Ultrasonics, Ferroelectrics, and Frequency Control*, *63*(3), 470–485. doi:10.1109/TUFFC.2016.2526670 PMID:26886981

Pizurica, A., Philips, W., Lemahieu, I., & Acheroy, M. (2003). A versatile wavelet domain noise filtration technique for medical imaging. *IEEE Transactions on Medical Imaging*, *22*(3), 323–331. doi:10.1109/TMI.2003.809588 PMID:12760550

Pizurica, A., Wink, A. M., Vansteenkiste, E., Philips, W., & Roerdink, B. J. (2006). A review of wavelet denoising in MRI and ultrasound brain imaging. *Current Medical Imaging Reviews*, *2*(2), 247–260. doi:10.2174/157340506776930665

Rabbani, H., Vafadust, M., Abolmaesumi, P., & Gazor, S. (2008). Speckle noise reduction of medical ultrasound images in complex wavelet domain using mixture priors. *IEEE Transactions on Biomedical Engineering*, *55*(9), 2152–2160. doi:10.1109/TBME.2008.923140 PMID:18713684

Ramos-Llordén, G., Vegas-Sánchez-Ferrero, G., Martin-Fernandez, M., Alberola-López, C., & Aja-Fernández, S. (2015). Anisotropic diffusion filter with memory based on speckle statistics for ultrasound images. *IEEE Transactions on Image Processing*, *24*(1), 345–358. doi:10.1109/TIP.2014.2371244 PMID:25415987

Saba, L., Acharya, U. R., Guerriero, S., & Suri, J. S. (Eds.). (2014). *Ovarian Neoplasm Imaging*. Springer Science & Business Media.

Seabra, J., Xavier, J., & Sanches, J. (2008, August). Convex ultrasound image reconstruction with log-euclidean priors. In *Engineering in Medicine and Biology Society, 2008. EMBS 2008. 30th Annual International Conference of the IEEE* (pp. 435-438). IEEE.

Seabra, J. C. R. (2011). *Medical ultrasound b-mode modeling, de-speckling and tissue characterization assessing the atherosclerotic disease* (Doctoral dissertation). Instituto Superior Técnico.

Shahdoosti, H. R., & Rahemi, Z. (2018). A maximum likelihood filter using non-local information for despeckling of ultrasound images. *Machine Vision and Applications, 29*(4), 689–702. doi:10.100700138-018-0929-8

Shao, D., Zhou, T., Liu, F., Yi, S., Xiang, Y., Ma, L., ... He, J. (2017). Ultrasound speckle reduction based on fractional order differentiation. *Journal of Medical Ultrasonics (2001), 44*(3), 227–237. doi:10.100710396-016-0763-4 PMID:28012088

Singh, K., Ranade, S. K., & Singh, C. (2017). A hybrid algorithm for speckle noise reduction of ultrasound images. *Computer Methods and Programs in Biomedicine, 148*, 55–69. doi:10.1016/j.cmpb.2017.06.009 PMID:28774439

Song, P., Manduca, A., Trzasko, J. D., & Chen, S. (2017). Ultrasound small vessel imaging with block-wise adaptive local clutter filtering. *IEEE Transactions on Medical Imaging, 36*(1), 251–262. doi:10.1109/TMI.2016.2605819 PMID:27608455

Soorajkumar, R., Krishnakumar, P., Girish, D., & Rajan, J. (2016). Coupled PDE for ultrasound despeckling using ENI classification. *Procedia Computer Science, 89*, 658–665. doi:10.1016/j.procs.2016.06.031

Sudeep, P. V., Palanisamy, P., Rajan, J., Baradaran, H., Saba, L., Gupta, A., & Suri, J. S. (2016). Speckle reduction in medical ultrasound images using an unbiased non-local means method. *Biomedical Signal Processing and Control, 28*, 1–8. doi:10.1016/j.bspc.2016.03.001

Suri, J. S. (2008). *Advances in diagnostic and therapeutic ultrasound imaging*. Artech House.

Tao, Z., Tagare, H. D., & Beaty, J. D. (2006). Evaluation of four probability distribution models for speckle in clinical cardiac ultrasound images. *IEEE Transactions on Medical Imaging, 25*(11), 1483–1491. doi:10.1109/TMI.2006.881376 PMID:17117777

Tay, P. C., Acton, S. T., & Hossack, J. A. (2006, April). A stochastic approach to ultrasound despeckling. In *Biomedical Imaging: Nano to Macro, 2006. 3rd IEEE International Symposium on* (pp. 221-224). IEEE. 10.1109/ISBI.2006.1624892

Tole, N. M., & Ostensen, H. (2005). *Basic physics of ultrasonographic imaging*. World Health Organization.

Tomasi, C., & Manduchi, R. (1998, January). Bilateral filtering for gray and color images. In *Computer Vision, 1998. Sixth International Conference on* (pp. 839-846). IEEE.

Trahey, G. E., Allison, J. W., Smith, S. W., & Von Ramm, O. T. (1986). A quantitative approach to speckle reduction via frequency compounding. *Ultrasonic Imaging, 8*(3), 151–164. doi:10.1177/016173468600800301 PMID:3548000

Uddin, M. S., Halder, K. K., Tahtali, M., Lambert, A. J., & Pickering, M. R. (2015, May). Speckle reduction and deblurring of ultrasound images using artificial neural network. In *Picture Coding Symposium (PCS)*, 2015 (pp. 105-108). IEEE. 10.1109/PCS.2015.7170056

Vedula, S., Senouf, O., Bronstein, A. M., Michailovich, O. V., & Zibulevsky, M. (2017). *Towards CT-quality Ultrasound Imaging using Deep Learning*. arXiv preprint arXiv:1710.06304

Vegas-Sanchez-Ferrero, G., Aja-Fernandez, S., Martín-Fernández, M., Frangi, A. F., & Palencia, C. (2010, September). Probabilistic-driven oriented speckle reducing anisotropic diffusion with application to cardiac ultrasonic images. In *International Conference on Medical Image Computing and Computer-Assisted Intervention* (pp. 518-525). Springer. 10.1007/978-3-642-15705-9_63

Vegas-Sánchez-Ferrero, G., Martín-Martínez, D., Aja-Fernández, S., & Palencia, C. (2010a, April). On the influence of interpolation on probabilistic models for ultrasonic images. In *Biomedical Imaging: From Nano to Macro, 2010 IEEE International Symposium on* (pp. 292-295). IEEE.

Wang, S., Huang, T. Z., Zhao, X. L., Mei, J. J., & Huang, J. (2018). Speckle noise removal in ultrasound images by first-and second-order total variation. *Numerical Algorithms*, *78*(2), 513–533. doi:10.100711075-017-0386-x

Wang, Z., Bovik, A. C., Sheikh, H. R., & Simoncelli, E. P. (2004). Image quality assessment: From error visibility to structural similarity. *IEEE Transactions on Image Processing*, *13*(4), 600–612. doi:10.1109/TIP.2003.819861 PMID:15376593

Wong, A., Mishra, A., Bizheva, K., & Clausi, D. A. (2010). General Bayesian estimation for speckle noise reduction in optical coherence tomography retinal imagery. *Optics Express*, *18*(8), 8338–8352. doi:10.1364/OE.18.008338 PMID:20588679

Yang, J., Fan, J., Ai, D., Wang, X., Zheng, Y., Tang, S., & Wang, Y. (2016). Local statistics and non-local mean filter for speckle noise reduction in medical ultrasound image. *Neurocomputing*, *195*, 88–95. doi:10.1016/j.neucom.2015.05.140

Yu, Y., & Acton, S. T. (2002). Speckle reducing anisotropic diffusion. *IEEE Transactions on Image Processing*, *11*(11), 1260–1270. doi:10.1109/TIP.2002.804276 PMID:18249696

Yu, Y., Dong, G., & Wang, J. (2011, June). Despeckling trilateral filter. In *IVMSP Workshop, 2011 IEEE 10th* (pp. 42-47). IEEE.

Zhang, J., Lin, G., Wu, L., Wang, C., & Cheng, Y. (2015a). Wavelet and fast bilateral filter based de-speckling method for medical ultrasound images. *Biomedical Signal Processing and Control*, *18*, 1–10. doi:10.1016/j.bspc.2014.11.010

Zhang, J., Wang, C., & Cheng, Y. (2015). Comparison of despeckle filters for breast ultrasound images. *Circuits, Systems, and Signal Processing*, *34*(1), 185–208. doi:10.100700034-014-9829-y

Zong, X., Laine, A. F., & Geiser, E. A. (1998). Speckle reduction and contrast enhancement of echocar-diograms via multiscale nonlinear processing. *IEEE Transactions on Medical Imaging*, *17*(4), 532–540. doi:10.1109/42.730398 PMID:9845309

Zukal, M., Beneš, R., Číka, P., & Říha, K. (2011). *Ultrasound image database*. Retrieved from http://splab.cz/en/download/databaze/ultrasound

ADDITIONAL READING

Caelli, T., & Bischof, W. F. (2013). *Machine learning and image interpretation*. Springer Science & Business Media.

Fenster, A., & Downey, D. B. (1996). 3-D ultrasound imaging: A review. *IEEE Engineering in Medicine and Biology Magazine*, *15*(6), 41–51. doi:10.1109/51.544511

Hossack, J. A., & Wang, J. S. (2000). *U.S. Patent No. 6,083,168*. Washington, DC: U.S. Patent and Trademark Office.

Litjens, G., Kooi, T., Bejnordi, B. E., Setio, A. A. A., Ciompi, F., Ghafoorian, M., ... Sánchez, C. I. (2017). A survey on deep learning in medical image analysis. *Medical Image Analysis*, *42*, 60–88. doi:10.1016/j.media.2017.07.005 PMID:28778026

Sonka, M. (2000). Medical image processing and analysis. Handbook of Medical Imaging, 2.

KEY TERMS AND DEFINITIONS

Adaptive Filtering: The filter whose parameters are adjusted iteratively to model the filter's input-output relationship in real time.

Anisotropic: The presence of directionally dependent characteristics (i.e., non-identical properties with directions).

Backscattering: The scattering direction changes towards its source.

Bhattacharya Coefficient: Dissimilarity measure between two distributions. It is considered a reliable measure of contrast between two patches in an image.

Coefficient of Variation: It gives the distribution of data around the expected value as the ratio of the standard deviation to the mean.

Fuzzy Logic: The multi-valued logic system, instead of the Boolean logic of '0' or '1', is called fuzzy logic.

Regularization: It is a method based on regression to avoid overfitting.

PSNR: It stands for peak signal-to-noise ratio.

SSIM: It stands for structural similarity index matrix.

Chapter 15
Prevalence of Musculoskeletal Disorders of Odisha Farmers in Selected Agricultural Tasks:
A Critical Analysis During Seeding, Fertilizing, and Weeding of Crops

Debesh Mishra
KIIT University (Deemed), India

Suchismita Satapathy
KIIT University (Deemed), India

ABSTRACT

In the chapter, there are dual main contributions. In the first phase, based on the extensive review of literature on the application of cuckoo search (CS) methodology, its application for the optimization of agricultural pesticide sprayers for maximum efficiency was suggested. In the second phase of study, 75 farmers of Odisha in India were considered to assess their musculoskeletal disorders (MSDs) during seeding, fertilizing, and weeding of crops using a Standardized Nordic Questionnaire with a five point rating scale (i.e., 1 = Very less, 2 =Less, 3 = Nil, 4 = Strong, 5 = Very Strong). Factor analysis was performed for "seeding, fertilizing, and weeding characteristics," "economical characteristics," and "tools and equipment characteristics of farmers." Then Pearson correlation coefficient matrix was generated for the seeding, fertilizing, and weeding characteristics of farmers, followed by regression analysis for the economic characteristics of farmers.

INTRODUCTION

Agriculture has been considered as the source of livelihood for most of the Indian families. Its contribution is about 18% of the gross domestic product in India (Department of Agriculture, Cooperation & Statistics, 2014). Similarly agricultural sectors in India also largely contribute to 49% of the total labor

DOI: 10.4018/978-1-5225-7796-6.ch015

force. Most of the Indian spends more than half of their income in food-preservation & security (NSSO, 2013). However, the growth rate of the agricultural sectors in India has been fluctuating and it depends primarily on the rainfall, as most of the cultivating area in India depends on rainfall (Dev, 2013). Farming is also greatly influenced by the techniques and tools used in various stages and activities involved. Though with the development of machinery and equipments, the farming process has become easier, more efficient and productive; still most of the farming activities are carried out by the conventional tools and techniques.

As most of the engineering problems are solved by optimization techniques where the goal is to determine either a maximum or a minimum value of the problem being solved generally known as the objective function. However, for solving the global optimization problems, the Cuckoo Search (CS) method is considered as the most powerful nature-inspired algorithm. It is inspired by the breeding behavior of some cuckoo species, and because of the simplicity & more performing efficiency, the Cuckoo Search method has been applied to various optimization problems in the engineering problems including the agricultural sectors.

Cuckoo Search Method

Cuckoo search is a meta-heuristic algorithm inspired by the bird Cuckoo; these are the "Brood parasites" birds. It never builds its own nest and lays their eggs in the nest of another host bird nest. Cuckoo is a best-known brood parasite. Some host birds can engage directly with the intruding cuckoo. If the host bird identifies the eggs that are not their egg then it will either throw that eggs away from its nest or simply rid its nest and build a new nest. Each egg in a nest represents a solution, and a cuckoo egg represents a new solution. The aim is to use the new and potentially better solutions (cuckoos) to replace a not-so-good solution in the nests. In the simplest form each nest has one egg of cuckoo, in which each nest will have multiple eggs representing a set of solutions.

CS is based on following idealized rules (Yang & Deb, 2009)

1. Each cuckoo lays one egg at a time, and dumps its egg in a randomly chosen nest;
2. The best nests with high quality of eggs will carry over to the next generation;
3. The number of available host's nests is fixed, and the egg laid by a cuckoo is discovered by the host bird with a probability P € (0, 1). Discovering operates on some set of worst nests, and discovered solutions dumped from farther calculations.
4. Levy Flight is used when new solution is derived from the old one to attain realistic approach.

Based on these rules, the possibility is the host bird can either throw the egg away or abandon the nest, and build a completely new nest. For simplicity, this last assumption can be approximated by the fraction P_a of the n nest is replaced by new nests (with new random solutions). An important issue of Cuckoo Search is the applications of Levy flights for generating new solutions, $X_{(t+1)}$ which is given by equation (1):

$$X_{(t+1)} = X_{(t)} + s\,E_{(t)} \quad (1)$$

where, $E_{(t)}$ is drawn from a standard normal distribution with zero mean and unity standard deviation for random walks, or drawn from Levy distribution for Levy flights. Then, the random walks can also be linked with the similarity between a cuckoo's egg and the host's egg which can be tricky in implementation. Then the step size *s* determines how far a random walker can go, for a fixed number of iterations. Additionally in certain condition where *s* is too large, then the new solution generated will be too far away from the old solution (or, even jump out side of the bounds). Then, such a move is unlikely to be accepted. If *s* is too small, the change is too small to be significant, and consequently such search is not efficient. So a proper step size is important to maintain the search to be as efficient as possible.

Cuckoo Search Algorithm

The algorithm can be extended to more complicated cases in which each nest has multiple eggs representing a set of solutions.

The pseudo code defined algorithm by Yang and Deb (2009) is as follows,

```
Generate initial population of n nests xi, i = (1, 2. . . n)
for i = 1: n
Determine fitness value Fi = (x i)
end for
while (stopping criterion is not satisfied)
Generate a cuckoo egg (xj) from random nest by L´evy flights
Determine fitness value Fj= (xj)
Select a random nest i
if Fj > Fi then
xi← xj
Fi← Fj
end if
Abandon a fraction pa of the worst nests
Build new nests by L´evy flights
Compare fitness of new nests and keep best nest
end while
```

Application of Cuckoo Search in Agricultural Pesticides Spraying

Pesticides are substances which are used mostly to protect plants or crops from weeds, insects or fungi in agricultural sectors. Most of the farmers use the pesticide sprayers to apply the pesticides and fertilizers on agricultural crops. As the farmers can't afford to lose their crops due to insects so they spray chemicals, pesticides, on them which repel the insects also prevent diseases from spreading. So using pesticides reduces the risk of losing crops of the season. One of the most important considerations when using the sprayer is optimization of the spray. As the Cuckoo search (CS) method, has been successfully used by different researchers and authors in different optimization applications which includes but not limited to systems design, electricity network operation, electricity generation, wireless communications routing and minimization of energy losses during electricity transmission (Belic et al., 2017; Koppel et al., 2017; Platonov, 2016; Das et al., 2017; Yan et al., 2017; & Parkinson et al., 2013). Figure 1 shows the use of Pesticides Sprayer in agricultural sectors.

Figure 1. Use of agricultural pesticides sprayer

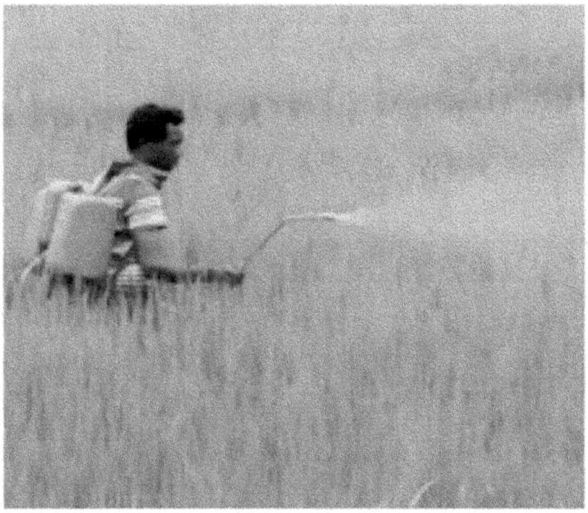

From the Figure 2, it is clear that the Cuckoo Search (CS) algorithm has been successfully applied in major categories such as in Engineering, followed by Pattern Recognition, Software Testing & Data Generation, Networking, Job Scheduling, and Data Fusion & Wireless Sensor Networks. Yildiz (2012) have used Cuckoo search (CS) method for selecting the most favorable parameters in milling-operation. Chifu (2012) have used Cuckoo search method to optimize semantic web-service composition process. Kumar et al. (2011) have obtained the optimum design for a 'reliable embedded-system'. Yang and Deb (2010) have proposed a new technique of Cuckoo Search to solve the engineering-design optimization problems, where the objective is to minimize the spring weight and overall fabrication cost, for springs & welded beam structures. Mareli et al. (2017) have investigated the CS algorithms performance by dynamically increasing switching parameters. They developed three CS algorithms using linear, exponential, and power increasing switching parameters, and tested them against the constant & linearly decreasing CS algorithms. It was found that the CS using exponential increasing switching parameter was more efficient than other CS algorithms.

Figure 2. Main categories in Cuckoo Search algorithm
Source: Mohamad et al, 2013

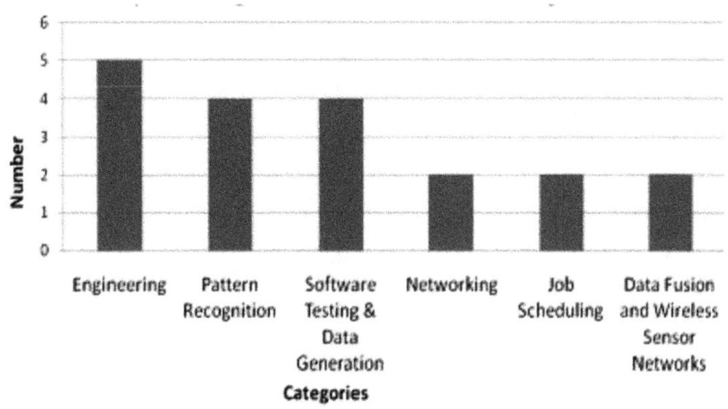

Figure 3. BCPC cumulative volumetric droplet size reference categories
Source: Hewitt, 2008

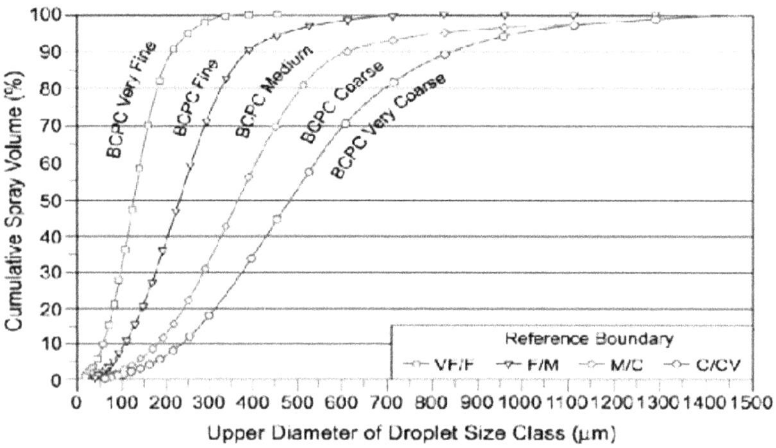

Hewitt (1997) have proposed that the optimal selection of droplet size of spray results in maximum efficiency and minimum drift. As the droplet size influences the spray performance and minimizes drift. So for the available range of nozzles for spray application, it is logical that sprays should be classified according to droplet size. The 'British Crop Protection Council (BCPC)' and 'American Society of Agricultural Engineers (ASAE)', have developed systems to classify the agricultural-sprays by its droplet size.

Figure 4. Cumulative volumetric droplet size spectra for different types of nozzles
Source: Hewitt, 2008

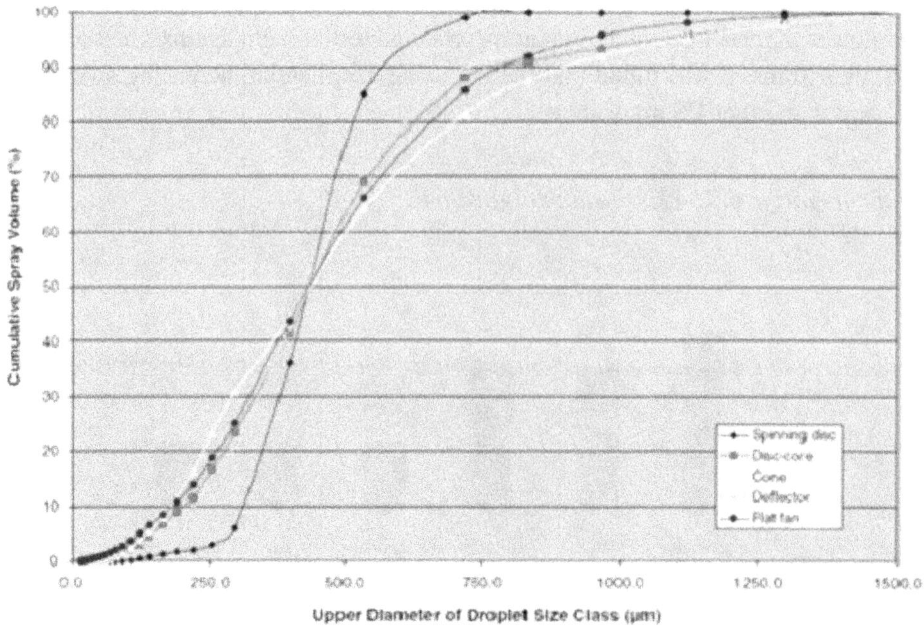

The spray classification system devised by 'BCPC nozzle classification scheme' in the mid 1980's is of five categories, such as "Very Fine, Fine, Medium, Coarse and Very-Coarse" (Doble et al., 1985).

Figure 3 shows the BCPC Cumulative Volumetric Droplet Size Reference Categories, and Figure 4 shows the cumulative volumetric droplet size spectra for different types of nozzle. As each egg in a nest, is a solution which is represented by one individual in the population, and an egg of the cuckoo is a new solution. So, if the nozzle of pesticide sprayer is considered as the egg and the droplet size is considered as Cuckoo egg with a new solution. And the objective functions as minimum drift. Then, determining the solution for minimum drift for a given nozzle with different droplet sizes and comparing the obtained solutions with previous best solutions, will provide the optimum value finally that will be retained. In this way the CS algorithm can be applied for the optimization and selection of sprayers, with maximum efficiency with minimum drift.

While designing the agricultural tools & equipments by considering its operational environment, it is mostly observed that the ergonomic considerations for user friendly tools are almost neglected. Thus the farmers dealing with the tools and techniques during farming suffer from various musculoskeletal disorders (MSDs) and injuries.

Musculoskeletal Disorders (MSDs) in Farming

It has been reported by many authors and researchers that the farmers engaged in agricultural sectors are highly affected by musculoskeletal disorders (MSDs) which not only cause harms but also is a threat to the health & life of them. For instance, lifting or carrying loads by hand and driving tractors were reported as risk factors for agricultural farmers (Parton et al., 1990; Murphy, 1992; Bobick et al., 1995). Most of the studies were carried out considering mechanized work applied in the work places. However the musculoskeletal disorders due to noise, vibrations produced by tractors and incorrect sitting postures of the operators were not considered, when using tractors in farming (Brookhuis et al., 2010). Pinzke et al. (2001) have reported that the body parts which are usually exposed to heavy loads are wrist, forearm, shoulder, neck and lumbar spine. Most of the jobs are designed considering the anthropometric dimensions of men and this result in lowering the productivity, increasing the discomfort level and the energy expenditure for women. Also it was reported that women's working continuously for eight hours, usually suffer from pain in hand, wrist, and neck (Jakob et al., 2009 and Stål et al., 2003). DeLuca (1997) has recommended the procedures to lift objects of unsymmetrical shapes based on his studies made on the musculoskeletal disorders due to handling, lifting, and transporting of objects by handcarts. Singh et al. (2010) have done an in depth literature review on musculoskeletal disorders of women agricultural farmers in India. Based on the conclusion of their study with musculoskeletal disorders with different body postures, they have recommended for ergonomically designed tools & equipments, and to have work rest periods for women. Kuta et al. (2015) have used surface electromyography system and job strain index method to analyze the muscle loads of fifteen farmers during milking, lifting, carrying a full bucket and in moving tractor. It was reported that maximum muscle force and tension occurred in the forearm muscle, while attaching teat cups to udder. Performance of work and associated work setting mainly causes the work related musculoskeletal disorders (Collins et al., 2011 and Punnett et al., 2004). Tinubu et al. (2010) and Smith et al. (2003) have reported that tenderness, disabilities, non-attendance, lower productivity and financial losses to the workers are caused mainly due to the musculoskeletal disorders in worldwide. The prolonged exposure to loads due to variable workloads results in musculoskeletal disorders (Kumar et al., 2013). High rate of doing work, repetitive work, forceful exertion, incorrect body postures and vibrations have been considered as the risk factors associated with the musculoskeletal disorders in the workplaces (NIOSH, 2002 and da Costa et al., 2010). Fabunmi et al. (2008), Schreuder et al. (2008), and Karahan et al. (2009) have reported that work is highly affected by musculoskeletal disorders, though its extent due to work is not clear. Also, the physiological and individual factors are more associated in developing the disorders. Mansi et al. (2013) and Arvidsson et al. (2012) have reported that repetitive movements, more application of forces, high working rates and incorrect postures for longer durations were found for the workers engaged in meat processing and performing various activities. The workers engaged in physical work are more affected by musculoskeletal disorders (Idowu et al., 2005). The hazards such as infection, lung cancer and knife related injuries are reported to be more evident in the case of butchers (Ola et al., 2008 and Corbin et al., 2011). Also, the butchers are more subjected to work related musculoskeletal disorders (Omokhodion et al., 2013). Pollack et al. (2007) have reported fatness and the excessive weight as the risk factors for occupational injuries. Janssen et al. (2011) have reported the natural means of musculoskeletal harms as altered step and stability, high forces in falls, high rate of sleep apneas & fatigues, and more susceptible to co-morbidities. Mishra et al. (2018) have considered ten farm women of Odisha in India and analyzed them while using plain and serrated sickles for cutting crops, and then an improved serrated sickle was recommended which resulted in reduction of the drudgery level in-comparison to the existing plain and serrated sickle. Pickett et al. (2015) have suggested that if the farmers feel inconvenience in their work due to fatness, then being self-employed they have the right and freedom to change or stop some sort of work. Bashir Kaka et al. (2016) have reported of high occurrence of work related musculoskeletal disorders between the butchers in Kano city and age was found to be the main risk factor. Also very few butchers only found to avail medical facilities. The musculoskeletal disorders (MSDs) was regarded as the most important public health related and work related problem, which varies from 15% to 42% (Hoogendoorn et al., 1999). Gallis (2006) has found that the maximum prevalence of MSDs occur in inexperienced laborers. The risk factors for MSDs were reported as physical, psychological, and socio-demographic characteristics (Devereux et al., 1999, 2002), various postural actions (Reid et al., 2010), faulty working postures (Scuffham et al., 2010), manually handling of materials (Yeung et al., 2002), standing and walking for longer durations (Andersen et al., 2007; Balasubramanian et al., 2009), prolonged shift works (Raanaas et al., 2008), distortion of trunk (Hartman et al., 2005), performing repetitive jobs (Juul-Kristensen et al., 2005), and poor work settings (Saurin et al., 2008). Meksawi et al. (2012) have reported of 52.9% of lower back pain for rubber tappers in Southern Thailand, which was found to be higher as compared to other regions. Ray et al. (2015) have suggested for improving the ergonomic performance of manual material handling tasks, based on their studies on the bio-mechanical assessment of manually material handling tasks of a construction site in India. It was reported that the compressive forces at some disc were above the limiting values for the construction workers. Kabir-Mokamelkhah et al. (2015) have considered the rice farmers in Iran and found the prevalence of musculoskeletal disorders in the lower limbs & the spinal sections. Luangwilai et al. (2014) have reported that MSDs are mainly associated with gender, education level, BMI, smoking habits, farming expertise and disease, if any. It was suggested that proper education and recommendations will improve the farming management system in rice farming. Gangopadhyay et al. (2010) have considered the stone-cutters and found significant work related disorders in the lower back, knees, and shoulders. Pascual et al. (2008) have reported that for assessment of work related musculoskeletal disorders (WMSDs), the National Institute of Occupational Safety and Health (NIOSH) used equations, and rapid upper limb assessment (RULA) or rapid entire body assessment (REBA), the certified-ergonomists used mostly Snook/Mital tables, while the Joint Health and Safety Committee (JHSC) used injury reports, and workers complaint. Dube et al. (2018) have analyzed different working postures of farmers of Odisha in India during seeding, fertilizing, and weeding, in agricultural field using RULA technique, and further it was suggested to give due attention to the present working techniques and methods. Das et al. (2012) have reported of major physiological loads and stresses between the female prawn seed collector of West Bengal in India, because of lengthy working hours in standing postures and more working pressures. Most of them were found suffering from musculoskeletal disorders in the lower back (98%), shoulders (75%), knees (88%), ankles (70%), and feet (67%), respectively. Similarly, the MSDs of the farmers of Kanpur in India were reported as lower back (60%), neck (10%), shoulder (22%), knee (39%), and highly afflicted chronically for nearly a year (Gupta et al. 2013).

Odisha is one of the prominent states in India, where most of the farmers prefer cultivation of rice. The farmers in the rural areas mainly prefer to use the traditional tools and techniques for farming purpose, and very few of them use the modern mechanized techniques. It has been found that most of the farmers undergo the musculoskeletal disorders (MSDs) because of a number of risk factors such as repetitive work, incorrect working postures, improper use of tools and techniques etc. Hence an attempt was made to collect and analyze the MSDs data for the farmers in Odisha while performing specific farming activities.

RESEARCH METHODOLOGY

Materials

The following materials were used for the present study:

1. Standard Nordic Questionnaire
2. Computer (Windows 7)
3. Statistical software (IBM SPSS 22.0 version)

Method

The primary activities involved in rice cultivation process are land preparation, seeding, fertilizing & weeding, harvesting and threshing processes. In the present study the farmers only in seeding, fertilizing, and weeding activities were considered. In Odisha, five villages were selected randomly where more than 60% population were from farming background. For collecting the information and data, a team comprising of three members was formulated and were well informed about the purpose and methods to collect data. Prior consent from the respective village heads or leaders was obtained. Using, a standardized nordic questionnaire the data regarding name, gender, age, other personal characteristics, socio-demographic characteristics, economical characteristics about the requirements, work setting characteristics and tools & equipment characteristics with a five point rating scale i.e. (1 = Very less, 2 =Less, 3 = Nil, 4 = Strong, 5 = Very Strong) as shown in Appendix, was collected from 75 selected farmers and considering 2 years period i.e. from 2015 to 2017.The body parameters which were considered to be associated with MSDs were neck, shoulder, upper back, lower back, elbow, wrist/hand, thigh, knees and ankles, respectively as illustrated in Figure 5.

Figure 5. Prevalence of MSDs in human body

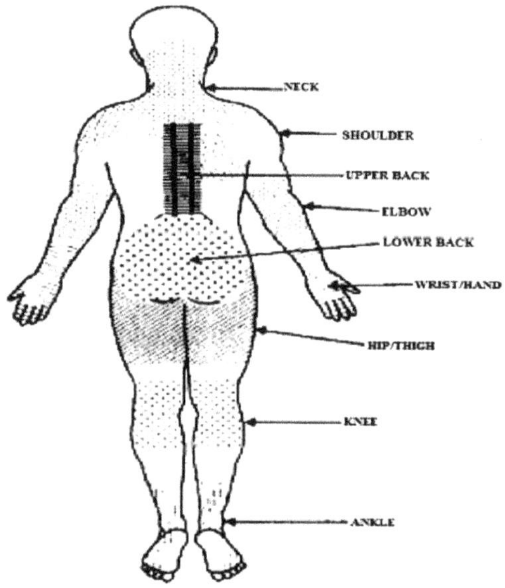

RESULTS AND DISCUSSION

From the socio-demographic characteristics of farmers (Table 1), it was observed that maximum musculoskeletal disorders of farmers were reported in lower back for age groups of <38 & in wrist for age groups of >38, in upper back of male farmers, in lower back and shoulder for female farmers. The disorders in shoulders were reported to be more, irrespective of "education levels, experiences, marital status, smoking habits, eating food habit per day, dominant hand, and previous weaknesses", respectively. The neck, upper back & lower back were reported to be highly affected for less than one year experienced farmers. Similarly, wrist & knee were reported to be more affected for 1-10 years & more than 10 years experienced farmers, respectively. Also, wrist was reported to be more affected irrespective of marital status, smoking habits, eating food habit per day, dominant hand, and previous weaknesses.

Similarly by considering the work-setting characteristics of farmers as shown in Table 2, higher occurrence of musculoskeletal disorders (MSDs) were found in "lower back & knees for sitting postures", and "neck, upper back, lower back, knees and ankles in squatting postures", and "upper back, lower back, wrist and knee in standing postures". The occurrence of MSDs in shoulder & wrist were more significant irrespective of working hours per day, working days per week and working time per day, respectively. Also it was observed that repetitive jobs produced more MSDs in neck, shoulder, elbow, wrist and knees. However, carrying heavy loads resulted in higher MSDs in shoulder, lower back & wrist, respectively.

Factor analysis was done using SPSS 22.0 for the "seeding, fertilizing and weeding characteristics of farmers', "economical characteristics of farmers", and 'risk level of different body parts of farmers by tools & equipments during seeding, fertilizing and weeding processes" to group different parameters under various dominant factors, as illustrated in Table 3, Table 4, and Table 5, respectively. By using the principal component analysis method with rotated component matrix, the variables with factor loading more than or equal to 0.5 were only considered. The "Kaiser's eigen value criteria" with eigen value greater than 1.00 were selected for subsequent factors selection (Kaiser, 1960). Factor analysis of seed-

Table 1. Socio-demographic characteristics of farmers (n=75)

Sl. No.	Parameters		No. of farmers reported of suffering of musculoskeletal disorders (MSDs)								
			Neck	Shoulder	Upper Back	Lower Back	Elbow	Wrist/ Hand	Thigh	Knee	Ankle
1.	Age	< 38	16	20	19	23	15	22	14	15	19
		> 38	16	14	21	20	19	22	15	15	13
2.	Gender	Male	15	19	24	15	15	15	20	15	15
		Female	18	25	18	25	16	20	14	20	15
3.	Education Level	Under primary	15	25	12	15	21	18	19	23	16
		primary to High school	12	24	15	07	15	19	21	13	20
		More than High school	12	25	13	17	15	14	12	16	16
4.	Experience	< 1 Year	25	25	25	25	22	24	21	21	22
		1-10 Years	18	25	16	15	18	25	15	13	13
		>10 Years	19	25	17	16	16	16	16	25	10
5.	Marital Status	Un-married	13	25	16	15	19	25	16	14	14
		Married	16	23	16	25	17	25	16	17	17
6.	Smoking habits	Non-Smoker	20	25	15	11	10	25	11	17	11
		Smoker	22	25	25	25	09	25	02	25	09
7.	Eating food habit per day	< 2	08	25	15	16	15	25	15	14	07
		> 2	12	25	17	17	19	25	14	15	18
8.	Handedness/ Dominant hand	Left-handed	16	25	19	22	17	25	17	16	14
		Right-handed	15	25	15	14	15	25	15	18	18
		Mixed-Handed	17	25	19	20	19	25	17	16	18
9.	Exposure to wet and humid soil	Low land	12	25	17	14	15	25	15	12	15
		Up land	18	25	16	21	22	25	20	18	17
		Wet land	13	25	15	15	15	25	15	15	12
		Dry land	11	25	16	18	15	25	15	15	12
		Horizontal/ Plain	21	25	19	22	18	25	15	21	09
		Sloped	15	25	21	20	22	25	15	15	16
10.	Previous weakness/injuries, if any		11	25	14	18	19	25	19	15	14

n= Total number of farmers

ing, fertilizing and weeding characteristics of farmers resulted in 6 dominant factors with cumulative % of variance of 72.82% (Table.3). In factor 1, the factor loading is high in "puncture from bamboo stick of seed containers" which was 0.79. Other variables in factor 1 with factor loading ≥ 0.5 included "exposure to loud noise of pesticide applying machines", and "symptoms from pesticide exposure". So the factor1 was named as "expose". Factor loading in factor 2 was high in "injuries from falling of pesticide applying machines", which was 0.93. Other variable in factor 2 was "musculoskeletal problems from seeding by machine". So the factor 2 was named as "machine". The factor loading in factor 3 was found

Table 2. Work-setting characteristics of farmers (n=75)

Sl. No.	Parameters		No. of farmers reported of suffering of musculoskeletal disorders (MSDs)								
			Neck	Shoulder	Upper Back	Lower Back	Elbow	Wrist/Hand	Thigh	Knee	Ankle
1.	Working posture(s)	Sitting	19	17	16	24	16	16	19	24	16
		Squatting	25	17	25	25	15	18	15	25	25
		Standing	17	17	25	25	17	25	17	25	18
2.	Working hours/day	< 3	15	24	25	15	24	17	17	16	21
		> 3	21	25	20	19	15	23	16	15	14
3.	Working days/week	< 4	16	25	18	17	16	25	18	16	16
		> 4	15	25	14	12	22	25	15	16	16
4.	Working time(s)/day	Before 8 A.M.	17	25	21	15	18	25	16	19	17
		8 A.M. – 12 P.M.	12	25	13	12	25	25	06	12	17
		After 12 P.M.	11	25	25	25	18	25	16	25	25
5.	Nature of job	Repetitive/forceful	25	25	20	17	25	25	19	25	20
		Carrying heavy loads	20	25	20	25	15	25	15	15	13

n= Total number of farmers

higher in "musculoskeletal problems from incorrect weeding postures", i.e. 0.85. The remaining variable in factor 3 was "exposure to vibration of pesticide applying machines". So the factor 3 was named as "discomfort". Factor loading in factor 4 was higher in 'nasal irritation from pesticide exposure", which was 0.75. And other variable in factor 4 was 'pesticides mixing and spraying processes". Hence, the factor 4 was named as "pesticide exposure". In factor 5, higher factor loading was found in "musculoskeletal problems from seeding by hand", which was 0.68. And the other variables in factor 5 were "exposure to wet and humid soil", "musculoskeletal problems from carrying heavy seed containers", "eye irritation from pesticide exposure". The factor 5 was named as "body". Further, the factor loading in factor 6 was obtained higher in "skin irritation from pesticide exposure", which was 0.84. Remaining variable in factor 6 was "musculoskeletal problems from carrying pesticides sprayer". Hence, the factor 6 was named as "pesticide spray".

Similarly, the factor analysis for "economical characteristics of farmers" resulted in 2 dominant factors and the factor analysis for "risk level of different body parts of farmers by tools and equipments during seeding, fertilizing and weeding processes", resulted in 15 dominant factors. In the factor analysis for "economical characteristics of farmers" (Table.4), the factor 1 was named as "manufacturing" and factor 2 as "farming", based on the requisite of manufacturer and farmers. In the factor analysis of "risk level of different body parts of farmers by tools and equipments during seeding, fertilizing and weeding processes" (Table 5), the factor 1 was named as "body-joint" as most of the body joint parts were involved. Similarly, factor 2 was named as "movement" as the MSDs in knees, ankles, & shoulder occur mainly due to movements. Subsequently, factor 3 was named as "discomfort" because the MSDs in neck, upper-back, & thigh results discomfort in work. Looking at the pain level of body parts, the factor 4 was named as "upper back pain", factor 5 as "shoulder pain", factor 6 as "wrist-ankle pain", factor 7 which included upper back, lower back & ankle, was named as "joint-pain", factor 8 including

Table 3. Seeding, fertilizing and weeding characteristics of farmers (n=75)

Parameters	Factor 1 (Expose)	Factor 2 (Machine)	Factor 3 (Discomfort)	Factor 4 (Pesticide exposure)	Factor 5 (Body)	Factor 6 (Pesticide Spray)
1.Exposure to wet and humid soil					0.64	
2.Musculoskeletal problems from carrying heavy seed containers					-0.59	
3.Puncture from bamboo stick of seed containers	0.79					
4.Musculoskeletal problems from seeding by hand					0.68	
5.Musculoskeletal problems from seeding by machine		0.73				
6.Pesticides-mixing and spraying processes				0.71		
7.Exposure to loud noise of pesticide applying machines	0.52					
8.Exposure to vibration of pesticide applying machines			-0.81			
9.Injuries from falling of pesticide applying machines		0.93				
10.Musculoskeletal problems from carrying pesticides sprayer						0.66
11.Musculoskeletal problems from incorrect weeding postures			0.85			
12.Symptoms from pesticide exposure: a) Vomiting	0.78					
b) Skin irritation						0.84
c) Nasal irritation				0.75		
d) Eye irritation					0.62	
e) Headache	-0.63					
Eigen value	02.88	02.48	01.94	01.68	01.44	01.20
Variance in %	18.00	15.53	12.17	10.53	09.04	07.51
Cumulative variance in %	18.00	33.54	45.71	56.25	65.30	72.82

n= Total number of farmers

knee, ankle, wrist & thigh was named as "hand-leg pain", factor 9 as "seeding pain" which comprised of neck, shoulder, elbow, wrist in seeding process, factor 10 as "weeding pain" comprising of neck & knee, factor 11 as "thigh-ankle pain", factor 12 as "thigh pain", factor 13 as "arm pain", factor 14 as "lower back pain", and factor 15 as "neck pain", respectively.

To illustrate the strength & linear relationship of various variables under consideration, the Pearson Correlation coefficients between various dominant factors in the "seeding, fertilizing and weeding characteristics of farmers" was obtained (Table 6). By using "pearson product moment correlation" in IBM SPSS 22.0 version, the correlation coefficient matrix was obtained. It was found that very high positive

Table 4. Economical characteristics of farmers (n=75)

Parameters	Factor 1 (Manufacturing)	Factor 2 (Farming)
1.Compliance with cost		-0.80
2.Cost reduction of existing Appliances	0.85	
3.Quality	0.84	
4.Service capability		0.69
5.Innovativeness		0.76
6.New use of technologies / modifications of design	0.62	
Eigen value	02.97	01.04
Variance in %	49.50	17.41
Cumulative variance in %	49.50	66.91

n= Total number of farmers

Table 5. Risk level of different body parts of farmers by tools and equipments during seeding, fertilizing and weeding processes (n=75)

Parameters[#]		Factors*														
		1	2	3	4	5	6	7	8	9	10	11	12	13	14	15
A	Neck			0.90												
	Shoulder					0.85										
	Upper Back				0.93											
	Lower back	0.85														
	Elbow	0.93														
	Wrist/Hand						0.50									
	Thighs												0.52			
	Knees		0.98													
	Ankles		0.67													
B	Neck			0.85												
	Shoulder					0.85										
	Upper Back				0.93											
	Lower back	0.85														
	Elbow	0.93														
	Wrist/Hand	0.52														
	Thighs	0.57														
	Knees		0.98													
	Ankles		0.66													

continued on following page

Table 5. Continued

Parameters[#]		Factors[*]														
		1	2	3	4	5	6	7	8	9	10	11	12	13	14	15
C	Neck									0.71						
	Shoulder									0.77						
	Upper Back			0.52												
	Lower back	0.66														
	Elbow									0.66						
	Wrist/Hand									0.71						
	Thighs	0.72														
	Knees	0.78														
	Ankles	0.85														
D	Neck			0.90												
	Shoulder															
	Upper Back				0.93											
	Lower back	0.79														
	Elbow	0.93														
	Wrist/Hand	0.66														
	Thighs												0.52			
	Knees		0.98													
	Ankles		0.67													
E	Neck			0.90												
	Shoulder					0.72										
	Upper Back				0.93											
	Lower back														0.67	
	Elbow	0.93														
	Wrist/Hand						0.50									
	Thighs												0.52			
	Knees		0.98													
	Ankles		0.67													
F	Neck			0.90												
	Shoulder					0.85										
	Upper Back				0.93											
	Lower back	0.85														
	Elbow	0.93														
	Wrist/Hand						0.50									
	Thighs			0.73												
	Knees		0.69													
	Ankles	-0.50														

continued on following page

Table 5. Continued

Parameters#		Factors*														
		1	2	3	4	5	6	7	8	9	10	11	12	13	14	15
G	Neck			0.90												
	Shoulder		0.98													
	Upper Back				0.93											
	Lower back	0.85														
	Elbow	0.93														
	Wrist/Hand						0.50									
	Thighs											0.76				
	Knees		0.98													
	Ankles											0.66				
H	Neck			0.87												
	Shoulder		0.98													
	Upper Back				0.93											
	Lower back	0.85														
	Elbow	0.93														
	Wrist/Hand						0.50									
	Thighs											0.79				
	Knees		0.98													
	Ankles											0.66				
I	Neck			0.90												
	Shoulder					0.85										
	Upper Back				0.93											
	Lower back	0.85														
	Elbow	0.93														
	Wrist/Hand						0.50									
	Thighs			0.66												
	Knees		0.98													
	Ankles						-0.66									
J	Neck	0.85														
	Shoulder	0.82														
	Upper Back	0.80														
	Lower back	0.78														
	Elbow	0.86														
	Wrist/Hand	0.85														
	Thighs	0.68														
	Knees								0.77							
	Ankles								0.58							

continued on following page

Table 5. Continued

Parameters[#]		Factors*														
		1	**2**	**3**	**4**	**5**	**6**	**7**	**8**	**9**	**10**	**11**	**12**	**13**	**14**	**15**
K	Upper Back	0.93														
	Lower back	0.95														
	Elbow	0.95														
	Wrist/Hand	0.95														
	Thighs	0.95														
	Knees	0.95														
	Ankles	0.93														
L	Neck			0.68												
	Shoulder	0.64														
	Upper Back	0.86														
	Lower back	0.95														
	Elbow	0.86														
	Wrist/Hand	0.95														
	Thighs	0.95														
	Knees	0.79														
	Ankles	0.93														
M	Neck										-0.60					
	Shoulder													0.77		
	Upper Back							0.68								
	Lower back							0.76								
	Elbow	0.87														
	Wrist/Hand								0.88							
	Thighs								0.65							
	Knees										0.92					
	Ankles							0.77								
N	Neck															0.56
	Shoulder													0.77		
	Upper Back							0.68								
	Lower back							0.72								
	Elbow	0.87														
	Wrist/Hand								0.88							
	Thighs								0.65							
	Knees										0.92					
	Ankles							0.77								

continued on following page

Table 5. Continued

Parameters#		Factors*														
		1	2	3	4	5	6	7	8	9	10	11	12	13	14	15
O	Neck	0.67														
	Shoulder	0.76														
	Upper Back			0.62												
	Lower back	0.95														
	Elbow	0.95														
	Wrist/Hand	0.95														
	Thighs	0.95														
	Knees	0.85														
	Ankles	0.95														
	Eigen value	58.07	16.16	12.11	08.11	07.79	06.49	04.90	03.95	02.85	02.51	02.01	01.81	01.57	01.34	01.15
	Variance in %	43.02	11.97	08.97	06.00	05.77	04.81	03.63	02.92	02.11	01.86	01.49	01.34	01.16	0.99	0.85
	Cumulative variance in %	43.02	54.99	63.97	69.97	75.75	80.56	84.19	87.12	89.23	91.10	92.59	93.93	95.09	96.09	96.94

***Factors:** 1-Body-joint, 2-Movement, 3-Discomfort, 4-Upper back pain, 5-Shoulder pain, 6-Wrist-Ankle pain, 7-Joint-pain, 8-Hand-leg pain, 9-Seeding pain, 10-Weeding pain, 11-Thigh-ankle pain, 12-Thigh pain, 13-Arm pain, 14-Lower back pain, 15-Neck pain.

#**Parameters:** A- Seeding/Planting (Completely Manual), B-Seeding/Planting (Partially Manual), C-Seeding/Planting (Completely Mechanical), D- Transplanting (Completely Manual), E- Transplanting (Partially Manual), F- Transplanting (Completely Mechanical), G- Holding, Mixing, Carrying of Sprayer (Completely Manual), H- Holding, Mixing, Carrying of Sprayer (Partially Manual), I- Holding, Mixing, Carrying of Sprayer (Completely Mechanical), J- Spraying pesticides process (Completely Manual), K- Spraying pesticides process (Partially Manual), L- Spraying pesticides process (Completely Mechanical), M- Weeding (Completely Manual), N- Weeding (Partially Manual), O- Weeding (Completely Mechanical).

n= Total number of farmers

correlation coefficient i.e. 0.599 was in between the parameters f-e, which was between "injuries from falling of pesticide applying machines" and "musculoskeletal problems from seeding by machine". Also, very high negative correlation coefficient value of -0.666 was obtained in between the parameters h-g, which was between "musculoskeletal problems from incorrect weeding postures" and 'exposure to vibration of pesticide applying machines". It was further found that non-linear relationships with correlation coefficient value of 0.000 existed between the parameters p-b & p-l, which was between 'symptoms from pesticide exposure (skin irritation) & exposure to loud noise of pesticide applying machines", and "symptoms from pesticide exposure (skin irritation) & musculoskeletal problems from carrying heavy seed containers", respectively.

The best fit linear regression equations between "innovativeness" and "other economic characteristics" were obtained by using regression analysis for the economic characteristics (Table 7). It was found that the economic parameters such as compliance with cost, and quality, were significant at $p < 0.05$. However, the parameters such as cost reduction of existing appliances, service capability, and innovativeness, were found significant at $p < 0.01$. The value of F indicated that the probability of the null hypothesis for the full-model was true and all of the regression coefficients were zero.

Table 6a. Correlation coefficient matrix for seeding, fertilizing and weeding characteristics

Parameters##	a	b	c	d	e
a	1.000				
b	0.314	1.000			
c	0.462*	0.462*	1.000		
d	-0.404*	-0.036	-0.364	1.000	
e	-0.017	0.299	0.129	-0.169	1.000
f	-0.272	0.320	0.128	0.014	0.599**
g	-0.302	-0.266	-0.292	0.119	-0.215
h	0.021	0.140	0.049	0.049	0.229
i	0.160	0.043	-0.015	-0.035	-0.073
j	0.042	-0.125	0.026	0.026	-0.132
k	0.141	0.101	0.100	-0.014	-0.064
l	0.341	0.063	0.139	-0.042	-0.117
m	0.119	0.169	0.140	-0.041	0.013
n	-0.220	-0.157	-0.124	0.071	-0.127
o	-0.116	-0.264	-0.025	0.098	-0.464*
p	-0.124	0.000	-0.143	0.163	-0.253

Table 6b. Correlation coefficient matrix for seeding, fertilizing and weeding characteristics

f	g	h	i	j	k	l	m	n	o	p
1.000										
-0.014	1.000									
-0.006	-0.666**	1.000								
-0.098	-0.317	0.233	1.000							
0.073	-0.026	-0.011	0.395	1.000						
-0.199	0.014	0.149	0.098	0.079	1.000					
-0.391	-0.256	0.202	0.155	0.172	-0.160	1.000				
0.104	0.119	-0.274	-0.192	-0.145	0.257	-0.282	1.000			
0.196	-0.071	-0.029	0.125	0.178	0.212	-0.415*	0.162	1.000		
-0.244	0.013	-0.133	0.411*	0.272	-0.376	0.067	-0.194	0.074	1.000	
-0.076	0.163	-0.270	-0.193	-0.179	-0.227	0.000	0.205	-0.193	0.439*	1.000

* Correlation is significant at $p < 0.05$

** Correlation is significant at $p < 0.01$

##**Parameters: a**- Puncture from bamboo stick of seed containers, **b**- Exposure to loud noise of pesticide applying machines, **c**- Symptoms from pesticide exposure (Vomiting), **d**- Symptoms from pesticide exposure (Headache), **e**- Musculoskeletal problems from seeding by machine, **f**- Injuries from falling of pesticide applying machines, **g**- Exposure to vibration of pesticide applying machines, **h**- Musculoskeletal problems from incorrect weeding postures, **i**- Pesticides-mixing and spraying processes, **j**- Symptoms from pesticide exposure (Nasal irritation), **k**- Exposure to wet and humid soil, **l**- Musculoskeletal problems from carrying heavy seed containers, **m**- Musculoskeletal problems from seeding by hand, **n**- Symptoms from pesticide exposure (Eye irritation, **o**- Musculoskeletal problems from carrying pesticides sprayer, **p**- Symptoms from pesticide exposure (Skin irritation).

Table 7. Best-Fit Linear Regression Equation between Innovativeness (X_5) and Other Economic Characteristics

Sl. No.	Parameters	Regression Equation	F
1	Compliance with cost(X_1)	$X_5 = 4.78\text{-}0.37X_1$	03.98*
2.	Cost reduction of existing Appliances(X_2)	$X_5 = 1.48+0.60X_2$	07.96**
3.	Quality(X_3)	$X_5 = 1.84+0.49X_3$	04.30*
4.	Service capability(X_4)	$X_5 = 1.00+0.75X_4$	27.05**
5.	Innovativeness(X_5)	$X_5= 1.19\text{-}0.21X_1+0.26X_2+0.08X_3+0.60X_4\text{-}0.14X_6$	06.29**
6.	New use of technologies/modifications of design(X_6)	$X_5 = 3.14+0.20X_6$	01.17

* Correlation is significant at $p < 0.05$

** Correlation is significant at $p < 0.01$

CONCLUSION

There were dual main contributions in the study. In the first phase of study the application of Cuckoo search algorithm for the optimum performance of pesticide sprayer was discussed based on the extensive literature review. As the pesticide sprayer has been frequently used by most of the farmers, hence the optimization and selection of sprayers with maximum efficiency and minimum drift could enhance the yield of crops. The Cuckoo search algorithm can be applied for determining the solution for minimum drift for a given nozzle with different droplet sizes and comparing the obtained solutions with previous best solutions. Thus the optimum value obtained finally will be retained.

In the second phase of study the musculoskeletal disorders (MSDs) of farmers were analyzed. From the socio-demographic characteristics of farmers, it was observed that maximum musculoskeletal disorders of farmers were reported in lower back for age groups of <38 & in wrist for age groups of >38, in upper back of male farmers, in lower back and shoulder for female farmers. The disorders in shoulders were reported to be more, irrespective of "education levels, experiences, marital status, smoking habits, eating food habit per day, dominant hand, and previous weaknesses", respectively. Similarly by considering the work-setting characteristics of farmers as shown, higher occurrence of MSDs were found in "lower back & knees for sitting postures", and "neck, upper back, lower back, knees and ankles in squatting postures", and "upper back, lower back, wrist and knee in standing postures". The occurrence of MSDs in shoulder & wrist were more significant irrespective of working hours per day, working days per week and working time per day, respectively. Also it was observed that repetitive jobs produced more MSDs in neck, shoulder, elbow, wrist and knees. However, carrying heavy loads resulted in higher MSDs in shoulder, lower back & wrist, respectively.

Further, from the correlation coefficient matrix it was found that very high positive correlation coefficient i.e. 0.599 was in between "injuries from falling of pesticide applying machines" and "musculoskeletal problems from seeding by machine". Also, very high negative correlation coefficient value of -0.666 was obtained in between "musculoskeletal problems from incorrect weeding postures" and 'exposure to vibration of pesticide applying machines". It was further found that non-linear relationships with correlation coefficient value of 0.000 existed between "symptoms from pesticide exposure (skin irritation) & exposure to loud noise of pesticide applying machines", and "symptoms from pesticide exposure (skin irritation) & musculoskeletal problems from carrying heavy seed containers", respectively.

Finally from the regression analysis for the economic characteristics it was found that the economic parameters such as compliance with cost, and quality, were significant at $p < 0.05$. However, the parameters such as cost reduction of existing appliances, service capability, and innovativeness, were found significant at $p < 0.01$.

Further MSDs analysis may be carried out considering more number of farmer populations and due considerations must be given in the ergonomic aspects of farming tools and equipment designs, such that the productivity, working efficiency of farmers can be enhanced and the drudgery can also be reduced to a significant level.

ACKNOWLEDGMENT

We would like to convey our sincere thanks to the farmers participated in the present survey and to KIIT (Deemed to be University) for continuous encouragement in carrying out such research work.

This research received no specific grants from any funding agency in the public, commercial, or not-for-profit sectors.

REFERENCES

Agricultural Statistics at a Glance. (2014). Department of Agriculture & Cooperation, & Statistics.

Andersen, J. H., Haahr, J. P., & Frost, P. (2007). Risk factors for more severe regional musculoskeletal symptoms: A two-year prospective study of a general working population. *Arthritis and Rheumatism*, *56*(4), 1355–1364. doi:10.1002/art.22513 PMID:17393441

Arvidsson, I., Balogh, I., Hansson, G. T., Ohlsson, K., Åkesson, I., & Nordander, C. (2012). Rationalization in meat cutting d consequences on physical workload. *Applied Ergonomics*, *43*(6), 1026–1032. doi:10.1016/j.apergo.2012.03.001 PMID:22475432

Balasubramanian, V., Adalarasu, K., & Regulapati, R. (2009). Comparing dynamic and stationary standing postures in an assembly task. *International Journal of Industrial Ergonomics*, *39*(5), 649–654. doi:10.1016/j.ergon.2008.10.017

Belic, E., Lukac, N., Dezelak, K., Zalik, B., & Stumberger, G. (2017). GPU-based online optimization of low voltage distribution network operation. *IEEE Transactions on Smart Grid*, *8*(3), 1460–1468.

Bobick, G., & Myers, J. R. (1995). *Back Injures in Agriculture: Occupations Affected*. Boca Raton, FL: CRC Press, Lewis Publishers.

Brookhuis, K. A., & de Waard, D. (2010). Monitoring drivers' mental workload in driving simulators using physiological measures. *Accident; Analysis and Prevention*, *42*(3), 898–903. doi:10.1016/j.aap.2009.06.001 PMID:20380918

Chifu, V., Pop, C., Salomie, I., Suia, D., & Niculici, A. (2012). Optimizing the Semantic Web Service Composition Process Using Cuckoo Search. *Intelligent Distributed Computing*, 93-102.

Collins, R. M., Janse van Rensburg, D. C., & Patricios, J. S. (2011). Common work-related musculoskeletal strains and injuries. *South African Family Practice*, *53*(3), 240–246. doi:10.1080/20786204.2011.10874091

Corbin, M., McLean, D., Mannetje, A., Dryson, E., Walls, C., McKenzie, F., ... Pearce, N. (2011). Lung cancer and occupation: A New Zealand cancer registry-based cased control study. *American Journal of Industrial Medicine*, *54*(2), 89–101. doi:10.1002/ajim.20906 PMID:20957667

da Costa, B. R., & Vieira, E. R. (2010). Risk factors for work-related musculoskeletal disorders: A systematic review of recent longitudinal Studies. *American Journal of Industrial Medicine*, *53*, 285–323. PMID:19753591

Das, B., Ghosh, T., & Gangopadhyay, S. (2012). Assessment of Ergonomic and Occupational Health-Related Problems Among Female Prawn Seed Collectors of Sunderbans, West Bengal, India. *International Journal of Occupational Safety and Ergonomics*, *18*(4), 531–540. doi:10.1080/10803548.2012.11076949 PMID:23294657

Das, S., Doppa, J. R., Pande, P. P., & Chakrabarty, K. (2017). Design-space exploration and optimization of an energy-efficient and reliable 3-D small-world network-on chip. *IEEE Transactions on Computer-Aided Design of Integrated Circuits and Systems*, *36*(5), 719–732. doi:10.1109/TCAD.2016.2604288

DeLuca, C. J. (1997). The use of surface electromyography in biomechanics. *Journal of Applied Biomechanics*, *13*(2), 135–163. doi:10.1123/jab.13.2.135

Dev, S. M. (2013). Small Farmers in India: Challenges and Opportunities. Mumbai: Academic Press.

Devereux, J. J., Buckle, P. W., & Vlachonikolis, I. G. (1999). Interactions between physical and psychosocial risk factors at work increase the risk of back disorders: An epidemiological approach. *Occupational and Environmental Medicine*, *56*(5), 343–353. doi:10.1136/oem.56.5.343 PMID:10472310

Devereux, J. J., Vlachonikolis, I. G., & Buckle, P. W. (2002). Epidemiological study to investigate potential interaction between physical and psychosocial factors at work that may increase the risk of symptoms of musculoskeletal disorder of the neck and upper limb. *Occupational and Environmental Medicine*, *59*(4), 269–277. doi:10.1136/oem.59.4.269 PMID:11934955

Doble, S. J., Matthews, G. A., Rutherford, I., & Southcombe, E. S. E. (1985). A System for Classifying Hydraulic Nozzles and Other Atomizers into Categories of Spray Quality/Pro. *1985 Bit. Crop Porf. Conf. –Weeds, 9*(A–6), 112.533.

Dube, B., Mishra, D., Satapathy, S., & Singh, S. (2018). Ergonomic evaluation of seeding, fertilizing and weeding postures in agricultural field. *International Journal of Pure and Applied Mathematics, 119*(10-Special Issue B), 1875-1880.

Fabunmi, A. A., Oworu, J. O., & Odunnaiya, N. E. (2008). Prevalence of musculoskeletal disorders among nurses in University College Hospital, Ibadan. *West Afr J Nurs.*, *19*, 21–25.

Gallis, C. (2006). Work-related prevalence of musculoskeletal symptoms among Greek forest workers. *International Journal of Industrial Ergonomics*, *36*(8), 731–736. doi:10.1016/j.ergon.2006.05.007

Gangopadhyay, S., Das, B., Das, T., Ghoshal, G., & Ghosh, T. (2010). An Ergonomics Study on Posture-Related Discomfort and Occupational-Related Disorders Among Stonecutters of West Bengal, India. *International Journal of Occupational Safety and Ergonomics*, *16*(1), 69–79. doi:10.1080/10803548.2010.11076830 PMID:20331920

Gupta, G. (2013). Prevalence of Musculoskeletal Disorders in Farmers of Kanpur Rural, India. *Journal of Community Medicine & Health Education*, *3*(07), 249. doi:10.4172/2161-0711.1000249

Hartman, E., Oude Vrielink, H. H. E., Metz, J. H. M., & Huirne, R. B. M. (2005). Exposure to physical risk factors in Dutch agriculture: Effect on sick leave due to musculoskeletal disorders. *International Journal of Industrial Ergonomics*, *35*(11), 1031–1045. doi:10.1016/j.ergon.2005.04.006

Hewitt, A. J. (1997). The Importance of Droplet Size in Agricultural Spraying. *Atomization and Sprays*, *7*(3), 235–244. doi:10.1615/AtomizSpr.v7.i3.10

Hewitt, A. J. (2008). Article. *The Environmentalist*, *28*(25). doi:10.100710669-007-9044-5

Hoogendoorn, W. E., van Poppel, M. N., Bongers, P. M., Koes, B. W., & Bouter, L. M. (1999). Physical load during work and leisure time as risk factors for back pain. *Scandinavian Journal of Work, Environment & Health*, *25*(5), 387–403. doi:10.5271jweh.451 PMID:10569458

Idowu, P. A., Adedoyin, R. A., & Adagunodo, R. E. (2005). Computer-related repetitive strain injuries. *J Nig Soc Physiother*, *15*, 13–15.

Jakob, M., & Liebers, F. (2009). Body posture variation during machine milking regarding weight of milking unit and working height—experimental study. *Bornimer Agrartechnische Berichte*, *66*, 31–37.

Janssen, I., Bacon, E., & Pickett, W. (2011). Obesity and Its Relationship with Occupational Injury in the Canadian Workforce. *Journal of Obesity*, *531403*. doi:10.1155/2011/531403 PMID:21773008

Juul-Kristensen, B., & Jensen, C. (2005). Self-reported workplace related ergonomic conditions as prognostic factors for musculoskeletal symptoms: The "BIT" follow up study on office workers. *Occupational and Environmental Medicine*, *62*(3), 188–194. doi:10.1136/oem.2004.013920 PMID:15723884

Kabir-Mokamelkhah, E. (2015). Rice Farming and Musculoskeletal Disorders. *Iranian Journal of Health, Safety and Environment*, *3*(1S), 489–494.

Kaiser, H. F. (1960). The application of electronic computers to factor analysis. *Educational and Psychological Measurement*, *20*(1), 141–151. doi:10.1177/001316446002000116

Kaka, Idowu, Fawole, Adeniyi, Ogwumike, & Toryila. (2016). WRMSDs among Butchers in Kano Metropolis. *Safety and Health at Work*, *7*, 218–224. doi:10.1016/j.shaw.2016.01.001 PMID:27630791

Karahan, A., Kar, S., Abbasogbu, A., & Dodan, N. (2009). Low back pain: Prevalence and associated factors among hospital staff. *Journal of Advanced Nursing*, *65*(3), 516–524. doi:10.1111/j.1365-2648.2008.04905.x PMID:19222649

Koppel, A., Sadler, B. M., & Ribeiro, A. (2017). Proximity without consensus in online multi agent optimization. *IEEE Transactions on Signal Processing*, *65*(12), 3062–3077. doi:10.1109/TSP.2017.2686368

Kumar, A., & Chakarverty, S. (2011). Design optimization for reliable embedded system using Cuckoo Search. *Electronics Computer Technology (ICECT), 2011 3rd International Conference IEEE,* (1), 264-268.

Kumar, V. K., Kumar, S. P., & Baliga, M. R. (2013). Prevalence of work-related musculoskeletal complaints among dentists in India: A national cross-sectional survey. *Indian Journal of Dental Research*, *24*(4), 428–438. doi:10.4103/0970-9290.118387 PMID:24047834

Kuta, L., Cieź, J., & Młotek, M. (2015). Musculoskeletal load assessment of farmers during selected agricultural works. *Procedia Manufacturing*, *3*, 1696–1703. doi:10.1016/j.promfg.2015.07.990

Luangwilai, T., Norkaew, S., & Siriwong, W. (2014). Factors associated with musculoskeletal disorders among rice farmers: Cross sectional study in Tarnlalord sub-district, Phimai district, Nakhonratchasima province, Thailand. *J Health Res.*, *28*(Suppl.), S85–S91.

Mansi, S., Milosavljevic, S., Tumilty, S., Hendrick, P., & Baxter, G. D. (2013). Use of pedometer driven walking to promote physical activity and improve health-related quality of life among meat processing workers: A feasibility trial. *Health and Quality of Life Outcomes*, *11*(1), 185. doi:10.1186/1477-7525-11-185 PMID:24175980

Mareli, M., & Twala, B. (2017). *An adaptive Cuckoo search algorithm for optimization*. Applied Computing and Informatics; doi:10.1016/j.aci.2017.09.001

Meksawi, S., Tangtrakulwanich, B., & Chongsuvivatwong, V. (2012). Musculoskeletal problems and ergonomic risk assessment in rubber tappers: A community-based study in southern Thailand. *International Journal of Industrial Ergonomics*, *42*(1), 129–135. doi:10.1016/j.ergon.2011.08.006

Mishra, D., & Satapathy, S. (2018). Drudgery Reduction of Farm Women of Odisha by Improved Serrated Sickle. *International Journal of Mechanical Engineering and Technology*, *9*(2), 53–61.

Mohamad, A., Zain, A. M., Nazira Bazin, N. E., & Udin, A. (2013). Cuckoo Search Algorithm for Optimization Problems – A literature Review. *Applied Mechanics and Materials*, *421*, 502–506. doi:10.4028/www.scientific.net/AMM.421.502

Murphy, D. J. (1992). *Safety and Health for Production Agriculture*. American Society of Agricultural Engineers, Books & Journals.

National Institute of Occupational Safety and Health (NIOSH). (2002). *Quality of work life questionnaire*. NIOSH.

Ola, S. O., Otegbayo, J. A., Yakubu, A., Odaibo, G. N., & Olaleye, D. O. (2008). Nigerian butchers and hepatitis B virus. *Tropical Gastroenterology*, *29*, 32–34. PMID:18564665

Omokhodion, F. O., & Adebayo, A. M. (2013). Occupational hazards and self-reported health problems of butchers in Ibadan, southwest Nigeria. *J Public Health (Germany)*, *21*(2), 131–134. doi:10.100710389-012-0528-5

Parkinson, A. R., Balling, R. J., & Hedengren, J. D. (2013). *Optimization Methods for Engineering Design: Applications and Theory* (5th ed.). Brigham Young University.

Parton, K. (1990). Back Injuries on farms: Regional variations in New South Wales. *Journal of Occup Health Safety-Aust NZ*, *6*, 53–59.

Pascual, S. A., & Naqvi, S. (2008). An Investigation of Ergonomics Analysis Tools Used in Industry in the Identification of Work-Related Musculoskeletal Disorders. *International Journal of Occupational Safety and Ergonomics*, *14*(2), 237–245. doi:10.1080/10803548.2008.11076755 PMID:18534158

Pickett, W., King, N., Lawson, J., Dosman, J. A., Trask, C., Brison, R. J., ... Janssen, I. (2015). Farmers, mechanized work, and links to obesity. *Preventive Medicine*, *70C*, 59–63. doi:10.1016/j.ypmed.2014.11.012 PMID:25448840

Pinzke, S., Stål, M., & Hansson, G.-A. (2001). Physical workload on upper extremities in various operations during machine milking. *Annals of Agricultural and Environmental Medicine*, *8*, 63–70. PMID:11426927

Platonov, A. (2016). Information theory and optimization of analog feedback communication systems. *IEEE International Black Sea Conference on Communications and Networking*. 10.1109/BlackSeaCom.2016.7901541

Pollack, K., Sorock, G., Slade, M., Cantley, L., Sircar, K., Taiwo, O., & Cullen, M. R. (2007). Association between body mass index and acute traumatic workplace injury in hourly manufacturing employees. *American Journal of Epidemiology*, *166*(2), 204–211. doi:10.1093/aje/kwm058 PMID:17485732

Punnett, L., & Wegman, D. H. (2004). Work-related musculoskeletal disorders: The epidemiologic evidence and the debate. *Journal of Electromyography and Kinesiology*, *14*(1), 13–23. doi:10.1016/j.jelekin.2003.09.015 PMID:14759746

Raanaas, R. K., & Anderson, D. (2008). A questionnaire survey of Norwegian taxi drivers' musculoskeletal health, and work-related risk factors. *International Journal of Industrial Ergonomics*, *38*(3-4), 280–290. doi:10.1016/j.ergon.2007.10.017

Ray, P., Parida, R., & Sarkar, S. (2015). Ergonomic analysis of construction jobs in India: A biomechanical modelling approach. *Procedia Manufacturing*, *3*, 4606–4612. doi:10.1016/j.promfg.2015.07.542

Reid, C. R., McCauley, B. P., Karwowski, W., & Durrani, S. K. (2010). Occupational postural activity and lower extremity discomfort: A review. *International Journal of Industrial Ergonomics*, *40*(3), 247–256. doi:10.1016/j.ergon.2010.01.003

Saurin, T. A., & de Macedo Guimaraes, L. B. (2008). Ergonomic assessment of suspended scaffolds. *International Journal of Industrial Ergonomics*, *38*(2), 238–246. doi:10.1016/j.ergon.2005.11.010

Schreuder, K. J., Roelen, C. A. M., Koopmans, A. C., & Groothoff, J. W. (2008). Job demands and health complaints in white and blue collar workers. *Work (Reading, Mass.)*, *31*, 425–432. PMID:19127013

Scuffham, A. M., Legg, S. J., Firth, E. C., & Stevenson, M. A. (2010). Prevalence and risk factors associated with musculoskeletal discomfort in New Zealand veterinarians. *Applied Ergonomics*, *41*(3), 444–453. doi:10.1016/j.apergo.2009.09.009 PMID:19857858

Singh, S., & Arora, R. (2010). Ergonomic Intervention for Preventing Musculoskeletal Disorders among Farm Women. *Journal of Agri. Science*, *1*(2), 61–71.

Smith, D. R., & Leggat, P. A. (2003). Musculoskeletal disorders in nursing. *Australian Nursing Journal*, *11*, 1–4.

Stål, M., Pinzke, S., & Hansson, G.-A. (2003). The effect on workload by using a support arm in parlour milking. *International Journal of Industrial Ergonomics*, *32*(2), 121–132. doi:10.1016/S0169-8141(03)00046-5

Tinubu, B. M. S., Mbada, C. E., Oyeyemi, A. L., & Fabunmi, A. A. (2010). Work-related musculoskeletal disorders among nurses in Ibadan, South-west Nigeria: A cross sectional. *BMC Musculoskeletal Disorders*, *11*(12). PMID:20089139

Yan, Z., Fan, J., & Wang, J. (2017). A collective neurodynamic approach to constrained global optimization. *IEEE Trans. Neural Learn. Syst*, *28*(5), 1206–1215. doi:10.1109/TNNLS.2016.2524619 PMID:27046909

Yang, X.-S., & Deb, S. (2009). *Cuckoo search via Levy flights*. IEEE Publications.

Yang, X. S., & Deb, S. (2010). Engineering optimisation by cuckoo search. *International Journal of Mathematical Modelling and Numerical Optimisation*, *1*(4), 330–343. doi:10.1504/IJMMNO.2010.035430

Yeung, S. S., Genaidy, A., Deddens, J., Alhemood, A., & Leung, P. C. (2002). Prevalence of musculoskeletal symptoms in single and multiple body regions and effects of perceived risk of injury among manual handling workers. *Spine*, *27*(19), 2166–2172. doi:10.1097/00007632-200210010-00017 PMID:12394933

Yildiz, A. R. (2012). Cuckoo search algorithm for the selection of optimal machining parameters in milling operations. *International Journal of Advanced Manufacturing Technology*, 1–7.

KEY TERMS AND DEFINITIONS

Agricultural Injury: It is the injury which occurs while doing some farm work or may occur while going to or from work.

Disorders: It is the disruption in the systematic functioning that retards the performance level.

Farming: Farming is the process of growing of crops or keeping animals by people for food and raw materials.

Injury: Injury is the damage to the body caused by some external forces. Different causes of injuries include accidents, falls, hits, weapons, and other factors.

Musculoskeletal Disorders: These are the disorders or injuries which affects the human body's movement and/or the musculoskeletal systems of body.

APPENDIX

Sample Questionnaire for Seeding, Fertilizing and Weeding Process

Place:
Date:

Please put (√) sign in your answer, where necessary:

Name (Optional):______________________________
Age: ______________________________
Sex: ______________________________
Left Handed () / Right Handed ()
Educational Level: ______________________
Land Holding: Own () / Rented () / Contract ()
Drought land () / Non-Drought land ()
Water source: Own () / External ()
Availability of Irrigation: Yes () / No ()
Water carrying facility: Manually () / Pump () / Both Manually and Pump () / others ()
Dependent on Rain water: No () / Partially () / Fully ()
Family Size (number and char): ____________
Address: ____________________________

Please put (√) in appropriate criteria option. *(Otherwise use any symbol as your own)*
NOTE: 1 indicates the least important and 5 indicates the most important
(1 = Very less, 2 = Less, 3 =Nil, 4 = Strong, 5 = Very Strong).

Musculoskeletal Risk Level During Seeding, Fertilizing and Weeding Process

Table 8.

SEEDING, FERTILIZING AND WEEDING PROCESS			1	2	3	4	5
1.	Exposure to wet and humid soil						
2.	Musculoskeletal problems from carrying heavy seed containers						
3.	Puncture from bamboo stick of seed containers						
4.	Musculoskeletal problems from seeding by hand						
5.	Musculoskeletal problems from seeding by machine						
6.	Pesticides-mixing and spraying processes						
7.	Exposure to loud noise of pesticide applying machines						
8.	Exposure to vibration of pesticide applying machines						
9.	Injuries from falling of pesticide applying machines						
10.	Musculoskeletal problems from carrying pesticides sprayer						
11.	Symptoms from pesticide exposure	a) Vomiting					
		b) Skin irritation					
		c) Nasal irritation					
		d) Eye irritation					
12.	Musculoskeletal problems from incorrect weeding postures						

Table 9.

ECONOMIC REQUIREMENT		1	2	3	4	5
1.	Compliance with cost					
2.	Cost reduction of existing Appliances					
3.	Quality					
4.	Service capability					
5.	Innovativeness					
6.	New use of technologies / modifications of design					

Table 10. Socio-Demographic Characteristics

Sl. No.	Parameters		Neck	Shoulder	Upper Back	Lower back	Elbow	Wrist/ Hand	Thighs	Knees	Ankles
1.	Age	< 38									
		> 38									
2.	Gender	Male									
		Female									
3.	Education Level	Under primary									
		primary to High school									
		More than High school									
4.	Experience	< 2 Yrs									
		2-10 Yrs									
		>10 Yrs									
5.	Marital Status	Un-married									
		Married									
6.	Smoking habits	Non-Smoker									
		Smoker									
7.	Eating food habit per day	< 2									
		> 2									
8.	Handedness/ Dominant hand	Left-handed									
		Right-handed									
		Mixed-Handed									
9.	Exposure to wet and humid soil	Low land									
		Up land									
		Wet land									
		Dry land									
		Horizontal/ Plain									
		Sloped									
10.	Previous weakness/injuries, if any										

Table 11. Work-setting characteristics

Sl. No.	Parameters		Neck	Shoulder	Upper Back	Lower back	Elbow	Wrist/ Hand	Thighs	Knees	Ankles
1.	Working posture(s)	Sitting									
		Squatting									
		Standing									
2.	Working hours/day	< 3									
		> 3									
3.	Working days/week	< 4									
		> 4									
4.	Working time(s)/ day	Before 8 A.M.									
		8 A.M. – 12 P.M.									
		After 12 P.M.									
5.	Nature of job	Repetitive/forceful									
		Carrying heavy loads									

Table 12. Tools and equipments characteristics

Sl. No.	Parameters		Neck	Shoulder	Upper Back	Lower back	Elbow	Wrist/ Hand	Thighs	Knees	Ankles
1.	Seeding/ Planting	Completely Manual									
		Partially Manual									
		Completely Mechanical									
2.	Transplanting	Completely Manual									
		Partially Manual									
		Completely Mechanical									
3.	Holding, Mixing, Carrying of Sprayer	Completely Manual									
		Partially Manual									
		Completely Mechanical									
4.	Spraying pesticides process	Completely Manual									
		Partially Manual									
		Completely Mechanical									
5.	Weeding	Completely Manual									
		Partially Manual									
		Completely Mechanical									

Compilation of References

AbdulRasool, D., & Sabra, S. (2011, June). Mobile-embedded smart guide for the blind. In *International Conference on Digital Information and Communication Technology and Its Applications* (pp. 571-578). Springer.

Abrahim, B. A., Mustafa, Z. A., Yassine, I. A., Zayed, N., & Kadah, Y. M. (2012). Hybrid total variation and wavelet thresholding speckle reduction for medical ultrasound imaging. *Journal of Medical Imaging and Health Informatics*, *2*(2), 114–124. doi:10.1166/jmihi.2012.1072

Acharya, U. R., Fujita, H., Oh, S. L., Hagiwara, Y., Tan, J. H., Adam, M., & Tan, R. S. (2018). Deep convolutional neural network for the automated diagnosis of congestive heart failure using ECG signals. *Applied Intelligence*, 1–12.

Acharya, U. R., Fujita, H., Sudarshan, V. K., Oh, S. L., Muhmmand, A., Koh, J. E., ... Tan, R. S. (2017). Application of empirical mode decomposition (EMD) for automated identification of congestive heart failure using heart rate signals. *Neural Computing & Applications*, *28*(10), 3073–3094. doi:10.100700521-016-2612-1

Acharya, U. R., Sree, S. V., Kulshreshtha, S., Molinari, F., Koh, J. E. W., Saba, L., & Suri, J. S. (2014). GyneScan: An improved online paradigm for screening of ovarian cancer via tissue characterization. *Technology in Cancer Research & Treatment*, *13*(6), 529–539. doi:10.7785/tcrtexpress.2013.600273 PMID:24325128

Achim, A., Bezerianos, A., & Tsakalides, P. (2001a). Ultrasound image denoising via maximum a posteriori estimation of wavelet coefficients. In *Engineering in Medicine and Biology Society, 2001. Proceedings of the 23rd Annual International Conference of the IEEE* (*Vol. 3*, pp. 2553-2556). IEEE. 10.1109/IEMBS.2001.1017300

Achim, A., Bezerianos, A., & Tsakalides, P. (2001). Novel Bayesian multiscale method for speckle removal in medical ultrasound images. *IEEE Transactions on Medical Imaging*, *20*(8), 772–783. doi:10.1109/42.938245 PMID:11513028

Acır, N. (2005). Classification of ECG beats by using a fast least square support vector machines with a dynamic programming feature selection algorithm. *Neural Computing & Applications*, *14*(4), 299–309. doi:10.100700521-005-0466-z

Adabi, S., Conforto, S., Clayton, A., Podoleanu, A. G., Hojjat, A., & Avanaki, M. R. (2016). An intelligent speckle reduction algorithm for optical coherence tomography images. In *4th International Conference on Photonics, Optics and Laser Technology (PHOTOPTICS), 2016* (pp. 1–6). IEEE.

Adabi, S., Rashedi, E., Clayton, A., Mohebbi-Kalkhoran, H., Chen, X. W., Conforto, S., & Nasiriavanaki, M. (2018). Learnable despeckling framework for optical coherence tomography images. *Journal of Biomedical Optics*, *23*(1), 016013. doi:10.1117/1.JBO.23.1.016013 PMID:29368458

Adler, D. C., Ko, T. H., & Fujimoto, J. G. (2004). Speckle reduction in optical coherence tomography images by use of a spatially adaptive wavelet filter. *Optics Letters*, *29*(24), 2878–2880. doi:10.1364/OL.29.002878 PMID:15645810

Afonso, M., & Sanches, J. M. (2015). Image reconstruction under multiplicative speckle noise using total variation. *Neurocomputing*, *150*, 200–213. doi:10.1016/j.neucom.2014.08.073

Agarwal & Bedi. (2016). *Implementation of hybrid image fusion technique for feature enhancement in medical diagnosis.* Springer.

Aggarwal, R., & Song, Y. (1997). Artificial neural networks in power systems. Part 1: General introduction to neural computing. *Power Engineering Journal, 11*(3), 129–134. doi:10.1049/pe:19970306

Agricultural Statistics at a Glance. (2014). Department of Agriculture & Cooperation, & Statistics.

Ahirwar, A. (2013). Study of Techniques used for Medical Image Segmentation and Computation of Statistical Test for Region Classification of Brain MRI. *International Journal Of Information Technology And Computer Science, 5*(5), 44–53. doi:10.5815/ijitcs.2013.05.06

Ahmed, T., Hoyle, R., Shaffer, P., Connelly, K., Crandall, D., & Kapadia, A. (2017). Understanding the Physical Safety, Security, and Privacy Concerns of People with Visual Impairments. *IEEE Internet Computing, 21*(3), 56–63. doi:10.1109/MIC.2017.77

Aitfares, W., Bouyakhf, E., Herbulot, A., Regragui, F., & Devy, M. (2013). Hybrid region and interest points-based active contour for object tracking. *Applied Mathematical Sciences, 7*, 5879–5899. doi:10.12988/ams.2013.38483

Aja-Fernández, S., & Alberola-López, C. (2006). On the estimation of the coefficient of variation for anisotropic diffusion speckle filtering. *IEEE Transactions on Image Processing, 15*(9), 2694–2701. doi:10.1109/TIP.2006.877360 PMID:16948314

Akinola, S. O., & Oyabugbe, O. J. (2015). Accuracies and training times of data mining classification algorithms: An empirical comparative study. *Journal of Software Engineering and Applications, 8*(09), 470–477. doi:10.4236/jsea.2015.89045

Alam, M. D. E., & Samanta, B. (2017). Empirical mode decomposition of EEG signals for brain computer interface. In SoutheastCon, 2017. IEEE. doi:10.1109/SECON.2017.7925341

Alexandridis, A., Chondrodima, E., & Sarimveis, H. (2013). Radial basis function network training using a nonsymmetric partition of the input space and particle swarm optimization. *IEEE Transactions on Neural Networks and Learning Systems, 24*(2), 219–230. doi:10.1109/TNNLS.2012.2227794 PMID:24808277

Algamal, Z. Y., Lee, M. H., Al-Fakih, A. M., & Aziz, M. (2017). High-dimensional QSAR classification model for anti-hepatitis C virus activity of thiourea derivatives based on the sparse logistic regression model with a bridge penalty. *Journal of Chemometrics, 31*(6), e2889. doi:10.1002/cem.2889

Alharbi, E. T., Rasheed, S., & Buhari, S. M. (2016). Feature selection algorithm for evoked EEG signal due to RGB colors. In *Image and Signal Processing, BioMedical Engineering and Informatics (CISP-BMEI), International Congress on*. IEEE.

Ali, H., Badshah, N., Chen, K., Khan, G., & Zikria, N. (2017). Multiphase segmentation based on new signed pressure force functions and one level set function. *Turkish Journal of Electrical Engineering and Computer Sciences, 25*, 2943–2955. doi:10.3906/elk-1606-260

Ali, H., Rada, L., & Badshah, N. (2018). Image Segmentation for Intensity Inhomogeneity in Presence of High Noise. *IEEE Transactions on Image Processing, 27*(8), 3729–3738. doi:10.1109/TIP.2018.2825101 PMID:29698205

Almonacid, M., Ibarrola, J., & Cano-Izquierdo, J.-M. (2016). Voting strategy to enhance multimodel EEG-based classifier systems for motor imagery BCI. *IEEE Systems Journal, 10*(3), 1082–1088. doi:10.1109/JSYST.2014.2360433

AL-Nabi, D. A., & Ahmed, S. S. (2013). Survey on classification algorithms for data mining: Comparison and evaluation. *International Journal of Computer Engineering and Intelligent Systems, 4*(8), 18–27.

Amancio, D. R., Comin, C. H., Casanova, D., Travieso, G., Bruno, O. M., Rodrigues, F. A., & da Fontoura Costa, L. (2014). A systematic comparison of supervised classifiers. *PLoS One*, *9*(4), e94137. doi:10.1371/journal.pone.0094137 PMID:24763312

American Academy of Sleep Medicine. (n.d.). Dates of insomnia day. *American Academy of Sleep Medicine.* Retrieved on July 13, 2018 available at https://aasm.org/

Amini, Z., & Rabbani, H. (2017). Optical coherence tomography image denoising using Gaussianization transform. *Journal of Biomedical Optics*, *22*(8), 086011. PMID:28853244

Amrouche, C., & Rejaiba, A. (2015). Navier-Stokes equations with Navier boundary condition. *Mathematical Methods in the Applied Sciences*, *39*(17), 5091–5112. doi:10.1002/mma.3338

Anantrasirichai, N., Nicholson, L., Morgan, J. E., Erchova, I., Mortlock, K., North, R. V., ... Achim, A. (2014). Adaptive-weighted bilateral filtering and other pre-processing techniques for optical coherence tomography. *Computerized Medical Imaging and Graphics*, *38*(6), 526–539. doi:10.1016/j.compmedimag.2014.06.012 PMID:25034317

Andersen, J. H., Haahr, J. P., & Frost, P. (2007). Risk factors for more severe regional musculoskeletal symptoms: A two-year prospective study of a general working population. *Arthritis and Rheumatism*, *56*(4), 1355–1364. doi:10.1002/art.22513 PMID:17393441

Anderson, T. W. (2003). *An introduction to multivariate statistical analysis* (3rd ed.). John Wiley & Sons, Inc.

Andrej, K., Janez, B., & Kos, A. (2011). Introduction to the Artificial Neural Networks. *Methodological Advances and Biomedical Applications.*

Anooj, P. K. (2011). Clinical decision support system: Risk level prediction of heart disease using weighted fuzzy rules and decision tree rules. *Central European Journal of Computer Science*, *1*(4), 482–498.

Antonelli, D., Baralis, E. M., Bruno, G., Cagliero, L., Cerquitelli, T., Chiusano, S. A., . . . Mahoto, N. A. (2015). MeTA: Characterization of medical treatments at different abstraction levels. *ACM Transactions on Intelligent Systems and Technology*, *6*(4), 1-25.

Antonelli, D., Baralis, E., Bruno, G., Chiusano, S., Mahoto, N. A., & Petrigni, C. (2012B). Analysis of diagnostic pathways for colon cancer. *Flexible Services and Manufacturing Journal*, *24*(4), 379-399.

Antonelli, D., Baralis, E., Bruno, G., Cerquitelli, T., Chiusano, S., & Mahoto, N. A. (2013). Analysis of diabetic patients through their examination history. *Expert Systems with Applications*, *40*(11), 4672–4678. doi:10.1016/j.eswa.2013.02.006

Antonelli, D., Baralis, E., Bruno, G., Chiusano, S., Mahoto, N. A., & Petrigni, C. (2012A). Extraction of medical pathways from electronic patient records. In *Medical Applications of Intelligent Data Analysis: Research Advancements* (pp. 273–289). IGI Global. doi:10.4018/978-1-4666-1803-9.ch018

Araki, T., Ikeda, N., Shukla, D., Londhe, N. D., Shrivastava, V. K., Banchhor, S. K., ... Suri, J. S. (2016). A new method for IVUS-based coronary artery disease risk stratification: A link between coronary & carotid ultrasound plaque burdens. *Computer Methods and Programs in Biomedicine*, *124*, 161–179. doi:10.1016/j.cmpb.2015.10.022 PMID:26707374

Archana, S., & Elangovan, K. (2014). Survey of classification techniques in data mining. *International Journal of Computer Science and Mobile Applications*, *2*(2), 65–71.

Aris, S. A. M., Jalil, S. Z. A., Bani, N. A., Kaidi, H. M., & Muhtazaruddin, M. N. (2016). EEG features extraction and k-NN classification during eyes closed. In *Biomedical Engineering and Sciences (IECBES), 2016 IEEE EMBS Conference on*. IEEE.

Arunachalam, S. P., Kapa, S., Mulpuru, S.K., Friedman, P.A., & Tolkacheva, E.G. (2016). Intelligent fractional-order pid (fopid) heart rate controller for cardiac pacemaker. In *Healthcare Innovation Point-Of- Care Technologies Conference (HI-POCT), 2016 IEEE*. IEEE.

Arvidsson, I., Balogh, I., Hansson, G. T., Ohlsson, K., Åkesson, I., & Nordander, C. (2012). Rationalization in meat cutting d consequences on physical workload. *Applied Ergonomics*, *43*(6), 1026–1032. doi:10.1016/j.apergo.2012.03.001 PMID:22475432

Asyali, M. H. (2003). Discrimination power of long-term heart rate variability measures. *Proceedings of the 25th Annual International Conference of the IEEE Engineering in Medicine and Biology Society* (pp. 200-203). Cancun, Mexico: IEEE. 10.1109/IEMBS.2003.1279568

Atkinson, J., & Campos, D. (2016). Improving BCI-based emotion recognition by combining EEG feature selection and kernel classifiers. *Expert Systems with Applications*, *47*, 35–41. doi:10.1016/j.eswa.2015.10.049

Attaran, N., Puranik, A., Brooks, J., & Mohsenin, T. (2018). Embedded Low-Power Processor for Personalized Stress Detection. *IEEE Transactions on Circuits and Wystems. II, Express Briefs*, 1. doi:10.1109/TCSII.2018.2799821

Aum, J., Kim, J. H., & Jeong, J. (2015). Effective speckle noise suppression in optical coherence tomography images using nonlocal means denoising filter with double Gaussian anisotropic kernels. *Applied Optics*, *54*(13), D43–D50. doi:10.1364/AO.54.000D43

Awang, R., & Palaniappan, S. (2007). Web based Heart Disease Decision Support System using Data Mining Classification Modeling techniques. In iiWAS, (pp. 177-187). Jakarta: Academic Press.

Ayat, S., & Khosravanian, A. (2014). Identification and classification of Coronary Artery disease patients using Neuro-Fuzzy Inference system. *Journal of Mathematics and Computer Science*, *13*(02), 136–141. doi:10.22436/jmcs.013.02.05

Aysal, T. C., & Barner, K. E. (2007). Rayleigh-maximum-likelihood filtering for speckle reduction of ultrasound images. *IEEE Transactions on Medical Imaging*, *26*(5), 712–727. doi:10.1109/TMI.2007.895484 PMID:17518065

Babar, A. H., Mahoto, N. A. (2018). Comparative Analysis of Classification Models for Healthcare Data Analysis. *International Journal of Computer and Information Technology, 7*(4), 170-175.

Babu, J. J. J., & Sudha, G. F. (2016). Adaptive speckle reduction in ultrasound images using fuzzy logic on Coefficient of Variation. *Biomedical Signal Processing and Control*, *23*, 93–103. doi:10.1016/j.bspc.2015.08.001

Bach, M., Meigen, T., & Strasburger, H. (1997). Raster-scan cathode-ray tubes for vision research-limits of resolution in space, time and intensity, and some solutions. *Spatial Vision*, *10*(4), 403–414. doi:10.1163/156856897X00311 PMID:9176948

Bagci, A. M., Shahidi, M., Ansari, R., Blair, M., Blair, N. P., & Zelkha, R. (2008). Thickness profiles of retinal layers by optical coherence tomography image segmentation. *American Journal of Ophthalmology*, *146*(5), 679–687. doi:10.1016/j.ajo.2008.06.010 PMID:18707672

Baghaie, A., D'souza, R. M., & Yu, Z. (2015, April). Sparse and low rank decomposition based batch image alignment for speckle reduction of retinal OCT images. In *12th International Symposium on Biomedical Imaging (ISBI), 2015 IEEE* (pp. 226-230). IEEE.

Balasubramanian, V., Adalarasu, K., & Regulapati, R. (2009). Comparing dynamic and stationary standing postures in an assembly task. *International Journal of Industrial Ergonomics*, *39*(5), 649–654. doi:10.1016/j.ergon.2008.10.017

Balocco, S., Gatta, C., Pujol, O., Mauri, J., & Radeva, P. (2010). SRBF: Speckle reducing bilateral filtering. *Ultrasound in Medicine & Biology*, *36*(8), 1353–1363. doi:10.1016/j.ultrasmedbio.2010.05.007 PMID:20691924

Banno, K., & Kryger, M. H. (2006). Comorbid insomnia. *Sleep Medicine Clinics*, *1*(3), 367–374. doi:10.1016/j.jsmc.2006.06.003

Banu, M. N., & Gomathy, B. (2014). Disease forecasting system using data mining methods. *International Conference on Intelligent Computing Applications (ICICA).* 10.1109/ICICA.2014.36

Baroni, M., Fortunato, P., & La Torre, A. (2007). Towards quantitative analysis of retinal features in optical coherence tomography. *Medical Engineering & Physics*, *29*(4), 432–441. doi:10.1016/j.medengphy.2006.06.003 PMID:16860587

Baselice, F. (2017). Ultrasound image despeckling based on statistical similarity. *Ultrasound in Medicine & Biology*, *43*(9), 2065–2078. doi:10.1016/j.ultrasmedbio.2017.05.006 PMID:28651920

Bashkansky, M., & Reintjes, J. (2000). Statistics and reduction of speckle in optical coherence tomography. *Optics Letters*, *25*(8), 545–547. doi:10.1364/OL.25.000545 PMID:18064106

Bawane, M. N., & Bhurchandi, K. M. (2014). Classification of Mental Task Based on EEG Processing Using Self Organising Feature Map. In *Intelligent Human-Machine Systems and Cybernetics (IHMSC), 2014 Sixth International Conference on* (Vol. 2). IEEE.

Begum, S., Chakraborty, D., & Sarkar, R. (2015, December). Data classification using feature selection and kNN machine learning approach. In *Computational Intelligence and Communication Networks (CICN), 2015 International Conference on* (pp. 811-814). IEEE.

Belic, E., Lukac, N., Dezelak, K., Zalik, B., & Stumberger, G. (2017). GPU-based online optimization of low voltage distribution network operation. *IEEE Transactions on Smart Grid*, *8*(3), 1460–1468.

Beneš, M., & Kučera, P. (2015). Solutions to the Navier-Stokes equations with mixed boundary conditions in two-dimensional bounded domains. *Mathematische Nachrichten*, *289*(2-3), 194–212. doi:10.1002/mana.201400046

Bernardes, R., Maduro, C., Serranho, P., Araújo, A., Barbeiro, S., & Cunha-Vaz, J. (2010). Improved adaptive complex diffusion despeckling filter. *Optics Express*, *18*(23), 24048–24059. doi:10.1364/OE.18.024048 PMID:21164752

Bhardwaj, A., Gupta, A., Jain, P., Rani, A., & Yadav, J. (2015). Classification of human emotions from EEG signals using SVM and LDA Classifiers. In *Signal Processing and Integrated Networks (SPIN), 2015 2nd International Conference on*. IEEE.

Bhardwaj, R., Nambiar, A. R., & Dutta, D. (2017, July). A Study of Machine Learning in Healthcare. In *Computer Software and Applications Conference (COMPSAC), 2017 IEEE 41st Annual* (Vol. 2, pp. 236-241). IEEE.

Bhargava, K., & Katarya, R. (2017, October). An improved lexicon using logistic regression for sentiment analysis. In *Computing and Communication Technologies for Smart Nation (IC3TSN), 2017 International Conference on* (pp. 332-337). IEEE.

Bhattacharjee, S., Mazumder, A., Das, Z., Kumar, L., Shree, K., & Neogi, B. (2013). Study on cardiovascular diseases with compression of generalized ECG signal to support biomedical advancement. *International Journal of Advanced Research in Electrical. Electronics and Instrumentation Engineering*, *2*(10), 5213–5219.

Bhattacharyya, A. (1943). On a measure of divergence between two statistical populations defined by their probability distributions. *Bulletin of the Calcutta Mathematical Society*, *35*, 99–109.

Bhuiyan, M. I. H., Ahmad, M. O., & Swamy, M. N. S. (2007, May). New spatially adaptive wavelet-based method for the despeckling of medical ultrasound images. In *Circuits and Systems, 2007. ISCAS 2007. IEEE International Symposium on* (pp. 2347-2350). IEEE.

Bian, L., Suo, J., Chen, F., & Dai, Q. (2015). Multiframe denoising of high-speed optical coherence tomography data using interframe and intraframe priors. *Journal of Biomedical Optics*, *20*(3), 036006. doi:10.1117/1.JBO.20.3.036006 PMID:25751163

Billi, M., Burzagli, L., Catarci, T., Santucci, G., Bertini, E., Gabbanini, F., & Palchetti, E. (2010). A unified methodology for the evaluation of accessibility and usability of mobile applications. *Universal Access in the Information Society*, *9*(4), 337–356. doi:10.100710209-009-0180-1

Bioucas-Dias, J. M., & Figueiredo, M. A. (2009, November). Total variation restoration of speckled images using a split-Bregman algorithm. In *Image Processing (ICIP), 2009 16th IEEE International Conference on* (pp. 3717-3720). IEEE.

Bioucas-Dias, J. M., & Figueiredo, M. A. (2010). Multiplicative noise removal using variable splitting and constrained optimization. *IEEE Transactions on Image Processing*, *19*(7), 1720–1730. doi:10.1109/TIP.2010.2045029 PMID:20215071

Biradar, N., Dewal, M. L., & Rohit, M. K. (2015). Speckle noise reduction in B-mode echocardiographic images: A comparison. *IETE Technical Review*, *32*(6), 435–453. doi:10.1080/02564602.2015.1031714

Biswas, R., Sarawadekar, K., Varna, S., & Banerjee, S. (2015). An FPGA-based architecture of DSC-SRI Units specially for motion blind ultrasound systems. *Journal of Real-Time Image Processing*, *10*(3), 573–595. doi:10.100711554-012-0289-y

Bobick, G., & Myers, J. R. (1995). *Back Injures in Agriculture: Occupations Affected.* Boca Raton, FL: CRC Press, Lewis Publishers.

Boegl, K., Adlassnig, K. P., Hayashi, Y., Rothenfluh, T. E., & Leitich, H. (2004). Knowledge acquisition in the fuzzy knowledge representation framework of a medical consultation system. *Artificial Intelligence in Medicine*, *30*(1), 1–26. doi:10.1016/S0933-3657(02)00073-8 PMID:14684262

Bogunović, H., Sonka, M., Kwon, Y. H., Kemp, P., Abràmoff, M. D., & Wu, X. (2014). Multi-surface and multi-field co-segmentation of 3-D retinal optical coherence tomography. *IEEE Transactions on Medical Imaging*, *33*(12), 2242–2253. doi:10.1109/TMI.2014.2336246 PMID:25020067

Boyer, K. L., Herzog, A., & Roberts, C. (2006). Automatic recovery of the optic nervehead geometry in optical coherence tomography. *IEEE Transactions on Medical Imaging*, *25*(5), 553–570. doi:10.1109/TMI.2006.871417 PMID:16689260

Breiman, L. (1996). Bagging predictors. *Machine Learning*, *24*(2), 123–140. doi:10.1007/BF00058655

Briggs, A., & Gray, A. (1999). Methods in health service research: Handling uncertainty in economic evaluations of health-care interventions. *BMJ (Clinical Research Ed.)*, *319*(7210), 635–638. doi:10.1136/bmj.319.7210.635 PMID:10473486

Brookhuis, K. A., & de Waard, D. (2010). Monitoring drivers' mental workload in driving simulators using physiological measures. *Accident; Analysis and Prevention*, *42*(3), 898–903. doi:10.1016/j.aap.2009.06.001 PMID:20380918

Cabena, P., Hadjinian, P., Stadler, R., Verhees, J., & Zanasi, A. (1997). Discovering data mining: from concept to implementation. Prentice Hall PTR.

Candes, E. J., & Donoho, D. L. (2005). Continuous curvelet transform: I. Resolution of the wavefront set. *Appl. Comput. Harmon.*, *19*(2), 162–197. doi:10.1016/j.acha.2005.02.003

Candes, E. J., & Donoho, D. L. (2005). Continuous curvelet transform: II. Discretization and frame. *Applied and Computational Harmonic Analysis*, *19*(2), 198–222. doi:10.1016/j.acha.2005.02.004

Candes, E., Demanet, L., Donoho, D., & Ying, L. (2006). Fast discrete curvelet transform. *Multiscale Modeling & Simulation*, *5*(3), 861–899. doi:10.1137/05064182X

Caponetti, L., Castellano, G., & Corsini, V. (2017). MR Brain Image Segmentation: A Framework to Compare Different Clustering Techniques. *Information*, *8*(4), 138. doi:10.3390/info8040138

Carlson. (2018). *National Comprehensive Cancer Network Clinical Practice Guidelines in Oncology (NCCN Guidelines)*. Retrieved from http://www.nccn.org

Carrasco, S., Nasr, M. B., Sergienko, A. V., Saleh, B. E., Teich, M. C., Torres, J. P., & Torner, L. (2006). Broadband light generation by noncollinear parametric downconversion. *Optics Letters*, *31*(2), 253–255. doi:10.1364/OL.31.000253 PMID:16441047

Casas, M. M., Avitia, R. L., Gonzalez-Navarro, F. F., Cardenas-Haro, J. A., & Reyna, M. A. (2018). Bayesian Classification Models for Premature Ventricular Contraction Detection on ECG Traces. *Journal of Healthcare Engineering*, *7*. doi:10.1155/2018/2694768 PMID:29861881

Castroa, V. G., Hernandeza, M. V., Armitageb, P. A., & Wardlawa, J. M. (2016). Texture-based classification for the automatic rating of the perivascular spaces in brain MRI. *Procedia Computer Science*, *90*, 9–14. doi:10.1016/j.procs.2016.07.003

Castro, V. J. F., & Malathi, R. (2018). Design of advanced control strategies for cardiovascular system. *Materials Today: Proceedings*, *5*(1), 1960–1966. doi:10.1016/j.matpr.2017.11.299

Cernazanu-Glavan, C., Todinca, D., & Precup, R. E. (2014, May). DeeDee-A mobile intelligent system able to assist a type 1 diabetic through the daily life. In *Applied Computational Intelligence and Informatics (SACI), 2014 IEEE 9th International Symposium on* (pp. 343-347). IEEE.

Chang, H. (2015). Book Review: Data-Driven Healthcare & Analytics in a Big Data World. *Healthcare Informatics Research*, *21*(1), 61. doi:10.4258/hir.2015.21.1.61

Chaparro-Vargas, R., Ahmed, B., Wessel, N., Penzel, T., & Cvetkovic, D. (2016). Insomnia Characterization: From Hypnogram to Graph Spectral Theory. *IEEE Transactions on Biomedical Engineering*, *63*(10), 2211–2219. doi:10.1109/TBME.2016.2515261 PMID:26742123

Chatterjee, H. K., Gupta, R., Bera, J. N., & Mitra, M. (2011). An FPGA implementation of Real Time QRS Detection. *International Conference on Computer and Communication Technology*, 274-279. 10.1109/ICCCT.2011.6075114

Chaudhry, M., Kamran, M., & Afzal, S. (2008). Speaking monuments—design and implementation of an RFID based blind friendly environment. In *Electrical Engineering, 2008. ICEE 2008. Second International Conference on* (pp. 1-6). IEEE.

Chaurasia, V. (2017). *Early prediction of heart diseases using data mining techniques*. Academic Press.

Chen, D. (2014). Image fusion method based on edge feature detection in electricalcapacitance tomography. *Int. J. Signal Process. Image Process. Pattern Recognit*, *7*(1), 67–76.

Chen, E. L., Chung, P. C., Chen, C. L., Tsai, H.-M., & Chang, C.-I. (1998). An Automatic Diagnostic System for CT Liver Image Classification. *IEEE Transactions on Biomedical Engineering*, *45*(6), 783–794. doi:10.1109/10.678613 PMID:9609943

Cheng, J., Duan, L., Wong, D. W. K., Akiba, M., & Liu, J. (2014, August). Speckle reduction in optical coherence tomography by matrix completion using bilateral random projection. In *36th Annual International Conference of the Engineering in Medicine and Biology Society (EMBC), 2014* (pp. 186-189). IEEE.

Chen, G., & Gao, Y. (2013). Multisource images adaptive fusion based on double density dual-tree complex wavelet transform. *J. Conv. Inf. Technol*, *8*(1), 548–557.

Chen, H., Fu, S., Wang, H., Lv, H., & Zhang, C. (2018). Speckle attenuation by adaptive singular value shrinking with generalized likelihood matching in optical coherence tomography. *Journal of Biomedical Optics*, *23*(3), 036014. doi:10.1117/1.JBO.23.3.036014 PMID:29595018

Chen, M.-S., Han, J., & Yu, P. S. (1996). Data mining: An overview from a database perspective. *IEEE Transactions on Knowledge and Data Engineering*, *8*(6), 866–883. doi:10.1109/69.553155

Chen, Q., de Sisternes, L., Leng, T., & Rubin, D. L. (2015). Application of improved homogeneity similarity-based denoising in optical coherence tomography retinal images. *Journal of Digital Imaging*, *28*(3), 346–361. doi:10.100710278-014-9742-8 PMID:25404105

Chen, Y., Huang, M., & Chen, S. (2013). Automatic Color Segmentation by Colormap and Edge Detection by Chan Vese Method for Tongue Image. *Journal of Applied Sciences (Faisalabad)*, *13*(18), 3676–3683. doi:10.3923/jas.2013.3676.3683

Chen, Z., Basarab, A., & Kouamé, D. (2016). Compressive deconvolution in medical ultrasound imaging. *IEEE Transactions on Medical Imaging*, *35*(3), 728–737. doi:10.1109/TMI.2015.2493241 PMID:26513780

Chifu, V., Pop, C., Salomie, I., Suia, D., & Niculici, A. (2012). Optimizing the Semantic Web Service Composition Process Using Cuckoo Search. *Intelligent Distributed Computing,* 93-102.

Chitchian, S., Fiddy, M. A., & Fried, N. M. (2009). Denoising during optical coherence tomography of the prostate nerves via wavelet shrinkage using dual-tree complex wavelet transform. *Journal of Biomedical Optics*, *14*(1), 014031. doi:10.1117/1.3081543 PMID:19256719

Chitra, R., & Seenivasagam, V. (2013). Review of heart disease prediction system using data mining and hybrid intelligent techniques. *ICTACT Journal on Soft Computing, 3*(4), 605-609.

Chiu, S. J., Li, X. T., Nicholas, P., Toth, C. A., Izatt, J. A., & Farsiu, S. (2010). Automatic segmentation of seven retinal layers in SDOCT images congruent with expert manual segmentation. *Optics Express*, *18*(18), 19413–19428. doi:10.1364/OE.18.019413 PMID:20940837

Choi, S. W., & Min, B. G. (2014). *Ventricular assist device cannula and ventricular assist device including the same*. US Patent 8,771,165.

Chouvarda, I., Grassi, A., Mendez, M. O., Bianchi, A. M., Parrino, L., Milioli, G., . . . Cerutti, S. (2013, July). Insomnia types and sleep microstructure dynamics. In *Engineering in Medicine and Biology Society (EMBC), 2013 35th Annual International Conference of the IEEE* (pp. 6167-6170). IEEE. 10.1109/EMBC.2013.6610961

Chouvarda, I., Papadelis, C., Domis, N., Staner, L., & Maglaveras, N. (2007, August). Insomnia treatment assessment based on physiological data analysis. In *Engineering in Medicine and Biology Society, 2007. EMBS 2007. 29th Annual International Conference of the IEEE* (pp. 6694-6696). IEEE.

Chouvarda, I., Mendez, M. O., Rosso, V., Bianchi, A. M., Parrino, L., Grassi, A., & Maglaveras, N. (2012). Cyclic alternating patterns in normal sleep and insomnia: Structure and content differences. *IEEE Transactions on Neural Systems and Rehabilitation Engineering*, *20*(5), 642–652. doi:10.1109/TNSRE.2012.2208984 PMID:22855235

Christodoulou, C. I., Loizou, C., Pattichis, C. S., Pantziaris, M., Kyriakou, E., Pattichis, M. S., . . . Nicolaides, A. (2002). De-speckle filtering in ultrasound imaging of the carotid artery. In *Engineering in Medicine and Biology, 2002. 24th Annual Conference and the Annual Fall Meeting of the Biomedical Engineering Society EMBS/BMES Conference, 2002. Proceedings of the Second Joint* (*Vol. 2*, pp. 1027-1028). IEEE. 10.1109/IEMBS.2002.1106259

Christopher, O. (2015). *Understanding LSTM Networks.* Retrieved from https://colah.github.io/posts/2015-08-Understanding-LSTMs/

Chua, C. K., Chandran, V., Acharya, R. U., & Min, L. C. (2009). Cardiac health diagnosis using higher order spectra and support vector machine. *The Open Medical Informatics Journal*, *3*(1), 1–8. doi:10.2174/1874431100903010001 PMID:19603098

Cios, K. J. (2000). From the guest editor medical data mining and knowledge discovery. *IEEE Engineering in Medicine and Biology Magazine*, *19*(4), 15–16. doi:10.1109/MEMB.2000.853477 PMID:10916728

Coast, D. A., Stern, R. M., Cano, G. G., & Briller, S. A. (1990). An approach to cardiac arrhythmia analysis using hidden Markov models. *IEEE Transactions on Biomedical Engineering*, *37*(9), 826–836. doi:10.1109/10.58593 PMID:2227969

Cohen, W. W. (1995). *Fast effective rule induction. In Machine Learning Proceedings 1995* (pp. 115–123). Elsevier. doi:10.1016/B978-1-55860-377-6.50023-2

Cohn, J. N., Ferrari, R., & Sharpe, N. (2000). Cardiac remodelling – concepts and clinical implications: A consensus paper from an international forum on cardiac remodeling. *Journal of the American College of Cardiology*, *35*(3), 569–582. doi:10.1016/S0735-1097(99)00630-0 PMID:10716457

Coifman, R. R., & Donoho, D. L. (1995). Translation-invariant de-noising. In *Wavelets and statistics* (pp. 125–150). New York, NY: Springer. doi:10.1007/978-1-4612-2544-7_9

Collins, R. M., Janse van Rensburg, D. C., & Patricios, J. S. (2011). Common work-related musculoskeletal strains and injuries. *South African Family Practice*, *53*(3), 240–246. doi:10.1080/20786204.2011.10874091

Cook, D. G., & Shaper, A. G. (1988). Breathlessness, lung function and the risk of heart attack. *European Heart Journal*, *9*(11), 1215–1222. doi:10.1093/oxfordjournals.eurheartj.a062432 PMID:3234413

Corbin, M., McLean, D., Mannetje, A., Dryson, E., Walls, C., McKenzie, F., ... Pearce, N. (2011). Lung cancer and occupation: A New Zealand cancer registry-based cased control study. *American Journal of Industrial Medicine*, *54*(2), 89–101. doi:10.1002/ajim.20906 PMID:20957667

Cososchi, S., Stungaru, R., Ungureanu, A., & Ugunureanu, M. (2006). EEG features extraction for motor imagery. In *Engineering in Medicine and Biology Society, 2006. EMBS'06. 28th Annual International Conference of the IEEE.* IEEE. 10.1109/IEMBS.2006.260004

Coughlan, J. M., & Miele, J. (2017). AR4VI: AR as an Accessibility Tool for People with Visual Impairments. In *Mixed and Augmented Reality (ISMAR-Adjunct), 2017 IEEE International Symposium on* (pp. 288-292). IEEE.

Coupé, P., Hellier, P., Kervrann, C., & Barillot, C. (2008, May). Bayesian non local means-based speckle filtering. In *Biomedical Imaging: From Nano to Macro, 2008. ISBI 2008. 5th IEEE International Symposium on* (pp. 1291-1294). IEEE. 10.1109/ISBI.2008.4541240

Coupé, P., Hellier, P., Kervrann, C., & Barillot, C. (2009). Nonlocal means-based speckle filtering for ultrasound images. *IEEE Transactions on Image Processing*, *18*(10), 2221–2229. doi:10.1109/TIP.2009.2024064 PMID:19482578

Cover, T., & Hart, P. (1967). Nearest neighbor pattern classification. *IEEE Transactions on Information Theory*, *13*(1), 21–27. doi:10.1109/TIT.1967.1053964

Cowie, M. R., Wood, D. A., Coats, A. J. S., Thompson, S. G., Suresh, V., Poole-Wilson, P. A., & Sutton, G. C. (2000). Survival of patients with a new diagnosis of heart failure: A population based study. *Heart (British Cardiac Society)*, *83*(5), 505–510. doi:10.1136/heart.83.5.505 PMID:10768897

Crasto, C. J., Marenco, L. N., Migliore, M., Mao, B., Nadkarni, P. M., Miller, P., & Shepherd, G. M. (2003). Text mining neuroscience journal articles to populate neuroscience databases. *Neuroinformatics*, *1*(3), 215–237. doi:10.1385/NI:1:3:215 PMID:15046245

Cuartas-Vélez, C., Restrepo, R., Bouma, B. E., & Uribe-Patarroyo, N. (2018). Volumetric non-local-means based speckle reduction for optical coherence tomography. *Biomedical Optics Express*, *9*(7), 3354–3372. doi:10.1364/BOE.9.003354 PMID:29984102

Cuesta–Frau, D., Miro-Martinez, P., Nunez, J. J., Oltra-Crespo, S., & Molina Pico, A. (2017). Noisy EEG signals classification based on entropy metrics. Performance assessment using first- and second-generation statistics. *Computers in Biology and Medicine*, *87*, 141–151. doi:10.1016/j.compbiomed.2017.05.028 PMID:28595129

Cui, Z., & Fan, Q. (2018). A "Nonconvex+Nonconvex" approach for image restoration with impulse noise removal. *Applied Mathematical Modelling*, *62*, 254–271. doi:10.1016/j.apm.2018.05.035

da Costa, B. R., & Vieira, E. R. (2010). Risk factors for work-related musculoskeletal disorders: A systematic review of recent longitudinal Studies. *American Journal of Industrial Medicine*, *53*, 285–323. PMID:19753591

Das, B., Ghosh, T., & Gangopadhyay, S. (2012). Assessment of Ergonomic and Occupational Health-Related Problems Among Female Prawn Seed Collectors of Sunderbans, West Bengal, India. *International Journal of Occupational Safety and Ergonomics*, *18*(4), 531–540. doi:10.1080/10803548.2012.11076949 PMID:23294657

Dash, D. P., & Kolekar, M. H. (2017, September). Epileptic seizure detection based on EEG signal analysis using hierarchy based Hidden Markov Model. In *International Conference on Advances in Computing, Communications and Informatics (ICACCI)*, (pp. 1114-1120). IEEE. 10.1109/ICACCI.2017.8125991

Das, S., Doppa, J. R., Pande, P. P., & Chakrabarty, K. (2017). Design-space exploration and optimization of an energy-efficient and reliable 3-D small-world network-on chip. *IEEE Transactions on Computer-Aided Design of Integrated Circuits and Systems*, *36*(5), 719–732. doi:10.1109/TCAD.2016.2604288

de Chazal, P., & Reilly, R. B. (2006). A patient-adapting heartbeat classifier using ECG morphology and heartbeat interval features. *IEEE Transactions on Biomedical Engineering*, *53*(12), 2535–2543. doi:10.1109/TBME.2006.883802 PMID:17153211

de León, F. S., Nicklin, P., Rhodesf, C., & Kwankam, S. Y. (2008). *Promoting appropriate eHealth technologies in the developing world: The Sharing eHealth Intellectual Property for Development (SHIPD) initiative*. World Health Organization.

de Oliveira, L. S., Andreão, R. V., & Sarcinelli-Filho, M. (2011, August). Premature ventricular beat classification using a dynamic Bayesian network. In *Annual International Conference of Engineering in Medicine and Biology Society, EMBC*, (pp. 4984-4987). IEEE. 10.1109/IEMBS.2011.6091235

De Souza Veriscimo, E., & Bernardes, J. L. (2015). A New 3D Interaction Technique Accessible to the Visually Impaired. In *2015 XVII Symposium on Virtual and Augmented Reality (SVR)* (pp. 208-211). IEEE. 10.1109/SVR.2015.37

Deepika, N. (2011). Association Rule for Classification of Heart Attack Patients. *IJAEST*, *11*(2), 253–257.

Del Cura, J. L., Seguí, P., & Nicolau, C. (Eds.). (2012). *Learning Ultrasound Imaging*. Springer Science & Business Media. doi:10.1007/978-3-642-30586-3

Delcourt, C., Korobelnik, J. F., Barberger-Gateau, P., Delyfer, M. N., Rougier, M. B., Le Goff, M., ... Dartigues, J. F. (2010). Nutrition and age-related eye diseases: The Alienor (Antioxydants, Lipides Essentiels, Nutrition et maladies OculaiRes) Study. *The Journal of Nutrition, Health & Aging*, *14*(10), 854–861. doi:10.100712603-010-0131-9 PMID:21125205

Deledalle, C. A., Denis, L., & Tupin, F. (2009). Iterative weighted maximum likelihood denoising with probabilistic patch-based weights. *IEEE Transactions on Image Processing*, *18*(12), 2661–2672. doi:10.1109/TIP.2009.2029593 PMID:19666338

DeLuca, C. J. (1997). The use of surface electromyography in biomechanics. *Journal of Applied Biomechanics, 13*(2), 135–163. doi:10.1123/jab.13.2.135

Derrac, J., Chiclana, F., García, S., & Herrera, F. (2016). Evolutionary fuzzy k-nearest neighbors algorithm using interval-valued fuzzy sets. *Information Sciences, 329*, 144–163. doi:10.1016/j.ins.2015.09.007

Desjardins, A. E., Vakoc, B. J., Tearney, G. J., & Bouma, B. E. (2006). Speckle reduction in OCT using massively-parallel detection and frequency-domain ranging. *Optics Express, 14*(11), 4736–4745. doi:10.1364/OE.14.004736 PMID:19516630

Determining the Appropriate Amount of Anesthetic Gas Using DWT and EMD Combined with Neural Network - Scientific Figure on ResearchGate. (n.d.). Retrieved June 2018, 15, from ResearchGate: https://www.researchgate.net/Artificial-neuron-model-43_fig2_275965841

Dev, S. M. (2013). Small Farmers in India: Challenges and Opportunities. Mumbai: Academic Press.

Devarapu, K. V., Murala, S., & Kumar, V. (2010, February). Denoising of ultrasound images using curvelet transform. In *Computer and Automation Engineering (ICCAE), 2010 The 2nd International Conference on* (Vol. 3, pp. 447-451). IEEE.

Devereux, J. J., Buckle, P. W., & Vlachonikolis, I. G. (1999). Interactions between physical and psychosocial risk factors at work increase the risk of back disorders: An epidemiological approach. *Occupational and Environmental Medicine, 56*(5), 343–353. doi:10.1136/oem.56.5.343 PMID:10472310

Devereux, J. J., Vlachonikolis, I. G., & Buckle, P. W. (2002). Epidemiological study to investigate potential interaction between physical and psychosocial factors at work that may increase the risk of symptoms of musculoskeletal disorder of the neck and upper limb. *Occupational and Environmental Medicine, 59*(4), 269–277. doi:10.1136/oem.59.4.269 PMID:11934955

Dhanasekar, A., & Mala, R. (2016). Analysis of Association Rule for Heart Disease Prediction from Large Datasets. *International Journal of Innovative Research in Science, Engineering and Technology, 5*(10), 18059-18063.

Dilsizian, S. E., & Siegel, E. L. (2014). Artificial intelligence in medicine and cardiac imaging: Harnessing big data and advanced computing to provide personalized medical diagnosis and treatment. *Current Cardiology Reports, 16*(1), 441. doi:10.100711886-013-0441-8 PMID:24338557

Dimitriou, N., & Delopoulos, A. (2013). Motion-based segmentation of objects using overlapping temporal windows. *Image and Vision Computing, 31*(9), 593–602. doi:10.1016/j.imavis.2013.06.005

Ding, J., Berleant, D., Nettleton, D., & Wurtele, E. (2001). Mining MEDLINE: Abstracts, sentences, or phrases? *InBiocomputing, 2002*, 326–337. PMID:11928487

Dissanyaka, C., Cvetkovic, D., Abdullah, H., Ahmed, B., & Penzel, T. (2016, December). Classification of healthy and insomnia subjects based on wake-to-sleep transition. In *Biomedical Engineering and Sciences (IECBES), 2016 IEEE EMBS Conference on* (pp. 480-483). IEEE.

Dixit, D., & Sahu, P. R. (2017, September). Outage Probability of Cooperative Relay Networks in eta-μ, kappa-μ, and Mixed Fading Channels. In *Vehicular Technology Conference (VTC-Fall), 2017 IEEE 86th* (pp. 1-5). IEEE. 10.1109/VTCFall.2017.8288003

Doble, S. J., Matthews, G. A., Rutherford, I., & Southcombe, E. S. E. (1985). A System for Classifying Hydraulic Nozzles and Other Atomizers into Categories of Spray Quality/Pro. *1985 Bit. Crop Porf. Conf. –Weeds, 9*(A–6), 112.533.

Dobre, O. A., Abdi, A., Bar-Ness, Y., & Su, W. (2007). Survey of automatic modulation classification techniques: Classical approaches and new trends. *IET Communications, 1*(2), 137–156. doi:10.1049/iet-com:20050176

Dolezal, J., Stastny, J., & Sovka, P. (2006). Modelling and recognition of movement related EEG signal. In *Applied Electronics, 2006. AE 2006. International Conference on*. IEEE.

Domingos, P., & Pazzani, M. (1997). On the optimality of the simple Bayesian classifier under zero-one loss. *Machine Learning*, *29*(2), 103–130. doi:10.1023/A:1007413511361

Dong, F., Guo, Q., Sun, S., Ren, X., Wang, L., Feng, S., & Gao, B. Z. (2013). Directional Weight Based Contourlet Transform Denoising Algorithm for Oct Image. *Intelligent Automation & Soft Computing*, *19*(4), 525–535. doi:10.1080/10798587.2013.869110

Dong, X., Wang, C., & Si, W. (2017). ECG beat classification via deterministic learning. *Neurocomputing*, *240*, 1–12. doi:10.1016/j.neucom.2017.02.056

Donoho, D. L., & Johnstone, J. M. (1994). Ideal spatial adaptation by wavelet shrinkage. *Biometrika, 81*(3), 425-455.

Drapikowski, P., & Domagała, Z. (2014). Semi-Automatic Segmentation of Ct/Mri Images Based on Active Contour Method for 3D Reconstruction of Abdominal Aortic Aneurysms. *Image Processing & Communications*, *19*(1), 13–19. doi:10.1515/ipc-2015-0002

Drexler, W., Morgner, U., Ghanta, R. K., Kärtner, F. X., Schuman, J. S., & Fujimoto, J. G. (2001, April). Ultrahigh-resolution ophthalmic optical coherence tomography. *Nature Medicine*, *7*(4), 502–507. doi:10.1038/86589 PMID:11283681

Dua, D., & Karra Taniskidou, E. (2017). *Statlog (Heart) Data Set.* Retrieved from UCI Machine Learning Repository: http://archive.ics.uci.edu/ml/datasets/Statlog+%28Heart%29

Duan, J., Lu, W., Tench, C., Gottlob, I., Proudlock, F., Samani, N. N., & Bai, L. (2016). Denoising optical coherence tomography using second order total generalized variation decomposition. *Biomedical Signal Processing and Control*, *24*, 120–127. doi:10.1016/j.bspc.2015.09.012

Duan, J., Tench, C., Gottlob, I., Proudlock, F., & Bai, L. (2015). New variational image decomposition model for simultaneously denoising and segmenting optical coherence tomography images. *Physics in Medicine and Biology*, *60*(22), 8901–8922. doi:10.1088/0031-9155/60/22/8901 PMID:26553577

Dube, B., Mishra, D., Satapathy, S., & Singh, S. (2018). Ergonomic evaluation of seeding, fertilizing and weeding postures in agricultural field. *International Journal of Pure and Applied Mathematics, 119*(10-Special Issue B), 1875-1880.

Dubey, A., Patel, R., & Choure, K. (2014). An efficient data mining and ant colony optimization technique (DMACO) for heart disease prediction. *International Journal of Advanced Technology and Engineering Exploration.*, *1*(1), 1–6.

Dubey, S. D. (1970). Compound gamma, beta and F distributions. *Metrika*, *16*(1), 27–31. doi:10.1007/BF02613934

Du, J., Li, W., Lu, K., & Xiao, B. (2016). An Overview of Multi-Modal Medical Image Fusion, *Elsevier*. *Neurocomputing*, *215*, 3–20. doi:10.1016/j.neucom.2015.07.160

Dunham, M. H. (2006). *Data mining: Introductory and advanced topics*. Pearson Education India.

Durairaj, M., & Meena, K. (2011). A Hybrid Prediction System using Rough Sets and Artificial Neural Network. *International Journal of Innovative Technology and Creative Engineering*, *1*(7), 16–23.

Du, Y., Liu, G., Feng, G., & Chen, Z. (2014). Speckle reduction in optical coherence tomography images based on wave atoms. *Journal of Biomedical Optics*, *19*(5), 056009. doi:10.1117/1.JBO.19.5.056009 PMID:24825507

El Majd, Y. A., El Ghazi, H., & Nahhal, T. (2017, November). PaRRT: Parallel rapidly-exploring random tree (RRT) based on MapReduce. In *Electrical and Information Technologies (ICEIT), 2017 International Conference on* (pp. 1-5). IEEE.

Elad, M., Starck, J. L., Querre, P., & Donoho, D. L. (2005). Simultaneous cartoon and texture image inpainting using morphological component analysis (MCA). *Applied and Computational Harmonic Analysis*, *19*(3), 340–358. doi:10.1016/j.acha.2005.03.005

El-Hoseny, El-Sayed, El Rabaie, Elrahman, & El-Samie. (2017). Medical Image Fusion Techniques Based on Combined Discrete Transform Domains. In *34th National Radio Science Conference*. IEEE.

Eliot, L. (2018, Jan 19). *Support Vector Machines (SVM) for AI Self-Driving Cars*. Retrieved from AITrends: https://aitrends.com/ai-insider/support-vector-machines-svm-ai-self-driving-cars/

Emiliani, P. L., & Stephanidis, C. (2005). Universal access to ambient intelligence environments: Opportunities and challenges for people with disabilities. *IBM Systems Journal*, *44*(3), 605–619. doi:10.1147j.443.0605

Eskin, E., & Pevzner, P. A. (2002). Finding composite regulatory patterns in DNA sequences. *Bioinformatics (Oxford, England)*, *18*(Suppl 1), 354–363. doi:10.1093/bioinformatics/18.suppl_1.S354 PMID:12169566

Espique, F. P. (2010). Notice of Retraction Provisions of computer technology in the learning development of students with visual impairment. In *Computer Engineering and Technology (ICCET), 2010 2nd International Conference on* (Vol. 7, pp. V7-547). IEEE.

Eun, S., Jung, E., & Park, D. (2017). Effective Brain Contour Segmentation based on Active Contour Model. *Journal Of Next-Generation Convergence Information Services Technology*, *6*(2), 75–88. doi:10.29056/jncist.2017.12.07

Fabritius, T., Makita, S., Miura, M., Myllylä, R., & Yasuno, Y. (2009). Automated segmentation of the macula by optical coherence tomography. *Optics Express*, *17*(18), 15659–15669. doi:10.1364/OE.17.015659 PMID:19724565

Fabunmi, A. A., Oworu, J. O., & Odunnaiya, N. E. (2008). Prevalence of musculoskeletal disorders among nurses in University College Hospital, Ibadan. *West Afr J Nurs.*, *19*, 21–25.

Fancott, T., & Wong, D. H. (1980). A minicomputer system for direct high speed analysis of cardiac arrhythmia in 24 h ambulatory ECG tape recordings. *IEEE Transactions on Biomedical Engineering*, *BME-27*(12), 685–693. doi:10.1109/TBME.1980.326593 PMID:7461643

Fang, L., Li, S., McNabb, R. P., Nie, Q., Kuo, A. N., Toth, C. A., ... Farsiu, S. (2013). Fast acquisition and reconstruction of optical coherence tomography images via sparse representation. *IEEE Transactions on Medical Imaging*, *32*(11), 2034–2049. doi:10.1109/TMI.2013.2271904 PMID:23846467

Fang, L., Li, S., Nie, Q., Izatt, J. A., Toth, C. A., & Farsiu, S. (2012). Sparsity based denoising of spectral domain optical coherence tomography images. *Biomedical Optics Express*, *3*(5), 927–942. doi:10.1364/BOE.3.000927 PMID:22567586

Fan, R., Zhong, M., Wang, S., Zhang, Y., Andrew, A., Karagas, M., ... Moore, J. (2011). Entropy-based information gain approaches to detect and to characterize gene-gene and gene-environment interactions/correlations of complex diseases. *Genetic Epidemiology*, *35*(7), 706–721. doi:10.1002/gepi.20621 PMID:22009792

Feng, R., & Jiang, H. (2010). Edge Based Level Set with Gaussian Filtering Regularized and its Application in Liver Segmentation. *Advanced Materials Research, 121-122*, 222-227. Retrieved from www.scientific.net/amr.121-122.222

Feng, W., Li, Y., Gao, S., Yan, Y., & Xue, J. (2016). A Novel Flame Edge Detection Algorithm via A Novel Active Contour Model. *International Journal Of Hybrid Information Technology*, *9*(9), 275–282. doi:10.14257/ijhit.2016.9.9.26

Ferguson, R. D., Hammer, D. X., Paunescu, L. A., Beaton, S., & Schuman, J. S. (2004). Tracking optical coherence tomography. *Optics Letters*, *29*(18), 2139–2141. doi:10.1364/OL.29.002139 PMID:15460882

Fernández, D. C., Villate, N., Puliafito, C. A., & Rosenfeld, P. J. (2004). Comparing total macular volume changes measured by optical coherence tomography with retinal lesion volume estimated by active contours. *Investigative Ophthalmology & Visual Science*, *45*(13), 3072–3072.

Fidele, B., Cheeneebash, J., Gopaul, A., & Goorah, S. S. (2009). Artificial neural network as a clinical decision-supporting tool to predict cardiovascular disease. *Trends in Applied Sciences Research*, *4*(1), 36–46. doi:10.3923/tasr.2009.36.46

Fisher, Y. (2012). *Fractal image compression: theory and application.* Springer Science & Business Media.

Fonseca-Delgado, R., & Gomez-Gil, P. (2013, September). An assessment of ten-fold and Monte Carlo cross validations for time series forecasting. In *Electrical Engineering, Computing Science and Automatic Control (CCE), 2013 10th International Conference on* (pp. 215-220). IEEE.

Forouzanfar, M., & Moghaddam, H. A. (2007, April). A directional multiscale approach for speckle reduction in optical coherence tomography images. In *International Conference on Electrical Engineering, 2007. ICEE'07.* (pp. 1-6). IEEE.

Forouzanfar, M., Moghaddam, H. A., & Dehghani, M. (2007, June). Speckle reduction in medical ultrasound images using a new multiscale bivariate Bayesian MMSE-based method. In Signal Processing and Communications Applications, 2007. SIU 2007. IEEE 15th (pp. 1-4). IEEE.

Forouzanfar, M., Moghaddam, H. A., & Gity, M. (2010). A new multiscale Bayesian algorithm for speckle reduction in medical ultrasound images. *Signal, Image and Video Processing*, *4*(3), 359–375. doi:10.100711760-009-0126-3

Franc, V., & Hlavác, V. (2002). Multi-class support vector machine. In *International Conference on Pattern Recognition* (Vol. 2, pp. 236-239). IEEE. 10.1109/ICPR.2002.1048282

Frazier, O. (1994). First use of an untethered, vented electric left ventricular assist device for long-term support. *Circulation*, *89*(6), 2908–2914. doi:10.1161/01.CIR.89.6.2908 PMID:8205707

Freitas, A. A., & Lavington, S. H. (1997). *Mining very large databases with parallel processing* (Vol. 9). Springer Science & Business Media.

Fritz, A., Percy, C., Jack, A., Shanmugaratnam, K., Sobin, L., Parkin, D. M., & Whelan, S. (2013). *WHO International Classification of Diseases for Oncology* (3rd ed.). ICD-O. Retrieved from www.who.int/classifications/icd/adaptations/oncology/

Frost, V. S., Stiles, J. A., Shanmugan, K. S., & Holtzman, J. C. (1982). A model for radar images and its application to adaptive digital filtering of multiplicative noise. *IEEE Transactions on Pattern Analysis and Machine Intelligence*, *PAMI-4*(2), 157–166. doi:10.1109/TPAMI.1982.4767223 PMID:21869022

Fujimoto, J., & Drexler, W. (2008). Introduction to optical coherence tomography. In *Optical coherence tomography* (pp. 1–45). Berlin: Springer. doi:10.1007/978-3-540-77550-8_1

Fukushima, K. (2013). Artificial vision by multi-layered neural networks: Neocognitron and its advances. *Neural Networks*, *37*, 103–119. doi:10.1016/j.neunet.2012.09.016 PMID:23098752

Fuller, A., Zawadzki, R., Choi, S., Wiley, D., Werner, J., & Hamann, B. (2007). Segmentation of three-dimensional retinal image data. *IEEE Transactions on Visualization and Computer Graphics*, *13*(6), 1719–1726. doi:10.1109/TVCG.2007.70590 PMID:17968130

Fu, X., Wang, Y., Chen, L., & Tian, J. (2015). An image despeckling approach using quantum-inspired statistics in dual-tree complex wavelet domain. *Biomedical Signal Processing and Control*, *18*, 30–35. doi:10.1016/j.bspc.2014.11.005

Gai, S., Zhang, B., Yang, C., & Yu, L. (2018). Speckle noise reduction in medical ultrasound image using monogenic wavelet and Laplace mixture distribution. *Digital Signal Processing*, *72*, 192–207. doi:10.1016/j.dsp.2017.10.006

Gallis, C. (2006). Work-related prevalence of musculoskeletal symptoms among Greek forest workers. *International Journal of Industrial Ergonomics*, *36*(8), 731–736. doi:10.1016/j.ergon.2006.05.007

Ganasala, P., & Kumar, V. (2015). Feature-Motivated Simplified Adaptive PCNN-Based Medical Image Fusion Algorithm in NSST Domain. *Journal of Digital Imaging*. PMID:26032980

Gangopadhyay, S., Das, B., Das, T., Ghoshal, G., & Ghosh, T. (2010). An Ergonomics Study on Posture-Related Discomfort and Occupational-Related Disorders Among Stonecutters of West Bengal, India. *International Journal of Occupational Safety and Ergonomics*, *16*(1), 69–79. doi:10.1080/10803548.2010.11076830 PMID:20331920

Gao, X. Z., Wang, J., Tanskanen, J. M. A., Bie, R., & Guo, P. (2012). BP neural networks with harmony search method-based training for epileptic EEG signal classification. In *Computational Intelligence and Security (CIS), 2012 Eighth International Conference on*. IEEE.

Gao, Y., Kikinis, R., Bouix, S., Shenton, M., & Tannenbaum, A. (2012). A 3D interactive multi-object segmentation tool using local robust statistics driven active contours. *Medical Image Analysis*, *16*(6), 1216–1227. doi:10.1016/j.media.2012.06.002 PMID:22831773

García, N., Ortiz, D., & Martínez, C. (2006). An alternative approach for neural network evolution with a genetic algorithm: Crossover by combinatorial optimization. *Neural Networks*, *19*(4), 514–528. doi:10.1016/j.neunet.2005.08.014 PMID:16343847

Garg, A. X., Adhikari, N. K., McDonald, H., Rosas-Arellano, M. P., Devereaux, P. J., Beyene, J., & Haynes, R. B. (2005). Effects of computerized clinical decision support systems on practitioner performance and patient outcomes: A systematic review. *Journal of the American Medical Association*, *293*(10), 1223–1238. doi:10.1001/jama.293.10.1223 PMID:15755945

Gargesha, M., Jenkins, M. W., Rollins, A. M., & Wilson, D. L. (2008). Denoising and 4D visualization of OCT images. *Optics Express*, *16*(16), 12313–12333. doi:10.1364/OE.16.012313 PMID:18679509

Garvin, M. K., Abràmoff, M. D., Kardon, R., Russell, S. R., Wu, X., & Sonka, M. (2008). Intraretinal layer segmentation of macular optical coherence tomography images using optimal 3-D graph search. *IEEE Transactions on Medical Imaging*, *27*(10), 1495–1505. doi:10.1109/TMI.2008.923966 PMID:18815101

Gaurav Bhatnagar, Q. M. (2015). A new contrast based multimodal medical image fusion framework, *Elsevier. Neurocomputing*, *157*, 143–152. doi:10.1016/j.neucom.2015.01.025

Ge, D., Srinivasan, N., & Krishnan, S. M. (2002). Cardiac arrhythmia classification using autoregressive modeling. *Biomedical Engineering Online*, *1*(1), 5. doi:10.1186/1475-925X-1-5 PMID:12473180

Gehrke, J., Ramakrishnan, R., & Ganti, V. (1998). *RainForest-A framework for fast decision tree construction of large datasets*. Paper presented at the VLDB.

Geman, O., & Chiuchisan, I. (2015). A health care self-monitoring system for patients with visual impairment using a network of sensors. In E-Health and Bioengineering Conference (EHB), 2015 (pp. 1-4). IEEE.

George, A., Dilienseger, J. L., Weber, M., & Pechereau, A. (2000, March). Optical coherence tomography image processing. In Investigative Ophthalmology & Visual Science (Vol. 41, No. 4, pp. S173-S173). Assoc Research Vision Ophthalmology Inc.

Ghaffari, A., Golbayani, H., & Ghasemi, M. (2008). A new mathematical based QRS detector using continuous wavelet transform. Computers and Electrical Engineering, 34, 81–91.

Ghosal, G., Darbar, R., Neogi, B., Das, A., & Tibarewala, D. N. (2012). Application of swarm intelligence computation techniques in pid controller tuning: A review. In *Proceedings of the International Conference on Information Systems Design and Intelligent Applications 2012 (INDIA 2012)*. Springer.

Girish, G. N., Kothari, A. R., & Rajan, J. (2017). Marker controlled watershed transform for intra-retinal cysts segmentation from optical coherence tomography b-scans. Pattern Recognition Letters. ISSN 0167-8655, https://doi.org/10.1016/j.patrec.2017.12.019

Girish, G. N., Anima, V. A., Kothari, A. R., Sudeep, P. V., Roychowdhury, S., & Rajan, J. (2018a). A benchmark study of automated intra-retinal cyst segmentation algorithms using optical coherence tomography B-scans. *Computer Methods and Programs in Biomedicine*, *153*, 105–114. doi:10.1016/j.cmpb.2017.10.010 PMID:29157443

Girish, G. N., Thakur, B., Chowdhury, S. R., Kothari, A. R., & Rajan, J. (2018 b). Segmentation of Intra-Retinal Cysts from Optical Coherence Tomography Images using a Fully Convolutional Neural Network Model. *IEEE Journal of Biomedical and Health Informatics*, 1. doi:10.1109/JBHI.2018.2810379 PMID:29994161

Gletsos, M., Mougiakakou, S. G., Matsopoulos, G. K., Nikita, K. S., Nikita, A. S., & Kelekis, D. (2003). A Computer-Aided Diagnostic System to Characterize CT Focal Liver Lesions: Design and Optimization of a Neural Network Classifier. *IEEE Transactions on Information Technology in Biomedicine*, *7*(3), 153–162. doi:10.1109/TITB.2003.813793 PMID:14518728

Global health aging report of the elderly population. (n.d.). Available at http://www.who.int/ageing/publications/global_health.pdf

Global health aging report of the total population. (n.d.). Available at http://www.who.int/ageing/publications/global_health.pdf

Gokulnath, C. B., & Shantharajah, S. P. (2018). An optimized feature selection based on genetic approach and support vector machine for heart disease. *Cluster Computing*, 1–11.

Goletsis, Y., Papaloukas, C., Fotiadis, D. I., Likas, A., & Michalis, L. (2004). Automated ischemic beat classification using genetic algorithm and multicriteria decision analysis. *IEEE Transactions on Biomedical Engineering*, *51*(10), 1717–1725. doi:10.1109/TBME.2004.828033 PMID:15490819

Gomathi, P. S., & Kalaavathi, B. (2016). Multimodal Medical Image Fusion in Non-Subsampled Contourlet Transform Domain" Scientific Research Publishing. *Circuits and Systems*, *7*(8), 1598–1610. doi:10.4236/cs.2016.78139

Goodman, J. W. (1975). Statistical properties of laser speckle patterns. In *Laser speckle and related phenomena* (pp. 9–75). Berlin: Springer.

Götzinger, E., Pircher, M., & Hitzenberger, C. K. (2005). High speed spectral domain polarization sensitive optical coherence tomography of the human retina. *Optics Express*, *13*(25), 10217–10229. doi:10.1364/OPEX.13.010217 PMID:19503236

Gregori, G., & Knighton, R. W. (2004). A robust algorithm for retinal thickness measurements using optical coherence tomography (Stratus OCT). *Investigative Ophthalmology & Visual Science*, *45*(13), 3007–3007.

Gregory, H., & Nejhdeh, G. (1998). A self-organizing estimator for hypoglycaemia monitoring in diabetic patients. *20th annual international conference of IEEE engineering in medicine and biology society, 20*(3), 23-29.

Gregory, R. L. (2015). *Eye and brain: The psychology of seeing*. Princeton University Press.

Guendouzi, F., & Attari, M. (2013). Polynomial modeling of the ECG signals. *IEEE 2013 International Conference on Computer Medical Applications (ICCMA)*, 1–5. 10.1109/ICCMA.2013.6506177

Guenther, D. A., & Walker, W. F. (2007). Optimal apodization design for medical ultrasound using constrained least squares part I: Theory. *IEEE Transactions on Ultrasonics, Ferroelectrics, and Frequency Control*, *54*(2). PMID:17328330

Guillonneau, X., Eandi, C. M., Paques, M., Sahel, J. A., Sapieha, P., & Sennlaub, F. (2017). On phagocytes and macular degeneration. *Progress in Retinal and Eye Research*, *61*, 98–128. doi:10.1016/j.preteyeres.2017.06.002 PMID:28602950

Gungor, M. A., & Karagoz, I. (2015). The homogeneity map method for speckle reduction in diagnostic ultrasound images. *Measurement*, *68*, 100–110. doi:10.1016/j.measurement.2015.02.047

Guo, K., Candra, H., Yu, H., Li, H., Hung, T., & Su, S. W. (2017). EEG-based emotion classification using innovative features and combined SVM and HMM classifier. In *Engineering in Medicine and Biology Society (EMBC), 2017 39th Annual International Conference of the IEEE*. IEEE.

Gupta, V., Chan, C. C., Poh, C. L., Chow, T. H., Meng, T. C., & Koon, N. B. (2008, May). Computerized automation of wavelet based denoising method to reduce speckle noise in OCT images. In *International Conference on Information Technology and Applications in Biomedicine, 2008* (pp. 120-123). IEEE.

Gupta, D., Anand, R. S., & Tyagi, B. (2015). Despeckling of ultrasound medical images using ripplet domain nonlinear filtering. *Signal, Image and Video Processing*, *9*(5), 1093–1111. doi:10.100711760-013-0540-4

Gupta, G. (2013). Prevalence of Musculoskeletal Disorders in Farmers of Kanpur Rural, India. *Journal of Community Medicine & Health Education*, *3*(07), 249. doi:10.4172/2161-0711.1000249

Gupta, M. P. (2016). *Retinal anatomy and pathology. In Retinal Pharmacotherapeutics* (Vol. 55, pp. 7–17). Karger Publishers. doi:10.1159/000431128

Gupta, S., Chauhan, R. C., & Saxena, S. C. (2005). Locally adaptive wavelet domain Bayesian processor for denoising medical ultrasound images using Speckle modelling based on Rayleigh distribution. *IEE Proceedings. Vision Image and Signal Processing*, *152*(1), 129–135. doi:10.1049/ip-vis:20050975

Gupta, S., Chauhan, R. C., & Sexana, S. C. (2004). Wavelet-based statistical approach for speckle reduction in medical ultrasound images. *Medical & Biological Engineering & Computing*, *42*(2), 189–192. doi:10.1007/BF02344630 PMID:15125148

Gutiérrez-Gnecchi, J. A., Morfin-Magana, R., Lorias-Espinoza, D., del Carmen Tellez-Anguiano, A., Reyes-Archundia, E., Méndez-Patiño, A., & Castañeda-Miranda, R. (2017). DSP-based arrhythmia classification using wavelet transform and probabilistic neural network. *Biomedical Signal Processing and Control*, *32*, 44–56. doi:10.1016/j.bspc.2016.10.005

Hadhoud, M. M., Eladawy, M. I., & Farag, A. (2006, November). Computer aided diagnosis of cardiac arrhythmias. In *International Conference on Computer Engineering and Systems*, (pp. 262-265). IEEE.

Haider, S. (2008). *U.S. Patent Application 12/192,216*. U.S. Patent and Trademark Office.

Hai-Ying, Z., & Kun-Mean, H. (2008). Embedded Real-Time QRS Detection Algorithm for Pervasive Cardiac Care System. *ICSP2008 Proceedings*, 2150- 2153.

Hall, M., Frank, E., Holmes, G., Pfahringer, B., Reutemann, P., & Witten, I. H. (2009). The WEKA data mining software: an update. *ACM SIGKDD Explorations Newsletter*, *11*(1), 10-18.

Hamida, S. T. B., Ahmed, B., & Penzel, T. (2015, December). A novel insomnia identification method based on Hjorth parameters. In *Signal Processing and Information Technology (ISSPIT), 2015 IEEE International Symposium on* (pp. 548-552). IEEE.

Hamilton, P. S., & Tompkins, W. J. (1986). Quantitative Investigation of QRS Detection Rules Using the MIT/BIH Arrhythmia Database. *IEEE Transactions on Biomedical Engineering*, *BME-33*(12), 1157–1165. doi:10.1109/TBME.1986.325695 PMID:3817849

Hand, D. (2009). Measuring classifier performance: A coherent alternative to the area under the ROC curve. *Machine Learning*, *77*(1), 103–123. doi:10.100710994-009-5119-5

Han, J., Pei, J., & Kamber, M. (2011). *Data mining: concepts and techniques*. Elsevier.

Harper, P. R. (2005). A review and comparison of classification algorithms for medical decision making. *Health Policy (Amsterdam)*, *71*(3), 315–331. doi:10.1016/j.healthpol.2004.05.002 PMID:15694499

Hartman, E., Oude Vrielink, H. H. E., Metz, J. H. M., & Huirne, R. B. M. (2005). Exposure to physical risk factors in Dutch agriculture: Effect on sick leave due to musculoskeletal disorders. *International Journal of Industrial Ergonomics*, *35*(11), 1031–1045. doi:10.1016/j.ergon.2005.04.006

Harvard Medical School. (n.d.). Retrieved from http://www.med.harvard.edu

Hee, M. R., Izatt, J. A., Swanson, E. A., Huang, D., Schuman, J. S., Lin, C. P., ... Fujimoto, J. G. (1995). Optical coherence tomography of the human retina. *Archives of Ophthalmology*, *113*(3), 325–332. doi:10.1001/archopht.1995.01100030081025 PMID:7887846

Herzog, A., Boyer, K. L., & Roberts, C. (2004). Robust extraction of the optic nerve head in optical coherence tomography. In *Computer Vision and Mathematical Methods in Medical and Biomedical Image Analysis* (pp. 395–407). Berlin: Springer. doi:10.1007/978-3-540-27816-0_34

Hewitt, A. J. (1997). The Importance of Droplet Size in Agricultural Spraying. *Atomization and Sprays*, *7*(3), 235–244. doi:10.1615/AtomizSpr.v7.i3.10

Hewitt, A. J. (2008). Article. *The Environmentalist*, *28*(25). doi:10.100710669-007-9044-5

Hii, P. C., & Chung, W. Y. (2011). A comprehensive ubiquitous healthcare solution on an Android™ mobile device. *Sensors (Basel)*, *11*(7), 6799–6815. doi:10.3390110706799 PMID:22163986

Hiremath, P. S., Akkasaligar, P. T., & Badiger, S. (2010). Speckle reducing contourlet transform for medical ultrasound images. *Int J Compt Inf Engg*, *4*(4), 284–291.

Hochreiter, S., Bengio, Y., Frasconi, P., & Schmidhuber, J. (2001). Gradient flow in recurrent nets: the difficulty of learning long-term dependencies. In S. C. Kremer & J. F. Kolen (Eds.), *A Field Guide to Dynamical Recurrent Neural Networks*. IEEE Press.

Hoogendoorn, W. E., van Poppel, M. N., Bongers, P. M., Koes, B. W., & Bouter, L. M. (1999). Physical load during work and leisure time as risk factors for back pain. *Scandinavian Journal of Work, Environment & Health*, *25*(5), 387–403. doi:10.5271jweh.451 PMID:10569458

Ho, T. K. (1998). The random subspace method for constructing decision forests. *IEEE Transactions on Pattern Analysis and Machine Intelligence*, *20*(8), 832–844. doi:10.1109/34.709601

Hu, F., Qiao, Y., Xie, G., Zhu, Y., Jia, Y., & Huang, P. (2017, October). Symptom Distribution Regulation of Core Symptoms in Insomnia Based on Informap-SA Algorithm. In *Distributed Computing and Applications to Business, Engineering and Science (DCABES), 2017 16th International Symposium on* (pp. 229-232). IEEE.

Huang, D., Swanson, E. A., Lin, C. P., Schuman, J. S., Stinson, W. G., Chang, W., ... & Puliafito, C. A. (1991). Optical coherence tomography. *Science, 254*(5035), 1178-1181.

Huang, G., & Pun, C. (2015). Robust Interactive Segmentation Using Color Histogram and Contourlet Transform. *International Journal Of Computer Theory And Engineering*, *7*(6), 489–494. doi:10.7763/IJCTE.2015.V7.1007

Huang, K., Yang, H., King, I., Lyu, M. R., & Chan, L. (2004). The Minimum Error Minimax Probability Machine. *Journal of Machine Learning Research*, *5*, 1253–1286.

Hughes, M., Spring, M., & Podoleanu, A. (2010). Speckle noise reduction in optical coherence tomography of paint layers. *Applied Optics*, *49*(1), 99–107. doi:10.1364/AO.49.000099 PMID:20062495

Huikuri, H. V., Castellanos, A., & Myerburg, R. J. (2001). Sudden death due to cardiac arrhythmias. *The New England Journal of Medicine*, *345*(20), 1473–1482. doi:10.1056/NEJMra000650 PMID:11794197

Hüllermeier, E. (2011). Fuzzy sets in machine learning and data mining. *Applied Soft Computing*, *11*(2), 1493–1505. doi:10.1016/j.asoc.2008.01.004

Human Heart Diagram. (n.d.). Retrieved May 21, 2018, from Dreamstime: https://www.dreamstime.com/stock-illustration-human-heart-diagram-illustration-image55185229

Idowu, P. A., Adedoyin, R. A., & Adagunodo, R. E. (2005). Computer-related repetitive strain injuries. *J Nig Soc Physiother*, *15*, 13–15.

Iftimia, N., Bouma, B. E., & Tearney, G. J. (2003). Speckle reduction in optical coherence tomography by. *Journal of Biomedical Optics*, *8*(2), 260–264. doi:10.1117/1.1559060 PMID:12683852

Isar, C. S. C. A. (n.d.). Optical Coherence Tomography Speckle Reduction in the Wavelets Domain. *Editorial Board*, 3.

Ishikawa, H., Stein, D. M., Wollstein, G., Beaton, S., Fujimoto, J. G., & Schuman, J. S. (2005). Macular segmentation with optical coherence tomography. *Investigative Ophthalmology & Visual Science*, *46*(6), 2012–2017. doi:10.1167/iovs.04-0335 PMID:15914617

Islam, M., & Murase, K. (2001). A new algorithm to design compact two-hidden-layer artificial neural networks. *Neural Networks*, *14*(9), 1265–1278. doi:10.1016/S0893-6080(01)00075-2 PMID:11718425

Isler, Y., & Kantalp, M. (2007). Combining classical HRV indices with wavelet entropy measures improves to performance in diagnosing congestive heart failure. *Computers in Biology and Medicine*, *37*(10), 1502–1510. doi:10.1016/j.compbiomed.2007.01.012 PMID:17359959

Izham, M., Fukui, T., & Morinishi, K. (2014). Simulation of three-dimensional homogeneous isotropic turbulence using the moment-based lattice Boltzmann method and LES-lattice Boltzmann method. *Journal of Fluid Science and Technology*, *9*(4). doi:10.1299/jfst.2014jfst0064

J. Ross Quinlan. (1993). *C4.5: Programs for Machine Learning*. San Francisco, CA: Morgan Kaufmann Publishers Inc.

Jakob, M., & Liebers, F. (2009). Body posture variation during machine milking regarding weight of milking unit and working height—experimental study. *Bornimer Agrartechnische Berichte*, *66*, 31–37.

Janssen, I., Bacon, E., & Pickett, W. (2011). Obesity and Its Relationship with Occupational Injury in the Canadian Workforce. *Journal of Obesity*, *531403*. doi:10.1155/2011/531403 PMID:21773008

Jarad, A., Katkar, R., Shaikh, A. R., & Salve, A. (2015). Intelligent Heart Disease Prediction System With MongoDB. *Future, 13*, 14.

Jáuregui, D. A. G., Castanier, C., Chang, B., Val, M., Cottin, F., Le Scanff, C., & Martin, J. C. (2017, October). Toward automatic detection of acute stress: Relevant nonverbal behaviors and impact of personality traits. In *Affective Computing and Intelligent Interaction (ACII), 2017 Seventh International Conference on* (pp. 354-361). IEEE.

Jensen, P. N., Gronroos, N. N., Chen, L. Y., Folsom, A. R., Heckbert, S. R., & Alonso, A. (2014). Incidence of and risk factors for sick sinus syndrome in the general population. *Journal of the American College of Cardiology, 64*(6), 531–538. doi:10.1016/j.jacc.2014.03.056 PMID:25104519

Jespersen, S. K., Wilhjelm, J. E., & Sillesen, H. (1998). Multi-angle compound imaging. *Ultrasonic Imaging, 20*(2), 81–102. doi:10.1177/016173469802000201 PMID:9691367

Jha, C. K., & Kolekar, M. H. (2015, December). Performance analysis of ECG data compression using wavelet based hybrid transform method. In *International Conference on Microwave, Optical and Communication Engineering (IC-MOCE)* (pp. 138-141). IEEE. 10.1109/ICMOCE.2015.7489709

Jha, C. K., & Kolekar, M. H. (2016, January). Efficient ECG data compression and transmission algorithm for telemedicine. In *International Conference on Communication Systems and Networks (COMSNETS)* (pp. 1-6). IEEE. 10.1109/COMSNETS.2016.7439988

Jha, C. K., & Kolekar, M. H. (2017). ECG data compression algorithm for tele-monitoring of cardiac patients. *International Journal of Telemedicine and Clinical Practices, 2*(1), 31–41. doi:10.1504/IJTMCP.2017.082106

Jha, C. K., & Kolekar, M. H. (2018). Classification and Compression of ECG Signal for Holter Device. In *Biomedical Signal and Image Processing in Patient Care* (pp. 46–63). IGI Global. doi:10.4018/978-1-5225-2829-6.ch004

Jha, C. K., & Kolekar, M. H. (2018). Electrocardiogram data compression using DCT based discrete orthogonal Stockwell transform. *Biomedical Signal Processing and Control, 46*, 174–181. doi:10.1016/j.bspc.2018.06.009

Jiang, H., Feng, R., & Gao, X. (2011). Level set based on signed pressure force function and its application in liver image segmentation. *Wuhan University Journal of Natural Sciences, 16*(3), 265–270. doi:10.100711859-011-0748-5

Jian, Z., Yu, L., Rao, B., Tromberg, B. J., & Chen, Z. (2010). Three-dimensional speckle suppression in optical coherence tomography based on the curvelet transform. *Optics Express, 18*(2), 1024–1032. doi:10.1364/OE.18.001024 PMID:20173923

Jian, Z., Yu, Z., Yu, L., Rao, B., Chen, Z., & Tromberg, B. J. (2009). Speckle attenuation in optical coherence tomography by curvelet shrinkage. *Optics Letters, 34*(10), 1516–1518. doi:10.1364/OL.34.001516 PMID:19448806

Jilani, T. A., Yasin, H., Yasin, M., & Ardil, C. (2009). Acute coronary syndrome prediction using data mining techniques-an application. *World Academy of Science, Engineering and Technology, 59*(4), 295–299.

Joachims, T. (1998). *Text categorization with support vector machines: Learning with many relevant features.* Paper presented at the European conference on machine learning. 10.1007/BFb0026683

John, G. H., & Langley, P. (1995). Estimating continuous distributions in Bayesian classifiers. *Proceedings of the Eleventh conference on Uncertainty in artificial intelligence.*

Jokic, S., Delic, V., Peric, Z., Krco, S., & Sakac, D. (2011). Efficient ECG modeling using polynomial functions. *Elektronika ir Elektrotechnika, 110*(4), 121–124. doi:10.5755/j01.eee.110.4.304

Jones, J., Xie, X., & Essa, E. (2014). Combining region-based and imprecise boundary-based cues for interactive medical image segmentation. *International Journal for Numerical Methods in Biomedical Engineering*, *30*(12), 1649–1666. doi:10.1002/cnm.2693 PMID:25377853

Jørgensen, T. M., Thomadsen, J., Christensen, U., Soliman, W., & Sander, B. A. (2007). Enhancing the signal-to-noise ratio in ophthalmic optical coherence tomography by image registration—method and clinical examples. *Journal of Biomedical Optics*, *12*(4), 041208. doi:10.1117/1.2772879 PMID:17867797

Jothi, R., Kayalvizhi, M., & Sagadevan, K. (2017). Smart walking stick for visually challenged people. *Asian J. Appl. Sci. Technol*, *1*, 274–276.

Juneja, P., & Kashyap, R. (2016). Optimal approach for CT image segmentation using improved energy based method. *International Journal of Control Theory and Applications*, *9*(41), 599–608.

Juul-Kristensen, B., & Jensen, C. (2005). Self-reported workplace related ergonomic conditions as prognostic factors for musculoskeletal symptoms: The "BIT" follow up study on office workers. *Occupational and Environmental Medicine*, *62*(3), 188–194. doi:10.1136/oem.2004.013920 PMID:15723884

Kabir-Mokamelkhah, E. (2015). Rice Farming and Musculoskeletal Disorders. *Iranian Journal of Health, Safety and Environment*, *3*(1S), 489–494.

Kachroo, S., Melek, W. W., & Kurian, C. (2013). *Evaluation of predictive learners for cancer incidence and mortality.* Paper presented at the E-Health and Bioengineering Conference (EHB). 10.1109/EHB.2013.6707388

Kafieh, R., Rabbani, H., Abramoff, M. D., & Sonka, M. (2013). Curvature correction of retinal OCTs using graph-based geometry detection. *Physics in Medicine and Biology*, *58*(9), 2925–2938. doi:10.1088/0031-9155/58/9/2925 PMID:23574790

Kafieh, R., Rabbani, H., & Selesnick, I. (2015). Three dimensional data-driven multi scale atomic representation of optical coherence tomography. *IEEE Transactions on Medical Imaging*, *34*(5), 1042–1062. doi:10.1109/TMI.2014.2374354 PMID:25934998

Kaiser, H. F. (1960). The application of electronic computers to factor analysis. *Educational and Psychological Measurement*, *20*(1), 141–151. doi:10.1177/001316446002000116

Kajić, V., Esmaeelpour, M., Považay, B., Marshall, D., Rosin, P. L., & Drexler, W. (2012). Automated choroidal segmentation of 1060 nm OCT in healthy and pathologic eyes using a statistical model. *Biomedical Optics Express*, *3*(1), 86–103. doi:10.1364/BOE.3.000086 PMID:22254171

Kajić, V., Považay, B., Hermann, B., Hofer, B., Marshall, D., Rosin, P. L., & Drexler, W. (2010). Robust segmentation of intraretinal layers in the normal human fovea using a novel statistical model based on texture and shape analysis. *Optics Express*, *18*(14), 14730–14744. doi:10.1364/OE.18.014730 PMID:20639959

Kaka, Idowu, Fawole, Adeniyi, Ogwumike, & Toryila. (2016). WRMSDs among Butchers in Kano Metropolis. *Safety and Health at Work*, *7*, 218–224. doi:10.1016/j.shaw.2016.01.001 PMID:27630791

Kakria, P., Tripathi, N. K., & Kitipawang, P. (2015). A real-time health monitoring system for remote cardiac patients using smartphone and wearable sensors. *International Journal of Telemedicine and Applications*, *2015*, 8. doi:10.1155/2015/373474 PMID:26788055

Kang, H., Kim, B., Lee, J., Shin, J., & Shin, Y. (2014). Automatic left and right heart segmentation using power watershed and active contour model without edge. *Biomedical Engineering Letters*, *4*(4), 355–361. doi:10.100713534-014-0164-9

Karahan, A., Kar, S., Abbasogbu, A., & Dodan, N. (2009). Low back pain: Prevalence and associated factors among hospital staff. *Journal of Advanced Nursing*, *65*(3), 516–524. doi:10.1111/j.1365-2648.2008.04905.x PMID:19222649

Karamata, B., Hassler, K., Laubscher, M., & Lasser, T. (2005). Speckle statistics in optical coherence tomography. *JOSA A*, *22*(4), 593–596. doi:10.1364/JOSAA.22.000593 PMID:15839265

Karaolis, M. A., Moutiris, J. A., Hadjipanayi, D., & Pattichis, C. P. (2010). Assessment of the Risk Factors of Coronary Heart Events Based on Data Mining With Decision Trees. *IEEE Transactions on Information Technology in Biomedicine*, *14*(3), 559–566. doi:10.1109/TITB.2009.2038906 PMID:20071264

Karthikeyan, C., & Ramadoss, B. (2016). Comparative Analysis of Similarity Measure Performance for Multimodality Image Fusion using DTCWT and SOFM with Various Medical Image Fusion Techniques. *Indian Journal of Science and Technology*, *9*(22). doi:10.17485/ijst/2016/v9i22/95298

Kashyap, R., & Piersson, A. (2018b). Big Data Challenges and Solutions in the Medical Industries. In Handbook of Research on Pattern Engineering System Development for Big Data Analytics. IGI Global. doi:10.4018/978-1-5225-3870-7.ch001

Kashyap, R., Gautam, P., & Tiwari, V. (2018). Management and Monitoring Patterns and Future Scope. In Handbook of Research on Pattern Engineering System Development for Big Data Analytics. IGI Global. doi:10.4018/978-1-5225-3870-7.ch014

Kashyap, R., & Gautam, P. (2015). Modified region based segmentation of medical images. *International Conference on Communication Networks (ICCN)*, 209–216. 10.1109/ICCN.2015.41

Kashyap, R., & Gautam, P. (2017). 'Fast Medical Image Segmentation Using Energy-Based Method', Biometrics. *Concepts, Methodologies, Tools, and Applications*, *3*(1), 1017–1042. doi:10.4018/978-1-5225-0983-7.ch040

Kashyap, R., & Piersson, A. (2018a). *Impact of Big Data on Security. In Handbook of Research on Network Forensics and Analysis Techniques* (pp. 283–299). IGI Global. doi:10.4018/978-1-5225-4100-4.ch015

Kashyap, R., & Tiwari, V. (2018). Active contours using global models for medical image segmentation. *International Journal of Computational Systems Engineering*, *4*(2/3), 195. doi:10.1504/IJCSYSE.2018.091404

Kasper, J. F., Mulley, J. A. Jr, & Wennberg, J. E. (1992). Developing shared decision-making programs to improve the quality of health care. *QRB. Quality Review Bulletin*, *18*(6), 183–190. doi:10.1016/S0097-5990(16)30531-0 PMID:1379705

Kaur, R., Albano, P. P., Cole, J. G., Hagerty, J., LeAnder, R. W., Moss, R. H., & Stoecker, W. V. (2015). Real-time supervised detection of pink areas in dermoscopic images of melanoma: Importance of color shades, texture and location. *Skin Research and Technology*, *21*(4), 466–473. doi:10.1111rt.12216 PMID:25809473

Kavitha, C. T., & Chellamuthu, C. (2014). Medical image fusion based on hybrid intelligence, *Elsevier. Applied Soft Computing*, *20*, 83–94. doi:10.1016/j.asoc.2013.10.034

Kavitha, C. T., & Chellamuthu, C. (2015). Fusion of SPECT and MRI images using integer wavelet transform in combination with curvelet transform. *Imaging Science Journal*, *63*(1), 17–23. doi:10.1179/1743131X14Y.0000000092

Keller, K. B., & Lemberg, L. (2006). The sick sinus syndrome. *American Journal of Critical Care*, *15*(2), 226–229. PMID:16501143

Keller, K. B., & Lemberg, L. (2007). Iatrogenic sick sinus syndrome. *American Journal of Critical Care*, *16*(3), 294–297. PMID:17460324

Kennedy, B. F., Hillman, T. R., Curatolo, A., & Sampson, D. D. (2010). Speckle reduction in optical coherence tomography by strain compounding. *Optics Letters*, *35*(14), 2445–2447. doi:10.1364/OL.35.002445 PMID:20634858

Ker, J., Wang, L., Rao, J., & Lim, T. (2018). Deep learning applications in medical image analysis. *IEEE Access: Practical Innovations, Open Solutions*, *6*, 9375–9389. doi:10.1109/ACCESS.2017.2788044

Khaing, T. T., & Aimmanee, P. (2017, May). Optic disk segmentation in retinal images using active contour model based on extended feature projection. In *2017 8th International Conference of Information and Communication Technology for Embedded Systems (IC-ICTES)* (pp. 1-6). IEEE.

Khalaf, A. F., Owis, M. I., & Yassine, I. A. (2015). A novel technique for cardiac arrhythmia classification using spectral correlation and support vector machines. *Expert Systems with Applications*, *42*(21), 8361–8368. doi:10.1016/j.eswa.2015.06.046

Khaled, E., Osama, B., & Tim, R. (2002). Predicting blood glucose levels in diabetes using feature extraction and artificial neural networks. *International Conference on Information and Communication Technologies*, 18-27.

Khan, M. N. H., Arovi, M. A. H., Mahmud, H., Hasan, M. K., & Rubaiyeat, H. A. (2015). Speech based text correction tool for the visually impaired. In *Computer and Information Technology (ICCIT), 2015 18th International Conference on* (pp. 150-155). IEEE.

Khare, A., Khare, M., Jeong, Y., Kim, H., & Jeon, M. (2010). Despeckling of medical ultrasound images using Daubechies complex wavelet transform. *Signal Processing*, *90*(2), 428–439. doi:10.1016/j.sigpro.2009.07.008

Khatibi, V., & Montazer, G. A. (2010). A fuzzy-evidential hybrid inference engine for coronary heart disease risk assessment. *Expert Systems with Applications*, *37*(12), 8536–8542. doi:10.1016/j.eswa.2010.05.022

Khemmarat, S., & Gao, L. (2015). Supporting drug prescription via predictive and personalized query system. In *Pervasive Computing Technologies for Healthcare (PervasiveHealth), 2015 9th International Conference on* (pp. 9-16). IEEE.

Kinsella, K., & He, W. (2009). *An aging world: 2008: International population reports*. US Government Printing Office.

Kishore, P. V. V., Kumar, K. V. V., Prasad, M. V. D., Goutham, E. N. D., Rahul, R., Krishna, C. V., & Sandeep, Y. (2015). Twofold processing for denoising ultrasound medical images. *SpringerPlus*, *4*(1), 775. doi:10.118640064-015-1566-6 PMID:26697285

Kleiger, R. E., Miller, J. P., Bigger, J. T. Jr, & Moss, A. J. (1987). Decreased heart rate variability and its association with increased mortality after acute myocardial infarction. *The American Journal of Cardiology*, *59*(4), 256–262. doi:10.1016/0002-9149(87)90795-8 PMID:3812275

Kolekar, M. H., & Dash, D. P. (2015). A nonlinear feature based epileptic seizure detection using least square support vector machine classifier. In IEEE Region 10 Conference TENCON (pp. 1-6). IEEE.

Kolekar, M. H. (2011). Bayesian belief network based broadcast sports video indexing. *Multimedia Tools and Applications*, *54*(1), 27–54. doi:10.100711042-010-0544-9

Kolekar, M. H., & Sengupta, S. (2015). Bayesian network-based customized highlight generation for broadcast soccer videos. *IEEE Transactions on Broadcasting*, *61*(2), 195–209. doi:10.1109/TBC.2015.2424011

Koozekanani, D., Boyer, K., & Roberts, C. (2001). Retinal thickness measurements from optical coherence tomography using a Markov boundary model. *IEEE Transactions on Medical Imaging*, *20*(9), 900–916. doi:10.1109/42.952728 PMID:11585207

Koppel, A., Sadler, B. M., & Ribeiro, A. (2017). Proximity without consensus in online multi agent optimization. *IEEE Transactions on Signal Processing*, *65*(12), 3062–3077. doi:10.1109/TSP.2017.2686368

Kovács, P. (2012). ECG signal generator based on geometrical features. *Annales Universitatis Scientarium Budapestinensis de Rolando Eötvös Nominatae Sectio Mathematica*, *37*, 247–260.

Koya, J. R., & Rao, S. P. V. M. (2015). Nano-fractal Electrodes Use in Electroencephalography (EEG) Array Generation to Map with Speech Signals. *Procedia Materials Science*, *10*, 693–698. doi:10.1016/j.mspro.2015.06.072

Krissian, K., Westin, C. F., Kikinis, R., & Vosburgh, K. G. (2007). Oriented speckle reducing anisotropic diffusion. *IEEE Transactions on Image Processing*, *16*(5), 1412–1424. doi:10.1109/TIP.2007.891803 PMID:17491469

Krithivasan, S., Wahal, S., & Ansumali, S. (2014). Diffused bounce-back condition and refill algorithm for the lattice Boltzmann method. *Physical Review. E*, *89*(3), 033313. doi:10.1103/PhysRevE.89.033313 PMID:24730973

Krogh, A. (1994). Hidden Markov models for labeled sequences. In *International Conference on Pattern Recognition* (pp. 140-144). Jerusalem: The IEEE Computer Society. 10.1109/ICPR.1994.576891

Kuan, D. T., Sawchuk, A. A., Strand, T. C., & Chavel, P. (1985). Adaptive noise smoothing filter for images with signal-dependent noise. *IEEE Transactions on Pattern Analysis and Machine Intelligence*, *PAMI-7*(2), 165–177. doi:10.1109/TPAMI.1985.4767641 PMID:21869255

Kumar, A., & Chakarverty, S. (2011). Design optimization for reliable embedded system using Cuckoo Search. *Electronics Computer Technology (ICECT), 2011 3rd International Conference IEEE,* (1), 264-268.

Kumar, S., & Arasu, G. T. (2017). Rough set theory and fuzzy logic based warehousing of heterogeneous clinical databases. *International Journal of Uncertainty, Fuzziness and Knowledge-based Systems*, *25*(3), 385–408. doi:10.1142/S0218488517500167

Kumar, V. K., Kumar, S. P., & Baliga, M. R. (2013). Prevalence of work-related musculoskeletal complaints among dentists in India: A national cross-sectional survey. *Indian Journal of Dental Research*, *24*(4), 428–438. doi:10.4103/0970-9290.118387 PMID:24047834

Kuncheva, L. I. (2004). *Combining pattern classifiers: methods and algorithms*. John Wiley & Sons. doi:10.1002/0471660264

Kuta, L., Cieź, J., & Młotek, M. (2015). Musculoskeletal load assessment of farmers during selected agricultural works. *Procedia Manufacturing*, *3*, 1696–1703. doi:10.1016/j.promfg.2015.07.990

Kutlu, Y., & Kuntalp, D. (2012). Feature extraction for ECG heartbeats using higher order statistics of WPD coefficients. *Computer Methods and Programs in Biomedicine*, *105*(3), 257–267. doi:10.1016/j.cmpb.2011.10.002 PMID:22055998

Kwon, O. Y., Shin, S. H., Shin, S. J., & Kim, W. S. (2010). Design of U-health system with the use of smart phone and sensor network. In *Ubiquitous Information Technologies and Applications (CUTE), 2010 Proceedings of the 5th International Conference on* (pp. 1-6). IEEE.

Lachenbruch, P. A., & Mickey, M. R. (1968). Estimation of Error Rate in Discriminant Analysis. *Technometrics*, *10*(1), 1–10. doi:10.1080/00401706.1968.10490530

Lakshmi, M. S., Haritha, D., & Srkit, V. (2016). Heart disease diagnosis using predictive data mining. *International Journal of Computer Science and Information Security*.

Langley, P., & Sage, S. (1994). *Induction of selective Bayesian classifiers. In Uncertainty Proceedings 1994* (pp. 399–406). Elsevier. doi:10.1016/B978-1-55860-332-5.50055-9

Lee, H. D., Mendesb, A. I., Spolaôra, N., Olivaa, J. T., Parmezana, A. R. S., Wua, F. C., & Fonseca-Pintob, R. (2018). Dermoscopic Assisted Diagnosis in Melanoma: Reviewing Results, Optimizing Methodologies and Quantifying Empirical Guidelines. *Knowledge-Based Systems*, *158*, 9–24. doi:10.1016/j.knosys.2018.05.016

Lee, H., Sheth, V., Bibi, M., Maconachie, G., Patel, A., McLean, R. J., ... Gottlob, I. (2013). Potential of handheld optical coherence tomography to determine cause of infantile nystagmus in children by using foveal morphology. *Ophthalmology*, *120*(12), 2714–2724. doi:10.1016/j.ophtha.2013.07.018 PMID:24161406

Lee, J. S. (1980). Digital image enhancement and noise filtering by use of local statistics. *IEEE Transactions on Pattern Analysis and Machine Intelligence*, *PAMI-2*(2), 165–168. doi:10.1109/TPAMI.1980.4766994 PMID:21868887

Lee, P. M., Khong, P., & Ghista, D. N. (2006). Impact of deficient healthcare service quality. *The TQM Magazine*, *18*(6), 563–571. doi:10.1108/09544780610707075

Lehto, T., Oinas-Kukkonen, H., Pätiälä, T., & Saarelma, O. (2013). Virtual health coaching for consumers: A persuasive systems design perspective. *International Journal of Networking and Virtual Organisations*, *13*(1), 24–41. doi:10.1504/IJNVO.2013.058440

Leonard, J. E., Colombe, J. B., & Levy, J. L. (2002). Finding relevant references to genes and proteins in Medline using a Bayesian approach. *Bioinformatics (Oxford, England)*, *18*(11), 1515–1522. doi:10.1093/bioinformatics/18.11.1515 PMID:12424124

Li, D., Han, H., Xu, X., Ling, Z., & Hong, B. (2017). Minimally invasive brain computer interface for fast typing. In *Neural Engineering (NER), 2017 8th International IEEE/EMBS Conference on*. IEEE.

Li, J., Zhang, R., Shi, L., & Wang, D. (2016). Automatic Whole-Heart Segmentation in Congenital Heart Disease Using Deeply-Supervised 3D FCN. In First International Workshops, RAMBO 2016 and HVSMR 2016.10129 (pp. 111-118). Athens: Reconstruction, Segmentation, and Analysis of Medical Images: LNCS.

Li, L., Wu, Y., & Ye, M. (2015). Experimental comparisons of multi-class classifiers. *Informatica*, *39*(1).

Li, X., Liu, X., Zhang, Z., Xia, Y., & Qian, S. (2010). Design of Health Eating System Based on Web Data Mining. In *Information Engineering (ICIE), 2010 WASE International Conference on* (Vol. 1, pp. 346-349). IEEE.

Li, Y., Xu, B., Chen, S., Liu, P., Ou, A., Xu, Y., . . . Zeng, L. (2011, November). A randomized, controlled study of efficacy and safety on mild to moderate insomnia intervened by Chinese medicine in the integrated program. In *Bioinformatics and Biomedicine Workshops (BIBMW), 2011 IEEE International Conference on* (pp. 732-739). IEEE.

Liang, W., Zhang, Y., Tan, J., & Li, Y. (2014). A novel approach to ECG classification based upon two-layered HMMs in body sensor networks. *Sensors (Basel)*, *14*(4), 5994–6011. doi:10.3390140405994 PMID:24681668

Lia, Y., Liu, X., Wei, F., Sima, D. M., Van Cauter, S., Himmelreich, U., ... Van Huffel, S. (2017). An advanced MRI and MRSI data fusion scheme for enhancing unsupervised brain tumor differentiation. *Elsevier. Computers in Biology and Medicine*, *8*, 121–129. doi:10.1016/j.compbiomed.2016.12.017

Li, D., He, Q., Chunli, L., & Hongjie, Y. (2017). Local Binary Fitting Segmentation by Cooperative Quantum Particle Optimization. *TELKOMNIKA*, *15*(1), 531. doi:10.12928/telkomnika.v15i1.3159

Lim, J. S. (1990). *Two-dimensional signal and image processing*. Englewood Cliffs, NJ: Prentice Hall.

Linh, T. H., Osowski, S., & Stodolski, M. (2003). On-line heart beat recognition using Hermite polynomials and neuro-fuzzy network. *IEEE Transactions on Instrumentation and Measurement*, *52*(4), 1224–1231. doi:10.1109/TIM.2003.816841

Lin, L. C., Yeh, Y. C., & Chu, T. Y. (2014). Feature Selection Algorithm for ECG Signals and Its Application on Heartbeat Case Determining. *International Journal of Fuzzy Systems*, *16*(4).

Li, P. C., & Chen, M. J. (2002). Strain compounding: A new approach for speckle reduction. *IEEE Transactions on Ultrasonics, Ferroelectrics, and Frequency Control*, *49*(1), 39–46. doi:10.1109/58.981382 PMID:11833890

Li, P., Wang, Y., He, J., Wang, L., Tian, Y., Zhou, T. S., ... Li, J. S. (2017). High-performance personalized heartbeat classification model for long-term ECG signal. *IEEE Transactions on Biomedical Engineering*, *64*(1), 78–86. doi:10.1109/10.650355 PMID:27046844

Liu, P., Yu, H., Xu, T., & Lan, C. (2017, December). Research on archives text classification based on Naive Bayes. In *Technology, Networking, Electronic and Automation Control Conference (ITNEC), 2017 IEEE 2nd Information* (pp. 187-190). IEEE.

Liu, Shi, Zhu, & Zhao. (2015). *Image fusion based on complex-shearlet domain with guided filtering,* Springer.

Liu, X., Yang, Z., & Wang, J. (2016, October). A novel noise reduction method for optical coherence tomography images. In *Image and Signal Processing, BioMedical Engineering and Informatics (CISP-BMEI), International Congress on* (pp. 167-171). IEEE.

Liu, X., Mei, W., & Du, H. (2017). Structure tensor and nonsubsampled sheasrlet transform based algorithm for CT and MRI image fusion, *Elsevier. Neurocomputing*, *235*, 131–139. doi:10.1016/j.neucom.2017.01.006

Liu, X., Wang, G., Gao, J., & Gao, Q. (2017). A Quantitative Analysis for EEG Signals Based on Modified Permutation-Entropy. *IRBM*, *38*(2), 71–77. doi:10.1016/j.irbm.2017.02.001

Liu, X., Wang, X., Su, Q., Zhang, M., Zhu, Y., Wang, Q., & Wang, Q. (2017). A Hybrid Classification System for Heart Disease Diagnosis Based on the RFRS Method. *Computational and Mathematical Methods in Medicine*. PMID:28127385

Li, X., Jiang, D., Shi, Y., & Li, W. (2015). Segmentation of MR image using local and global region based geodesic model. *Biomedical Engineering Online*, *14*(1), 8. doi:10.1186/1475-925X-14-8 PMID:25971306

Li, Y., & Shen, L. (2018). Skin Lesion Analysis towards Melanoma Detection Using Deep Learning Network. *Sensors (Basel)*, *18*(556), 2–16. PMID:29439500

Li, Z., Liu, G., & Li, Q. (2017). Nonparametric Knn estimation with monotone constraints. *Econometric Reviews*, 1–19. doi:10.1080/07474938.2017.1310080

Li, Z., Zeng, L., Xu, Y., Chen, J., & Yan, B. (2016). Level set method for image segmentation based on local variance and improved intensity inhomogeneity model. *IET Image Processing*, *10*(12), 1007–1016. doi:10.1049/iet-ipr.2016.0352

Lodh, T., Subramaniam, A., & Paswan, A. K. (2016). Ultrasound based assistive mobility devices for the visually-impaired. In *Power India International Conference (PIICON), 2016 IEEE 7th* (pp. 1-6). IEEE.

Loizou, C. P., Pattichis, C. S., Christodoulou, C. I., Istepanian, R. S., Pantziaris, M., & Nicolaides, A. (2014a). *Image despeckle filtering (IDF) toolbox*. Retrieved from http://www.medinfo.cs.ucy.ac.cy/doc/toolboxes/IDF.zip

Loizou, C. P., & Pattichis, C. S. (2015). Despeckle filtering for ultrasound imaging and video, Volume I: Algorithms and software. *Synthesis Lectures on Algorithms and Software in Engineering*, *7*(1), 1–180. doi:10.2200/S00641ED1V01Y201504ASE014

Loizou, C. P., Pattichis, C. S., Christodoulou, C. I., Istepanian, R. S., Pantziaris, M., & Nicolaides, A. (2005). Comparative evaluation of despeckle filtering in ultrasound imaging of the carotid artery. *IEEE Transactions on Ultrasonics, Ferroelectrics, and Frequency Control*, *52*(10), 1653–1669. doi:10.1109/TUFFC.2005.1561621 PMID:16382618

Loizou, C. P., Theofanous, C., Pantziaris, M., & Kasparis, T. (2014). Despeckle filtering software toolbox for ultrasound imaging of the common carotid artery. *Computer Methods and Programs in Biomedicine, 114*(1), 109–124. doi:10.1016/j.cmpb.2014.01.018 PMID:24560276

Lopes, A., Touzi, R., & Nezry, E. (1990). Adaptive speckle filters and scene heterogeneity. *IEEE Transactions on Geoscience and Remote Sensing, 28*(6), 992–1000. doi:10.1109/36.62623

Luan, F., & Wu, Y. (2013). Application of RPCA in optical coherence tomography for speckle noise reduction. *Laser Physics Letters, 10*(3), 035603. doi:10.1088/1612-2011/10/3/035603

Luangwilai, T., Norkaew, S., & Siriwong, W. (2014). Factors associated with musculoskeletal disorders among rice farmers: Cross sectional study in Tarnlalord sub-district, Phimai district, Nakhonratchasima province, Thailand. *J Health Res., 28*(Suppl.), S85–S91.

Lu, J. Y., Zou, H., & Greenleaf, J. F. (1994). Biomedical ultrasound beam forming. *Ultrasound in Medicine & Biology, 20*(5), 403–428. doi:10.1016/0301-5629(94)90097-3 PMID:7941100

Lüscher, T. F., & Templin, C. (2016). Is takotsubo syndrome a microvascular acute coronary syndrome? Towards a new definition. *European Heart Journal, 37*(37), 2816–2820. doi:10.1093/eurheartj/ehw057 PMID:26966148

Luukka, P., & Lampinen, J. (2010). A Classification method based on principal component analysis and differential evolution algorithm applied for prediction diagnosis from clinical EMR heart data sets. In Y. Tenne & C. K. Goh (Eds.), *Computational Intelligence in Optimization. Adaptation, Learning, and Optimization* (pp. 263–283). Springer. doi:10.1007/978-3-642-12775-5_11

Lv, H., Fu, S., Zhang, C., & Zhai, L. (2018). Speckle noise reduction for optical coherence tomography based on adaptive 2D dictionary. *Laser Physics Letters, 15*(5), 055401. doi:10.1088/1612-202X/aaaeb0

Mahmoodabadi, S. Z., Ahmadian, A., & Abolhasani, M. D. (2005). ECGFeature Extraction using Daubechies Wavelets. *2005 IEEE Engineering in Medicine and Biology 27th Annual Conference.*

Mahoto, N. A., Shaikh, A., & Khuhawar, F. (2014). CliTA: Discovering Knowledge from Clinical Data. *Sindh University Research Journal, 46*(4), 539-546.

Mahoto, N. A., Shaikh, F. K., & Ansari, A. Q. (2014). Exploitation of Clustering Techniques in Transactional Healthcare Data. *Mehran University Research Journal of Engineering & Technology, 33*(1), 77-92.

Mahoto, N. A., Shaikh, F. K., & Chowdhry, B. S. (2015). Innovative Architecture to Enhance Quality of Service for Laboratory Management Information System. In *Laboratory Management Information Systems: Current Requirements and Future* (pp. 242–256). IGI Global. doi:10.4018/978-1-4666-6320-6.ch012

Maillo, J., Ramírez, S., Triguero, I., & Herrera, F. (2017). kNN-IS: An Iterative Spark-based design of the k-Nearest Neighbors classifier for big data. *Knowledge-Based Systems, 117*, 3–15. doi:10.1016/j.knosys.2016.06.012

Ma, M., Manuel, J., & Tavares, R. S. (2017). Effective features to classify skin lesions in dermoscopic images. *Expert Systems with Applications, 84*, 92–101. doi:10.1016/j.eswa.2017.05.003

Mangalagowri, S. G., & Prasanna Raj, P. C. (2016). EEG feature extraction and classification using feed forward backpropogation algorithm for emotion detection. In *Electrical, Electronics, Communication, Computer and Optimization Techniques (ICEECCOT), 2016 International Conference on.* IEEE.

Mangasarian, O. L., & Wolberg, W. H. (1990a). Cancer diagnosis via linear programming. *SIAM News, 23*(5).

Mangasarian, O. L., & Wolberg, W. H. (1990b). Multisurface method of pattern separation for medical diagnosis applied to breast cytology. *Proceedings of the National Academy of Sciences of the United States of America*, *87*(23), 9193–9196. doi:10.1073/pnas.87.23.9193 PMID:2251264

Manogaran, G., Varatharajan, R., & Priyan, M. K. (2018). Hybrid Recommendation System for Heart Disease Diagnosis based on Multiple Kernel Learning with Adaptive Neuro-Fuzzy Inference System. *Multimedia Tools and Applications*, *77*(4), 4379–4399. doi:10.100711042-017-5515-y

Mansi, S., Milosavljevic, S., Tumilty, S., Hendrick, P., & Baxter, G. D. (2013). Use of pedometer driven walking to promote physical activity and improve health-related quality of life among meat processing workers: A feasibility trial. *Health and Quality of Life Outcomes*, *11*(1), 185. doi:10.1186/1477-7525-11-185 PMID:24175980

Mantzaris, D., Anastassopoulos, G., & Adamopoulos, A. (2011). Genetic algorithm pruning of probabilistic neural networks in medical disease estimation. *Neural Networks*, *24*(8), 831–835. doi:10.1016/j.neunet.2011.06.003 PMID:21723704

Mareli, M., & Twala, B. (2017). *An adaptive Cuckoo search algorithm for optimization*. Applied Computing and Informatics; doi:10.1016/j.aci.2017.09.001

Marks, D. L., Ralston, T. S., & Boppart, S. A. (2005). Speckle reduction by I-divergence regularization in optical coherence tomography. *JOSA A*, *22*(11), 2366–2371. doi:10.1364/JOSAA.22.002366 PMID:16304722

Mar, T., Zaunseder, S., Martínez, J. P., Llamedo, M., & Poll, R. (2011). Optimization of ECG classification by means of feature selection. *IEEE Transactions on Biomedical Engineering*, *58*(8), 2168–2177. doi:10.1109/TBME.2011.2113395 PMID:21317067

Martín-Smith, P., Ortega, J., Ascenio-Cubero, J., Gan, J. Q., & Ortiz, A. (2017). A supervised filter method for multi-objective feature selection in EEG classification based on multi-resolution analysis for BCI. *Neurocomputing*, *250*, 45–56. doi:10.1016/j.neucom.2016.09.123

Martis, R. J., Acharya, U. R., Mandana, K. M., Ray, A. K., & Chakraborty, C. (2013). Cardiac decision making using higher order spectra. *Biomedical Signal Processing and Control*, *8*(2), 193–203. doi:10.1016/j.bspc.2012.08.004

Martis, R. J., Acharya, U. R., & Min, L. C. (2013). ECG beat classification using PCA, LDA, ICA and discrete wavelet transform. *Biomedical Signal Processing and Control*, *8*(5), 437–448. doi:10.1016/j.bspc.2013.01.005

Martis, R. J., Chakraborty, C., & Ray, A. K. (2009). A two-stage mechanism for registration and classification of ECG using Gaussian mixture model. *Pattern Recognition*, *42*(11), 2979–2988. doi:10.1016/j.patcog.2009.02.008

Martis, R. J., Krishnan, M. M. R., Chakraborty, C., Pal, S., Sarkar, D., Mandana, K. M., & Ray, A. K. (2012). Automated screening of arrhythmia using wavelet based machine learning techniques. *Journal of Medical Systems*, *36*(2), 677–688. doi:10.100710916-010-9535-7 PMID:20703662

Masud, M., Adel Serhani, M., & Navaz, A. (2017). Resource-Aware Mobile-Based Health Monitoring. *IEEE Journal of Biomedical and Health Informatics*, *21*(2), 349–360. doi:10.1109/JBHI.2016.2525006 PMID:26863682

Mauldin, F. W., Lin, D., & Hossack, J. A. (2011). The singular value filter: A general filter design strategy for PCA-based signal separation in medical ultrasound imaging. *IEEE Transactions on Medical Imaging*, *30*(11), 1951–1964. doi:10.1109/TMI.2011.2160075 PMID:21693416

Mayer, M. A., Borsdorf, A., Wagner, M., Hornegger, J., Mardin, C. Y., & Tornow, R. P. (2012). Wavelet denoising of multiframe optical coherence tomography data. *Biomedical Optics Express*, *3*(3), 572–589. doi:10.1364/BOE.3.000572 PMID:22435103

Mayer, M. A., Tornow, R. P., Bock, R., Hornegger, J., & Kruse, F. E. (2008). Automatic nerve fiber layer segmentation and geometry correction on spectral domain OCT images using fuzzy C-means clustering. *Investigative Ophthalmology & Visual Science*, *49*(13), 1880–1880.

McCall, J. (2005). Genetic algorithms for modelling and optimisation. *Journal of Computational and Applied Mathematics*, *184*(1), 205–222. doi:10.1016/j.cam.2004.07.034

McLaughlin, C., & Fitzgerald, C. (2001). Converging genetics and information technologies and the emerging healthcare system. *International Journal of Healthcare Technology and Management*, *3*(5/6), 498. doi:10.1504/IJHTM.2001.001125

Meiniel, W., Gan, Y., Olivo-Marin, J. C., & Angelini, E. (2017, August). A sparsity-based simplification method for segmentation of spectral-domain optical coherence tomography images. In *Wavelets and Sparsity XVII* (Vol. 10394, p. 1039406). International Society for Optics and Photonics. doi:10.1117/12.2274126

Meissimilly, G., Rodriguez, J., Rodriguez, G., Gonzalez, R., & Caiiizares, M. (2003). Microcontroller-Based Real-Time QRS Detector for Ambulatory Monitoring. *Proceedings of the 25 Annual International Conference of the IEEE EMBS*, 2881-2884. 10.1109/IEMBS.2003.1280520

Meksawi, S., Tangtrakulwanich, B., & Chongsuvivatwong, V. (2012). Musculoskeletal problems and ergonomic risk assessment in rubber tappers: A community-based study in southern Thailand. *International Journal of Industrial Ergonomics*, *42*(1), 129–135. doi:10.1016/j.ergon.2011.08.006

Melgani, F., & Bazi, Y. (2008). Classification of electrocardiogram signals with support vector machines and particle swarm optimization. *IEEE Transactions on Information Technology in Biomedicine*, *12*(5), 667–677. doi:10.1109/TITB.2008.923147 PMID:18779082

Mert, A., Kılıç, N., & Akan, A. (2014). Evaluation of bagging ensemble method with time-domain feature extraction for diagnosing of arrhythmia beats. *Neural Computing & Applications*, *24*(2), 317–326. doi:10.100700521-012-1232-7

Meyer, U., & Scheich, H. (1997). Artificial implementation of auditory neurons: A comparison of biologically motivated models and a new transfer function oriented model. *Biological Cybernetics*, *77*(2), 123–130. doi:10.1007004220050373 PMID:9323861

Miao, J., Huang, T., Zhou, X., Wang, Y., & Liu, J. (2018). Image segmentation based on an active contour model of partial image restoration with local cosine fitting energy. *Information Sciences*, *447*, 52–71. doi:10.1016/j.ins.2018.02.007

Mishra, D., Chaudhury, S., Sarkar, M., & Soin, A. S. (2018). *Unsupervised Despeckling*. arXiv preprint arXiv:1801.03318

Mishra, A., Wong, A., Bizheva, K., & Clausi, D. A. (2009). Intra-retinal layer segmentation in optical coherence tomography images. *Optics Express*, *17*(26), 23719–23728. doi:10.1364/OE.17.023719 PMID:20052083

Mishra, D., & Satapathy, S. (2018). Drudgery Reduction of Farm Women of Odisha by Improved Serrated Sickle. *International Journal of Mechanical Engineering and Technology*, *9*(2), 53–61.

Mohamad, A., Zain, A. M., Nazira Bazin, N. E., & Udin, A. (2013). Cuckoo Search Algorithm for Optimization Problems – A literature Review. *Applied Mechanics and Materials*, *421*, 502–506. doi:10.4028/www.scientific.net/AMM.421.502

Mohs, R., Wescourt, K., & Atkinson, R. (1973). Effects of short-term memory contents on short-and long-term memory searches. *Memory & Cognition*, *1*(4), 443–448. doi:10.3758/BF03208906 PMID:24214639

Moin, A., Bhateja, V., & Srivastava, A. (2016). Weighted-PCA Based Multimodal Medical Image Fusion in Contourlet Domain. *Proceedings of the International Congress on Information and Communication Technology, Advances in Intelligent Systems and Computing*, 439.

Moody, G. B., & Mark, R. G. (2001). The impact of the MIT-BIH arrhythmia database. *IEEE Engineering in Medicine and Biology Magazine*, *20*(3), 45–50. doi:10.1109/51.932724 PMID:11446209

Moody, J., & Darken, C. J. (1989). Fast learning in networks of locally-tuned processing units. *Neural Computation*, *1*(2), 281–294. doi:10.1162/neco.1989.1.2.281

Morin, C. M., Belleville, G., Bélanger, L., & Ivers, H. (2011). The Insomnia Severity Index: Psychometric indicators to detect insomnia cases and evaluate treatment response. *Sleep*, *34*(5), 601–608. doi:10.1093leep/34.5.601 PMID:21532953

Mosadeghrad, A. M. (2014). Factors influencing healthcare service quality. *International Journal of Health Policy and Management*, *3*(2), 77–89. doi:10.15171/ijhpm.2014.65 PMID:25114946

Motinath, V. A., Jha, C. K., & Kolekar, M. H. (2016). A novel ECG data compression algorithm using best mother wavelet selection. In *International Conference on Advances in Computing, Communications and Informatics (ICACCI)* (pp. 682-686). IEEE. 10.1109/ICACCI.2016.7732125

Muftuoglu, I. K., Ramkumar, H. L., Bartsch, D. U., Meshi, A., Gaber, R., & Freeman, W. R. (2018). Quantitative analysis of the inner retinal layer thicknesses in age-related macular degeneration using corrected optical coherence tomography segmentation. *Retina (Philadelphia, Pa.)*, *38*(8), 1478–1484. doi:10.1097/IAE.0000000000001759 PMID:28650925

Mulaffer, L., Shahin, M., Glos, M., Penzel, T., & Ahmed, B. (2017, July). Comparing two insomnia detection models of clinical diagnostic techniques. In *Engineering in Medicine and Biology Society (EMBC), 2017 39th Annual International Conference of the IEEE* (pp. 3749-3752). IEEE.

Müller, K.-R., Krauledat, M., Dornhege, G., Curio, G., & Blankertz, B. (2004). *Machine learning techniques for brain-computer interfaces*. Retrieved from: http://doc.ml.tu-berlin.de/bbci/publications/MueKraDorCurBla04.pdf

Muramatsu, S., Choi, S., & Kawamura, T. (2015, December). 3-D OCT data denoising with nonseparable oversampled lapped transform. In *Signal and Information Processing Association Annual Summit and Conference (APSIPA), 2015 Asia-Pacific* (pp. 901-906). IEEE.

Murphy, D. J. (1992). *Safety and Health for Production Agriculture*. American Society of Agricultural Engineers, Books & Journals.

Murugappan, M., Rizon, M., Nagarajan, R. & Yaacob, S. (2007). EEG feature extraction for classifying emotions using FCM and FKM. *International Journal of Computers and Communications, 1*(2), 21-25.

Muthukarupan, S., & Erib, M. J. (2012). A hybrid PSO based fuzzy expert system for the diagnosis of Coronary heart system. *Expert Systems with Applications*, *39*, 11657–11665. doi:10.1016/j.eswa.2012.04.036

Naegel, B., & Passat, N. (2014). Interactive Segmentation Based on Component-trees. *Image Processing On Line*, *4*, 89–97. doi:10.5201/ipol.2014.71

Nagai, T. (2000). Artificial neural networks estimate the contribution of taste neurons to coding. *Physiology & Behavior*, *69*(1-2), 107–113. doi:10.1016/S0031-9384(00)00194-3 PMID:10854922

Nahar, J., Imam, T., Tickle, K. S., & Chen, Y.-P. P. (2013). Association rule mining to detect factors which contribute to heart disease in males and females. *Expert Systems with Applications*, *40*(4), 1086–1093. doi:10.1016/j.eswa.2012.08.028

Naidu, A. (2009). Factors affecting patient satisfaction and healthcare quality. *International Journal of Health Care Quality Assurance*, *22*(4), 366–381. doi:10.1108/09526860910964834 PMID:19725209

Nalavade, K. C., Bharmal, F., Deore, T., & Patil, A. (2014). Use of ultrasonic sensors, GPS and GSM technology to implement alert and tracking system for blind man. *Proceedings of the International Conference of Advance Research and Innovation (ICARI)*, 272-274.

Nambiar, R., Bhardwaj, R., Sethi, A., & Vargheese, R. (2013). A look at challenges and opportunities of big data analytics in healthcare. In *Big Data, 2013 IEEE International Conference on* (pp. 17-22). IEEE.

Naraballobh, J., Thanapatay, D., Chinrungrueng, J., & Nishihara, A. (2015). Effect of auditory stimulus in EEG signal using a Brain-Computer Interface. In *Electrical Engineering/Electronics, Computer, Telecommunications and Information Technology (ECTI-CON), 2015 12th International Conference on*. IEEE.

Naraei, P., Abhari, A., & Sadeghian, A. (2016). *Application of multilayer perceptron neural networks and support vector machines in classification of healthcare data*. Paper presented at the Future Technologies Conference (FTC). 10.1109/FTC.2016.7821702

Narasimha Murthy, K. N., & Kusuma, J. (2017). Fusion of Medical Image Using STSVD. *Proceedings of the 5th International Conference on Frontiers in Intelligent Computing: Theory and Applications, 516*, 69-79.

Nasrin Amini, E. (2015). MRI-PET image fusion based on NSCT transform using local energy and local variance fusion rules. *Journal of Medical Engineering & Technology, 38*(4), 211–219. doi:10.3109/03091902.2014.904014 PMID:24758393

National Institute of Occupational Safety and Health (NIOSH). (2002). *Quality of work life questionnaire*. NIOSH.

National Sleep Foundation. (n.d.). *Types of Insomnia*. National Sleep Foundation. Available at https://sleepfoundation.org/insomnia/content/what-are-different-types-insomnia

Negrato, C., Cobas, R., & Gomes, M. (2012). Temporal changes in the diagnosis of type 1 diabetes by diabetic ketoacidosis in Brazil: A nationwide survey. *Diabetic Medicine, 29*(9), 1142–1147. doi:10.1111/j.1464-5491.2012.03590.x PMID:22269058

Neikrug, A. B., & Ancoli-Israel, S. (2010). Sleep disorders in the older adult–a mini-review. *Gerontology, 56*(2), 181–189. doi:10.1159/000236900 PMID:19738366

Nevill-Manning, C. G., Holmes, G., & Witten, I. H. (1995). The development of Holte's 1R classifier. *Proceedings of the Second New Zealand International Two-Stream Conference*.

Nguyen, D., Tran, D., Sharma, D., & Ma, W. (2017). Investigating the Impact of Epilepsy on EEG-Based Cryptographic Key Generation Systems. *Procedia Computer Science, 112*, 177–185. doi:10.1016/j.procs.2017.08.015

Nikolic, K. (2015). Stochastic Search Algorithms for Identification, Optimization, and Training of Artificial Neural Networks. *Advances in Artificial Neural Systems, 2015*, 1–16. doi:10.1155/2015/931379

Nirschl, J. J., Janowczyk, A., Peyster, E. G., Frank, R., Margulies, K. B., Feldman, M. D., & Madabhushi, A. (2018). A deep-learning classifier identifies patients with clinical heart failure using whole-slide images of H&E tissue. *PLoS One, 13*(4), e0192726. doi:10.1371/journal.pone.0192726 PMID:29614076

Nugrahaeni, R. A., & Mutijarsa, K. (2016, August). Comparative analysis of machine learning KNN, SVM, and random forests algorithm for facial expression classification. In *Technology of Information and Communication (semantic), International Seminar on Application for* (pp. 163-168). IEEE.

O'day, B. L., Killeen, M., & Iezzoni, L. I. (2004). Improving health care experiences of persons who are blind or have low vision: Suggestions from focus groups. *American Journal of Medical Quality, 19*(5), 193–200. doi:10.1177/106286060401900503 PMID:15532911

Ocampo, M. G., Leal, E. H., Cadavid, J. M., Gómez, D. E., & Méndez, N. D. (2016). Application of a technical tool to support the inclusion process of people with visual impairment in an educational web platform. In *Learning Objects and Technology (LACLO), Latin American Conference on* (pp. 1-5). IEEE.

Ogier, A., Hellier, P., & Barillot, C. (2006, March). Restoration of 3D medical images with total variation scheme on wavelet domains (TVW). In Medical Imaging 2006: Image Processing (Vol. 6144, p. 61441E). International Society for Optics and Photonics.

Ogorodnikov, V., Sereseva, O., & Kargapolova, N. (2016). Stochastic models of piecewise-constant and piecewise-linear non-Gaussian processes based on Poisson flows. *Russian Journal of Numerical Analysis and Mathematical Modelling*, *31*(3). doi:10.1515/rnam-2016-0018

Olabarriaga, S., & Smeulders, A. (2001). Interaction in the segmentation of medical images: A survey. *Medical Image Analysis*, *5*(2), 127–142. doi:10.1016/S1361-8415(00)00041-4 PMID:11516707

Ola, S. O., Otegbayo, J. A., Yakubu, A., Odaibo, G. N., & Olaleye, D. O. (2008). Nigerian butchers and hepatitis B virus. *Tropical Gastroenterology*, *29*, 32–34. PMID:18564665

Omokhodion, F. O., & Adebayo, A. M. (2013). Occupational hazards and self-reported health problems of butchers in Ibadan, southwest Nigeria. *J Public Health (Germany)*, *21*(2), 131–134. doi:10.100710389-012-0528-5

Onan, A. (2016). Classifier and feature set ensembles for web page classification. *Journal of Information Science*, *42*(2), 150–165. doi:10.1177/0165551515591724

Ordonez, C. (2006). Association rule discovery with the train and test approach for heart disease prediction. *IEEE Transactions on Information Technology in Biomedicine*, *10*(2), 334–343. doi:10.1109/TITB.2006.864475 PMID:16617622

Ordonez, C., Omincenski, E., de Braal, L., Santana, C. A., Ezquerra, N., Taboada, J. A., ... Garcia, E. V. (2001). Mining Constraint Association Rules to Predict Heart Disease. In *IEEE International Conference of Data Mining* (pp. 433-440). San Jose, CA: IEEE.

Orhan, U., Hekim, M., & Ozer, M. (2011). EEG signals classification using the K-means clustering and a multilayer perceptron neural network model. *Expert Systems with Applications*, *38*(10), 13475–13481. doi:10.1016/j.eswa.2011.04.149

Ortiz, S. H. C., Chiu, T., & Fox, M. D. (2012). Ultrasound image enhancement: A review. *Biomedical Signal Processing and Control*, *7*(5), 419–428. doi:10.1016/j.bspc.2012.02.002

Ozcan, A., Bilenca, A., Desjardins, A. E., Bouma, B. E., & Tearney, G. J. (2007). Speckle reduction in optical coherence tomography images using digital filtering. *JOSA A*, *24*(7), 1901–1910. doi:10.1364/JOSAA.24.001901 PMID:17728812

Ozcift, A., & Gulten, A. (2011). Classifier ensemble construction with rotation forest to improve medical diagnosis performance of machine learning algorithms. *Computer Methods and Programs in Biomedicine*, *104*(3), 443–451. doi:10.1016/j.cmpb.2011.03.018 PMID:21531475

Pace, D. F. D. A. (2015). Interactive Whole-Heart Segmentation in Congenital Heart Disease. In MICCAI 2015.9351 (pp. 80-88). Munich, Germany: LNCS Springer.

Palaniappan, S., & Awang, R. (2008). Intelligent heart disease prediction system using data mining techniques. *IEEE/ACS International Conference on Computer Systems and Applications, AICCSA 2008*. 10.1109/AICCSA.2008.4493524

Palaniappan, S., & Awang, R. (2008). Intelligent heart disease prediction system using data mining techniques. *International Journal of Computer Science and Network Security*, *8*(8), 108–115.

Pal, S., & Mitra, M. (2010). Detection of ECG characteristic points using multiresolution wavelet analysis based selective coefficient method. *Measurement*, *43*(2), 255–261. doi:10.1016/j.measurement.2009.10.004

Pandey, P. S. (2017, July). Machine learning and iot for prediction and detection of stress. In *Computational Science and Its Applications (ICCSA), 2017 17th International Conference on* (pp. 1-5). IEEE.

Pang, Z., Li, J., Ji, H., & Li, M. (2016). A new approach for EEG feature extraction for detecting error-related potentials. In *Progress in Electromagnetic Research Symposium (PIERS)*. IEEE.

Panin, G., & Knoll, A. (2006). Fully Automatic Real-Time 3D Object Tracking using Active Contour and Appearance Models. *Journal of Multimedia*, *1*(7). doi:10.4304/jmm.1.7.62-70

Pan, J., & Tompkins, W. J. (1985). A real-time QRS detection algorithm. *IEEE Transactions on Biomedical Engineering*, *32*(3), 230–236. doi:10.1109/TBME.1985.325532 PMID:3997178

Papadimitriou, S., Mavroudi, S., Vladutu, L., & Bezerianos, A. (2001, May). Ischemia detection with a self-organizing map supplemented by supervised learning. *IEEE Transactions on Neural Networks*, *12*(3), 503–515. doi:10.1109/72.925554 PMID:18249884

Papaloukas, C., Fotiadis, D. I., Likas, A., & Michalis, L. K. (2002). An expert system for ischemia detection based on parametric modeling and artificial neural networks. *Processings of the European Medical Biological Engineering Conference.*

Papaloukas, C., Fotiadis, D. I., Likas, A., Liavas, A. P., & Michalis, L. K. (2001). A knowledge-based technique for automated detection of ischemic episodes in long duration electrocardiograms. *Medical & Biological Engineering & Computing*, *39*(1), 105–112. doi:10.1007/BF02345273 PMID:11214261

Papaloukas, C., Fotiadis, D. I., Likas, A., & Michalis, L. K. (2002). An ischemia detection method based on artificial neural networks. *Artificial Intelligence in Medicine*, *24*(2), 167–178. doi:10.1016/S0933-3657(01)00100-2 PMID:11830369

Park, H. (2006). Part 2: Multilayer perceptron and natural gradient learning. *New Generation Computing*, *24*(1), 79–95. doi:10.1007/BF03037294

Parkinson, A. R., Balling, R. J., & Hedengren, J. D. (2013). *Optimization Methods for Engineering Design: Applications and Theory* (5th ed.). Brigham Young University.

Parthiban, L., & Subramanian, R. (2006, December). Speckle noise removal using contourlets. In *Information and Automation, 2006. ICIA 2006. International Conference on* (pp. 250-253). IEEE. 10.1109/ICINFA.2006.374121

Parton, K. (1990). Back Injuries on farms: Regional variations in New South Wales. *Journal of Occup Health Safety-Aust NZ*, *6*, 53–59.

Pascual, S. A., & Naqvi, S. (2008). An Investigation of Ergonomics Analysis Tools Used in Industry in the Identification of Work-Related Musculoskeletal Disorders. *International Journal of Occupational Safety and Ergonomics*, *14*(2), 237–245. doi:10.1080/10803548.2008.11076755 PMID:18534158

Patil, S. B., & Kumaraswamy, Y. S. (2009). Intelligent and effective heart attack prediction system using data mining and artificial neural network. *European Journal of Scientific Research*, *31*(4), 642–656.

Patro, V. M., & Patra, M. R. (2015). *A Novel Approach to Compute Confusion Matrix for Classification of n-Class Attributes with Feature Selection.* doi:10.14738/tmlai.32.1108

Pattnaik, S., Dash, M., & Sabut, S. K. (2016). DWT-based feature extraction and classification for motor imaginary EEG signals. In *Systems in Medicine and Biology (ICSMB), 2016 International Conference on.* IEEE.

Pazzani, M. J., & Ratanamahatana, C. A. (2005). Exact indexing of dynamic time warping. *Knowledge and Information Systems*, *7*(3), 358–386. doi:10.100710115-004-0154-9

Peng, Y., Zhu, Y., & Wang, Y. (2016). A fast medical image segmentation method of based on initial contour forecast segmentation model. *International Journal Of Computing Science And Mathematics*, *7*(3), 212. doi:10.1504/IJCSM.2016.077863

Peretto, P. (1992). *An Introduction to the Modeling of Neural Networks*. Cambridge, UK: Cambridge University Press. doi:10.1017/CBO9780511622793

Perona, P., & Malik, J. (1990). Scale-space and edge detection using anisotropic diffusion. *IEEE Transactions on Pattern Analysis and Machine Intelligence*, *12*(7), 629–639. doi:10.1109/34.56205

Perperidis, A. (2016). Postprocessing approaches for the improvement of cardiac ultrasound B-mode images: A review. *IEEE Transactions on Ultrasonics, Ferroelectrics, and Frequency Control*, *63*(3), 470–485. doi:10.1109/TUFFC.2016.2526670 PMID:26886981

Phyu, T. N. (2009). Survey of classification techniques in data mining. *Proceedings of the International MultiConference of Engineers and Computer Scientists.*

Pickett, W., King, N., Lawson, J., Dosman, J. A., Trask, C., Brison, R. J., ... Janssen, I. (2015). Farmers, mechanized work, and links to obesity. *Preventive Medicine*, *70C*, 59–63. doi:10.1016/j.ypmed.2014.11.012 PMID:25448840

Pinzke, S., Stål, M., & Hansson, G.-A. (2001). Physical workload on upper extremities in various operations during machine milking. *Annals of Agricultural and Environmental Medicine*, *8*, 63–70. PMID:11426927

Pircher, M., Götzinger, E., Leitgeb, R. A., Fercher, A. F., & Hitzenberger, C. K. (2003). Speckle reduction in optical coherence tomography by frequency compounding. *Journal of Biomedical Optics*, *8*(3), 565–570. doi:10.1117/1.1578087 PMID:12880365

Pitas, I., Strintzis, M. G., Grippas, S., & Xerostylides, C. (1983). Machine classification of ischemic electrocardiograms. Presented at the *IEEE Mediterranean Electrotechnical Conf.*, Athens, Greece.

Pittman, P. (2010). Health Services Research in 2020: data and methods needs for the future. *Health Services Research, 45*(5), 1431-1441.

Pizurica, A., Jovanov, L., Huysmans, B., Zlokolica, V., De Keyser, P., Dhaenens, F., & Philips, W. (2008). Multiresolution denoising for optical coherence tomography: A review and evaluation. *Current Medical Imaging Reviews*, *4*(4), 270–284. doi:10.2174/157340508786404044

Pizurica, A., Philips, W., Lemahieu, I., & Acheroy, M. (2003). A versatile wavelet domain noise filtration technique for medical imaging. *IEEE Transactions on Medical Imaging*, *22*(3), 323–331. doi:10.1109/TMI.2003.809588 PMID:12760550

Pizurica, A., Wink, A. M., Vansteenkiste, E., Philips, W., & Roerdink, B. J. (2006). A review of wavelet denoising in MRI and ultrasound brain imaging. *Current Medical Imaging Reviews*, *2*(2), 247–260. doi:10.2174/157340506776930665

Platonov, A. (2016). Information theory and optimization of analog feedback communication systems. *IEEE International Black Sea Conference on Communications and Networking*. 10.1109/BlackSeaCom.2016.7901541

Polat, K., & Gunes, S. (2009). A new feature selection method on classification of medical datasets: Kernel F-score feature selection. *Expert Systems with Applications*, *36*(7), 10367–10373. doi:10.1016/j.eswa.2009.01.041

Pollack, K., Sorock, G., Slade, M., Cantley, L., Sircar, K., Taiwo, O., & Cullen, M. R. (2007). Association between body mass index and acute traumatic workplace injury in hourly manufacturing employees. *American Journal of Epidemiology, 166*(2), 204–211. doi:10.1093/aje/kwm058 PMID:17485732

Portet, F., Hernandez, A. I., & Carrault, G. (2005). Evaluation of realtime QRS detection algorithms in variable contexts. *Medical & Biological Engineering & Computing, 43*(3), 379–385. doi:10.1007/BF02345816 PMID:16035227

Pourghassem, H., & Ghassemian, H. (2008). Content-based medical image classification using a new hierarchical merging scheme. *Computerized Medical Imaging and Graphics, 32*(8), 651–661. doi:10.1016/j.compmedimag.2008.07.006 PMID:18789648

Povazay, B., Bizheva, K., Unterhuber, A., Hermann, B., Sattmann, H., Fercher, A. F., ... Russell, P. S. J. (2002). Submicrometer axial resolution optical coherence tomography. *Optics Letters, 27*(20), 1800–1802. doi:10.1364/OL.27.001800 PMID:18033368

Power, D. J., Sharda, R., & Burstein, F. (2013). Decision support systems. John Wiley & Sons, Ltd.

Pradhan, L., Taneja, N. A., Dixit, C., & Suhag, M. (2017). *Comparison of Text Classifiers on News Articles.* Academic Press.

Pradhan, M., Ranjit, & Sahu, K. (2011). Predict the onset of diabetes disease using Artificial Neural Network (ANN). *International Journal of Computer Science & Emerging Technologies, 2.*

Prakash, S., Chakravarthy, T., & Kaveri, E. (2015). Statistically weighted reviews to enhance sentiment classification. *Karbala International Journal of Modern Science, 1*(1), 26–31. doi:10.1016/j.kijoms.2015.07.001

Prasad, A., Belwin Edward, J., & Ravi, K. (n.d.). A review on fault classification methodologies in power transmission systems: Part—I. *Journal of Electrical Systems and Information Technology.* doi:10.1016/j.jesit.2017.01.004

Pueyo, E., Sörnmo, L., & Laguna, P. (2008). QRS Slopes for Detection and Characterization of Myocardial Ischemia. *IEEE Transactions on Biomedical Engineering, 55*(2), 468–477. doi:10.1109/TBME.2007.902228 PMID:18269981

Punnett, L., & Wegman, D. H. (2004). Work-related musculoskeletal disorders: The epidemiologic evidence and the debate. *Journal of Electromyography and Kinesiology, 14*(1), 13–23. doi:10.1016/j.jelekin.2003.09.015 PMID:14759746

Puvanathasan, P., & Bizheva, K. (2009). Interval type-II fuzzy anisotropic diffusion algorithm for speckle noise reduction in optical coherence tomography images. *Optics Express, 17*(2), 733–746. doi:10.1364/OE.17.000733 PMID:19158887

Qin, B., Xia, Y., Prabhakar, S., & Tu, Y. (2009). *A rule-based classification algorithm for uncertain data.* Paper presented at the Data Engineering, 2009. ICDE'09. IEEE 25th International Conference on.

Quellec, G., Lee, K., Dolejsi, M., Garvin, M. K., Abramoff, M. D., & Sonka, M. (2010). Three-dimensional analysis of retinal layer texture: Identification of fluid-filled regions in SD-OCT of the macula. *IEEE Transactions on Medical Imaging, 29*(6), 1321–1330. doi:10.1109/TMI.2010.2047023 PMID:20363675

Qu, G., Zhang, D., & Yan, P. (2002). Information measure for performance of image fusion. *Electronics Letters, 38*(7), 313–315. doi:10.1049/el:20020212

Quigley, D. D., Elliott, M. N., Setodji, C. M., & Hays, R. D. (2018). Quantifying Magnitude of Group-Level Differences in Patient Experiences with Health Care. *Health Services Research, 53*, 3027–3051. doi:10.1111/1475-6773.12828 PMID:29435975

Raanaas, R. K., & Anderson, D. (2008). A questionnaire survey of Norwegian taxi drivers' musculoskeletal health, and work-related risk factors. *International Journal of Industrial Ergonomics, 38*(3-4), 280–290. doi:10.1016/j.ergon.2007.10.017

Rabbani, H., Sonka, M., & Abramoff, M. D. (2013). Optical coherence tomography noise reduction using anisotropic local bivariate Gaussian mixture prior in 3D complex wavelet domain. *Journal of Biomedical Imaging*, *2013*, 22. PMID:24222760

Rabbani, H., Vafadust, M., Abolmaesumi, P., & Gazor, S. (2008). Speckle noise reduction of medical ultrasound images in complex wavelet domain using mixture priors. *IEEE Transactions on Biomedical Engineering*, *55*(9), 2152–2160. doi:10.1109/TBME.2008.923140 PMID:18713684

Radiopaedia. (n.d.). Retrieved from https://radiopaedia.org

Raghavendra, U., Acharya, U. R., Gudigar, A., Shetty, R., Krishnananda, N., Pai, U., ... Nayak, C. (2017). Automated screening of congestive heart failure using variational mode decomposition and texture features extracted from ultrasound images. *Neural Computing & Applications*, *28*(10), 2869–2878. doi:10.100700521-017-2839-5

Rajabi, H., & Zirak, A. (2016). Speckle noise reduction and motion artifact correction based on modified statistical parameters estimation in OCT images. *Biomedical Physics & Engineering Express*, *2*(3), 035012. doi:10.1088/2057-1976/2/3/035012

Rajalingam, B., & Priya, R. (2017a). A Novel approach for Multimodal Medical Image Fusion using Hybrid Fusion Algorithms for Disease Analysis. *International Journal of Pure and Applied Mathematics*, *117*(15), 599–619.

Rajalingam, B., & Priya, R. (2017b). Multimodality Medical Image Fusion Based on Hybrid Fusion Techniques. *International Journal of Engineering and Manufacturing Science*, *7*(1).

Rajalingam, B., & Priya, R. (2018a). Hybrid Multimodality Medical Image Fusion based on Guided Image Filter with Pulse Coupled Neural Network. *International Journal of Scientific Research in Science. Engineering and Technology*, *5*(3), 86–100.

Rajalingam, B., & Priya, R. (2018b). Hybrid Multimodality Medical Image Fusion Technique for Feature Enhancement in Medical Diagnosis. *International Journal of Engineering Science Invention*, *2*, 52–60.

Rajalingam, B., & Priya, R. (2018c). Combining Multi-Modality Medical Image Fusion Based on Hybrid Intelligence for Disease Identification. *International Journal of Advanced Research Trends in Engineering and Technology*, *5*(12), 862–887.

Rajalingam, B., & Priya, R. (2018d). Enhancement of Hybrid Multimodal Medical Image Fusion Techniques for Clinical Disease Analysis. *International Journal of Computer Vision and Image Processing*, *8*(3), 17–40. doi:10.4018/IJCVIP.2018070102

Rajalingam, B., & Priya, R. (2018e). Multimodal Medical Image Fusion based on Deep Learning Neural Network for Clinical Treatment Analysis. *International Journal of Chemtech Research*, *11*(6), 160–176.

Rajalingam, B., & Priya, R. (2018f). Multimodal Medical Image Fusion Using Various Hybrid Fusion Techniques For clinical Treatment Analysis. *Smart Construction Research*, *2*(2), 1–20.

Rajalingam, B., & Priya, R. (2018g). Review of Multimodality Medical Image Fusion Using Combined Transform Techniques for Clinical Application. *International Journal of Scientific Research in Computer Science Applications and Management Studies*, *7*(3).

Rajeeb, D., Vaibhav, B., Gagan, G., & Barnali, D. (2008). *Application of artificial neural network technique for diagnosing diabetes mellitus. In IEEE Region 10 Colloquium and the Third ICIIS* (pp. 18–23). Kharagpur: IEEE.

Rajendran, P., & Madheswaran, M. (2010). Hybrid Medical Image Classification Using Association Rule Mining with Decision Tree Algorithm. *Journal of Computers*, *2*(1), 127–136.

Raj, S., & Ray, K. C. (2017). ECG signal analysis using DCT-based DOST and PSO optimized SVM. *IEEE Transactions on Instrumentation and Measurement*, *66*(3), 470–478. doi:10.1109/TIM.2016.2642758

Ramos-Llordén, G., Vegas-Sánchez-Ferrero, G., Martin-Fernandez, M., Alberola-López, C., & Aja-Fernández, S. (2015). Anisotropic diffusion filter with memory based on speckle statistics for ultrasound images. *IEEE Transactions on Image Processing*, *24*(1), 345–358. doi:10.1109/TIP.2014.2371244 PMID:25415987

Ramrath, L., Moreno, G., Mueller, H., Bonin, T., Huettmann, G., & Schweikard, A. (2008, September). Towards multi-directional OCT for speckle noise reduction. In *International Conference on Medical Image Computing and Computer-Assisted Intervention* (pp. 815-823). Springer. 10.1007/978-3-540-85988-8_97

Ranawana, R., & Palade, V. (2006). Multi-classifier systems: Review and a roadmap for developers. *International Journal of Hybrid Intelligent Systems*, *3*(1), 35–61. doi:10.3233/HIS-2006-3104

Rangnath, R., Perotte, A., Elhadad, N., & Blei, D. (2016). Deep Survival Analysis. In *Proceedings of the 1st Machine Learning in Health Care*, (pp. 101-114). Los Angeles, CA: Academic Press.

Raschka, S. (2014). *Naive bayes and text classification i-introduction and theory*. arXiv preprint arXiv:1410.5329

Rashid, T. A., Abdulla, S. M., & Abdulla, R. M. (2016). Decision support system for diabetes mellitus through machine learning techniques. *Database, 7.*

Rashid, T. A., & Abdullah, S. M. (2018). A Hybrid of Artificial Bee Colony, Genetic Algorithm, and Neural Network for Diabetic Mellitus Diagnosing. *ARO-The Scientific Journal of Koya University*, *6*(1), 55–64. doi:10.14500/aro.10368

Rashid, T. A., Abdullah, S. M., & Abdullah, R. M. (2016). An intelligent approach for diabetes classification, prediction, and description. In *Innovations in Bio-Inspired Computing and Applications* (pp. 323–335). Cham: Springer. doi:10.1007/978-3-319-28031-8_28

Rashid, T. A., Abdullah, S. M., & Abdullah, R. M. (2016). *An Intelligent Approach for Diabetes Classification*. Cham: Prediction and Description.

Rasku, J., Juhola, M., Toppila, E., & Pyykko, I. (2007). Recognition of balance signals between healthy subjects and otoneurological patients with hidden Markov models. *Biomedical Signal Processing and Control*, *2*(1), 1–8. doi:10.1016/j.bspc.2006.12.005

Ravı, D., Wong, C., Deligianni, F., Berthelot, M., Andreu-Perez, J., Lo, B., & Yang, G. Z. (2017). Deep learning for health informatics. *IEEE Journal of Biomedical and Health Informatics*, *21*(1), 4–21. doi:10.1109/JBHI.2016.2636665 PMID:28055930

Ray, P., Parida, R., & Sarkar, S. (2015). Ergonomic analysis of construction jobs in India: A biomechanical modelling approach. *Procedia Manufacturing*, *3*, 4606–4612. doi:10.1016/j.promfg.2015.07.542

Reid, C. R., McCauley, B. P., Karwowski, W., & Durrani, S. K. (2010). Occupational postural activity and lower extremity discomfort: A review. *International Journal of Industrial Ergonomics*, *40*(3), 247–256. doi:10.1016/j.ergon.2010.01.003

Rejer, I., & Górski, P. (2017). Independent component analysis in a motor imagery brain computer interface. In *Smart Technologies, IEEE EUROCON 2017-17th International Conference on*. IEEE.

Ren, H., Qin, L., & Zhu, X. (2016). Speckle reduction and cartoon-texture decomposition of ophthalmic optical coherence tomography images by variational image decomposition. *Optik-International Journal for Light and Electron Optics*, *127*(19), 7809–7821. doi:10.1016/j.ijleo.2016.05.088

Riza, L. S., Janusz, A., Bergmeir, C., Cornelis, C., Herrera, F., Śle¸zak, D., & Benítez, J. M. (2014). Implementing algorithms of rough set theory and fuzzy rough set theory in the R package "RoughSets". *Information Sciences*, *287*, 68–89. doi:10.1016/j.ins.2014.07.029

Robinson, V., & Varghese, E. B. (2016). A novel approach for ensuring the privacy of EEG signals using application-specific feature extraction and AES algorithm. In *Inventive Computation Technologies (ICICT), International Conference on* (Vol. 2). IEEE.

Rogowska, J., & Brezinski, M. E. (2002). Image processing techniques for noise removal, enhancement and segmentation of cartilage OCT images. *Physics in Medicine and Biology*, *47*(4), 641–655. doi:10.1088/0031-9155/47/4/307 PMID:11900196

Rokach, L. (2010). Ensemble-based classifiers. *Artificial Intelligence Review*, *33*(1-2), 1–39. doi:10.100710462-009-9124-7

Ryba, T., & Zelezny, M. (2015). An automatic image segmentation algorithm involving shortest path basins. *Pattern Recognition and Image Analysis*, *25*(1), 89–95. doi:10.1134/S1054661815010162

Saba, L., Acharya, U. R., Guerriero, S., & Suri, J. S. (Eds.). (2014). *Ovarian Neoplasm Imaging*. Springer Science & Business Media.

Saddichaa, S. (2010). Information about acute insomnia. *Annals of Indian Academy of Neurology*, *13*(2). Available at https://www.ncbi.nlm.nih.gov/pmc/articles/PMC2924526/

Sadh, A. S., & Shukla, N. (2013). Association rules Optimization: A survey. *International Journal of Advanced Computer Research*, *3*(9), 111–115.

Sahoo, S., Kanungo, B., Behera, S., & Sabut, S. (2017). Multiresolution wavelet transform based feature extraction and ECG classification to detect cardiac abnormalities. *Measurement*, *108*, 55–66. doi:10.1016/j.measurement.2017.05.022

Sahu, S., & Mehtre, B. M. (2015). Network intrusion detection system using J48 Decision Tree. *International Conference on Advances in Computing Communication Information*, *2015*, 2023–2026. doi:10.1109/icacci.2015.7275914

Sakai, M. (2013). Kernel Nonnegative Matrix Factorization with Constraint Increasing the Discriminability of Two Classes for the EEG Feature Extraction. In *Signal-Image Technology & Internet-Based Systems (SITIS), 2013 International Conference on*. IEEE.

Saktheeswari, R., & Adalarasu, K. (2017). Survey on signal processing techniques for diagnoising cardiovascular diseases. *2017 International Conference on Innovations in Information, Embedded and Communication Systems (ICIIECS)*. 10.1109/ICIIECS.2017.8276116

Salazar-Varas, R., & Gutiérrez, D. (2015). Feature extraction for multi-class BCI using EEG coherence. In *Neural Engineering (NER), 2015 7th International IEEE/EMBS Conference on*. IEEE.

Salinas, H. M., & Fernández, D. C. (2007). Comparison of PDE-based nonlinear diffusion approaches for image enhancement and denoising in optical coherence tomography. *IEEE Transactions on Medical Imaging*, *26*(6), 761–771. doi:10.1109/TMI.2006.887375 PMID:17679327

Salzberg, S. L. (1994). C4. 5: Programs for machine learning by j. ross quinlan. *Machine Learning*, *16*(3), 235–240. doi:10.1007/BF00993309

Samagaio, G., Estévez, A., de Moura, J., Novo, J., Fernandez, M. I., & Ortega, M. (2018). Automatic Macular Edema Identification and Characterization Using OCT Images. *Computer Methods and Programs in Biomedicine*, *163*, 47–63. doi:10.1016/j.cmpb.2018.05.033 PMID:30119857

Saminu, S., Özkurt, N., & Karaye, I. A. (2008). Wavelet Feature Extraction for ECG Beat Classification. *2014 IEEE 6th International Conference on Adaptive Science & Technology (ICAST).*

Sander, B., Larsen, M., Thrane, L., Hougaard, J. L., & Jørgensen, T. M. (2005). Enhanced optical coherence tomography imaging by multiple scan averaging. *The British Journal of Ophthalmology, 89*(2), 207–212. doi:10.1136/bjo.2004.045989 PMID:15665354

Sannino, G., & De Pietro, G. (2011). A smart context-aware mobile monitoring system for heart patients. *IEEE International Conference on Bioinformatics and Biomedicine Workshops (BIBMW).* 10.1109/BIBMW.2011.6112448

Saqlain, S. M., Sher, M., Shah, F. A., Khan, I., Ashraf, M. U., Awais, M., & Ghani, A. (2018). Fisher score and Matthews correlation coefficient-based feature subset selection for heart disease diagnosis using support vector machines. *Knowledge and Information Systems*, 1–29.

Sasakawa, T., Hu, J., & Hirasawa, K. (2007). A brainlike learning system with supervised, unsupervised, and reinforcement learning. *Electrical Engineering in Japan, 162*(1), 32–39. doi:10.1002/eej.20600

Sau, A., & Bhakta, I. (2017) Predicting anxiety and depression in elderly patients using machine learning technology. Healthcare Technology Letters, 4(6), 238-243.

Saurin, T. A., & de Macedo Guimaraes, L. B. (2008). Ergonomic assessment of suspended scaffolds. *International Journal of Industrial Ergonomics, 38*(2), 238–246. doi:10.1016/j.ergon.2005.11.010

Schirrmacher, F., Köhler, T., Husvogt, L., Fujimoto, J. G., Hornegger, J., & Maier, A. K. (2017, September). Quasi: Quantile sparse image prior for spatio-temporal denoising of retinal oct data. In *International Conference on Medical Image Computing and Computer-Assisted Intervention* (pp. 83-91). Springer. 10.1007/978-3-319-66185-8_10

Schmidhuber, J. (1997). Discovering neural nets with low Kolmogorov complexity and high generalization capability. *Neural Networks, 10*(5), 857–873. doi:10.1016/S0893-6080(96)00127-X PMID:12662875

Schmidhuber, J., Wierstra, D., Gagliolo, M., & Gomez, F. (2007). Training Recurrent Networks by Evolino. *Neural Computation, 19*(3), 757-779.

Schmitt, J. M. (1999). Optical coherence tomography (OCT): A review. *IEEE Journal of Selected Topics in Quantum Electronics, 5*(4), 1205–1215. doi:10.1109/2944.796348

Schmitt, J. M., & Knüttel, A. (1997). Model of optical coherence tomography of heterogeneous tissue. *JOSA A, 14*(6), 1231–1242. doi:10.1364/JOSAA.14.001231

Schmitt, J. M., Xiang, S. H., & Yung, K. M. (1999). Speckle in optical coherence tomography. *Journal of Biomedical Optics, 4*(1), 95–106. doi:10.1117/1.429925 PMID:23015175

Schreuder, K. J., Roelen, C. A. M., Koopmans, A. C., & Groothoff, J. W. (2008). Job demands and health complaints in white and blue collar workers. *Work (Reading, Mass.), 31*, 425–432. PMID:19127013

Scuffham, A. M., Legg, S. J., Firth, E. C., & Stevenson, M. A. (2010). Prevalence and risk factors associated with musculoskeletal discomfort in New Zealand veterinarians. *Applied Ergonomics, 41*(3), 444–453. doi:10.1016/j.apergo.2009.09.009 PMID:19857858

Seabra, J. C. R. (2011). *Medical ultrasound b-mode modeling, de-speckling and tissue characterization assessing the atherosclerotic disease* (Doctoral dissertation). Instituto Superior Técnico.

Seabra, J., Xavier, J., & Sanches, J. (2008, August). Convex ultrasound image reconstruction with log-euclidean priors. In *Engineering in Medicine and Biology Society, 2008. EMBS 2008. 30th Annual International Conference of the IEEE* (pp. 435-438). IEEE.

Seetharaman, K., & Krishnamoorthi, R. (2007). A Statistical Framework Based on A Family of Full Range Autoregressive Models for Edge Extraction. *Pattern Recognition Letters*, *28*(7), 759–770. doi:10.1016/j.patrec.2006.11.003

Seetharaman, K., & Palanivel, N. (2013). Texture Characterization, Representation, Description and Classification Based on a Family of Full Range Gaussian Markov Random Field Model. *International Journal of Image and Data Fusion*, *4*(4), 342–362. doi:10.1080/19479832.2013.804007

Sekar, B. D., & Dong, M. (2014). Function Formula Oriented Construction of Bayesian Inference Nets for Diagnosis of Cardiovascular Disease. *BioMed Research International*. PMID:25247174

Serhani, M. A., El Menshawy, M., Benharref, A., & Navaz, A. N. (2015). Real time EEG compression for energy-aware continous mobile monitoring. In *Microelectronics (ICM), 2015 27th International Conference on*. IEEE.

Setiawan, N. A., Venkatachalam, P. A., & Hani, A. F. (2009). Diagnosis of coronary artery disease using artificial intelligence based decision support system. In *International Conference on Man-Machine Systems*, (pp. 1-5). Batu Ferringhi, Penang: Academic Press.

Shadmand, S., & Mashoufi, B. (2016). A new personalized ECG signal classification algorithm using block-based neural network and particle swarm optimization. *Biomedical Signal Processing and Control*, *25*, 12–23. doi:10.1016/j.bspc.2015.10.008

Shah, H., Meghji, A. F., & Mahoto, N. A. (2018). Healthcare Services in Developing Countries of the South Asian Region: Present and Future Perspectives. In Design and Development of Affordable Healthcare Technologies. IGI Global. Doi:10.4018/978-1-5225-4969-7.ch001

Shahdoosti, H. R., & Rahemi, Z. (2018). A maximum likelihood filter using non-local information for despeckling of ultrasound images. *Machine Vision and Applications*, *29*(4), 689–702. doi:10.100700138-018-0929-8

Shahidi, M., Wang, Z., & Zelkha, R. (2005). Quantitative thickness measurement of retinal layers imaged by optical coherence tomography. *American Journal of Ophthalmology*, *139*(6), 1056–1061. doi:10.1016/j.ajo.2005.01.012 PMID:15953436

Shahin, M., Ahmed, B., Hamida, S. T. B., Mulaffer, F. L., Glos, M., & Penzel, T. (2017). Deep Learning and Insomnia: Assisting Clinicians With Their Diagnosis. *IEEE Journal of Biomedical and Health Informatics*, *21*(6), 1546–1553. doi:10.1109/JBHI.2017.2650199 PMID:28092583

Shah, S. (2009). Blindness and visual impairment due to retinal diseases. *Community Eye Health*, *22*(69), 8. PMID:19506713

Shaikh, A., Mahoto, N., Khuhawar, F., & Memon, M. (2015). Performance evaluation of classification methods for heart disease dataset. *Sindh University Research Journal-SURJ (Science Series)*, *47*(3).

Shaikhina, T., Lowe, D., Daga, S., Briggs, D., Higgins, R., & Khovanova, N. (2017). Decision tree and random forest models for outcome prediction in antibody incompatible kidney transplantation. *Biomedical Signal Processing and Control*. doi:10.1016/j.bspc.2017.01.012

Shanker, M. (1996). Using Neural Networks to Predict the Onset of Diabetes Mellitus. *Journal of Chemical Information and Computer Sciences*, *36*(1), 35–41. doi:10.1021/ci950063e PMID:8576289

Shao, D., Zhou, T., Liu, F., Yi, S., Xiang, Y., Ma, L., ... He, J. (2017). Ultrasound speckle reduction based on fractional order differentiation. *Journal of Medical Ultrasonics (2001)*, *44*(3), 227–237. doi:10.100710396-016-0763-4 PMID:28012088

Shao, G., & Sang, N. (2017). Regularized max-min linear discriminant analysis. *Pattern Recognition*, *66*, 353–363. doi:10.1016/j.patcog.2016.12.030

Shatovskaya, T., Repka, V., & Good, A. (2006). Application of the Bayesian Networks in the informational modeling. *International conference: Modern problems of radio engineering, telecommunications, and computer science* (p. 108). Lviv-Slavsko, Ukraine: Academic Press.

Shaw, L. J., Bugiardini, R., & Merz, C. N. B. (2009). Women and ischemic heart disease: Evolving knowledge. *Journal of the American College of Cardiology*, *54*(17), 1561–1575. doi:10.1016/j.jacc.2009.04.098 PMID:19833255

Shepp, L. A., & Logan, B. F. (1974). The Fourier reconstruction of a head section. *IEEE Transactions on Nuclear Science*, *21*(3), 21–43. doi:10.1109/TNS.1974.6499235

Shi, H., & Liu, Y. (2011). Naïve Bayes vs. Support Vector Machine: Resilience to Missing Data. In *International Conference on Artificial Intelligence and Computational Intelligence* (pp. 680-687). Chengdu, China: LNCS, Springer. 10.1007/978-3-642-23887-1_86

Shrivas, A. K. & R. K. Y. (2017). An Effective Prediction Factors for Coronary Heart Disease using Data Mining based Classification Technique. *International Journal on Recent and Innovation Trends in Computing and Communication*, *5*(5).

Siegel, C. (2014). Re: Fully Automated Prostate Segmentation on MRI: Comparison with Manual Segmentation Methods and Specimen Volumes. *The Journal of Urology*, *192*(3), 767. doi:10.1016/j.juro.2014.06.025

Sierra, B., Lazkano, E., Irigoien, I., Jauregi, E., & Mendialdua, I. (2011). K Nearest Neighbor Equality: Giving equal chance to all existing classes. *Information Sciences*, *181*(23), 5158–5168. doi:10.1016/j.ins.2011.07.024

Sietsma, J., & Dow, R. (1991). Creating artificial neural networks that generalize. *Neural Networks*, *4*(1), 67–79. doi:10.1016/0893-6080(91)90033-2

Silveira, M., Nascimento, J. C., Marques, J. S., Marçal, A. R. S., Mendonça, T., Yamauchi, S., ... Rozeira, J. (2009). Comparison of Segmentation Methods for Melanoma Diagnosis in Dermoscopy Images. *IEEE Journal of Selected Topics in Signal Processing*, *3*(1), 35–45. doi:10.1109/JSTSP.2008.2011119

Singh, P. P., Prasad, S., Das, B., Poddar, U., & Choudhury, D. R. (2018). Classification of Diabetic Patient Data Using Machine Learning Techniques. Singapore: Academic Press. doi:10.1007/978-981-10-7386-1_37

Singh, K., Ranade, S. K., & Singh, C. (2017). A hybrid algorithm for speckle noise reduction of ultrasound images. *Computer Methods and Programs in Biomedicine*, *148*, 55–69. doi:10.1016/j.cmpb.2017.06.009 PMID:28774439

Singh, S., & Arora, R. (2010). Ergonomic Intervention for Preventing Musculoskeletal Disorders among Farm Women. *Journal of Agri. Science*, *1*(2), 61–71.

Singh, S., & Sachdeva, G. (2012). Yagi-Uda Antenna Design Optimization for Maximum Gain using different BBO Migration Variants. *International Journal of Computers and Applications*, *58*(5), 14–18. doi:10.5120/9278-3471

Siuly, S., & Li, Y. (2012). Improving the separability of motor imagery EEG signals using a cross correlation-based least square support vector machine for brain–computer interface. *IEEE Transactions on Neural Systems and Rehabilitation Engineering*, *20*(4), 526–538. doi:10.1109/TNSRE.2012.2184838 PMID:22287252

Sivan, S., & Darsan, G. (2016). Computer Vision based Assistive Technology for Blind and Visually Impaired People. In *Proceedings of the 7th International Conference on Computing Communication and Networking Technologies* (p. 41). ACM. 10.1145/2967878.2967923

Skaer, T. L. (n.d.). *Treatment of Insomnia with Comorbid Mental Illness.* Retrieved from http://cdn.intechopen.com/pdfs/32274.pdf

Smith, D. R., & Leggat, P. A. (2003). Musculoskeletal disorders in nursing. *Australian Nursing Journal, 11*, 1–4.

Snae, C., & Brueckner, M. (2008). Personal health assistance service expert system (PHASES). *International Journal of Biological and Medical Sciences, 1*(2), 109–112.

Song, P., Manduca, A., Trzasko, J. D., & Chen, S. (2017). Ultrasound small vessel imaging with block-wise adaptive local clutter filtering. *IEEE Transactions on Medical Imaging, 36*(1), 251–262. doi:10.1109/TMI.2016.2605819 PMID:27608455

Soni, J., Ansari, U., Sharma, D., & Soni, S. (2011). Predictive data mining for medical diagnosis: An overview of heart disease prediction. *International Journal of Computers and Applications, 17*(8), 43–48. doi:10.5120/2237-2860

Sony, J., Ansari, U., Sharma, D., & Sony, S. (2011). "Predictive data mining for medical diagnosis: an overview of heart disease prediction" International Journal of Computer Science and Engineering, vol. 3. Ahmad, P., Qamar, S. & Rizvi, S.Q.A. (2015) Techniques of data mining in healthcare: A review. *International Journal of Computers and Applications, 120*(15).

Soorajkumar, R., Krishnakumar, P., Girish, D., & Rajan, J. (2016). Coupled PDE for ultrasound despeckling using ENI classification. *Procedia Computer Science, 89*, 658–665. doi:10.1016/j.procs.2016.06.031

Sreelakshmi, T.G., & Paul, S. (2015). *An Accurate ECG Feature Extraction Method for Detecting Multiple Cardiovascular Diseases.* Retrieved from: http://www.ijiset.com/v1s9/IJISET_V1_I9_08.pdf

Srinivasan, V. J., Monson, B. K., Wojtkowski, M., Bilonick, R. A., Gorczynska, I., Chen, R., ... Fujimoto, J. G. (2008). Characterization of outer retinal morphology with high-speed, ultrahigh-resolution optical coherence tomography. *Investigative Ophthalmology & Visual Science, 49*(4), 1571–1579. doi:10.1167/iovs.07-0838 PMID:18385077

Srivastava, R., Prakash, O., & Khare, A. (2016). Local energy-based multimodal medical image fusion in curvelet domain. *IET Computer Vision*, 1–16.

Stål, M., Pinzke, S., & Hansson, G.-A. (2003). The effect on workload by using a support arm in parlour milking. *International Journal of Industrial Ergonomics, 32*(2), 121–132. doi:10.1016/S0169-8141(03)00046-5

Stankiewicz, A., Marciniak, T., Dąbrowski, A., Stopa, M., Rakowicz, P., & Marciniak, E. (2017). Denoising methods for improving automatic segmentation in OCT images of human eye. *Bulletin of the Polish Academy of Sciences. Technical Sciences, 65*(1), 71–78. doi:10.1515/bpasts-2017-0009

Steinwachs, D. M., & Hughes, R. G. (2008). *Health services research: Scope and significance.* Academic Press.

Subhani, A. R., Mumtaz, W., Saad, M. N. B. M., Kamel, N., & Malik, A. S. (2017). Machine learning framework for the detection of mental stress at multiple levels. *IEEE Access: Practical Innovations, Open Solutions, 5*, 13545–13556. doi:10.1109/ACCESS.2017.2723622

Sudeep, P. V., Niwas, S. I., Palanisamy, P., Rajan, J., Xiaojun, Y., Wang, X., ... Liu, L. (2016). Enhancement and bias removal of optical coherence tomography images: An iterative approach with adaptive bilateral filtering. *Computers in Biology and Medicine, 71*, 97–107. doi:10.1016/j.compbiomed.2016.02.003 PMID:26907572

Sudeep, P. V., Palanisamy, P., Rajan, J., Baradaran, H., Saba, L., Gupta, A., & Suri, J. S. (2016). Speckle reduction in medical ultrasound images using an unbiased non-local means method. *Biomedical Signal Processing and Control, 28*, 1–8. doi:10.1016/j.bspc.2016.03.001

Sudharsan, B., Peeples, M., & Shomali, M. (2014). Hypoglycemia Prediction Using Machine Learning Models for Patients With Type 2 Diabetes. *Journal of Diabetes Science and Technology*, *9*(1), 86–90. doi:10.1177/1932296814554260 PMID:25316712

Sujith, B., & Safeeda, V. (2014). Computer Vision-Based Aid for the Visually Impaired Persons-A Survey and Proposing New Framework. *International Journal of Innovative Research in Computer and Communication Engineering.*

Suleiman, A.-B. R., & Fatehi, T. A.-H. (2007). Features extraction techniqes of EEG signal for BCI applications. Faculty of Computer and Information Engineering Department College of Electronics Engineering, University of Mosul.

Sun, J., & Reddy, C. K. (2013, August). Big data analytics for healthcare. In *Proceedings of the 19th ACM SIGKDD international conference on Knowledge discovery and data mining* (pp. 1525-1525). ACM. 10.1145/2487575.2506178

Suri, J. S. (2008). *Advances in diagnostic and therapeutic ultrasound imaging.* Artech House.

Susanti, S. P., & Azizah, F. N. (2017, November). Imputation of missing value using the dynamic Bayesian network for multivariate time series data. In *Data and Software Engineering (ICoDSE), 2017 International Conference on* (pp. 1-5). IEEE.

Syed, Z., & Guttag, J. (2011). Unsupervised Similarity-Based Risk Stratification for Cardiovascular Events Using Long-Term Time-Series Data. *Journal of Machine Learning Research*, *12*, 999–1024.

Tan, K. C., Teoh, E. J., Yu, Q., & Goh, K. C. (2009). A hybrid evolutionary algorithm for attribute selection in data mining. *Expert Systems with Applications*, *36*(4), 8616–8630. doi:10.1016/j.eswa.2008.10.013

Tao, Z., Tagare, H. D., & Beaty, J. D. (2006). Evaluation of four probability distribution models for speckle in clinical cardiac ultrasound images. *IEEE Transactions on Medical Imaging*, *25*(11), 1483–1491. doi:10.1109/TMI.2006.881376 PMID:17117777

Tarikm, A. R. (2016). Decision Support System for Diabetes Mellitus through Machine Learning Techniques. *International Journal of Advanced Computer Science and Applications*, *7*(7). doi:10.14569/IJACSA.2016.070724

Tay, P. C., Acton, S. T., & Hossack, J. A. (2006, April). A stochastic approach to ultrasound despeckling. In *Biomedical Imaging: Nano to Macro, 2006. 3rd IEEE International Symposium on* (pp. 221-224). IEEE. 10.1109/ISBI.2006.1624892

terBraack, E. M., de Jonge, B., & van Putten, M. J. A. M. (2013). Reduction of TMS induced artifacts in EEG using principal component analysis. *IEEE Transactions on Neural Systems and Rehabilitation Engineering*, *21*(3), 376–382. doi:10.1109/TNSRE.2012.2228674 PMID:23359012

Thapliyal, H., Khalus, V., & Labrado, C. (2017). Stress detection and management: A survey of wearable smart health devices. *IEEE Consumer Electronics Magazine*, *6*(4), 64–69. doi:10.1109/MCE.2017.2715578

Thomas, M., Das, M. K., & Ari, S. (2015). Automatic ECG arrhythmia classification using dual tree complex wavelet based features. *AEÜ. International Journal of Electronics and Communications*, *69*(4), 715–721. doi:10.1016/j.aeue.2014.12.013

Ting, K. M., & Witten, I. H. (1997). *Stacking bagged and dagged models.* Academic Press.

Tinubu, B. M. S., Mbada, C. E., Oyeyemi, A. L., & Fabunmi, A. A. (2010). Work-related musculoskeletal disorders among nurses in Ibadan, South-west Nigeria: A cross sectional. *BMC Musculoskeletal Disorders*, *11*(12). PMID:20089139

Tole, N. M., & Ostensen, H. (2005). *Basic physics of ultrasonographic imaging.* World Health Organization.

Tomar, D., & Agarwal, S. (2013). A survey on Data Mining approaches for Healthcare. *International Journal of Bio-Science and Bio-Technology*, *5*(5), 241–266. doi:10.14257/ijbsbt.2013.5.5.25

Tomasi, C., & Manduchi, R. (1998, January). Bilateral filtering for gray and color images. In *Computer Vision, 1998. Sixth International Conference on* (pp. 839-846). IEEE.

Tong, W., Kan, C., & Yang, H. (2018, March). Sensitivity analysis of wearable textiles for ECG sensing. In *Biomedical & Health Informatics (BHI), 2018 IEEE EMBS International Conference on* (pp. 157-160). IEEE.

Trahey, G. E., Allison, J. W., Smith, S. W., & Von Ramm, O. T. (1986). A quantitative approach to speckle reduction via frequency compounding. *Ultrasonic Imaging*, *8*(3), 151–164. doi:10.1177/016173468600800301 PMID:3548000

Tsai, D.-Y., Lee, Y., Sekiya, M., & Ohkubo, M. (2004). Medical image classification using genetic algorithm based fuzzy-logic approach. *Journal of Electronic Imaging*, *13*(4), 780–788. doi:10.1117/1.1786607

Tsipouras, M. G., Exarchos, T. P., Fotiadis, D. I., Kotsia, A. P., Vakalis, K. V., Naka, K. K., & Michalis, L. K. (2008). Automated Diagnosis of Coronary Artery Disease Based on Data Mining and Fuzzy Modeling. *IEEE Transactions on Information Technology in Biomedicine*, *12*(4), 447–458. doi:10.1109/TITB.2007.907985 PMID:18632325

Turabieh, H. (2016). A Hybrid ANN-GWO Algorithm for Prediction of Heart Disease. *American Journal of Operations Research*, *6*(02), 136–146. doi:10.4236/ajor.2016.62016

Ubeda, A., Ianez, E., Azor'in, J. M., Sabater-Navarro, J. M., & Fernandez, E. (2013). Classification method for BCIs based on the correlation of EEG maps. *Neurocomputing*, *114*, 98–106. doi:10.1016/j.neucom.2012.08.040

Übeyli, E. D. (2007). ECG beats classification using multiclass support vector machines with error correcting output codes. *Digital Signal Processing*, *17*(3), 675–684. doi:10.1016/j.dsp.2006.11.009

UCI Machine Learning Repository. (2018). *Cleveland Heart Disease Dataset*. Retrieved from https://archive.ics.uci.edu/ml/datasets/Heart+Disease

Uddin, M. S., Halder, K. K., Tahtali, M., Lambert, A. J., & Pickering, M. R. (2015, May). Speckle reduction and deblurring of ultrasound images using artificial neural network. In *Picture Coding Symposium (PCS)*, 2015 (pp. 105-108). IEEE. 10.1109/PCS.2015.7170056

Uguz, H. (2012). Adaptive neuro-fuzzy inference system for diagnosis of the heart valve diseases using wavelet transform with entropy. *Neural Computing & Applications*, *21*(7), 1617–1628. doi:10.100700521-011-0610-x

United Nations. (2010). World population data available at United Nations. *World Population Prospects: The 2010.* Retrieved on July 13, 2018 available at http://esa.un.org/unpd/wpp

Utyuzh, O., Wilk, G., & Wodarczyk, Z. (2007). Numerical symmetrization of state of identical particles. *Brazilian Journal of Physics*, *37*(2c). doi:10.1590/S0103-97332007000500007

Vafaie, M. H., Ataei, M., & Koofigar, H. R. (2014). Heart diseases prediction based on ECG signals' classification using agenetic-fuzzy system and dynamical model of ECG signals. *Biomedical Signal Processing and Control*, *14*, 291–296. doi:10.1016/j.bspc.2014.08.010

Valeriani, D., Cinel, C., & Poli, R. (2017). Augmenting Group Performance in Target-Face Recognition via Collaborative Brain-Computer Interfaces for Surveillance Applications. 2017 *8th International IEEE/EMBS Conference on Neural Engineering (NER).*

Vapnik, V. (2013). *The nature of statistical learning theory*. Springer science & business media.

Varnousfaderani, E. S., Vogl, W. D., Wu, J., Gerendas, B. S., Simader, C., Langs, G., . . . Schmidt-Erfurth, U. (2016, March). Geodesic denoising for optical coherence tomography images. In Medical Imaging 2016: Image Processing (Vol. 9784, p. 97840K). International Society for Optics and Photonics.

Vedula, S., Senouf, O., Bronstein, A. M., Michailovich, O. V., & Zibulevsky, M. (2017). *Towards CT-quality Ultrasound Imaging using Deep Learning.* arXiv preprint arXiv:1710.06304

Vegas-Sánchez-Ferrero, G., Martín-Martínez, D., Aja-Fernández, S., & Palencia, C. (2010, April). On the influence of interpolation on probabilistic models for ultrasonic images. In *Biomedical Imaging: From Nano to Macro, 2010 IEEE International Symposium on* (pp. 292-295). IEEE.

Vegas-Sánchez-Ferrero, G., Martín-Martínez, D., Aja-Fernández, S., & Palencia, C. (2010a, April). On the influence of interpolation on probabilistic models for ultrasonic images. In *Biomedical Imaging: From Nano to Macro, 2010 IEEE International Symposium on* (pp. 292-295). IEEE.

Vegas-Sanchez-Ferrero, G., Aja-Fernandez, S., Martín-Fernández, M., Frangi, A. F., & Palencia, C. (2010, September). Probabilistic-driven oriented speckle reducing anisotropic diffusion with application to cardiac ultrasonic images. In *International Conference on Medical Image Computing and Computer-Assisted Intervention* (pp. 518-525). Springer. 10.1007/978-3-642-15705-9_63

Velázquez, R. (2010). Wearable assistive devices for the blind. In *Wearable and autonomous biomedical devices and systems for smart environment* (pp. 331–349). Berlin: Springer. doi:10.1007/978-3-642-15687-8_17

W.H.O. (2018). Retrieved from http://www.who.int/mediacentre/factsheets/fs310.pdf

Wahbeh, A. H., Al-Radaideh, Q. A., Al-Kabi, M. N., & Al-Shawakfa, E. M. (2011). A comparison study between data mining tools over some classification methods. *International Journal of Advanced Computer Science and Applications*, *8*(2), 18–26.

Wang, J., Gao, X. Z., Tanskanen, J. M. A., & Guo, P. (2012). Epileptic EEG Signal Classification with ANFIS based on Harmony Search Method. In *Computational Intelligence and Security (CIS), 2012 Eighth International Conference on*. IEEE.

Wang, L., Zhang, H., He, K., Chang, Y., & Yang, X. (2015). Active Contours Driven by Multi-Feature Gaussian Distribution Fitting Energy with Application to Vessel Segmentation. *PLoS One*, *10*(11), e0143105. doi:10.1371/journal.pone.0143105 PMID:26571031

Wang, M. (2005). Extension Neural Network-Type 2 and Its Applications. *IEEE Transactions on Neural Networks*, *16*(6), 1352–1361. doi:10.1109/TNN.2005.853334 PMID:16342480

Wang, Q., Garrity, G. M., Tiedje, J. M., & Cole, J. R. (2007). Naive Bayesian classifier for rapid assignment of rRNA sequences into the new bacterial taxonomy. *Applied and Environmental Microbiology*, *73*(16), 5261–5267. doi:10.1128/AEM.00062-07 PMID:17586664

Wang, S., Huang, T. Z., Zhao, X. L., Mei, J. J., & Huang, J. (2018). Speckle noise removal in ultrasound images by first- and second-order total variation. *Numerical Algorithms*, *78*(2), 513–533. doi:10.100711075-017-0386-x

Wang, Y., Shu, C., & Yang, L. (2016). Boundary condition-enforced immersed boundary-lattice Boltzmann flux solver for thermal flows with Neumann boundary conditions. *Journal of Computational Physics*, *306*, 237–252. doi:10.1016/j.jcp.2015.11.046

Wang, Z., & Bovik, A. C. (2002). A universal image quality index. *IEEE Signal Processing Letters*, *9*(3), 81–84. doi:10.1109/97.995823

Wang, Z., Bovik, A. C., Sheikh, H. R., & Simoncelli, E. P. (2004). Image quality assessment: From error visibility to structural similarity. *IEEE Transactions on Image Processing*, *13*(4), 600–612. doi:10.1109/TIP.2003.819861 PMID:15376593

Waoo, N., Kashyap, R., & Jaiswal, A. (2010). DNA nano array analysis using hierarchical quality threshold clustering. *2010 2nd IEEE International Conference on Information Management and Engineering*, 81–85.

Weston, J., & Watkins, C. (1998). *Multi-class support vector machines*. Technical Report CSD-TR-98-04, Department of Computer Science, Royal Holloway, University of London.

Whan Lee, J., Kim, S. K., Lee, B., Lee, B., & Lee, M. H. (2002). A Real Time QRS Detection Using DelayCoordinate Mapping for the Microcontroller Implementation. *Annals of Biomedical Engineering*, *30*(9), 1140–1151. doi:10.1114/1.1523030 PMID:12502225

Wickramasinghe, N. (2010). The Role for Knowledge Management in Modern Healthcare Delivery. *International Journal of Healthcare Delivery Reform Initiatives*, *2*(2), 1–9. doi:10.4018/jhdri.2010040101

William, H. W. (1995). General Surgery Dept. University of Wisconsin, Clinical Sciences Center.

Wilson, J., Coleman, R., & Turkington, T. (2011). Variable-time positron emission tomography leg protocol to equalize noise for positron emission tomography/computed tomography acquisitions. *Nuclear Medicine Communications*, *32*(9), 868–872. doi:10.1097/MNM.0b013e328347f1a3 PMID:21799371

Winston, W. T. (2018). *TNM Classification for Malignant Melanoma: TNM Classification for Malignant Melanoma*. Retrieved from https://emedicine.medscape.com/article/2007147-overview

Witten, Hall, & Pal. (2016). *Data Mining: Practical machine learning tools and techniques*. Academic Press.

Wong, A., Mishra, A., Bizheva, K., & Clausi, D. A. (2010). General Bayesian estimation for speckle noise reduction in optical coherence tomography retinal imagery. *Optics Express*, *18*(8), 8338–8352. doi:10.1364/OE.18.008338 PMID:20588679

World Health Organization. (2017). *Cardiovascular diseases (CVDs)*. Retrieved October 17 May 2017, from http://www.who.int/news-room/fact-sheets/detail/cardiovascular-diseases-(cvds)

Wu, M., Chen, Q., He, X., Li, P., Fan, W., Yuan, S., & Park, H. (2018). Automatic Subretinal fluid segmentation of retinal SD-OCT images with neurosensory retinal detachment guided by enface fundus imaging. *IEEE Transactions on Biomedical Engineering*, *65*(1), 87–95. doi:10.1109/TBME.2017.2695461 PMID:28436839

Wu, X., Kumar, V., Ross Quinlan, J., Ghosh, J., Yang, Q., Motoda, H., ... Steinberg, D. (2008). Top 10 algorithms in data mining. *Knowledge and Information Systems*, *14*(1), 1–37. doi:10.100710115-007-0114-2

Xin, Z., & Chen, W. (2014). Medical image fusion based on weighted Contourlet transformation coefficients. *J. Image Graphics*, *19*(1), 133–140.

Xu, X. J., Wang, Y. R., & Chen, S. (2014). Novel image fusion method based on down sampling fractional wavelet transform. *Yiqi Yibiao Xuebao*, *35*(9), 2061–2069.

Xu, X., Wang, Y., & Chen, S. (2016). Medical image fusion using discrete fractional wavelet transform, *Elsevier. Biomedical Signal Processing and Control*, *27*, 103–111. doi:10.1016/j.bspc.2016.02.008

Xydeas, C. S., & Petrovic, V. (2000). Objective image fusion performance measure. *Electronics Letters*, *36*(4), 308–309. doi:10.1049/el:20000267

Yan, B., Wang, Y., Li, Y., Gong, Y., Guan, L., & Yu, S. (2016). An EEG signal classification method based on sparse auto-encoders and support vector machine. In *Communications in China (ICCC), 2016 IEEE/CIC International Conference on*. IEEE.

Yang, X. B., Yan, S. X., Zhou, Z. Y., Li, G. Z., Li, Y., & Guo, X. F. (2011, November). Balance-bagging-PRFS algorithm for feature optimization on insomnia data intervened by traditional Chinese Medicine. In *Bioinformatics and Biomedicine Workshops (BIBMW), 2011 IEEE International Conference on* (pp. 854-857). IEEE.

Yang, G., Xie, L., Mäntysalo, M., Zhou, X., Pang, Z., Da Xu, L., ... Zheng, L. R. (2014). A health-IoT platform based on the integration of intelligent packaging, unobtrusive bio-sensor, and intelligent medicine box. *IEEE Transactions on Industrial Informatics, 10*(4), 2180–2191. doi:10.1109/TII.2014.2307795

Yang, J., Fan, J., Ai, D., Wang, X., Zheng, Y., Tang, S., & Wang, Y. (2016). Local statistics and non-local mean filter for speckle noise reduction in medical ultrasound image. *Neurocomputing, 195*, 88–95. doi:10.1016/j.neucom.2015.05.140

Yang, J.-G., Kim, J. K., Kang, U. G., & Lee, Y. H. (2014). Coronary heart disease optimization system on adaptive-network-based fuzzy inference system and linear discriminant analysis (ANFIS–LDA). *Personal and Ubiquitous Computing, 18*(6), 1351–1362. doi:10.100700779-013-0737-0

Yang, X. S., & Deb, S. (2010). Engineering optimisation by cuckoo search. *International Journal of Mathematical Modelling and Numerical Optimisation, 1*(4), 330–343. doi:10.1504/IJMMNO.2010.035430

Yang, X.-S., & Deb, S. (2009). *Cuckoo search via Levy flights*. IEEE Publications.

Yan, Z., Fan, J., & Wang, J. (2017). A collective neurodynamic approach to constrained global optimization. *IEEE Trans. Neural Learn. Syst, 28*(5), 1206–1215. doi:10.1109/TNNLS.2016.2524619 PMID:27046909

Yatollahi, A. A., Jafarnia Dabanloo, N., McLemon, D., Johari Majd, V., & Zhang, H. (2005). A comprehensive model using modified Zeeman model for generating ECG sig-nals. *Iran. J. Electr. Electron. Eng., 1*, 88–93.

Yeh, Y. C., Wang, W. J., & Chiou, C. W. (2009). Cardiac arrhythmia diagnosis method using linear discriminant analysis on ECG signals. *Measurement, 42*(5), 778–789. doi:10.1016/j.measurement.2009.01.004

Yen, H., Zheng, J., Jiang, Y., Peng, C., & Xaio, S. (2008). Selecting critical clinical features for heart diseases diagnosis with a real-coded genetic algorithm. *Applied Soft Computing, 8*(2), 1105–1111. doi:10.1016/j.asoc.2007.05.017

Yeung, S. S., Genaidy, A., Deddens, J., Alhemood, A., & Leung, P. C. (2002). Prevalence of musculoskeletal symptoms in single and multiple body regions and effects of perceived risk of injury among manual handling workers. *Spine, 27*(19), 2166–2172. doi:10.1097/00007632-200210010-00017 PMID:12394933

Yildiz, A. R. (2012). Cuckoo search algorithm for the selection of optimal machining parameters in milling operations. *International Journal of Advanced Manufacturing Technology*, 1–7.

Ying, K., Ameri, A., Trivedi, A., Ravindra, D., Patel, D., & Mozumdar, M. (2015, November). Decision tree-based machine learning algorithm for in-node vehicle classification. In *Green Energy and Systems Conference (IGESC)* (pp. 71-76). IEEE. 10.1109/IGESC.2015.7359454

Yorston, D. (2003). Retinal diseases and vision 2020. *Community Eye Health, 16*(46), 19–20. PMID:17491850

Yosipof, A., Guedes, R. C., & García-Sosa, A. T. (2018). Data Mining and Machine Learning Models for Predicting Drug Likeness and Their Disease or Organ Category. *Frontiers in Chemistry, 6*, 162. doi:10.3389/fchem.2018.00162 PMID:29868564

Yu, Y., & Acton, S. T. (2002). Speckle reducing anisotropic diffusion. *IEEE Transactions on Image Processing, 11*(11), 1260–1270. doi:10.1109/TIP.2002.804276 PMID:18249696

Yu, Y., Dong, G., & Wang, J. (2011, June). Despeckling trilateral filter. In *IVMSP Workshop, 2011 IEEE 10th* (pp. 42-47). IEEE.

Zabidi, A., Mansor, W., Lee, Y. K., & Che Wan Fadzal, C. W. N. F. (2012). Short-time Fourier Transform analysis of EEG signal generated during imagined writing. In *System Engineering and Technology (ICSET), 2012 International Conference on*. IEEE.

Zachary, C., & Lipton, D. (2017). *Learning to Diagnose with LSTM Recurrent Neural Networks*. Cornell University Library.

Zadeh, A. E., Khazaee, A., & Ranaee, V. (2010). Classification of the electrocardiogram signals using supervised classifiers and efficient features. *Computer Methods and Programs in Biomedicine, 99*(2), 179-194.

Zeeman, E. C. (1972). *Differential Equations for the Heartbeat and Nerve Impulse*. Coventry, UK: Math-ematics Institute, University of Warwick.

Zengyou, H. (2015). *Data mining for bioinformatics applications*. Woodhead Publishing.

Zeraatkar, E., & Kermani, S. (2010) Improving QRS Detection for Artifacts Reduction. *Proceedings of the 17th Iranian Conference of Biomedical Engineerin (ICBME2010)*, 978-981.

Zhang, J. A., Mo, G., & Zhang, K. (2017, October). The design and clinical application of sleep disorder treatment system. In *Image and Signal Processing, Biomedical Engineering and Informatics (CISP-BMEI), 2017 10th International Congress on* (pp. 1-5). IEEE.

Zhang, L. (2017). Real-time feature extraction for multi-channel EEG signals time-frequency analysis. In *Neural Engineering (NER), 2017 8th International IEEE/EMBS Conference on*. IEEE.

Zhang, L., Li, J., Han, H., Liu, B., Yang, J., & Wang, Q. (2017, May). Automatic cataract detection and grading using Deep Convolutional Neural Network. In *Networking, Sensing and Control (ICNSC), 2017 IEEE 14th International Conference on* (pp. 60-65). IEEE.

Zhang, J., Lin, G., Wu, L., Wang, C., & Cheng, Y. (2015a). Wavelet and fast bilateral filter based de-speckling method for medical ultrasound images. *Biomedical Signal Processing and Control, 18*, 1–10. doi:10.1016/j.bspc.2014.11.010

Zhang, J., Wang, C., & Cheng, Y. (2015). Comparison of despeckle filters for breast ultrasound images. *Circuits, Systems, and Signal Processing*, *34*(1), 185–208. doi:10.100700034-014-9829-y

Zhang, K., Song, H., & Zhang, L. (2010). Active contours driven by local image fitting energy. *Pattern Recognition*, *43*(4), 1199–1206. doi:10.1016/j.patcog.2009.10.010

Zhang, S., McClean, S. I., Nugent, C. D., Donnelly, M. P., Galway, L., Scotney, B. W., & Cleland, I. (2014). A predictive model for assistive technology adoption for people with dementia. *IEEE Journal of Biomedical and Health Informatics*, *18*(1), 375–383. doi:10.1109/JBHI.2013.2267549 PMID:24403437

Zhang, T., & Chen, W. (2017). LMD based features for the automatic seizure detection of EEG signals using SVM. *IEEE Transactions on Neural Systems and Rehabilitation Engineering*, *25*(8), 1100–1108. doi:10.1109/TNSRE.2016.2611601 PMID:27662677

Zhang, X., Wen, X., Xu, H., & Meng, Q. (2016). Synthetic aperture radar image segmentation based on edge-region active contour model. *Journal of Applied Remote Sensing*, *10*(3), 036014. doi:10.1117/1.JRS.10.036014

Zhang, Y., Cao, G., Li, X., & Wang, B. (2018). Cascaded Random Forest for Hyperspectral Image Classification. *IEEE Journal of Selected Topics in Applied Earth Observations and Remote Sensing*, *11*(4), 1082–1094. doi:10.1109/JSTARS.2018.2809781

Zhao, C. J., Sun, Y. X., Zhu, H. Q., & Liu, X. X. (2015). Axial suspension fuzzy pid control for axial artificial heart pump. *Applied Mechanics and Materials, 703*, 323–326.

Zhao, F., Liang, H., Wu, X., & Ding, D. (2017). Region-based Active Contour Segmentation Model with Local Discriminant Criterion. *International Journal Of Security And Its Applications*, *11*(7), 73–86. doi:10.14257/ijsia.2017.11.7.06

Zhao, Q., & Zhan, L. (2005). ECG Feature Extraction and Classification Using Wavelet Transform and Support Vector Machines. *2005 International Conference on Neural Networks and Brain.*

Zhengzhong, G., Fanxue, K., & Xu, Z. (2011). Accurate and Rapid QRS Detection for Intelligent ECG Monitor. *2011 Third International Conference on Measuring Technology and Mechatronics Automation*, 1, 298-301. 10.1109/ICMTMA.2011.76

Zhou, Q., Zhao, M., & Bian, G. (2017, December). An HFC-based Bayesian Network Structure Learning Algorithm. In *2017 International Conference on Industrial Informatics-Computing Technology, Intelligent Technology, Industrial Information Integration (ICIICII)* (pp. 104-107). IEEE.

Zhuang, M., Dierckx, R., & Zaidi, H. (2016). Generic and robust method for automatic segmentation of PET images using an active contour model. *Medical Physics*, *43*(8Part1), 4483–4494. doi:10.1118/1.4954844 PMID:27487865

Zhu, J., He, L., & Gao, Z. (2014). Feature extraction from a novel ECG model for arrhythmia diagnosis. *Bio-Medical Materials and Engineering*, *24*(6), 2883–2891. PMID:25226994

Zifan, A., & Gharibzadeh, S. (2006). The chaotic nature of temper in humans: A long short-term memory recurrent neural network model. *Medical Hypotheses*, *67*(3), 658–661. doi:10.1016/j.mehy.2006.02.032 PMID:16624500

Zlokolica, V., Jovanov, L., Pižurica, A., De Keyser, P., Dhaenens, F., & Philips, W. (2007, October). Wavelet-based denoising for 3D OCT images. In *Applications of Digital Image Processing XXX* (Vol. 6696, p. 66960P). International Society for Optics and Photonics. doi:10.1117/12.734286

Zong, X., Laine, A. F., & Geiser, E. A. (1998). Speckle reduction and contrast enhancement of echocardiograms via multiscale nonlinear processing. *IEEE Transactions on Medical Imaging*, *17*(4), 532–540. doi:10.1109/42.730398 PMID:9845309

Zukal, M., Beneš, R., Číka, P., & Říha, K. (2011). *Ultrasound image database.* Retrieved from http://splab.cz/en/download/databaze/ultrasound

About the Contributors

Chinmay Chakraborty is Assistant Professor in the Department of Electronics and Communication Engineering, Birla Institute of Technology, Jharkhand, India. His primary areas of research include Wireless Body Area Network, Internet of Medical Things, Energy-Efficient Wireless Communications and Networking, Point-of-Care Diagnosis. Prior to BIT Mesra, he worked at Faculty of Science and Technology, ICFAI University, Tripura, India. He worked as a Research Consultant in Coal India project at Industrial Engineering & Management, IIT Kharagpur, project coordinator in the Indo-US project at IIT Kharagpur, and also worked as a Network Engineer in System Administration at MISPL, India. He received his Ph.D. in Electronics & Communication from BIT Mesra, India. He did his Masters in Telecommunication Engineering from G. S. Sanyal School of Telecommunication, IIT Kharagpur, India. He did his B. Tech. in Electronics and Communication Engineering from MAKAUT (formerly, WBUT), India. He has published more than 30 technical papers in various journals, book, book chapter, and conferences. He has also been an Editor for a book published by a reputed international publisher. He is an Editorial Board Member in Journal of Wireless Communication Technology and also a member of International Advisory Board for Malaysia Technical Scientist Congress, and Machine Intelligence Research Labs. He got Outstanding Researcher Award from TESFA, 2016 and also got Young Faculty Award from VIFA 2018.

* * *

Geetha Mary A. received her Ph.D. from VIT University, Vellore, India. She has completed M.Tech. in Computer Science and Engineering from VIT University and B.E. from University of Madras, Tamil Nadu, India. She is working for VIT University as Associate Professor. She was awarded Merit Scholarship for her best academic performance for the year 2007-2008 during her M.Tech. study. She has authored more than 20 journal and conference papers. She has authored book chapters in the area of data mining and artificial intelligence. Her research interests include security for data mining, databases and intelligent systems. She works to empower healthcare management using computer science. Dr. Geetha Mary is associated with many professional bodies like IACSIT, CSTA and IAENG.

Ravinder Ahuja was born in Hansi, Haryana, India in 1985. He received his B.Tech in Computer Science and Engineering from Kurukshetra University, Kurukshetra in 2005 and M.Tech in Computer Science and Engineering from Indian Institute of Technology Roorkee Uttrakhand, India in 2011. From 2005 to 2009, he was a Lecturer with Jind Institute of Engineering and Technology, Jind Haryana. Since 2012, he has been an Assistant Professor in Computer Science and Engineering in Jaypee Educational Group, Noida.

Siddhartha Arjaria specializes in supervised learning algorithms. Completed Ph.D from NIT, Bhopal in Computer Science and Engineering and currently working as Assistant Professor in REC Banda, India.

B. Rajalingam graduated B.Tech (IT) in Alpha College of Engineering Affiliated by Anna University, Chennai, Tamilnadu in 2010. He got ME (CSE) degree from Annamalai University, Chidambaram, Tamilnadu in 2012. He has worked as assistant professor at Aksheyaa college of Engineering, Maduranthakam, Tamilnadu from 2012 to 2016. Currently he is pursuing his Ph.D. in Department of Computer Science and Engineering at Annamalai University. He has published 11 papers in international journals and presented 10 papers in the national and international conferences. His research interest includes Medical Image Processing, Pattern Recognition and Artificial Intelligence.

Anoop B. N. received his B.Tech degree from Cochin University of Science and Technology, Kerala, India and M.Tech degrees from NIT Calicut, Kerala, India. Currently, he is pursuing PhD from the department of computer science and engineering, National Institute of Technology Karnatka, Surathkal, India. His areas of interest include Medical Image Analysis and Machine Learning.

Abdul Hafeez Babar is student of Masters of Engineering at Department of Software Engineering, Mehran University of Engineering and Technology, Jamshoro, Sindh, Pakistan. He received his B.E degree from the Mehran UET. His research interests are in the field of data mining, machine learning and data engineering. He is member of Pakistan Engineering Counsel (PEC).

Alisha Banga was born in Hansi, Haryana, India in 1988. He received his B.Tech degree in Electronics and Communication Engineering from Maharshi Dayanand University, Rohtak in 2009 and M.Tech in Electrical and Electronics Engineering from same university in 2009. She is currently pursuing PhD in EID department at Thapar Institute of Engineering and Technology, Patiala, Punjab. She has teaching experience of around 7 years and currently working as Assistant Professor in ECE department at Satyug darshan Institute of Engineering and Technology Faridabad.

Soumyendu Bhattacharjee is pursuing Ph.D from Maulana Abul Kalam Azad University of Technology (WBUT) and attached with Kanad Institute of Engineering & Management as a Head of the Department of Electronics & Communication Engineering. He completed his M.E. degree in VLSI Design from Bengal Engineering and Science University, Shibpur in 2009. He did his B.Tech degree in the Department of Electronics & Communication Engineering from JIS College of Engineering in 2005.

R. Bhavani received her B.E. degree in Computer Science and Engineering from Regional Engineering College, Trichy in 1989. She received her M.E. degree in Computer Science and Engineering from Regional Engineering College, Trichy in 1992. She worked at Mookambigai College of Engineering, Keeranur from 1990 to 1994. She has been with Annamalai University, since 1994. She received her Ph.D. degree in Computer Science and Engineering at Annamalai University, in the year 2007. She presented 45 papers in International Conferences, 19 papers in National Conferences and published 46 papers in National and International Journals. She also published 1 Book and 5 Book Chapters. Her research area includes Image processing, Image Segmentation, Image Compression, Image Classification, Stenography, Pattern Classification, Medical Imaging, Content Based Image Retrieval and Software metrics.

Manika Chandna was born in Haridwar, Uttrakhand, India in 1997. She has completed her higher secondary from Haldwani, Uttrakhand. She is currently pursuing her B.Tech (IVth year) in CSE Dept. from Jaypee Institute of Information Technology, Noida, India.

Kym Fraser is a business management academic. Before joining the University of Kurdistan Hewlêr he spent 15 years at the University of South Australia in Adelaide. He also holds adjunct professorships at the University of Brawijaya in Indonesia and Aalborg University in Denmark. He has a PhD in Manufacturing Management and holds degrees in accounting, economics, business and engineering. Before becoming an academic he spent 25 years in practice, holding senior management positions in both government and private enterprises, specialising in service and operations management. Due to a keen interest in other cultures and a global perspective he has visited over 150 countries, which includes university teaching assignments in 10 countries. He currently collaborates with five research universities in Japan, Denmark, Indonesia, USA, and Singapore, and has published over 80 research articles in internationally refereed books, journals and conferences.

Girish G. N. is a research scholar at Department of Computer Science and Engineering, National Institute of Technology Karnataka, India. He received his B.E. degree in Computer Science and Engineering in 2012, followed by M.Tech. in Computer Science and Engineering in 2014 from the Visvesvaraya Technological University (VTU), Karnataka, India. His research interests include biometrics, object recognition and tracking, computer vision, image processing, ophthalmic image analysis, and medical image analysis.

Subham Ghosh is pursuing B.Tech degree from JIS College of Engineering in the Department of Electronics & Communication Engineering.

Bharat Gupta is attached with educational and research from last 15 years and Senior Member of IEEE (USA). Presently, Dr. Gupta is working as an Assistant Professor in the Department of Electronics & Communication Engineering, National Institute of Technology Patna, India. He received his Bachelors of Engineering in Electronics and Telecommunication from Govt. Engineering College, Ujjain, India and a Master of Technology from Birla Institute of Technology, Ranchi, India. Dr. Gupta has completed his doctorate in Wireless Communication from University of Rome, Tor Vergata, Italy. He has delivered many talks in International & National conferences and workshops. He has acted as reviewer of many conferences & Journals. His works is published in renowned National and International Journals. He was a TPC member of ICDECOM and reviewers of standard conferences like ICDECOM, Wireless VITAE, ISABEL, etc. He was an Advisory Committee in National Conference on "Emerging Trends in Electronics and Telecommunication Engineering" and has also chaired many sessions in conferences. He has organized the workshops at national and international level. His research area covers mainly Wireless Body Area Network, Routing and MAC protocol for Medical Wireless Communication, ICT for Healthcare, FM-UWB communication technology, etc.

Mohammed Kamal Hassan has bachelor degree in computer science with extensive experience and management skills and working in a company that provides financial solution to the customer as an IT specialists. As a senior software engineer, he is responsible of all software and IT related issues in his working place. He has Master degree in software engineering from the university of Kurdistan-Hawler (2018).

Chandan Kumar Jha is currently pursuing Ph.D. from Indian Institute of Technology Patna in the Department of Electrical Engineering. He worked as an Assistant Professor of Electronics and Communication Engineering at Institute of Information Technology and Management, Gwalior from March 2013 to December. 2014. He received his Master degree with distinction in Electronics and Communication Engineering from Birla Institute of Technology Mesra in 2012. He received his Bachelor Degree in Electronics and Communication Engineering from the West Bengal University of Technology Kolkata in 2010. His research interests include biomedical signal processing, ECG signal analysis, and telemedicine.

Priya Kandan received her B.E. degree in Computer Science and Engineering from Thiagarajar College of Engineering, Madurai in 1997. She received her M.E. degree in Computer Science and Engineering from Annamalai University, Chidambaram in the year 2005. She has been with Annamalai University, since 1999 with 19 years of experience. She received her Ph.D. degree in Computer Science and Engineering at Annamalai University, in the year 2014. She has published 47 papers in international conferences and journals. Her research interest includes Medical Image processing and Pattern Classification Methods. Life member of the Indian Society for Technical Education (ISTE) and a member of Computer Society of India (C.S.I).

Venkatram Kari is a PhD scholar in the School of Computer Science and Engineering (SCOPE) in VIT University, Vellore, Tamilnadu, India. He received master's degree in Software Engineering from BITS Pilani. He is currently working as delivery manager at Tech Mahindra Limited, India. His research interests in Big Data, Distributed computing, Data Analytics, Digital technologies and Machine Learning areas.

Ramgopal Kashyap's areas of interest are image processing, pattern recognition, and machine learning. He has published many quality research papers, and book chapters in international journals and conferences like Springer, Inderscience, Elsevier, ACM, and IGI-Global indexed by Science Citation Index (SCI) and Scopus (Elsevier). He has Reviewed Research Papers in the Science Citation Index Expanded, Springer Journals and Editorial Board Member and conferences programme committee member of the IEEE, Springer international conferences and journals held in countries: Czech Republic, Switzerland, UAE, Australia, Hungary, Poland, Taiwan, Denmark, India, USA, UK, Austria, and Turkey. He has written many book chapters published by IGI Global, USA.

Maheshkumar H. Kolekar is working as an Associate Professor in the Department of Electrical Engineering, Indian Institute of Technology Patna since March 2010. He worked as Head in Department of Electrical Engineering, IIT Patna during January 2013 to December 2013. Since January 2014, he is Head of the Centre for Advanced Systems Engineering at IIT Patna. He received his Ph.D. degree in Electronics and Electrical Communication Engineering from Indian Institute of Technology Kharagpur in 2007. During 2008-2009, he was Post-Doctoral Research Fellow in the Department of Computer Science, University of Missouri, Columbia, USA. His research interests are in the digital image and video processing, video surveillance and biomedical image and signal processing. He was a recipient of the Best Paper Award from the Computer Society of India for his research paper. In 2012, he was an Organizing Chair of the IEEE Sponsored International Conference on Signal, Image and Video Processing at the IIT Patna, a Guest Editor of the Journal of Medical Imaging and Health Informatics (American Scientific) for Special Issue on Biomedical Signal and Image Processing, a Tutorial Chair of the 4th IEEE International Conference on Intelligent Human Computer Interaction, a keynote speaker of the International Conference on Biomedical Systems, Signals and Images at the IIT Madras, an editorial board member of the American Journal of Signal Processing (Scientific and Academic). In 2014, he successfully organized Special Session on Intelligent Video Surveillance Systems at the International Conference on Systems Engineering, Las Vegas, NV, USA.

Seetharaman Krishnamoorthy received his M.Sc. degree in Statistics, the Ph.D. in Computer Science and Engineering from Annamalai University, India, in 1990 and 2006 respectively; the M.S. degree in Software Systems from Birla Institute of Technology and Science, Pilani, India, in 1995; and the M.Tech. degree in Computer and Information Technology from Manonmaniam Sundaranar University, India, in 2013. He is currently working as Associate Professor in the Department of Computer and Information Sciences, Annamalai University. His research interests include Statistical Pattern Recognition, Image and Video Retrieval, Digital Image Analysis includes medical image, Data Mining and Knowledge Discovery, and Big Data Analytics. He is actively involved in professional activities, viz. reviewer in the journals: IET Image Processing, Pattern Recognition (Elsevier), Swarm and Evolutionary Computation (Elsevier), Knowledge–Based SYSTEMS (Elsevier), Computer and Electronics in Agriculture (Elsevier). He is currently serving as an Associate Editor of the Aloy Journal of Soft Computing and Applications, which is an International Journal, and Editorial Board Member of the International Journal of Information Technology and Management Sciences. He is also the member of the professional societies – IEEE, ACM, IAENG, and Indian Science Congress Association. He has received R & D Major Research Project funds from funding agencies, such as University Grants Commission (UGC) and DST, India. He has authored the book entitled 'Image Processing: Stochastic Model Based Approach'; published more than 75 articles in journals of the Elsevier, Springer, Taylor and Francis, IEEE, etc. He has successfully supervised 11 Ph.D. scholars and 7 M.Phil. Scholars. He has received Outstanding Scientist in Image Processing. He has delivered more than Fifty Speech includes the Key Note Speech, Special Lecture, and served as Chairpersonat various forums of the Computer Science.

Naeem Ahmed Mahoto received Master degree in Computer Engineering from Mehran University of Engineering and Technology, Pakistan and Ph.D in Information and System Engineering from Politecnico di Torino, Italy in 2013. He is currently working as Associate Professor at Department of Software Engineering, Mehran UET Pakistan. His research interests are focused in the field of data mining and bioinformatics. His research activities are also devoted to summarization of web documents, sentiment analysis, data visualization and educational data mining. He is member of IEEE Computer society and Pakistan Engineering Council (PEC).

Mokhtar Mohammadi received the B.S. degree in Computer Engineering (Hardware) from Shahed University, Tehran, Iran, in 2003. He received the M.S. degree in Computer Engineering (Computer Architecture) from Shahid Beheshti University, Tehran, Iran, in 2012. He received the Ph.D degree in Artificial Intelligence from Shahrood University of Technology, Shahrood, Iran, in 2018. Currently, he is with the Department of Information Technology, University of Human Development, Sulaimanyah, Iraq. His current research interests include signal processing, time–frequency analysis, and machine learning.

Biswarup Neogi is presently attached with JIS College of Engineering (JIS Group, India) as an Associate Professor of ECE Dept. and In-Charge of CII Centre for Innovation, JISCE. He associated as a Coordinator (Technology Transfer Vertical) with Centre for Excellency (Russian Federation) JIS Group. He is the Executive Council Member of West Bengal University of Technology (Govt. of WB). He awarded AICTE Career Award for Young Teacher (CAYT) 2014-15 (Government of India). He received his PhD (Engineering) degree from Jadavpur University, WB, India before that M.Tech degree in Electronics & Comm. Engineering from Kalyani Government Engineering College, WB, India in 2007. He obtained B.E in ECE from UIT, The University of Burdwan in 2005. Previously, he was associated as a faculty with several institutions as like HIT, DIATM, KGEC in India. He have achieved several funds from Government of India with successful outcome completed research project. He involved with Product Design research and filed 20 number of Patent as an Inventor in India. He published several numbers of research article in reputed journals.

Sudeep P. V. received his B.Tech and M.Tech degrees from the University of Kerala, India and the PhD from National Institute of Technology, Tiruchirappalli, India. Currently, he is working as Assistant Professor in the Department of Electronics and Communication Engineering, National Institute of Technology Calicut, Kerala. His area of interest includes Medical Image Analysis and Machine Learning.

P. Palanisamy received his BE from Bharathiar University, Coimbatore and his ME and PhD degrees from National Institute of Technology, Tiruchirappalli, India. Currently, he is working as Professor in the Department of Electronics and Communication Engineering, National Institute of Technology, Tiruchirappalli. His area of interest includes Signal Processing, Medical Image Analysis and Data and Image compression.

Anudeep Peddi was born in Guntur, India, in 1989. He received the B.Tech degree in Electronics and Communication Engineering from Jawaharlal Nehru Technological University, Kakinada (JNTUK), India, in 2010, and the M.Tech in VLSI Design from GITAM University, Visakhapatnam, India, in 2012. In 2012, he joined for the Department of Electronics and Communication Engineering, MLR Institute of Technology, as an Assistant Professor and in 2015, he moved to VNR Vignana Jyothi Institute of Engineering and Technology, Hyderabad, India. His current research interests include Neuromorphic Engineering, Sound stream segregation and auditory scene analysis. He is a Life Member of the Indian Society for Technical Education (ISTE).

Jeny Rajan received his M.Tech degree from the University of Kerala, India and the PhD from the University of Antwerp, Belgium. He is currently working as an Assistant Professor at the Department of Computer Science and Engineering, National Institute of Technology Karnataka. His main research interests are MRI, OCT and Ultrasound image processing.

Sravanth Kumar Ramakuri received his Bachelor's degree in Electronics and Communications Engineering from JNTU University Hyderabad and Master's degree in RF and Microwave Engineering from GITAM University, Visakhapatnam. He is pursuing PhD from Birla Institute of Technology, Mesra. Presently, he is working as an Assistant Professor in VNRVJIET, Hyderabad. His area of interest is bio-medical signal processing, sensor networks, and Brain-Computer Interface.

Tarik Ahmed Rashid received his Ph.D. in Computer Science and Informatics degree from College of Engineering, Mathematical and Physical Sciences, University College Dublin (UCD) in 2001-2006. He pursued his Post-Doctoral Follow at the Computer Science and Informatics School, College of Engineering, Mathematical and Physical Sciences, University College Dublin (UCD) from 2006-2007. He was a Professor at Salahaddin University-Erbil, Hawler, Kurdistan. He Joined the University of Kurdistan Hewlêr (UKH) in 2017.

Megha Rathi completed Ph.D from Banasthali University, Rajasthan. Completed M.Tech in computer science from the Banasthali University, Rajasthan in the year 2010 (I Ranker and Scholarship Holder) and received the B.Tech degree in computer science from U.P. Technical University. Total 10 years of Teaching experience. Presently working with Jaypee Institute of Information Technology, Noida (UP). During my teaching career, I have taught subjects like Data Mining, R Programming, Advanced Java, Software engineering, Database Systems, Operating System and Data Structure. I had supervised various projects at graduate levels. I have completed many projects including research project of Xform generator at NIC, Delhi. Have experience in Software development. Worked as Project Associate at IIT Delhi. Research areas include: Data Mining, Data Analytics, Health Science, Machine Learning, and Data Science.

Abhishek Rathore is currently working in the field of Machine Learning. Complete PhD from National Institute of Technology, Bhopal, India on Topic Models.

Suchismita Satapathy obtained her PhD from NIT Rourkela, and is working as an associate professor in mechanical engineering department at KIIT Deemed to be University, bhubaneswar, Odisha, India. She has published more than 25 research articles in different reputed journals.

Shikha Singhal is an aspiring teacher, and completed her M.TECH in Computer Science from Jaypee Institute of Information Technology, Noida. She is also assisting teachers with Teacher's assistantship program at JIIT, gaining on-ground experience with the students of B.Tech. She loves teaching and doing research work, with a special affinity towards wireless communication and Cognitive Science. She excelled her GATE Score and has done several projects practicing the core principles of computing. She is constantly looking for the opportunities of learning and contributing to the society.

Adwitiya Sinha has received Doctor of Philosophy from Jawaharlal Nehru University (JNU), New Delhi, India in 2015. She has obtained Master of Technology in Computer Science and Technology in 2010 from JNU, New Delhi, India. She has also completed Master and Bachelor of Computer Applications in 2008 and 2006, respectively. She is a recipient of Senior Research Fellowship from Council of Scientific & Industrial Research, New Delhi, India and also awarded with UGC Research Scholarship for her research in data analytics across social and wireless domains. Presently, she is working as an Assistant Professor in Jaypee Institute of Information Technology, UP, India. She has delivered MOOC on Networks & Graphs organized by CEC, UGC, New Delhi, India. Her research area includes performance analysis of wireless sensor & ad hoc networks, cognitive networks, data aggregation & prediction techniques, confluence of sensor-based applications with social networking (social sensing).

Shivani Virmani was born in Kota, Rajasthan, India in 1996. She has completed her higher secondary from Kota. She is currently pursuing her B.Tech (III rd year) in CSE dept. from Jaypee Institute of Information Technology, Noida, India.

Vishal Vivek was born in Motihari, Bihar, India in 1996. He has completed his higher secondary from Motihari. He is currently pursuing his B.Tech (III rd year) in CSE Dept. from Jaypee Institute of Information Technology, Noida, India.

Index

T

V

W

www.ingramcontent.com/pod-product-compliance
Lightning Source LLC
LaVergne TN
LVHW062110300926
849161LV00010B/2421